2021

CODING EXAM REVIEW

The Physician and Facility Certification Step

Jackie L. Koesterman, CPC
Lead Technical Collaborator
Coding and Reimbursement Specialist
JDK Medical Coding EDU, LLC
Grand Forks, North Dakota

BUCK'S

ELSEVIER

Elsevier
3251 Riverport Lane
St. Louis, Missouri 63043

Notice

Practitioners and researchers must always rely on their own experience and knowledge in evaluating and using any information, methods, compounds or experiments described herein. Because of rapid advances in the medical sciences, in particular, independent verification of diagnoses and drug dosages should be made. To the fullest extent of the law, no responsibility is assumed by Elsevier, authors, editors or contributors for any injury and/or damage to persons or property as a matter of products liability, negligence or otherwise, or from any use or operation of any methods, products, instructions, or ideas contained in the material herein.

Senior Content Strategist: Brandi Graham
Senior Content Development Manager: Luke E. Held
Senior Content Development Specialist: Joshua S. Rapplean
Publishing Services Manager: Julie Eddy
Senior Project Manager: Abigail Bradberry
Senior Book Designer: Maggie Reid

Printed in Canada

Last digit is the print number: 9 8 7 6 5 4 3 2 1

Working together
to grow libraries in
developing countries

www.elsevier.com • www.bookaid.org

To coding instructors,
who each day strive to enhance the lives
of their students and provide the next generation
of knowledgeable medical coders.

Carol J. Buck
Jackie L. Koesterman

About the Authors

Carol J. Buck, MS, is a leading coding author and educator. Her *Step* series of textbooks were the first in the market to help coders and coding students develop their skills to advanced and specialized levels. Carol has dedicated herself to the growth and advancement of the coding profession.

Carol has a Master's degree in Education. She began authoring textbooks when she was Program Director of the Medical Secretarial programs at Northwest Technical College in Minnesota, recognizing the need for classroom texts that could be used to teach medical coding. It was then that she began developing classroom lectures, abstracting medical reports, and compiling materials to prepare her students for careers as medical coders. These materials later became *Buck's Step-by-Step Medical Coding*.

Carol expanded on the original text with a line of annual products for advanced coding, certification, specialization, and reference manuals, providing quality educational materials from the first day of a coding program to preparation for national certification.

Jackie L. Koesterman, CPC, has been a Certified Professional Coder and Medical Assistant for over 25 years. Jackie has also served as an instructor at the Minnesota Northland Technical College in the medical clerical and medical assistant programs. Jackie is employed by a large medical health system as a Senior Coder III and Reimbursement Specialist, specializing in multispecialty coding and multipayer denial review in both the inpatient and outpatient settings. She also serves as a trainer and mentor to the coders. Jackie performs audits for multispecialties for private practice clinics in her area.

Since the inception of *Buck's Step-by-Step Medical Coding*, Jackie has been involved in the development and review of the texts, serving as a technical collaborator, reviewer, and author.

Acknowledgments

There are so many, many people who participated in the development of this text, and only through the effort of all of the team members has it been possible to publish this text.

Patricia Cordy Henricksen, Query Manager, who graciously lends her amazing knowledge and attention to detail to the query process. Her dedication to excellence consistently improves this work.

Brandi Graham, Senior Content Strategist, who maintains an excellent sense of humor and is a valued member of the team who can always be depended upon for reasoned judgment. **Josh Rapplean,** Senior Content Development Specialist, who assumed the responsibility of shepherding this project with steady fortitude. **Megan Chandler and Mauri Loemker,** Senior Project Managers at Graphic World, who assumed responsibility for many projects while maintaining a high degree of professionalism. The employees of Elsevier have participated in the publication of this text and demonstrated exceptional professionalism and competence.

Preface

Thank you for purchasing *Coding Exam Review 2021: The Physician and Facility Certification Step,* the latest guide to the physician and facility coding certification exams. This 2021 edition has been carefully reviewed and updated with the latest content, making it the most current guide for your review. The author and publisher have made every effort to equip you with skills and tools you will need to succeed on the exam. To this end, this review guide presents essential information about all health care coding systems, anatomy, terminology, and pathophysiology, as well as sample examinations for practice. No other review guide on the market brings together such thorough coverage of all necessary examination material in one source.

Organization of This Textbook

Following a basic outline approach, this text takes a practical approach to assisting you with your examination preparations. The text is divided into seven parts—Anatomy, Terminology, and Pathophysiology; Physician-based Reimbursement Issues; Facility-based Reimbursement Issues; CPT and HCPCS Coding; ICD-10-CM and ICD-10-PCS Coding; Physician-based Examinations; and Facility-based Examinations—and there are several appendices for your reference. Additionally, Part 4 includes Practice Exercises, while examinations are provided on the companion Evolve website to help assist you in your preparation.

> ### NOTE
>
> Some of the CPT code descriptions for physician services include physician extender services. Physician extenders, such as nurse practitioners, physician assistants, and nurse anesthetists, etc., provide medical services typically performed by a physician. Within this educational material the term "physician" may include "and other qualified health care professionals" depending on the code. Refer to the official CPT® code descriptions and guidelines to determine codes that are appropriate to report services provided by non-physician practitioners.

Part 1, Anatomy, Terminology, and Pathophysiology, covers all the essential body systems and terms you'll need to get certified. Organized by body systems to follow the CPT codes, the sections also include illustrations to review each major anatomical area and quizzes to check your understanding and recall. (Answers are located in Appendix B.)

Part 2, Physician-based Reimbursement Issues, and Part 3, Facility-based Reimbursement Issues, provide a review of important insurance and billing information to help you review the connections between medical coding, insurance, billing, and reimbursement.

Part 4, CPT and HCPCS Coding, and Part 5, ICD-10-CM and ICD-10-PCS Coding, contain comprehensive coverage of the different coding systems and their applications, making other references unnecessary! Simplified text and clear examples are the highlights of these parts, and illustrations are included to clarify difficult concepts.

Part 6, Physician-based Examinations, and Part 7, Facility-based Examinations, outline the Practice Examination options on Evolve that simulate the experience of taking the actual coding exams, allowing you to assess your strengths and weaknesses in order to develop a plan for focused study.

About the Certification Examinations

The American Academy of Professional Coders (AAPC, www.aapc.com) and the American Health Information Management Association (AHIMA, www.ahima.org) offer many coding certifications. Among the most prominent are:

AAPC CPC® (Certified Professional Coder)
AHIMA CCS® (Certified Coding Specialist)
AHIMA CCS-P® (Certified Coding Specialist-Physician)
AAPC: The choice of date and location to take the examination is to be made from the AAPC website at www.aapc.com/certification.
AHIMA: The choice of date and location to take the examination is to be made from the AHIMA website at www.ahima.org/certification.

About the Practice Examinations

The companion Evolve website contains valuable resources to assist with preparation for both the Physician and Facility coding certification examinations. (To access the Exams along with your free Evolve resources, follow the instructions located on the inside front cover of this book.) For the purposes of this text, three practice exam formats have been developed. It's recommended that the learner focus on the exam format that most closely resembles the certification exam they've chosen:

Physician Exam (Format A)
Pre-/Post-Examination (150 multiple-choice questions)
Final Examination (150 multiple-choice questions)

Physician Exam (Format B)
Pre-/Post-Examination (97 multiple-choice and 8 cases)
Final Examination (97 multiple-choice and 8 cases)
Facility Exam (Format C)
Pre-/Post-Examination (97 multiple-choice and 8 cases)
Final Examination (97 multiple-choice and 8 cases)

The Pre-Examination on the Evolve website should be completed at the start of your study, and the Post-Examination, also on the Evolve website, should be taken after your study is complete. By comparing the results of these examinations, you can see your improvement after using the review guide! Once you check your scores, you are ready to take the Final Examination.

Exam Sessions Screen

After choosing your exam format, the Exam Sessions screen serves as home base. Here you can find information relating to your progress and performance in different subject areas. From this screen, you can choose an examination mode, submit an examination, check your progress, and review your results.

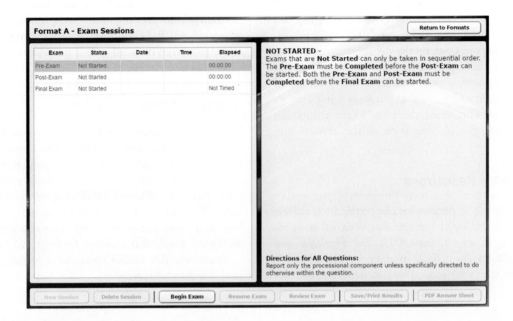

In addition to displaying your scores for completed sections and tracking the total elapsed time, this screen also shows the total, attempted, and correct questions in each subsection. You can return to the Exam Sessions screen at any point while taking or reviewing an examination, and all information related to your answers and position is saved.

Taking the Examination

While taking the examination, click on the letter of your answer choice, and the circle will appear in red to the left. Click on the "Next" button at the bottom of the screen to proceed to the next question. At the top of the screen, the

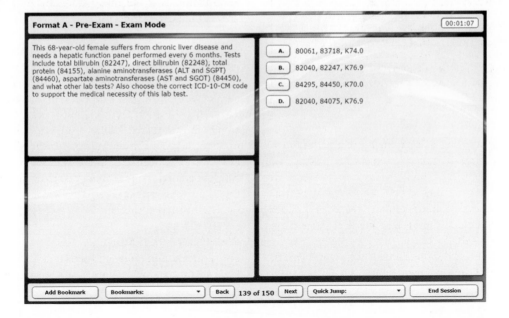

Quick Jump feature is a pull-down menu that allows you to jump to any question in the current section. Additionally, the Bookmark button at the bottom of the screen allows you to mark questions for later reference.

Reviewing Your Results

Once you have taken the Post-Examination on the companion Evolve website, you have the option to review all the Pre- and Post-Examination questions with rationales, even the ones you answered correctly, by clicking the "Review Exam" button at the bottom of the summary screen. The correct answer is shown for each question, and a rationale is given for each answer option. Or, if you prefer, you can review the answers and rationales using a PDF answer sheet. You can also compare your results on the Pre- and Post-Examinations by clicking on each exam on the Exam Sessions screen and viewing your results in the "Completed Exams" on the right or by printing out your results.

Once you have completed the Final Examination, the software will then provide you with all the answers and rationales.

Supplemental Resources

However you decide to prepare for the certification examination, we have developed supplements designed to complement *Coding Exam Review 2021: The Physician and Facility Certification Step*. Each of these supplements has been developed with the needs of both students and instructors in mind.

Instructor's Electronic Resource

No matter what your level of teaching experience, this total-teaching solution, located on the companion Evolve website, will help you plan your lessons with ease, and the author has developed all the curriculum materials necessary to use the textbook in the classroom. This includes extra quizzes, a course calendar and syllabus, lesson plans, ready-made tests for easy assessment, and PDF files with the questions and answers for the Pre-/Post- and Final Examinations. Also included is a comprehensive PowerPoint collection for the entire text, and ExamView test banks. The PowerPoint slides can be easily customized to support your lectures or formatted as handouts for student note-taking. The ExamView test generator will help you quickly and easily prepare quizzes and exams from the ready-made test questions, and the test banks can be customized to your specific teaching methods.

Additional Evolve Resources

The Evolve companion website offers many resources that will extend your studies beyond the classroom. Mobile-optimized quick quizzes offer on-the-go practice and review with 380 additional medical terminology, pathophysiology, CPT, ICD-10-CM, and HCPCS questions. Related Web links offer you the opportunity to expand your knowledge base and stay current with this ever-changing field, and additional material is available for help and practice.

Access the free Evolve resources at http://evolve.elsevier.com/Buck/examreview/.

Reviewers

Advisory Board

Contents

Success Strategies, xv

Part 1: Anatomy, Terminology, and Pathophysiology, 1

1 Integumentary System, 2

ANATOMY AND TERMINOLOGY, 2
Layers, 2
Two Layers Make Up Skin: Epidermis and Dermis, 2
Nails, 2
Glands, 3
Anatomy and Terminology Quiz, 4

PATHOPHYSIOLOGY, 5
Lesions and Other Abnormalities (Fig. 1.2), 5
Inflammatory Disorders, 7
Skin Infections, 10
Tumors of Skin, 12
Pathophysiology Quiz, 13

2 Musculoskeletal System, 14

ANATOMY AND TERMINOLOGY, 14
Skeletal System, 14
Structure, 14
Muscular System, 17
Muscle Tissue Types, 17
Muscle Action, 18
Anatomy and Terminology Quiz, 23

PATHOPHYSIOLOGY, 23
Injuries, 23
Bone Disorders, 24
Joint Disorders, 25
Tendon, Muscle, and Ligament Disorders, 25
Tumors, 25
Pathophysiology Quiz, 26

3 Respiratory System, 27

ANATOMY AND TERMINOLOGY, 27
Upper Respiratory Tract (URT), 27
Lower Respiratory Tract (LRT), 27
Anatomy and Terminology Quiz, 31

PATHOPHYSIOLOGY, 32
Signs and Symptoms of Pulmonary Disorders, 32
Pulmonary Diseases and Disorders, 32

Lower Respiratory Infection (LRI), 33
Pathophysiology Quiz, 34

4 Cardiovascular System, 35

ANATOMY AND TERMINOLOGY, 35
Blood (Function Is to Maintain a Constant Environment), 35
Vessels—Circulatory System, 35
Heart, 35
Heartbeat, 38
Anatomy and Terminology Quiz, 40

PATHOPHYSIOLOGY, 41
Vascular Disorders, 41
Heart Disorders, 43
Valvular Heart Disease, 43
Heart Wall Disorders, 44
Cardiomyopathies, 44
Congenital Heart Defects, 44
Pathophysiology Quiz, 45

5 Female Genital System and Pregnancy, 46

ANATOMY AND TERMINOLOGY, 46
Terminology, 46
Accessory Organs (Fig. 5.2), 46
Menstruation and Pregnancy, 46
Anatomy and Terminology Quiz, 50

PATHOPHYSIOLOGY, 50
Menstrual and Hormonal Disorders, 50
Infection, Inflammation, and Sexually Transmitted Diseases, 51
Benign Lesions, 52
Malignant Lesions, 53
Pregnancy, 54
Pathophysiology Quiz, 57

6 Male Genital System, 58

ANATOMY AND TERMINOLOGY, 58
Essential Organs, 58
Accessory Organs, 58
Anatomy and Terminology Quiz, 60

PATHOPHYSIOLOGY, 60
Male Genital System Disorders, 60
Pathophysiology Quiz, 64

7   Urinary System, 66

ANATOMY AND TERMINOLOGY, 66
Organs (Fig. 7.1), 66
Anatomy and Terminology Quiz, 69

PATHOPHYSIOLOGY, 69
Renal Failure, 69
Urinary Tract Infections (UTI), 70
Glomerular Disorders, 71
Urinary Tract Obstructions, 71
Vascular Disorders, 72
Congenital Disorders, 72
Pathophysiology Quiz, 73

8   Digestive System, 74

ANATOMY AND TERMINOLOGY, 74
Mouth (Fig. 8.1), 74
Teeth, 74
Salivary Glands (Fig. 8.3), 74
Pharynx or Throat (Fig. 8.4), 74
Esophagus, 74
Stomach, 74
Small Intestine, 74
Large Intestine, 74
Accessory Organs, 74
Peritoneum, 76
Anatomy and Terminology Quiz, 78

PATHOPHYSIOLOGY, 79
Disorders of Oral Cavity, 79
Esophageal Disorders, 79
Stomach and Duodenum Disorders, 80
Intestinal Disorders, 81
Disorders of Liver, Gallbladder, and Pancreas, 84
Pathophysiology Quiz, 86

9   Mediastinum and Diaphragm, 87

ANATOMY AND TERMINOLOGY, 87
Mediastinum, 87
Diaphragm, 87
Anatomy and Terminology Quiz, 87

10   Hemic and Lymphatic System, 89

ANATOMY AND TERMINOLOGY, 89
Lymph, 89
Lymph Vessels, 89
Lymph Organs, 89
Hematopoietic Organ, 89
Anatomy and Terminology Quiz, 91

PATHOPHYSIOLOGY, 92
Anemia, 92
Granulocytosis, 93
Eosinophilia, 93
Basophilia, 93

Monocytosis, 93
Leukocytosis, 93
Leukocytopenia, 93
Infectious Mononucleosis, 93
Leukemia, 93
Chronic Lymphocytic Leukemia (CLL), 94
Lymphadenopathy, 94
Malignant Lymphoma, 94
Myeloma, 95
Pathophysiology Quiz, 95

11   Endocrine System, 96

ANATOMY AND TERMINOLOGY, 96
Endocrine Glands (Fig. 11.1), 96
Anatomy and Terminology Quiz, 98

PATHOPHYSIOLOGY, 99
Diabetes Mellitus, 99
Pituitary Disorders, 99
Thyroid Disorders, 100
Parathyroid Disorders, 101
Adrenal Gland Disorders, 101
Pathophysiology Quiz, 102

12   Nervous System, 103

ANATOMY AND TERMINOLOGY, 103
Cells of the Nervous System (Fig. 12.1), 103
Divisions of Central Nervous System (CNS)
    (Fig. 12.2), 103
Peripheral Nervous System (PNS), 104
Autonomic Nervous System (ANS)—Housed Within
    Both PNS and CNS, 104
Anatomy and Terminology Quiz, 106

PATHOPHYSIOLOGY, 106
Dementias—Classified by Causative
    Factor, 106
Congenital Neurologic Disorders, 108
Mental Disorders, 108
Central Nervous System (CNS) Disorders, 109
Pathophysiology Quiz, 112

13   Senses, 114

ANATOMY AND TERMINOLOGY, 114
Sight: Three Layers of Eye (Fig. 13.1), 114
Hearing, Three Divisions of Ear, 114
Smell, 115
Taste, 115
Touch, 115
Anatomy and Terminology Quiz, 118

PATHOPHYSIOLOGY, 118
Eye, 118
Ear, 120
Pathophysiology Quiz, 121

Part 2: Physician-based Reimbursement Issues, 122

14   Physician-based Reimbursement Issues, 123
Medicare, 123
National Correct Coding Initiative (NCCI), 125
Federal Register, 125
Quality Improvement Organizations (QIO), 125
Resource-Based Relative Value
    Scale (RBRVS), 125
Medicare Fraud and Abuse, 127
Managed Health Care, 127
Reimbursement Quiz, 130

Part 3: Facility-based Reimbursement Issues, 132

15   Facility-based Reimbursement Issues, 133
Medicare, 133
National Correct Coding Initiative (NCCI), 137
Prospective Payment Systems (PPS), 137
Ambulatory Payment Classifications (APCs), 137
Medicare Severity Diagnosis-Related Groups
    (MS-DRGs), 142
Post Acute Transfer, 147
Present on Admission Indicator (POA), 148
Hospital-Acquired Conditions (HAC), 149
Revenue Codes, 150
Data Quality, 150
Office of the Inspector General (OIG), 151
Managed Health Care, 152
Reimbursement Quiz, 154

Part 4: CPT and HCPCS Coding, 156

16   Introduction to CPT, 157
Introduction to Medical Coding, 157
CPT, 157
Types of CPT Codes, 157
CPT Codes, 157
CPT Format, 157
Two Types of Code Descriptions, 159
Modifiers Add Information, 159
Unlisted Services, 159
Category II Codes—Supplemental Tracking
    Codes, 159
Category III Codes—New Technology, 160
The Index, 160
Appendices of CPT, 160

**17   Evaluation and Management (E/M) Section
(99202-99499), 161**
Integral Factors When Selecting E/M Codes, 161
Levels of E/M Service Based On, 161
Levels of 99202-99215 Based Only On, 161
E/M Levels Divided Based On, 161
Key Components, 162
Physician and Patient Dialogue, 162
Practice Exercises, 172

18   Anesthesia Section (00100-01999), 176
Anesthesiologist, 176
CRNA, 176
Uses of Anesthesia, 176
Analgesia, 176
Some Methods of Anesthesia, 176
Patient-Controlled Analgesia (PCA), 176
Moderate (Conscious) Sedation, 176
Anesthesia Formula, 176
Practice Exercises, 177

**19   CPT/HCPCS Level I Modifiers
(-22 to -99), 180**
HCPCS Level II Modifiers, 183
Practice Exercises, 184

20   Surgery Section (10004-69990), 188
General Subsection (10004-10021), 188
Integumentary System Subsection
    (10040-19499), 189
Practice Exercises, 193
Musculoskeletal System Subsection
    (20100-29999), 195
Practice Exercises, 198
Respiratory System Subsection (30000-32999), 201
Cardiovascular System Subsection, 203
Cardiovascular in Surgery Section
    (33016-37799), 203
Cardiovascular in Medicine Section
    (92920-93799), 206
Cardiovascular in Radiology Section
    (75557-75774), 208
Hemic and Lymphatic System Subsection
    (38100-38999), 208
Mediastinum and Diaphragm Subsection
    (39000-39499), 209
Practice Exercises, 209
Digestive System Subsection (40490-49999), 212
Practice Exercises, 213
Urinary System Subsection (50010-53899), 216
Male Genital System Subsection
    (54000-55899), 216
Reproductive System Procedures (55920), 217
Intersex Surgery Subsection (55970-55980), 217
Female Genital System Subsection
    (56405-58999), 217
Maternity Care and Delivery Subsection
    (59000-59899), 218
Practice Exercises, 220
Endocrine System Subsection (60000-60699), 223
Nervous System Subsection (61000-64999), 223

Eye and Ocular Adnexa Subsection
(65091-68899), 224
Auditory System Subsection (69000-69979), 225
Operating Microscope Subsection (+69990), 225
Practice Exercises, 225

21 **Radiology Section (70010-79999), 228**
Diagnostic Radiology Subsection
(70010-76499), 229
Diagnostic Ultrasound Subsection
(76506-76999), 230
Radiologic Guidance Subsection
(77001-77022), 230
Breast Mammography Subsection
(77046-77063), 230
Bone/Joint Studies Subsection (77071-77086), 230
Radiation Oncology Subsection (77261-77799), 230
Nuclear Medicine Subsection (78012-79999), 231
Practice Exercises, 232

22 **Pathology and Laboratory Section
(80047-89398, 0001U-0138U), 234**
Practice Exercises, 237

23 **Medicine Section (90281-99607), 239**
Practice Exercises, 244

24 **HCPCS Coding, 247**
One of Two Levels of Codes, 247
Format, 247
Temporary Codes, 247
HCPCS National Level II Index, 247
Table of Drugs, 247

**Part 5: ICD-10-CM and ICD-10-PCS Coding,
248**

25 **ICD-10-CM Overview, 249**
Introduction, 249
Format, 249
Alphabetic Index, 250
Table of Neoplasms, 251
Table of Drugs and Chemicals, 251
Tabular List, 252

26 **Using ICD-10-CM, 253**
General Guidelines, 253
Steps to Diagnosis Coding, 253
Diagnosis and Services, 254
Late Effects (Sequela), 254

27 **ICD-10-CM Chapters 1-10, 255**
Chapter 1, Certain Infectious and Parasitic
Diseases, 255
Chapter 2, Neoplasms, 256

Chapter 3, Diseases of the Blood and
Blood-Forming Organs and Certain Disorders
Involving the Immune Mechanism, 256
Chapter 4, Endocrine, Nutritional, and Metabolic
Diseases, 256
Chapter 5, Mental, Behavioral, and
Neurodevelopmental Disorders, 257
Chapter 6, Diseases of Nervous System, 257
Chapter 7, Diseases of Eye and Adnexa, 257
Chapter 8, Diseases of Ear and Mastoid
Process, 257
Chapter 9, Diseases of Circulatory System, 257
Chapter 10, Diseases of Respiratory System, 258

28 **ICD-10-CM Chapters 11-14, 259**
Chapter 11, Diseases of Digestive System, 259
Chapter 12, Diseases of Skin and Subcutaneous
Tissue, 259
Chapter 13, Diseases of Musculoskeletal System
and Connective Tissue, 259
Chapter 14, Diseases of Genitourinary System, 259

29 **ICD-10-CM Chapters 15-22, 261**
Chapter 15, Pregnancy, Childbirth, and
the Puerperium, 261
Chapter 16, Certain Conditions Originating in
the Perinatal Period, 261
Chapter 17, Congenital Malformations,
Deformations, and Chromosomal
Abnormalities, 262
Chapter 18, Symptoms, Signs, and Abnormal
Clinical and Laboratory Findings, Not Elsewhere
Classified, 262
Chapter 19, Injury, Poisoning, and Certain Other
Consequences of External Causes, 262
Chapter 20, External Causes of Morbidity, 262
Chapter 21, Factors Influencing Health Status and
Contact With Health Services, 263
Chapter 22, Codes for Special Purposes, 264

30 **Outpatient Coding, 265**
OGCR Section IV, Diagnostic Coding and Reporting
Guidelines for Outpatient Services, 265

31 **ICD-10-PCS, Reporting Inpatient
Procedures, 267**
Table of Contents, 267
Alphabetic Index, 267
Tabular List, 267
Index, 267
Guidelines, 267
Bundling, 268

Part 6: Physician-based Examinations, 270

32 **Physician-based Examinations, 271**
Pre-Examination and Post-Examination, 271

Final Examination, 272
Physician Exam (Format A)—Final Examination
    Answer Sheet, 273
Physician Exam (Format A)—Final Examination, 274

Part 7: Facility-based Examinations, 292

33   Facility-based Examinations, 293
Pre-Examination and Post-Examination, 293
Final Examination, 294

Figure Credits, 295

Appendix A   Resources, 296

Appendix B   Answers, 297
Part 1 Quiz Answers, 297
Part 2 Quiz Answers, 300
Part 3 Quiz Answers, 300
Part 4 Practice Exercise Answers and
    Rationales, 300

Appendix C   Medical Terminology, 311

Appendix D   Combining Forms, 324

Appendix E   Prefixes, 327

Appendix F   Suffixes, 328

Appendix G   Abbreviations, 329

Appendix H   Further Text Resources, 332

Appendix I   Pharmacology Review, 335

Index, 345

Success Strategies

This review was developed to help you as you prepare for your certification examination. First, congratulations on your initiative. Preparing for a certification examination can seem like a daunting and formidable task. You have already taken the first and hardest step: you have made a commitment. Your steely determination and organizational skills are your best tools as you prepare to complete this exciting journey successfully.

How do you prepare for a certification examination? The answers to that question are as varied as the persons preparing for it. Each person comes to the preparation with different educational, coding, and personal experiences. Therefore, each must develop a plan that meets his or her individual needs and preferences. Success Strategies will help you to develop your individual plan.

The Certification Examination

This text has been developed to serve as a tool in your preparation for the outpatient (physician-based) certification examination.

AAPC: For AAPC, the CPC® (Certified Professional Coder) certification examination consists of a total of 150 multiple-choice questions covering medical terminology, anatomy, pathophysiology, CPT, ICD-10-CM, HCPCS, coding guidelines, and compliance and regulatory. You have 5 hours and 40 minutes to complete the examination. Exam results are reported with scores and your top three areas of weakness. Visit the AAPC website (www.aapc.com/certification/cpc) for the latest information on the CPC® examination.

AHIMA: For AHIMA, the CCS-P® (Certified Coding Specialist-Physician) and CCS® (Certified Coding Specialist) certification examinations both consist of 105 questions: 97 multiple-choice and 8 coding scenarios. Questions cover medical terminology, anatomy, pathophysiology, coding for CPT, ICD-10-CM/PCS, and HCPCS, and reimbursement and health information management concepts. You will have 4 hours to complete the examination. Exam results are reported with score percentages for each "domain" tested, as well as the total possible score and the individual's score. Visit the AHIMA website (www.ahima.org/certification) for the latest information on the CCS-P® and CCS® exams.

To be successful on either certification examination, you will have to know how to assign medical codes to patient services and diagnoses. This textbook focuses on providing you with that coding practice as well as anatomy, terminology, pathophysiology, reimbursement, and health information management concepts in preparation for the examination.

Date and Location

Although every journey begins with the first step, you have to know where you are going to make a plan to get there.

- Choose the **date and location** for taking the certification examination.

    AAPC: The website www.aapc.com/certification contains detailed information about examination sites and dates. The exams are sponsored by local chapters or instructors licensed through AAPC. You may choose from those listed. The test is administered on paper.

    AHIMA: The website www.ahima.org/certification contains detailed information about applying for the examination.

- **AAPC:** The AAPC has information that can be downloaded from their website at www.aapc.com/certification or by calling (877)-290-0440.

- **AHIMA:** The American Health Information Management Association has a Candidate Guide that includes eligibility requirements, information on applying for the examination, test center restrictions, and sample examination screens. The Candidate Guide can be downloaded from their website at www.ahima.org/certification.

- After you have obtained the candidate information and examination materials, read all the information carefully. Review all competencies outlined in the material to ensure that your study plan contains strategies to address each of these competencies. Check for the latest information on acceptable forms of identification, coding rules to follow, and passing scores.

- The questions within this textbook are not the same questions that are in the certification examination, but the skill and knowledge that you gain through analysis, coding, and recall will increase your ability to be successful on examination day.

Managing Your Time

Role strain! That is what you get when you have so many different roles in your life and you cannot find time for all of them! Know that feeling? Are you a daughter/son, mother/father, wife/husband, student, friend, worker, volunteer, hobbyist—the list is endless. Each takes time from your schedule, and somehow you now need to fit into the role of successful learner. Because you have only 24 hours in your day, being a successful learner requires a time-balancing act. Maybe you will have to be satisfied with dust bunnies under your bed, dishes in your kitchen sink, or fewer visits with your friends. Whatever you have to do to juggle the time around to give yourself ample time to devote to this important task of examination preparation, you must do and make a plan for in advance; otherwise, life just takes over and you find you do not have adequate study time.

If you are planning a big event in your life—moving, a trip, and so on—think about postponing it until after the examination. Your focus right now has to be on yourself. Make your motto **"It's All About Me!"** Sounds self-centered, I know, and most likely very different from who you are, but just this once, you need to carve out the time you need to accomplish this important goal. This time is for yourself. Make it happen for yourself. Move everything you can out of the way, focus on this preparation, and give this preparation your best effort.

Schedule

Each person has an individual learning style. The coding profession seems to attract those most influenced by logic and facts. The best way for a logical and factual person to learn is to problem-solve and apply the information. Hands-on practice is how you will build your skill and confidence for the examination.

- Choose a location to be your Study Central.
- Gather into Study Central the following study resources:
  - Certification packet or handbook from the certifying organization
  - CPT, designated edition
  - ICD-10-CM, designated edition
  - ICD-10-PCS, designated edition (facility exams only)
  - HCPCS, designated edition
  - ICD-10-CM/PCS *Official Guidelines for Coding and Reporting* (can be accessed by following the Evolve Resources link provided in Appendix A of this text)
  - Medical dictionary
  - Coding textbooks, professional journals, and magazines
  - Terminology, anatomy, or pathology text, as needed
  - See Appendix H for Further Text Resources

Make Study Central your special place where you can get away from all other responsibilities. Make it a quiet, calm getaway, even if it is a corner of your bedroom. In this quiet place have a comfortable chair, adequate lighting, supplies, and sufficient desktop surface to use all your coding books. This is your place to focus all your attention on preparation for the examination, without distractions.

- Plan your **schedule** from now until the certification examination using a calendar. Make weekly goals so that you have definite tasks to accomplish each week and you can check the tasks off—a great feeling of accomplishment comes from being able to check off a task. In this way, you can see your progress on your countdown to success.
- Choose a specific **time** each day or several times a week when you are going to study and mark them on your calendar. Make this commitment in writing. After each study session, you should check off that date on the calendar as a visual reminder that you are sticking to your plan and are one step closer to your goal.
- You should plan your study time in advance, know what you are going to be studying the next session, and **be prepared** for that upcoming study session. This will greatly increase the amount of material you are able to cover during the session. At the end of each session, decide what you are going to study next session and ensure that you have all the material and references you will need readily available. At the end of each session, you should be ready for the next study session.
- Your plan should include those areas where you know you will need improvement. For example, when is the last time you read, not referenced or reviewed, but really read, the CPT Anesthesia Guidelines? You probably do not code anesthesia services often, if ever, and as such are not familiar with the information in these guidelines. That is an area of improvement, and your plan should include a thorough reading of all the CPT section guidelines.
- **DO THIS BEFORE YOU BEGIN YOUR STUDY: Assess** your strengths and weaknesses. By making this assessment, you will know where to concentrate your efforts and where to focus your study schedule. You know those areas where you already have strong skills and knowledge and will not need to spend as much time preparing in these areas. The **Pre-Examination,** found on the Evolve website, is an examination that you can use as a tool to assess your current skill level. This examination should be taken before you begin your study and then again (as the Post-Examination) immediately after you have completed your entire study schedule. Do not analyze the questions by reviewing the Pre-Examination rationales (located on the Evolve website); rather, wait until after you have completed your studies and have taken this same examination a second time as the Post-Examination. If you review the rationales after the first time you take the examination, you will know the answers too well to provide a valid comparison between examinations. See Parts 6 and 7 of this textbook for further information.
- After you have completed your course of study, take the **Post-Examination** on the companion Evolve website. You should plan to cover the examination in the same amount of time as will be given for the certification examination you are going to take. Compare your scores to those from the first time you took this examination. Note the areas where you did not demonstrate sufficient skills and knowledge.
- Develop a **second plan** to improve the specific areas where you believe you need further study.

- You are now ready to take the **Final Examination**. Take the examination in the same amount of time that will be allocated for the certification examination. It is best if you do this final in one sitting, thereby mimicking the actual examination. If your schedule does not allow for taking the examination in one sitting, plan to take it in several sessions, but always keep track of the time used to ensure that you take the examination in the same amount of time allowed for the official examination. Learning to work within the time allocated is part of the skill you are developing. Remember the certification examinations assess not only your coding knowledge but also your efficiency in completing the examination within the allocated time.

Using This Text

This text is divided into:
- Success Strategies
- Part 1, Anatomy, Terminology, and Pathophysiology
- Part 2, Physician-based Reimbursement Issues
- Part 3, Facility-based Reimbursement Issues
- Part 4, CPT and HCPCS Coding
- Part 5, ICD-10-CM and ICD-10-PCS Coding
- Part 6, Physician-based Examinations
- Part 7, Facility-based Examinations
- Appendix A, Resources (Web-Based)
- Appendix B, Answers
- Appendix C, Medical Terminology
- Appendix D, Combining Forms
- Appendix E, Prefixes
- Appendix F, Suffixes
- Appendix G, Abbreviations
- Appendix H, Further Text Resources
- Appendix I, Pharmacology Review

Appendices C–G are combined lists of Medical Terminology, Combining Forms, Prefixes, Suffixes, and Abbreviations used within Part 1, Anatomy, Terminology, and Pathophysiology.

The material in this review features the following:
- Comprehensive guide in outline format
- Photos and drawings to illustrate key points
- Practice examinations

  For the purposes of this text, three practice exam formats have been developed so you can focus on the exam format that most closely resembles the certification exam you've chosen to take:

  Physician Exam (Format A)
  Pre-/Post-Examination (150 multiple-choice questions)
  Final Examination (150 multiple-choice questions)

  Physician Exam (Format B)
  Pre-/Post-Examination (97 multiple-choice and 8 case scenarios)
  Final Examination (97 multiple-choice and 8 case scenarios)

  Facility Exam (Format C)
  Pre-/Post-Examination (97 multiple-choice and 8 cases)
  Final Examination (97 multiple-choice and 8 cases)

- **Part 1** is a review of the anatomy, terminology, and pathophysiology by organ systems designed to provide you with a quick review of that organ system. In addition, there is a list of combining forms, prefixes, suffixes, and abbreviations that are often used in that organ system. At the end of each organ system, there is a quiz that will give you an opportunity to assess your knowledge. (Answers are located in Appendix B.)
- **Part 2 and Part 3** review reimbursement issues and terminology. A quiz is located at the end of each part to assess your knowledge. (Answers are located in Appendix B.)
- **Part 4 and Part 5** review CPT, HCPCS, ICD-10-CM, and ICD-10-PCS. The CPT and ICD-10-CM material follows the order of the manuals. Practice exercises are located throughout this part. (Answers are located in Appendix B.)
- **Part 6 and Part 7** contain instructions regarding the practice examinations, including the Final Examination for Physician Exam (Format A).

> **NOTE**
>
> To enable the learner to calculate an examination score, the minimum of 70% has been identified as "passing" within this text; however, this may not be the percentage identified by the certifying organization as a "passing" grade. It is your responsibility to review all certification information published by the certifying organization.

There are many ways you could use this text. However you decide to prepare, you should take the Pre-Examination before you begin your study to ensure that you develop a study plan that includes time and activities that will increase your knowledge in those areas where your test scores indicate areas of weakness. You could then take the parts in the order they are presented, or you may want to review the anatomy, terminology, and pathophysiology for a body system and then review the CPT material for that body system. There is no one best way to approach the use of this text because each individual will have a personal learning style and preferences that will direct how the material is used. Your skills may be very strong in one or more coding or knowledge areas, and you will want to delete those areas from your individual study plan.

This text is not meant to be the only study source but only one tool of many that you will use. For example, if your terminology skills need a complete overhaul, the brief overview in this text may not meet your needs. You may want to supplement this text with a terminology text and an in-depth study of terminology.

- **Appendices** are a resource for you as you prepare your study plan.
  - **Appendix A,** Resources, is an Evolve Resources link (web-based) to the *ICD-10-CM Official Guidelines for Coding and Reporting*. This link provides the rules for use of ICD-10-CM codes and will be referenced

in Part 4 when reviewing the use of ICD-10-CM codes.

- **Appendix B,** Answers, Parts 1-3 Quiz Answers, and Part 4 Practice Exercises Answers and Rationales.
- **Appendix C,** Medical Terminology, is a complete alphabetic list of all the medical terms listed in the Medical Terminology portion of the organ system reviews used in Part 1.
- **Appendix D,** Combining Forms, is a complete alphabetic list of the combining forms used in Part 1.
- **Appendix E,** Prefixes, is a complete alphabetic list of the prefixes used in Part 1.
- **Appendix F,** Suffixes, is a complete alphabetic list of the suffixes used in Part 1.
- **Appendix G,** Abbreviations, is a complete list of the abbreviations referenced in Part 1.
- **Appendix H,** Further Text Resources, is a list of texts that you may want to obtain to supplement your study plan.
- **Appendix I,** Pharmacology Review, contains a list of drugs with generic name, trade/registered brand name, and therapeutic use and/or medication action.

Day Before the Examination

- No cramming! Your study time is now over, and cramming the day before the test is not a good idea because it just increases your anxiety level. This day is your day to prepare yourself. Do some things you enjoy this day. Take your mind off the examination. Pamper yourself: you deserve it.
- Review the examination requirements one last time to ensure that you have all the required material.
- Listen to the weather and traffic reports. Plan your route to the examination site. If it is in a new location, drive to the location before the big day.
- Eat a light supper and get to bed early. Set the alarm in plenty of time to arrive at the site early. It is a good idea to have a friend or family member give you an early wake-up call to ensure that you do not oversleep.
- Bring a copy of any official errata associated with your CPT, HCPCS, or ICD-10-CM manual.
- **AAPC:** Prepare pencils (no. 2), erasers, picture identification, CPT (AMA standard or professional version only), ICD-10-CM, HCPCS code manuals, and examination admission card. For a paper/pencil examination, take a ruler so that if you skip a question and want to mark that question to return to later, you can use the ruler to make certain you return to the correct question.
- **AAPC:** Although writing, sticky notes, labels, etc., are allowed in your code books, make sure to check the AAPC examination information to ensure that your books meet the specifications identified by the testing organization.
- **AAPC:** Pack quiet snacks and bottled water sufficient for 5 hours and 40 minutes.

- **AHIMA:** Bring two forms of ID. One must be a government-issued picture ID. The other may be a credit card or acceptable ID with the candidate's signature (reference the Candidate Guide for the latest list of acceptable IDs). Your identification will be checked multiple times during your exam experience.
- **AHIMA:** Your test will be administered at a computer terminal. If you wear special glasses when working on a computer, plan to bring them.
- **AHIMA:** No food or snacks will be permitted at the exam. Everything except your code books and identification will be stowed in a locker.
- **AHIMA:** Plan to bring your examination confirmation form with you to the exam.
- **AHIMA:** AHIMA designates the year of CPT, HCPCS, ICD-10-PCS, and ICD-10-CM code books used for the exam. Be sure you possess the right year. You are also allowed to bring a medical dictionary into the exam, and you should plan to do so. You will still be admitted to the exam if you do not have a medical dictionary, but you must have all three designated-year code books. The code books must be free of excessive writing, additional papers, or sticky notes.

Day of the Examination

- Wear comfortable clothes and be prepared for any room temperature. A short-sleeved shirt with a sweater is a good plan. Dress in layers so you can ensure that you will be comfortable in any environment.
- Eat a good breakfast. Avoid caffeine because it initially stimulates you, but in the long run will decrease your concentration.
- Arrive early. The doors are locked to those who arrive late. This is a day to be early.
- Ensure that you have the correct room for your examination. Often there are several examinations being administered at one time, so be certain you are in the correct room for your examination.
- **AAPC:** Bring a watch with you so that you can pace yourself during the exam. Phones are prohibited in the exam room.
- **AHIMA:** No phones or watches are allowed into the exam room but should be left at home or placed in the locker provided to you. The computer will have a clock embedded in it so you can manage your time during the test.

The Certification Examination

You are ready for this! You have planned your work and have worked your plan. Now it is time to reap the rewards for all that hard work.

- **AAPC:** Choose a good location in which to sit. Choose a location that will not get a lot of traffic from those leaving the room. Place all your supplies on the table.
- **AHIMA:** You will be taken to an assigned seat to begin your exam. Have all your books available to you. The

exam table is small, so plan how best to access your books quickly in this space.

- Have faith in yourself, and visualize yourself being successful. Say to yourself "I can do this," and then take several deep breaths before you begin to help relax you.
- **AAPC:** Some prefer to take the parts of the examination out of order, taking those questions they are most confident of first. Others prefer to start at the beginning and work through all questions in order. The approach that you use will depend on your individual test-taking style.
- **AAPC:** When you come to a question for which you are unsure of the answer, you may wish to skip over and come back to all those ones you were unsure of at the end of the examination, depending on the time available. Or you may want to attempt each question and note those you are unsure of to return to when you have finished the exam section. Again, the approach you will use depends on your individual style.
- **AHIMA:** One question will be displayed at a time. You must answer a question before moving to the next. If the answer is not immediately apparent to you, select your "best guess" and flag this question for review once you have completed the entire exam. In this way, you will be able to manage your time more effectively.
- Read the directions. This may sound too simple, but many persons do not completely read the directions, only to find that the directions gave specific directions about what or what not to code on a certain case (for example, "code only this certain portion of the procedure"). Yet the choices for answers included the full coding of the case as a selection; if you did not read all the directions, you would choose the response with codes for all the items listed in the report. For example, the question may have directed you to code the service only, not the diagnosis, and yet one of the choices would be the correct service and diagnosis codes, which of course would be an incorrect answer based on the directions. So read all of the directions.
- Your speed and accuracy are being tested. You do not have time to labor over each question for a long time if you intend to complete all the questions. Read the directions, read the question, put down your best assessment of the answer, and then move on to the next question.
- Words such as *always, every, never,* and *all* generally indicate broad terms that, with true/false questions, usually indicate a false question.

- If you do not know the answer to the question, try eliminating those that you know are incorrect first and then select that answer that seems more likely to be correct.
- Judge the time as you are moving through the examination. Keep assessing whether you are making sufficient progress or whether you can slow down or need to speed up.
- **AAPC:** Answer all questions. Even if you have to guess quickly, at least fill in an answer. The best situation is that you answer all questions and have time left to go back over the questions about which you are in doubt.
- Use every minute of the test time, but it is not a good idea to begin second-guessing yourself. Do not return to those questions for which you did not have serious doubts about the correct answer. Usually, your first answer is the best.
- **AAPC:** When the time is finished and you've submitted your examination, pat yourself on the back! You have done an excellent job.
- **AHIMA:** When your time is up, report to the test center staff to receive your score. You will know that day whether you passed the exam.
- Now it is time to go get a good supper and a good night's sleep.

Days After the Examination

- You will miss the preparation! Okay, maybe not miss it exactly, but your life will be different now without that constant preparation.
- **AAPC:** Relax and await the results in confidence. You have done your best. That is always good enough!
- **Be proud of yourself;** this was no small undertaking, and you did it.

Our personal best wishes to you as you prepare for your certification. You can do this!

Best regards,

Carol J. Buck, MS

Jackie L. Koesterman, CPC

Our goals can only be reached through a vehicle of a plan, in which we must fervently believe, and upon which we must vigorously act. There is no other route to success.

—*Stephen A. Brennen*

PART 1

Anatomy, Terminology, and Pathophysiology

1

Integumentary System

The skin and accessory organs (nails, hair, and glands)

Layers

(Fig. 1.1)

Two Layers Make Up Skin: Epidermis and Dermis

Epidermis. Outermost layer; containing keratin
Stratum corneum, most superficial layer of four layers called stratum
Basal layer, deepest region of epidermis (stratum germinativum or stratum basale), is growth layer
Dermis. The second layer of skin

Two layers are papillary and reticulary and contain:

Fibrous connective tissue or skin appendages
Blood vessels
Nerves
Hair
Nails
Glands
Subcutaneous Tissue or Hypodermis. Not considered a layer of skin
Contains fat tissue and fibrous connective tissue
AKA: superficial fascia
Connects skin to underlying muscle

Nails

Keratin plates covering dorsal surface of each finger and toe
Lunula—semilunar or half-moon

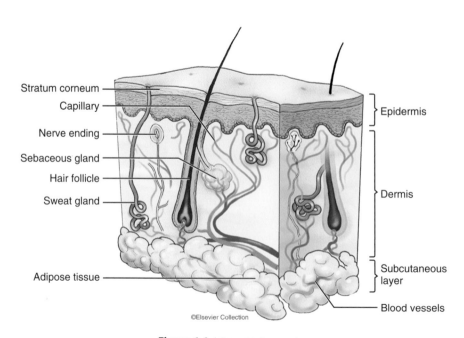

Stratum corneum
Capillary
Nerve ending
Sebaceous gland
Hair follicle
Sweat gland
Adipose tissue

Epidermis
Dermis
Subcutaneous layer
Blood vessels

©Elsevier Collection

• **Figure 1.1** Integumentary system.

White area at base of nail plate is growth area
  Thickens and lengthens nail
Eponychium or cuticle: narrow band of epidermis at base
  and sides of nail
Paronychium: soft tissue around nail border

Glands

Sebaceous glands located in dermal layer
  Secrete sebum that lubricates skin/hair
  Influenced by sex hormones so they hypertrophy in adolescence and atrophy in old age
Sudoriferous glands originate in dermis. See Fig. 1.1.
  AKA: sweat glands
  Extend up through epidermis opening as pores
  Secrete mostly water and salts to cool body

TABLE 1-1
Combining Forms

Combining Form	Meaning
1. aden/o	in relationship to a gland
2. adip/o	fat
3. albin/o	white
4. aut/o	self
5. bi/o	life
6. caus/o	burning sensation
7. cauter/o	burn
8. crypt/o	hidden
9. cutane/o	skin
10. cyan/o	blue
11. derm/o, dermat/o	skin
12. diaphor/o	profuse sweating
13. eosin/o	rosy
14. erythem/o	red
15. erythr/o	red
16. heter/o	different
17. hidr/o	sweat
18. ichthy/o	dry/scaly
19. jaund/o	yellow
20. kerat/o	hard
21. leuk/o	white
22. lip/o	fat
23. lute/o	yellow
24. melan/o	black
25. myc/o	fungus
26. necr/o	death
27. onych/o	nail
28. pachy/o	thick
29. phyt/o	plant
30. pil/o	hair
31. poli/o	gray matter
32. py/o	pus
33. rhytid/o	wrinkle
34. rube/o	red
35. seb/o	sebum/oil
36. staphyl/o	clusters
37. steat/o	fat
38. strept/o	twisted chain
39. squam/o	flat/scalelike
40. trich/o	hair
41. ungu/o	nail
42. xanth/o	yellow
43. xer/o	dry

TABLE 1-2
Prefixes

Prefix	Meaning
1. epi-	on/upon
2. hyper-	over
3. hypo-	under
4. intra-	within
5. para-	beside
6. per-	through
7. peri-	surrounding
8. sub-	under

TABLE 1-3
Suffixes

Suffix	Meaning
1. -coccus	spherical bacterium
2. -ectomy	removal
3. -ia	condition
4. -malacia	softening
5. -opsy	view of
6. -plasty	surgical repair
7. -rrhea	discharge
8. -tome	an instrument to cut
9. -tomy	to cut

TABLE 1-4
Medical Abbreviations

Abbreviation	Meaning
1. bx	biopsy
2. ca	cancer
3. derm	dermatology
4. I&D	incision and drainage
5. subcu, subq, SC, SQ	subcutaneous
6. PPD	tuberculin skin test

TABLE 1-5

Medical Terms

Term	Meaning	Term	Meaning
Absence	Without	Hematoma	A localized collection of blood, usually result of a break in a blood vessel
Adipose	Fatty		
Albinism	Lack of color pigment		
Allograft	Homograft, same species graft	Homograft	Allograft, same species graft
Alopecia	Condition in which hair falls out	Ichthyosis	Skin disorder characterized by scaling
Anhidrosis	Deficiency of sweat		
Autograft	From patient's own body	Incise	To cut into
Avulsion	Ripping or tearing away of part either surgically or accidentally	Island pedicle flap	Contains a single artery and vein that remains attached to origin temporarily or permanently
Biopsy	Removal of a small piece of living tissue for diagnostic purposes		
		Leukoderma	Depigmentation of skin
Causalgia	Burning pain	Leukoplakia	White patch on mucous membrane
Collagen	Protein substance of skin	Lipocyte	Fat cell
Debridement	Cleansing of or removal of dead tissue from a wound	Lipoma	Fatty tumor
		Melanin	Dark pigment of skin
Delayed flap	Pedicle of skin with blood supply that is separated from origin over time	Melanoma	Tumor of epidermis, malignant and black in color
Dermabrasion	Planing of skin by means of sander, brush, or sandpaper	Mohs surgery or Mohs micrographic surgery	Removal of skin cancer in layers by a surgeon who also acts as a pathologist during surgery
Dermatologist	Physician who treats conditions of skin	Muscle flap	Transfer of muscle from origin to recipient site
Dermatoplasty	Surgical repair of skin	Neurovascular flap	Contains artery, vein, and nerve
Electrocautery	Cauterization by means of heated instrument	Pedicle	Growth attached with a stem
		Pilosebaceous	Pertains to hair follicles and sebaceous glands
Epidermolysis	Loosening of epidermis		
Epidermomycosis	Superficial fungal infection	Sebaceous gland	Secretes sebum
Epithelium	Surface covering of internal and external organs of body	Seborrhea	Excess sebum secretion
		Sebum	Oily substance
Erythema	Redness of skin	Split-thickness graft	All epidermis and some of dermis
Escharotomy	Surgical incision into necrotic (dead) tissue	Steatoma	Fat mass in sebaceous gland
		Stratified	Layered
Fissure	Cleft or groove	Stratum (strata)	Layer
Free full-thickness graft	Graft of epidermis and dermis that is completely removed from donor area	Subungual	Beneath nail
		Xanthoma	Tumor composed of cells containing lipid material, yellow in color
Furuncle	Nodule in skin caused by *Staphylococcus* entering through hair follicle	Xenograft	Different species graft
		Xeroderma	Dry, discolored, scaly skin

Chapter 1: Anatomy and Terminology Quiz

(Quiz Answers Are Located in Appendix B)

1. This is the outermost layer of skin:
   a. basal
   b. dermis
   c. epidermis
   d. subcutaneous

2. Which of the following is/are NOT a part of skin or accessory organs?
   a. sudoriferous glands
   b. sebaceous gland
   c. nail
   d. arterioles

3. This prefix means beside:
   a. para-
   b. intra-
   c. per-
   d. epi-

4. This combining form means hair:
   a. xanth/o
   b. trich/o
   c. ichthy/o
   d. kerat/o

5. Lunula is the:
   a. narrow band of epidermis at base of nail
   b. opening of pores
   c. outermost layer of epidermis
   d. white area at base of nail plate

6. Subcutaneous tissue is also known as:
   a. dermal
   b. adipose
   c. hypodermis
   d. stratum corneum

7. Which of the following combining forms does NOT refer to a color?
   a. cyan/o
   b. jaund/o
   c. eosin/o
   d. pachy/o

8. This medical term means surgical incision into dead tissue:
   a. onychomycosis
   b. escharotomy
   c. keratotomy
   d. curettage

9. This suffix means surgical repair:
   a. -opsy
   b. -rrhea
   c. -plasty
   d. -tome

10. Soft tissue around nail border is the:
   a. cuticle
   b. lunula
   c. paronychium
   d. corium

PATHOPHYSIOLOGY

Lesions and Other Abnormalities (Fig. 1.2)

Macule

Flat area of color change (mostly reddened)
No elevation or depression
Example: flat moles, freckles

Papule

Solid elevation
Less than 1.0 cm in diameter
May run together and form plaques
Example: warts, lichen planus, elevated mole

Nodule

Solid elevation 1-2 cm in diameter
Extends deeper into dermis than papule
Example: lipoma, erythema nodosum, enlarged lymph nodes

Pustule

Elevated area
Filled with purulent fluid
Example: pimple, impetigo, abscess

Tumor

Solid mass
Uncontrolled, progressive growth of cells
Example: hemangioma, neoplasm, lipoma

Plaque

Flat, elevated surface
Equal or greater than 1.0 cm
Example: psoriasis, seborrheic keratosis

Wheal

Temporary localized elevation of skin
Results in transient edema in dermis
Example: insect bite, allergic reaction

Vesicle

Small blister
Less than 1 cm in diameter
Filled with serous fluid in epidermis
Example: herpes zoster (shingles), varicella (chickenpox)

Bulla

Large blister
Greater than 1.0 cm in diameter
Example: blister

Scales

Flakes of cornified skin layer
Example: dry skin

Crust

Dried exudate on skin
Example: scab

MACULE
Flat area of color change; no elevation or depression

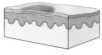
©Elsevier Collection

PAPULE
Solid elevation; less than 1.0 cm in diameter

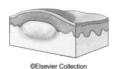
©Elsevier Collection

NODULE
Solid elevation 1-2 cm in diameter; extends deeper into dermis than papule

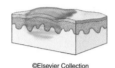
©Elsevier Collection

PUSTULE
Elevated, superficial lesion; similar to a vesicle but filled with purulent fluid

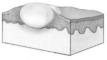
©Elsevier Collection

TUMOR
Solid mass; larger than 2.0 cm

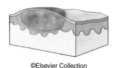
©Elsevier Collection

PLAQUE
Flat elevated surface found where papules, nodules, or tumors cluster

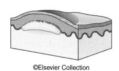
©Elsevier Collection

WHEAL
Temporary localized elevation of the skin; result is transient edema in dermis

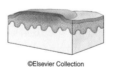
©Elsevier Collection

VESICLE
Small blister; fluid within or under epidermis

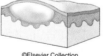
©Elsevier Collection

BULLA
Larger blister; greater than 1.0 cm in diameter

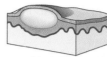
©Elsevier Collection

SCALES
Flakes of cornified skin layer

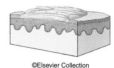
©Elsevier Collection

CRUST
Dried exudate on skin

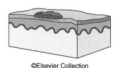
©Elsevier Collection

FISSURE
Cracks in skin

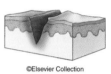
©Elsevier Collection

EROSION
Loss of epidermis that does not extend into dermis

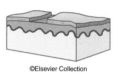
©Elsevier Collection

SCAR
Excess collagen production following injury

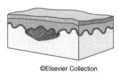
©Elsevier Collection

ATROPHY
Loss of some portion of the skin

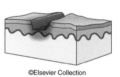
©Elsevier Collection

ULCER
Area of destruction of entire epidermis

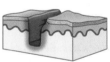
©Elsevier Collection

• **Figure 1.2** Lesions of skin.

Fissure

Cracks in skin
Example: athlete's foot, openings in corners of mouth

Erosion

Loss of epidermis
Does not extend into dermis
Example: blisters

Scar

Excess collagen production following surgery or trauma
Example: healed surgical wound

Atrophy

Loss of some portion of skin and appears translucent
Example: aged skin
• Not a lesion, but a physiologic response in aging process

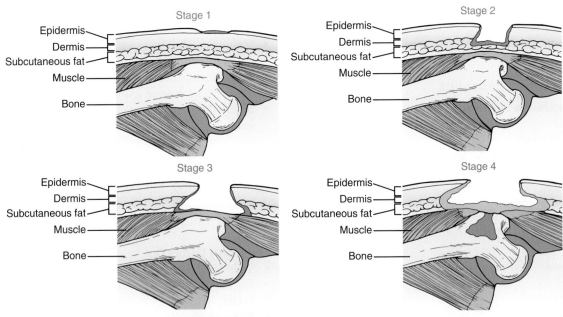

Figure 1.3 Stages 1, 2, 3, and 4 of pressure ulcers.

Ulcer

Area of destruction of entire epidermis
Example: missing tissue on heel, decubitus bedsore (pressure sore)

Pressure Ulcer (Decubitus Ulcer) *(Fig. 1.3)*

Result of Pressure or Force
Occludes blood flow, causing ischemia and tissue death
Develops over bony prominence

Locations
- Coccygeal (end of spine)
- Sacral (between hips)
- Heel
- Elbow
- Ischial (lower hip)
- Trochanteric (outer hip)

Staging or Classification System
- Stage 1: erythema (redness) of skin
- Stage 2: partial loss of skin (epidermis or dermis)
- Stage 3: full-thickness loss of skin (up to but not through fascia)
- Stage 4: full-thickness loss (extensive destruction and necrosis)
  Deep ulcers may require surgical debridement

Keloids

Sharply elevated, irregularly shaped scars that progressively enlarge
Due to excessive collagen in corneum during connective tissue repair
Result of tissue repair or trauma
Familial tendency for formation

Cicatrix

Normal scar left after wound healing

Inflammatory Disorders

Atopic Dermatitis

Unknown etiology
  Exogenous (External) Causes Include
Irritant dermatitis
  Allergic contact dermatitis
  Endogenous (Internal) Cause Includes
Seborrheic dermatitis
  Results in Activation Of
- Mast cells
- Eosinophils
- T lymphocytes
- Monocytes

Greater in Those With Family History Of
- Asthma
- Dry skin
- Eczema
- Allergic rhinitis

Common In
- Children
- Infants

Results In
- Chronic inflammation
- Scratching
- Erythema
- Thickened, leathery skin (lichenification)
- Secondary *Staphylococcus aureus* infection

Treatment
- Topical steroid
- Antibiotic for secondary infection
- Antihistamines

Allergic Contact Dermatitis

Most common in infants and children

Potential Causes
- Hypersensitivity to allergens
  - Microorganisms
  - Drugs
  - Foreign proteins
  - Chemicals
  - Latex
  - Metals
  - Plants

Manifestations
- Scaling
- Lichenification (leathery, thickened skin)
- Erythema
- Itching (pruritus)
- Vesicular lesions
- Edema

Diagnosis and Treatment
- Check medical history
- Patch test
- Avoidance of irritant
- Skin lubrication and hydration
- Steroids
  - Topical
  - Systemic
- Topical tacrolimus (immunosuppressive agent)

Irritant Contact Dermatitis

Response To
- Chemical
- Exposure to irritant

Treatment
- Removal of irritant
- Topical agents

Stasis Dermatitis

Usually on the legs from venous stasis

Associated With
- Phlebitis
- Vascular trauma
- Varicosities

Progress
- Begins with erythema and pruritus
- Progresses to scaling, hyperpigmentation, petechiae (small hemorrhagic areas)
- Lesion becomes ulcerated

Treatment
- Elevate legs
- Reduce standing
- No constricting clothes
- Eliminate external compression
- Antibiotics for acute lesions
- Silver nitrate or Burow's solution dressings for chronic lesions

Seborrheic Dermatitis

Common chronic inflammation of sebaceous glands—cause unknown

Periods of remission and exacerbation

Commonly Occurs On
- Scalp (cradle cap in infants)
- Ear canals
- Eyelids
- Eyebrow
- Nose
- Axillae
- Chest
- Groin

Lesions Are
- Scaly (dry or greasy)
- White or yellowish
- Mildly pruritic

Treatment of Mild Cases
- Soap/shampoo of
  - Coal tar
  - Sulfur
  - Salicylic acid

Treatment of More Severe Cases
- Corticosteroid

Papulosquamous Disorders

Conditions Associated With
- Scales
- Papules
- Plaque
- Erythema

Three Types
- Psoriasis
- Pityriasis
- Lichen planus

Psoriasis

Chronic, relapsing, proliferating skin disorder
   Usually begins by age 20

Cause Unknown, Suggested to Be
- Exacerbated by anxiety; appears to run in families
- Immunologic

- Biochemical alterations
- Triggering agent

Commonly Occurs On
- Face
- Scalp
- Forearms and elbows
- Knees and legs

Results In
- Thickened dermis and epidermis
- Well-demarcated plaque
- Cell hyperproliferation/scaly
- Inflammation (pruritus)
- Deep red lesions

Treatment
- Only palliative (treatment of symptoms)

Mild cases
- Keratolytic agents
- Corticosteroids
- Emollients

Moderate cases
- Interleukin-2 inhibitors
- Psoralens and ultraviolet A (PUVA) light therapy
- Coal tar
- Cyclosporin
- Vitamin D analogs

Severe cases
- Topical agents
- Systemic corticosteroids
- Antimetabolic
- Hospitalization

Pityriasis Rosea

Unknown cause
Self-limiting inflammatory disorder
Occurs most often in young adults

Primary Lesion
- Begins with herald patch 3 to 4 cm
- Salmon-pink colored
- Circular and well-defined lesions

Secondary Lesions
- 14 to 21 days

Trunk and upper extremities
- Oval lesions
- Severe pruritus

Diagnosis
May be confused with
- Secondary syphilis
- Seborrheic dermatitis
- Psoriasis

Treatment
- Antipruritics

- Antihistamines
- Corticosteroids
- Ultraviolet light
- Sunlight

Lichen Planus

Occurs on skin and mucous membranes
Unknown cause (idiopathic)
Autoimmune inflammatory disorder
Onset ages 30 to 70

Lesions
- Begin as pink lesions that turn into violet-colored pruritic papules
- Result in hyperpigmentation
- 2- to 10-mm flat lesions with central depression
- Last 12 to 18 months
- Tend to recur

Treatment
- Antihistamines
- Corticosteroids
  Topical
  Systemic

Acne Vulgaris

Site of lesion is sebaceous (pilosebaceous) follicles

Primarily on face and upper trunk
Occurs in 85% of the population between the ages of 12 and 25
Exact cause: unknown
Causative factor: sebum accumulation/inflammation in pores of skin

Types
Noninflammatory acne
- Whiteheads
- Blackheads

Inflammatory acne
- Follicle walls rupture
- Sebum expels into dermis
- Inflammation begins
- Pustules, cysts, and papules result

Cause
Unknown

Treatment
Topical
- Antibiotics
- Salicylic acid
- Benzoyl peroxide
- Tretinoin

Systemic
- Antibiotic
- Hormones
- Corticosteroids
- Isotretinoin

Diaper Dermatitis

Variety of disorders

Causes
Urine
Feces
Plastic diaper cover
Allergic reaction
Secondary *Candida albicans* infection

Treatment
Clean, dry area
Expose to air
Topical antifungal medications
Topical steroids

Pruritus (Itching)

Symptom of skin disorder/dermatitis

Can be localized or generalized and is a condition, not an inflammation
Results from stimulation of nerves of skin reacting to an allergen or irritation from substances in blood or foreign bodies

Causes
Primary skin disorder
 Example: eczema or lice
 Systemic disease
 Example: chronic renal failure
 Opiates
 Allergic reaction

Treatment Is for Underlying Condition
Antihistamines
Minor tranquilizers
Application of emollients (lotions)
Topical steroids

Skin Infections

Bacterial

Impetigo

Most common in infants and children

Usually on face and begins as small vesicles
Caused primarily by *Staphylococcus*
 • Sometimes by group A beta-hemolytic *Streptococcus*
It is a highly contagious pyoderma

Treatment in Mild Cases
Topical antibiotics
Topical antiseptics

Treatment in Moderate Cases
Systemic antibiotics

Local compresses
Analgesics

Cellulitis

Caused primarily by *Staphylococcus*
Often secondary to an injury

Results In
Erythema, usually of lower trunk and legs
Fever
Localized pain
Lymphangitis

Treatment
Systemic antibiotics
Burow's soaks for pain relief

Furuncles (Boils)

Infected hair follicle

Usually caused by *Staphylococcus*
Developed boil drains pus and necrotic tissue
Squeezing spreads infection
Collection of furuncles that have merged is a carbuncle

Folliculitis

Infection of hair follicles

Results In
Erythema
Pustules

Causes
Skin trauma, such as irritation or friction
Poor hygiene
Excessive skin moisture

Treatment
Cleansing of area
Topical antibiotics

Erysipelas

Infection of skin

Cause
Group A beta-hemolytic *Streptococcus*
Common occurrence: face, ears, lower legs
Prior to outbreak, presents with
 • Fever
 • Malaise
 • Chills

Lesions Appear As
Bright red and hot
 • Develop raised borders
 • Itching

- Burning
- Tenderness

Acute Necrotizing Fasciitis

Flesh-Eating Disease
Virulent strain of gram-positive, group A beta-hemolytic *Streptococcus*
  Mortality rate of over 40%

Causes
Skin trauma
Skin infection

Areas Secrete Tissue-Destroying Enzyme, Proteases
Extreme inflammation and pain

Rapidly increasing
Dermal gangrene develops

Systemic Toxicity May Develop With
Fever
Disorientation
Hypotension
Tachycardia (fast heart rate)
  May lead to organ failure

Treatment
Antimicrobial therapy
Fluid replacement
Removal of areas of infection

Viral

Herpes Simplex (Cold Sores)

Causes
Herpes simplex virus type 1 (HSV-1)
- Most common type
- Results in fever blisters or cold sores on or near lips or canker sores of the mouth
Herpes simplex virus type 2 (HSV-2)
- Genital and oral type
- Prominent sexually transmitted disease
  Primary infections may show no symptoms (asymptomatic)
  Virus remains in nerve tissue to later reactivate

Reactivation May Be Triggered By
Stress
Common cold
Exposure to sun

Presents With
Burning or tingling

Develops Painful Vesicles That Rupture
Causes spreading
  May cause secondary infection of eye

- Episode lasts several weeks
- Treatment may include antiviral medication
  - No permanent cure exists

Herpes Zoster (Shingles)
Usually older adult

Caused by Varicella-Zoster Virus (VZV)
Virus was dormant and then reactivates
Result of varicella or chickenpox, usually in childhood

Affects
One cranial nerve or one dermatome (an area of skin supplied with afferent nerve fibers by a posterior spinal root)

Results In
Pain
Rash (unilateral)
Paresthesia (abnormal touch sensation, such as burning)

Course
Several weeks
Pain may continue even after lesion disappears

Treatment
Clears spontaneously
Antiviral medications provide symptomatic relief
Sedatives
Analgesic
Antipruritics

Warts (Verrucae)
Verruca vulgaris (common wart)

Caused by human papillomavirus (HPV)
- Numerous types of HPV
Spread by contact
Appear anywhere on body
Present with a grayish appearance
Variety of shapes and sizes
Transmitted by touch
Plantar warts (verrucae) are located on pressure points of body (such as feet; *plantar* means the bottom surface of foot)
Painful when pressure is applied
Juvenile warts occur on feet and hands of children
Venereal warts occur on genitals/anus

Treatment
Liquid nitrogen
Topical keratolytics
Laser
Electrocautery
Often persist even with treatment

Fungal (Mycoses)
Usually superficial dermatophytes (fungus)
  Fungus lives off dead cells

Tinea
Superficial skin infections

Tinea capitis
- Infection of scalp
- Common in children
- Treatment with oral antifungal medication

Tinea corporis (ringworm)
- Infection of body
- Presents as a red ring
- Produces burning sensation and pruritus
- Treatment with topical antifungal medication

Tinea pedis (athlete's foot)
- Involves feet and toes
- Produces pain, inflammation, fissures, and foul odor
- Treatment with topical antifungal medication

Tinea unguium (onychomycosis)
- Nail infection
- Usually toenails
- Nail turns white then brown, thickens and cracks
- Spreads to other nails

Candidiasis
Caused by *Candida albicans*

Normally on mucous membranes of gastrointestinal tract and vagina

Poor health and certain conditions predispose individuals to overarching infection by *Candida*
- Antibiotic therapy, which changes the balance of the normal flora in the body

Treatment is topical or oral antifungal medications

Tumors of Skin

Benign Tumors
Keratosis(es)

Seborrheic Keratosis
Proliferation of basal cells
Dark-colored lesion
Found on trunk and face

Actinic Keratosis
Pigmented, scaly patch
Often caused by exposure to sun
Often in fair-skinned individuals
Premalignant lesion
May develop into squamous cell carcinoma
 Treatment with cryosurgery (freezing area) or excision

Keratoacanthoma
Occurs in hair follicles
Usually in those over 60

Often on face, neck, back of hands, and other locations exposed to the sun
Resolve spontaneously or are excised

Moles (Nevi)
Located on any body part
Various shapes and sizes
May become malignant
- Especially if located in area of continual irritation

Malignant Tumors
Squamous Cell Carcinoma
Similar to basal cell carcinoma
 Grows wherever squamous epithelium is located (skin, mouth, pharynx, esophagus, lungs, bladder)

Most often appears in areas exposed to sun (actinic keratosis—precancerous)
Scaly appearance
Rarely metastatic (spreading)
Easily treated with good prognosis
Surgical excision
 Cryotherapy
 Curettage
 Electrodesiccation
 Radiotherapy

Basal Cell Carcinoma
Common type of skin cancer
 Developed in deeper skin layers (basal cells) than squamous cell carcinoma
 Often occurs with sun exposure in fair-skinned individuals
 Shiny appearance and slow growing
 Easily treated with good prognosis

Malignant Melanoma
Originates in cells that produce pigment (melanocytes) or nevi

Increased Incidence With
Sun exposure
Fair hair and skin, freckles
Genetic predisposition
Skin nevus (mole) often brown and evenly colored with irregular borders
Grow downward into tissues
- Metastasize quickly

Treatment is removal with extensive border excision
- Depending on extent, chemotherapy or radiation therapy may be used

Kaposi's Sarcoma
Rare form of vascular skin cancer

Associated With

Human immunodeficiency virus (HIV)

Acquired immunodeficiency syndrome (AIDS)

Herpes virus may be found in lesions

Cells originate from endothelium in small blood vessels

Painful lesions develop rapidly, appearing as purple papules; spread quickly to lymph nodes and internal organs

Treatment

Radiation

Chemotherapy

Merkel Cell Carcinoma

Neuroendocrine carcinoma of skin

Rare and very aggressive

Associated With

Sun-exposed skin in elderly patients

Treatment with excision, radiation, and chemotherapy

Chapter 1: Pathophysiology Quiz

(Quiz Answers Are Located in Appendix B)

1. A pimple is an example of a:
   a. papule
   b. vesicle
   c. pustule
   d. nodule
2. A Stage III pressure ulcer involves:
   a. erythema of skin
   b. partial loss of epidermis and dermis
   c. full thickness loss of skin up to but not through fascia
   d. full thickness loss of skin with extensive destruction and necrosis
3. This type of dermatitis may be exogenous or endogenous and is common in children and infants:
   a. atopic
   b. irritant contact
   c. stasis
   d. seborrheic
4. Psoriasis, pityriasis, and lichen planus are three types of this disorder:
   a. dermatitis
   b. inflammatory
   c. acne
   d. papulosquamous
5. This condition begins with a herald spot:
   a. psoriasis
   b. pityriasis
   c. lichen planus
   d. dermatitis
6. This skin infection is caused by group A beta-hemolytic *Streptococcus*, and the lesions appear as firm red spots with itching, burning, and tenderness:
   a. furuncles
   b. folliculitis
   c. erysipelas
   d. fasciitis
7. This type of herpes produces cold sores:
   a. herpes zoster
   b. shingles
   c. VZV
   d. herpes simplex
8. This condition is caused by human papillomavirus:
   a. mycoses
   b. verrucae
   c. shingles
   d. folliculitis
9. This type of tumor occurs in hair follicles:
   a. keratoses
   b. nevi
   c. Kaposi's sarcoma
   d. keratoacanthoma
10. This type of superficial carcinoma is rarely metastatic:
    a. squamous cell
    b. basal cell
    c. melanoma
    d. Kaposi's sarcoma

2

Musculoskeletal System

ANATOMY AND TERMINOLOGY

Skeletal System

Comprises 206 bones, cartilage, and ligaments
Provides organ protection, movement, framework, stores calcium, hematopoiesis (formation of blood cells)

Classification of Bones

Long Bones (Tubular)
Length exceeds width of bone
Broad at ends, such as thigh, lower leg, upper arm, and lower arm

Short Bones (Cuboidal)
Cubelike bones, such as carpals (wrist) and tarsals (ankle)

Flat
Thin—flattened with curved surfaces
Cover body parts, such as skull, scapula, sternum, ribs

Irregular
Varied shapes, such as zygoma of face or vertebrae

Sesamoid
Rounded
Found near joint, such as patella (kneecap)
Patella is largest sesamoid bone in body

Structure

Long Bones (Fig. 2.1)
Diaphysis: shaft

Epiphysis: both ends of long bones—bulbular shape with muscle attachments
  • Articular cartilage covers epiphyses and serves as a cushion
Epiphyseal line or plate: growth plate that disappears when fully grown
Metaphysis: flared portion of bone near epiphyseal plate
Periosteum: dense, white outer covering (fibrous)
Cortical or compact bone: hard bone beneath periosteum mainly found in shaft

  • Medullary cavity contains yellow marrow (fatty bone marrow)
Cancellous bones: spongy or trabecular
  • Contains red bone marrow (blood cell development)
Endosteum is thin epithelial membrane lining medullary cavity of long bone

Two Skeletal Divisions
Axial (trunk)
Appendicular (appendages)

Axial Skeleton, Comprised of 80 Bones
Skull, hyoid bone, vertebral column, sacrum, ribs, and sternum

Skull
(Fig. 2.2)

Cranial
Frontal (forehead)
Parietal (sides and top)
Temporal (lower sides)
Occipital (posterior of cranium)

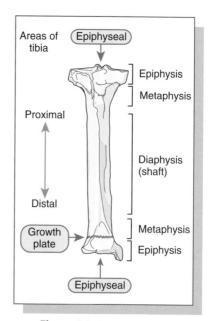

• **Figure 2.1** Structure of bones.

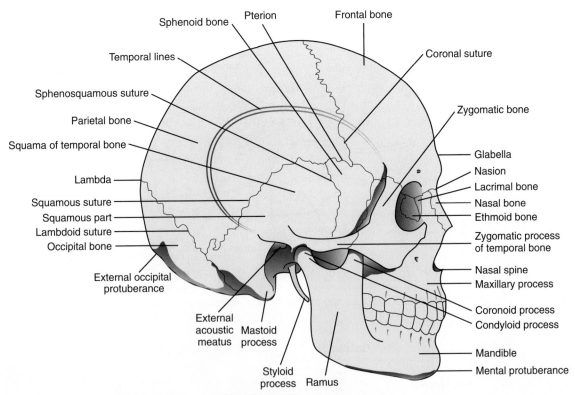

• **Figure 2.2** Lateral view of skull.

Sphenoid (floor of cranium)
Ethmoid (area between orbits and nasal cavity)
Styloid process (below ear)
Zygomatic process (cheek)

Middle Ear Bones (Fig. 2.3)
Malleus (hammer)
Incus (anvil)
Stapes (stirrup)

Face (Fig. 2.4)
Nasal (bridge of nose)
Maxilla (upper jaw)
Zygomatic (arch of cheekbone)
Mandible (lower jawbone)
Lacrimal (near orbits)
Palate (separates oral and nasal cavities)
Vomer (base, nasal septum)
Nasal conchae (turbinates)
   Interior
   Middle
   Superior

Hyoid
Supports tongue
   U-shaped
   Attached by ligaments and muscles to larynx and skull

Spine (33 Vertebrae) (Fig. 2.5)
Cervical vertebrae (7)
• C1-7

• (C1)-atlas
• (C2)-axis
Thoracic vertebrae (12) (T1-12)
Lumbar vertebrae (5) (L1-5)
Sacrum (5)—fused in adults
Coccyx (4)—fused in adults

Thorax (Fig. 2.6)
Ribs, 12 pairs
• True ribs, 1-7
• False ribs, 8-10
• Floating ribs, 11 and 12
Sternum

Appendicular Skeleton, Comprised of 126 Bones (Fig. 2.7)

Shoulder, Girdle, Pelvic Girdle, and Extremities, Pelvis
Ilium (uppermost part), wing shaped
• Acetabulum, depression on lateral hip surface into which head of femur fits
   Ischium (posterior part)
   Pubis (anterior part)
   Pubis symphysis (cartilage between pubic bones)

Lower Extremities, Femur (Thighbone)
Trochanter (processes at neck of femur)
   Head fits into acetabulum
   Patella (kneecap)
   Tibia (shinbone)
   Fibula (smaller lateral bone in lower leg)

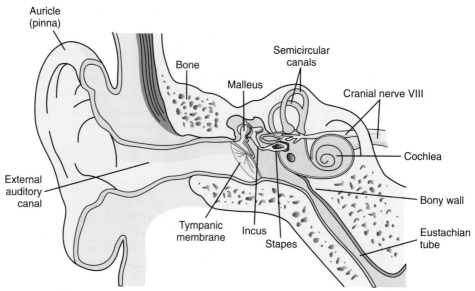

• **Figure 2.3** Structure of ear and three divisions of external, middle, and inner ear.

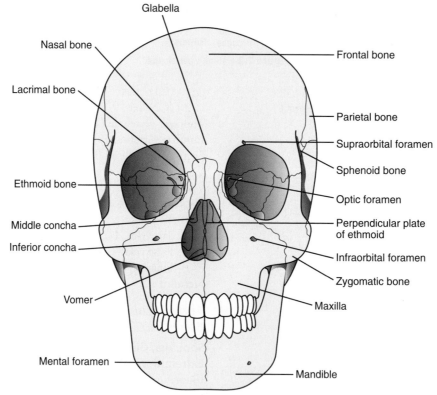

• **Figure 2.4** Frontal view of skull.

Talus (ankle bone)
Calcaneus (heel bone)
Metatarsals (foot instep)
Phalanges (toes)
Lateral malleolus (lower part of fibula)
Medial malleolus (lower part of tibia)

Upper Extremities
Clavicle (collarbone)
  Scapula (shoulder blade)

Humerus (upper arm)
Radius (forearm, thumb side)
Ulna (forearm, little finger side)
Olecranon (projection of ulna at elbow)
Carpals (wrist)—eight bones bound by ligaments in two
  rows with four bones in each
Metacarpals (hand)—framework or palm of hand (five
  bones)
Phalanges (finger)
Olecranon (tip of elbow)

Joints (Articulations)

Condyle, rounded end of bone
   Classified by degree of movement
- Synarthrosis (immovable and fibrous)
   Example: joint between cranial bones
- Amphiarthrosis (slightly movable and cartilaginous)

Example: intervertebral (joint between bodies of vertebra)
- Diarthrosis (considerably movable and synovial)
   Types
- Uniaxial—hinge and pivot joints
   Example—elbow (hinge and pivot) and cervical 2 (axis) (pivot)
- Biaxial—saddle and condyloid joints
   Example—thumb and joints between radius and carpal bones
- Multiaxial—ball and socket, gliding
   Example—shoulder and hip joints between articular surfaces of vertebrae
   Example: elbow, hip
- Bursa, sac of synovial fluid located in the tissues to prevent friction

Muscular System

Functions

Heat production
   Movement
   Posture
   Protection
   Shape

Muscle Tissue Types

Skeletal—600 Muscles Constituting 40% to 50% of Body Weight

Striated (cross-striped) (Figs. 2.8 and 2.9)
Move body
Voluntary
Attaches to bones
- Most attach to two bones with a joint in between
- Origin, point where muscle attaches to stationary bone
- Insertion, where muscle attaches to movable bone
- Body of muscle, main part of muscle

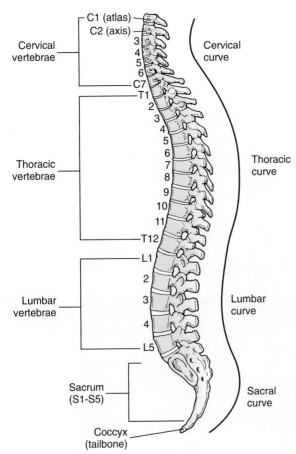

- **Figure 2.5** Anterior view of vertebral column.

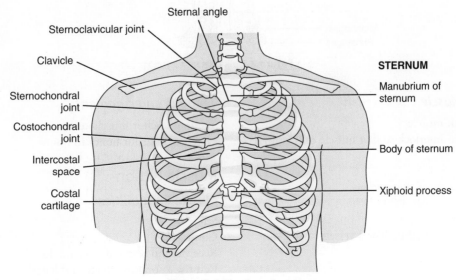

- **Figure 2.6** The thoracic cage.

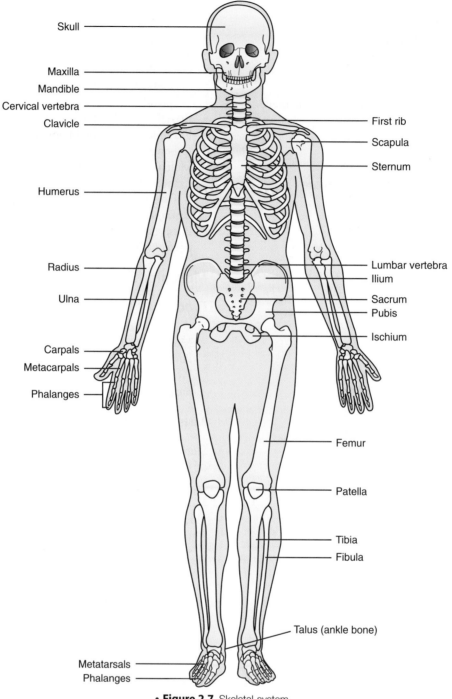

Skull

Maxilla
Mandible
Cervical vertebra
Clavicle

First rib
Scapula
Sternum

Humerus

Radius

Ulna

Lumbar vertebra
Ilium
Sacrum
Pubis
Ischium

Carpals
Metacarpals

Phalanges

Femur

Patella

Tibia
Fibula

Talus (ankle bone)

Metatarsals
Phalanges

• **Figure 2.7** Skeletal system.

Cardiac/Heart Muscle

Striated and smooth muscle
Specialized cells that interlock so that muscle cells contract
   together
Involuntary
Moves blood by means of contractions

Smooth/Visceral

Linings such as bowel, urethra, blood vessels
Nonstriated
Involuntary

Tendons and Ligaments

Tendons anchor muscle to bone
Ligaments anchor bones to bones

Muscle Action

Muscle Capabilities

Stretches
Contracts
Receives and responds to stimulus
Returns to original shape and length

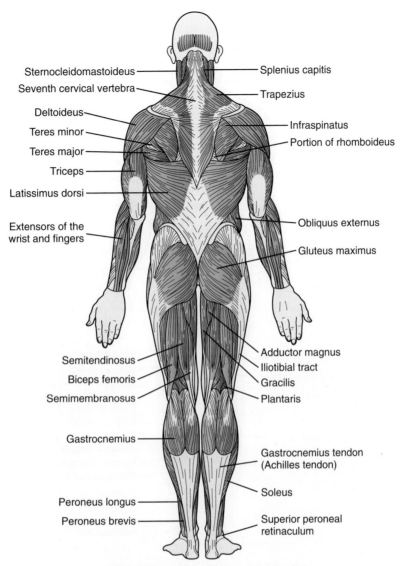

Sternocleidomastoideus
Seventh cervical vertebra
Deltoideus
Teres minor
Teres major
Triceps
Latissimus dorsi
Extensors of the wrist and fingers
Semitendinosus
Biceps femoris
Semimembranosus
Gastrocnemius
Peroneus longus
Peroneus brevis

Splenius capitis
Trapezius
Infraspinatus
Portion of rhomboideus
Obliquus externus
Gluteus maximus
Adductor magnus
Iliotibial tract
Gracilis
Plantaris
Gastrocnemius tendon (Achilles tendon)
Soleus
Superior peroneal retinaculum

• **Figure 2.8** Muscular system, posterior view.

Muscle Movement

Prime mover, responsible for movement (agonist)
  Synergist, assists prime mover
  Antagonist, relaxes as prime mover and synergists contract, resulting in movement
  Fixator, acts as joint stabilizer

Terms of Movement—From Midline of Body

Flexion (bend)
Extension (straighten)
Abduction (away)
Adduction (toward)
Rotation (turn on axis)
Circumduction (circular)
Supination (turning palm upward or forward [anteriorly] or lying down with face upward)
Pronation (turning palm downward or backward or act of lying face down)
Hyperextension (overextension)
Inversion (inward)
Eversion (outward)

Names of Muscles

Head and Neck

Facial expression
• Occipitofrontalis (raises eyebrows and wrinkles forehead horizontally)
• Corrugator supercilii (wrinkles forehead vertically)
• Orbicularis oris (opens mouth)
• Zygomaticus (elevates corners of mouth)
• Orbicularis oculi (opens and closes eyelid)
• Buccinator (smiling and blowing)
Mastication (chewing)

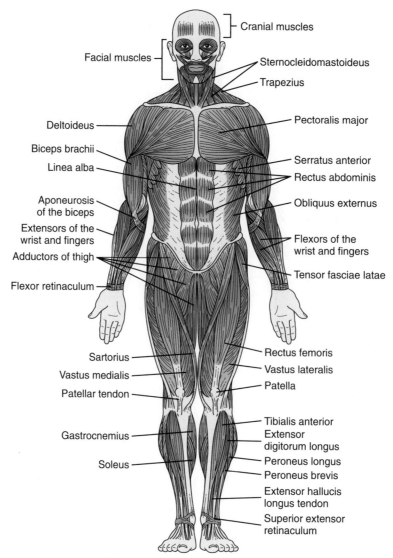

• **Figure 2.9** Muscular system, anterior view.

- Masseter (used to chew closing jaw)
- Temporalis (closes jaw)
- Pterygoids (grates teeth)

Muscles moving head
- Sternocleidomastoid (flexes head)
- Semispinalis capitis (complexus) (extends head)
- Splenius capitis (extends head, bends and rotates head to side where muscle is contracting)
- Longissimus capitis (trachelomastoid muscle) (extends head, bends and rotates to contracting side)
- Trapezius (extends head)

Upper Extremities
Biceps brachii (flexes elbow)
Triceps brachii and anconeus (extends elbow)
Brachialis (flexes prone forearm)
Brachioradialis (flexes semi-prone/supinated forearm)
Deltoid (abducts upper arm)
Latissimus dorsi (extends upper arm)

Pectoralis major (flexes upper arm)
Trapezius (raises/lowers shoulder)

Trunk
External oblique (compresses abdomen)
Internal oblique (compresses abdomen)
Transversus abdominis (compresses abdomen)
Rectus abdominis (flexes trunk)
Quadratus lumborum (flexes vertebral column laterally)

Respiratory
Diaphragm (enlarges thorax/inspiration)
External intercostals (raise ribs)
Internal intercostal (depress ribs)

Lower Extremities
Thigh
- Gluteus group, maximus, medius, minimus (abducts thigh)

TABLE 2-1

Combining Forms

Combining Form	Meaning	Combining Form	Meaning
1. acetabul/o	hip socket	32. myel/o	bone marrow
2. ankyl/o	bent, fused	33. my/o, muscul/o	muscle
3. aponeur/o	tendon type	34. olecran/o	olecranon (elbow)
4. arthr/o	joint	35. orth/o	straight
5. articul/o	joint	36. oste/o	bone
6. burs/o	fluid-filled sac in a joint	37. patell/o	patella (kneecap)
7. calc/o, calci/o	calcium	38. pelv/i	pelvis (hip)
8. calcane/o	calcaneus (heel)	39. perone/o	fibula
9. carp/o	carpals (wrist bones)	40. petr/o	stone
10. chondr/o	cartilage	41. phalang/o	phalanges (finger or toe)
11. clavic/o, clavicul/o	clavicle (collar bone)	42. plant/o	sole of foot
12. cost/o	rib	43. pub/o	pubis
13. crani/o	cranium (skull)	44. rachi/o	spine
14. disc/o	intervertebral disc	45. radi/o	radius (lower arm)
15. femor/o	thighbone	46. rhabdomy/o	skeletal (striated muscle)
16. fibul/o	fibula	47. rheumat/o	watery flow (collection of fluids in joints)
17. humer/o	humerus (upper arm bone)		
18. ili/o	ilium (upper pelvic bone)	48. sacr/o	sacrum
19. ischi/o	ischium (posterior pelvic bone)	49. scapul/o	scapula (shoulder)
20. kinesi/o	movement	50. scoli/o	bent
21. kyph/o	hump	51. spondyl/o	vertebra
22. lamin/o	lamina	52. stern/o	sternum (breast bone)
23. lord/o	curve	53. synovi/o	synovial joint membrane
24. lumb/o	lower back	54. tars/o	tarsal (ankle/foot)
25. malleol/o	malleolus (process on lateral ankle)	55. ten/o	tendon
26. mandibul/o	mandible (lower jawbone)	56. tend/o	tendon (connective tissue)
27. maxill/o	maxilla (upper jawbone)	57. tendin/o	tendon (connective tissue)
28. menisc/o	meniscus	58. tibi/o	shin bone
29. menisci/o	meniscus	59. uln/o	ulna (lower arm bone)
30. metacarp/o	metacarpals (hand)	60. vertebr/o	vertebra
31. metatars/o	metatarsals (foot)		

- Tensor fasciae latae (abducts thigh)
- Abductor group, brevis, longus, magnus (adducts thigh)
- Gracilis (adducts thigh)
- Iliopsoas (flexes thigh)
- Rectus femoris (flexes thigh)
  Hamstring group, biceps femoris, semitendinosus, semi-membranosus (extends thigh)
  Quadriceps group, rectus femoris, vastus lateralis, vastus medialis, vastus intermedius (extends lower leg)
  Sartorius (flexes, abducts, and rotates leg)
  Lower leg
  Tibialis anterior (dorsiflexes foot)
  Peroneus group, longus, brevis, tertius (everts foot)
  Gastrocnemius (calf, with soleus extends foot, also flexes knee)

TABLE 2-2

Prefixes

Prefix	Meaning
1. inter-	between
2. supra-	above
3. sym-	together
4. syn-	together

Soleus (calf, extends foot)
Extensor digitorum longus (extends toes, flexes foot)
Achilles tendon (largest tendon, extending from gastrocnemius to calcaneus)

TABLE 2-3

Suffixes

Suffix	Meaning
1. -asthenia	weakness
2. -blast	embryonic
3. -clast, -clasia, -clasis	break
4. -desis	bind together
5. -listhesia	slipping
6. -malacia	softening
7. -physis	to grow
8. -porosis	passage, cavity formation
9. -schisis	split
10. -stenosis	narrowing
11. -tome	instrument that cuts
12. -tomy	incision

TABLE 2-4

Medical Abbreviations

Abbreviation	Meaning
1. ACL	anterior cruciate ligament
2. AKA	above-knee amputation
3. BKA	below-knee amputation
4. C1-C7	cervical vertebrae
5. CTS	carpal tunnel syndrome
6. fx	fracture
7. L1-L5	lumbar vertebrae
8. OA	osteoarthritis
9. RA	rheumatoid arthritis
10. T1-T12	thoracic vertebrae
11. TMJ	temporomandibular joint

TABLE 2-5

Medical Terms

Term	Meaning
Arthrocentesis	Injection and/or aspiration of joint
Arthrodesis	Surgical immobilization of a joint
Arthrography	Radiography of joint
Arthroplasty	Reshaping or reconstruction of a joint
Arthroscopy	Use of scope to view inside joint
Arthrotomy	Incision into a joint
Articular	Pertains to a joint
Aspiration	Use of a needle and a syringe to withdraw fluid
Atrophy	Wasting away
Bunion	Hallux valgus, abnormal increase in size of metatarsal head that results in displacement of great toe
Bursitis	Inflammation of bursa (joint sac)
Carpal tunnel syndrome	Compression of medial nerve
Chondral	Referring to the cartilage
Closed fracture repair	Not surgically opened with/without manipulation and with/without traction
Closed treatment	Fracture site that is not surgically opened and visualized
Colles' fracture	Fracture at lower end of radius that displaces bone posteriorly
Dislocation	Placement in a location other than original location
Endoscopy	Inspection of body organs or cavities using a lighted scope that may be inserted through an existing opening or through a small incision
Fasciectomy	Removal of band of fibrous tissue
Fissure	Groove
Fracture	Break in a bone
Ganglion	Knot or knotlike mass
Internal/External fixation	Application of pins, wires, screws, placed externally or internally to immobilize a body part
Kyphosis	Humpback
Lamina	Flat plate
Ligament	Fibrous band of tissue that connects cartilage or bone
Lordosis	Anterior curvature of the spine
Lumbodynia	Pain in lumbar area
Lysis	Releasing
Manipulation or reduction	Alignment of a fracture or joint dislocation to normal position
Open fracture repair	Surgical opening (incision) over or remote opening as access to a fracture site
Osteoarthritis	Degenerative condition of articular cartilage
Osteoclast	Absorbs or removes bone
Osteotomy	Cutting into bone
Percutaneous	Through skin
Percutaneous fracture repair	Repair of a fracture by means of pins and wires inserted through the fracture site
Percutaneous skeletal fixation	Considered neither open nor closed; fracture is not visualized, but fixation is placed across fracture site under x-ray imaging

TABLE 2-5

Medical Terms—cont'd

Term	Meaning	Term	Meaning
Reduction	Replacement to normal position	Synchondrosis	Union between two bones (connected by cartilage)
Scoliosis	Lateral curvature of the spine	Tendon	Attaches a muscle to a bone
Skeletal traction	Application of pressure to bone by means of pins and/or wires inserted into bone	Tenodesis	Suturing of a tendon to a bone
		Tenorrhaphy	Suture repair of tendon
Skin traction	Application of pressure to bone by means of tape applied to the skin	Traction	Application of pressure to maintain normal alignment
Spondylitis	Inflammation of vertebrae	Trocar needle	Needle with a cannula that can be removed; used to puncture and withdraw fluid from a cavity
Subluxation	Partial dislocation		
Supination	Supine position—lying on back, face upward		

Chapter 2: Anatomy and Terminology Quiz

(Quiz Answers Are Located in Appendix B)

1. Tubular is another name for these bones:
   a. short
   b. long
   c. flat
   d. irregular
2. These bones are found near joints:
   a. irregular
   b. flat
   c. sesamoid
   d. broad
3. Zygoma is an example of this type of bone:
   a. irregular
   b. flat
   c. sesamoid
   d. broad
4. Diaphysis is this part of bone:
   a. end
   b. surface
   c. shaft
   d. marrow
5. Which is NOT a part of the cranium?
   a. condyle
   b. sphenoid
   c. ethmoid
   d. parietal

6. This is NOT an ear bone:
   a. malleus
   b. stapes
   c. incus
   d. styloid
7. This term describes growth plate:
   a. endosteum
   b. epiphyseal
   c. metaphysis
   d. periosteum
8. This is a depression on lateral hip surface into which head of femur fits:
   a. ilium
   b. ischium
   c. patella
   d. acetabulum
9. Tip of elbow is the:
   a. olecranon
   b. trapezium
   c. humerus
   d. tarsal
10. This term describes an immovable joint:
    a. amphiarthrosis
    b. diarthrosis
    c. synarthrosis
    d. ischium

PATHOPHYSIOLOGY

Injuries

Fractures

Classification of Fractures

Open/Closed

Open (compound): broken bone penetrates skin
Closed (simple): broken bone does not penetrate skin

Complete/Incomplete

Complete: bone is broken all the way through
Example: oblique, linear, spiral, and transverse
Incomplete: bone is not broken all the way through
Example: greenstick, bowing, torus, stress, and transchondral

Treatment

Closed reduction (realignment of bone fragments by manipulation)

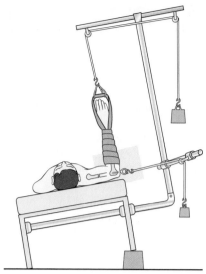

• **Figure 2.10** Skeletal traction uses patient's bones to secure internal devices to which traction is attached.

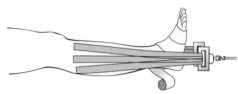

• **Figure 2.11** Skin traction utilizes strapping, wraps, or tape to which traction is attached.

Reduction (the returning of the bone to normal alignment)

Immobilization (returns to normal alignment and holds in place)

Traction (application of pulling force to hold bone in alignment)
- Skeletal traction uses internal devices (pins, screws, wires, etc.) inserted into bone with ends sticking out through skin for attachment of traction device (Fig. 2.10)
- Skin traction is use of strapping, elastic wrap, or tape attached to skin to which weights are attached (Fig. 2.11)

Improper Union
Nonunion: failure of bone ends to grow together
Malunion: incorrect alignment of bone ends
Delayed union: delay of bone union 8 or 9 months

Dislocations
Bone and soft tissue damage usually caused by trauma
Any part of bone is displaced
Can result in nerve and tissue damage

Treatment
Reduction
Immobilization

Sprains and Strains
Soft tissue damage usually caused by trauma to tendons and ligaments
Strain: partial tear of a tendon
Sprain: results from overuse or overextension/tearing or rupture of some part of musculature

Bone Disorders

Osteomyelitis
Bone infection
Usually caused by bacteria
- Exogenous osteomyelitis is caused by bacteria that enter from outside body
- Hematogenous osteomyelitis (endogenous) is caused by a bacterial infection within body

Osteoporosis
Common disorder in postmenopausal women and elderly and most common metabolic disease
- Malabsorption of calcium and magnesium; certain trace elements and vitamins C and D contribute to bone loss
- Decreased bone mass and density
- Fractures more common due to decrease in strength of bone

Treatment
Increased intake of calcium, magnesium, and vitamin D
Increased weight-bearing activity

Osteomalacia and Rickets
Osteomalacia is softened adult bones, whereas rickets is softened growing bones in children
Caused by vitamin D and phosphate deficiency

Osteitis Deformans (Paget's Disease)
Abnormal bone remodeling and resorption resulting in enlarged, soft bones
Unknown cause but strong genetic considerations

Treatment
Calcitonin and biophosphates

Spinal Curvatures
Lordosis: swayback
- Inward curvature of spine
  Kyphosis: humpback
- Outward curvature of spine
  Scoliosis
- Lateral curvature of spine

Spina Bifida
Congenital abnormality in which vertebrae do not close correctly around the spinal cord

Joint Disorders

Bursitis: inflammation of bursa (joint sac)
Arthritis: inflammation of joints

Osteoarthritis (OA)

This is degenerative or wear/tear arthritis
- DJD, degenerative joint disease
  Chronic inflammation of joint
  Increased pain on weightbearing or movement
  Affects weight-bearing joints
- Loss of articular cartilage
- Sclerosis of bone—eburnation
  Turning bone into ivorylike mass—polished
- Osteophytes (bone spurs)

Symptoms

Pain and stiffness
Crepitation (bone on bone creates characteristic grinding sound)

Classifications

Primary (idiopathic)
- No known cause
  Secondary
- Associated with joint instability, joint stress, or congenital abnormalities

Treatment

Symptomatic
  Arthroplasty

Rheumatoid Arthritis (RA)

Progressive inflammatory connective tissue disease of the joints

Systemic autoimmune disease
- Can invade arteries, lungs, skin, and other organs with inflammation or nodules
Affects small joints
- Destroys synovial membrane, articular cartilage, and surrounding tissues
Leads to loss of function due to fixation and deformity

Treatment

Pharmaceuticals to modify autoimmune and inflammatory processes
Gene therapy and stem cell transplantation are being researched
Symptomatic
Arthroplasty

Infectious and Septic Arthritis

Infectious process

Usually affects single joint
Without antimicrobial intervention, permanent joint damage results
Example: Lyme disease

Treatment

Antibiotics—early intervention

Gout (Gouty Arthritis)

Inflammatory arthritis
  Often affects the joint of the great toe
  Caused by excessive amounts of uric acid that crystallizes in connective tissue of joints
  Leads to inflammation and destruction of joint

Treatment

Pharmaceuticals—nonsteroidal anti-inflammatory drugs

Ankylosing Spondylitis (AS)

Inflammatory disease that is progressive
Affects vertebral joints and insertion points of ligaments, tendons, and joint capsules
Leads to rigid spinal column and sacroiliac joints

Treatment

Nonsteroidal anti-inflammatory drugs relieve symptoms
Analgesics for pain

Tendon, Muscle, and Ligament Disorders

Muscular Dystrophy—Familial Disorder

Progressive degenerative muscle disorder
Multiple types of muscular dystrophy
Most often affects boys
- Genetic predisposition—Duchenne muscular dystrophy

Primary Fibromyalgia Syndrome

Symptoms

Generalized aching and pain
Tender points
Fatigue
Depression

Usually Appears in

Middle-aged women

Polymyositis

General muscle inflammation causing weakness
- With skin rash = dermatomyositis

Tumors

Bone Tumors

Origin of Bone Tumors

Osteogenic (bone cells)

Chondrogenic (cartilage cell)
Collagenic (fibrous tissue cell)
Myelogenic (marrow cell)

Osteoma
Benign
Abnormal outgrowth of bone

Chondroblastoma
Rare
Usually benign

Osteosarcoma
Malignant tumor of long bones
Usually in young adults
Typically causes bone pain

Multiple Myeloma
Malignant plasma cells in skeletal system and soft tissue
Progressive and generally fatal
Usually in those over 40

Chondrosarcoma
Malignant cartilage tumor
Usually in middle-aged and older individuals
In late stages, symptoms include local swelling and pain
  • Worsens with time
Surgical excision is usually treatment of choice
If diagnosed in early stages, it is treatable with long-term survival possible

Muscle Tumors
Rare
• Rhabdomyosarcoma
• Aggressive, invasive carcinoma with widespread metastasis

Chapter 2: Pathophysiology Quiz

(Quiz Answers Are Located in Appendix B)

1. A compound fracture is also known as:
   a. complete
   b. incomplete
   c. closed
   d. open
2. This is a common bone disorder in postmenopausal women resulting from lower levels of calcium and potassium:
   a. Paget's disease
   b. lordosis
   c. osteoporosis
   d. rheumatoid arthritis
3. This inflammatory disease is progressive and leads to a rigid spinal column:
   a. polymyositis
   b. ankylosing spondylitis
   c. primary fibromyalgia syndrome
   d. septic arthritis of spine
4. This type of tumor arises from bone cells:
   a. osteogenic
   b. chondrogenic
   c. collagenic
   d. myelogenic
5. This type of tumor is the most common type of malignant bone tumor that occurs in those over 40 and is progressive and generally fatal:
   a. rhabdomyosarcoma
   b. chondrosarcoma
   c. osteosarcoma
   d. multiple myeloma
6. A general muscle inflammation with an accompanying skin rash is:
   a. muscular dystrophy
   b. dermatologic arthritis
   c. ankylosing spondylitis
   d. dermatomyositis
7. A cartilage tumor that usually occurs in middle-aged and older individuals:
   a. chondrosarcoma
   b. osteosarcoma
   c. chondroblastoma
   d. rhabdomyosarcoma
8. Returning of bone to normal alignment is:
   a. immobilization
   b. traction
   c. reduction
   d. manipulation
9. Result of overuse or overextension of a ligament is:
   a. strain
   b. sprain
   c. fracture
   d. displacement
10. Primary osteoarthritis is also known as:
    a. secondary
    b. functional
    c. congenital
    d. idiopathic

3

Respiratory System

ANATOMY AND TERMINOLOGY

Supplies oxygen to body and helps clean body of waste (carbon dioxide)
Two tracts (Fig. 3.1A)
- Upper respiratory tract (nose, pharynx, and larynx)
- Lower respiratory tract (trachea, bronchial tree, and lungs)

Lined with ciliated mucosa
- Purifies air by trapping irritants
- Warms and humidifies air

Upper Respiratory Tract (URT)

Nose

Sense of smell (olfactory)
Moistens and warms air
Nasal septum divides interior

Sinuses (Paranasal or Accessory Sinuses) (4 Pair)

Frontal
Ethmoid
Maxillary
Sphenoid

Turbinates (Conchae)

Bones on inside of nose
Divided into inferior, middle, and superior (Fig. 3.1B)
Warms and humidifies air

Pharynx (Throat)

Passageway for both food and air
Nasopharynx contains adenoids
Oropharynx contains tonsils
Laryngopharynx leads to larynx

Larynx (Voice Box) (Opening to Trachea)

Contains vocal cords
- Cartilages of larynx, thyroid, epiglottis, and arytenoid

Lower Respiratory Tract (LRT)

Trachea (Windpipe)—Air-Conducting Structure

Mucus-lined tube with C-shaped cartilage rings to hold windpipe open

Segmental Bronchi

Trachea divides into right and left main bronchus, which further divide into lobar bronchii—3 on right, 2 on left

Bronchioles

Branches divide into secondary bronchi, then smaller bronchioles

Alveolar Ducts (Minute Branches of Bronchial Tree)

End in alveoli (sacs) of simple squamous cells
- Primary gas-exchange units

Surrounded by capillaries and where exchange of oxygen and carbon dioxide takes place

Lungs

Covered by pleura
Cone-shaped organs filling thoracic cavity
Base rests on diaphragm and apex (top of lungs) extends to above clavicles
Hilum is medial surface of lung where pulmonary artery, pulmonary veins, nerves, lymphatics, and bronchial tubes enter and exit
Left lung contains two lobes divided by fissures
Right lung contains three lobes

Respiration

Inspiration—oxygen moves in, downward movement of lungs enlarging thoracic cavity
Expiration—carbon dioxide moves out, upward movement of diaphragm decreasing lung space

Upper Respiratory Tract

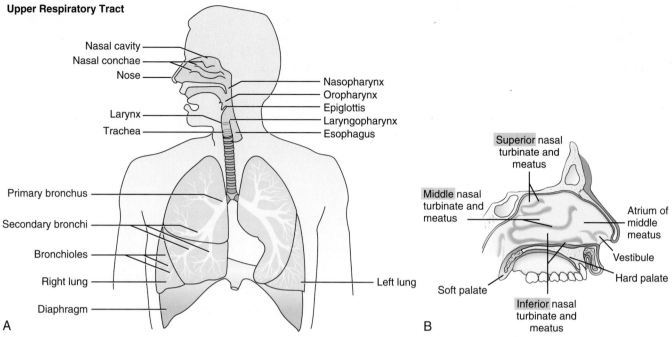

• **Figure 3.1 A.** Upper and lower respiratory system. **B.** Superior, inferior, and middle nasal turbinates.

TABLE 3-1

Combining Forms

Combining Form	Meaning	Combining Form	Meaning
1. adenoid/o	adenoid	20. pector/o	chest
2. alveol/o	alveolus	21. pharyng/o	pharynx
3. atel/o	incomplete	22. phon/o	voice
4. bronch/o	bronchus	23. phren/o	diaphragm
5. bronchi/o	bronchus	24. pleur/o	pleura
6. bronchiol/o	bronchiole	25. pneum/o	lung/air
7. capn/o	carbon dioxide	26. pneumat/o	air
8. coni/o	dust	27. pneumon/o	lung/air
9. cyan/o	blue	28. pulmon/o	lung
10. diaphragmat/o	diaphragm	29. py/o	pus
11. epiglott/o	epiglottis	30. rhin/o	nose
12. laryng/o	larynx	31. sept/o	septum
13. lob/o	lobe	32. sinus/o	sinus
14. mediastin/o	mediastinum	33. spir/o	breath
15. muc/o	mucus	34. tel/o	complete
16. nas/o	nose	35. thorac/o	thorax
17. orth/o	straight	36. tonsill/o	tonsil
18. ox/o	oxygen	37. trache/o	trachea
19. oxy/o	oxygen		

TABLE 3-2

Prefixes

Prefix	Meaning
1. a-	not
2. an-	not
3. endo-	within
4. eu-	good
5. dys-	difficult
6. pan-	all
7. poly-	many

TABLE 3-3

Suffixes

Suffix	Meaning
1. -algia	pain
2. -ar	pertaining to
3. -ary	pertaining to
4. -capnia	carbon dioxide
5. -centesis	puncture to remove (drain)
6. -dynia	pain
7. -eal	pertaining to
8. -ectasis	stretching
9. -emia	blood
10. -gram	record
11. -graph	recording instrument
12. -graphy	recording process
13. -itis	inflammation
14. -meter	measurement or instrument that measures
15. -metry	measurement of
16. -osmia	smell
17. -oxia	oxygen
18. -pexy	fixation
19. -phonia	sound
20. -pnea	breathing
21. -ptysis	spitting
22. -rrhage, -rrhagia	abnormal, excessive flow
23. -scopy	to examine
24. -spasm	contraction of muscle
25. -sphyxia	pulse
26. -stenosis	blockage, narrowing
27. -stomy	opening
28. -thorax	chest
29. -tomy	cutting, incision

TABLE 3-4

Medical Abbreviations

Abbreviation	Meaning
1. ABG	arterial blood gas
2. AFB	acid-fast bacillus
3. ARDS	adult respiratory distress syndrome
4. BiPAP	bi-level positive airway pressure
5. COPD	chronic obstructive pulmonary disease
6. CPAP	continuous positive airway pressure
7. DLCO	diffuse capacity of lungs for carbon monoxide
8. FEF	forced expiratory flow
9. FEV_1	forced expiratory volume in 1 second
10. FEV_1: FVC	maximum amount of forced expiratory volume in 1 second
11. FRC	functional residual capacity
12. FVC	forced vital capacity
13. HHN	handheld nebulizer
14. IPAP	inspiratory positive airway pressure
15. IRDS	infant respiratory distress syndrome
16. MDI	metered-dose inhaler
17. MVV	maximum voluntary ventilation
18. PAWP	pulmonary artery wedge pressure
19. PCWP	pulmonary capillary wedge pressure
20. PEAP	positive end-airway pressure
21. PEEP	positive end-expiratory pressure
22. PFT	pulmonary function test
23. PND	paroxysmal nocturnal dyspnea
24. RDS	respiratory distress syndrome
25. RSV	respiratory syncytial virus
26. RV	respiratory volume
27. RV: TLC	ratio of respiratory volume to total lung capacity
28. TLC	total lung capacity
29. TLV	total lung volume
30. URI	upper respiratory infection
31. V/Q	ventilation/perfusion scan

TABLE 3-5

Medical Terms

Term	Meaning	Term	Meaning
Ablation	Removal or destruction by cutting, chemicals, or electrocautery	Laryngoscopy	Direct visualization and examination of interior of larynx with a laryngoscope
Adenoidectomy	Removal of adenoids	Laryngotomy	Incision into larynx
Apnea	Cessation of breathing	Lavage	Washing out
Asphyxia	Lack of oxygen	Lobectomy	Surgical excision of a lobe of lung
Asthma	Shortage of breath caused by contraction of bronchi	Nasal button	Synthetic circular disc used to cover a hole in the nasal septum
Atelectasis	Incomplete expansion of lung, collapse	Orthopnea	Difficulty in breathing, relieved by assuming upright position
Auscultation	Listening to sounds, such as to lung sounds	Percussion	Tapping with sharp blows as a diagnostic technique
Bacilli	Plural of bacillus, a rod-shaped bacteria	Pertussis	Whooping cough—highly contagious bacterial infection of pharynx, larynx, and trachea
Bilobectomy	Surgical removal of two lobes of a lung	Pharyngolaryngectomy	Surgical removal of pharynx and larynx
Bronchiole	Smaller division of bronchial tree	Pleura	Covers lungs and lines thoracic cavity
Bronchoplasty	Surgical repair of bronchi	Pleurectomy	Surgical excision of pleura
Bronchoscopy	Inspection of bronchial tree using a bronchoscope	Pleuritis	Inflammation of pleura
Catheter	Tube placed into body to put fluid in or take fluid out	Pneumocentesis/ pneumonocentesis	Surgical puncturing of a lung to withdraw fluid
Cauterization	Destruction of tissue by use of cautery	Pneumonia	Inflammation of lungs with consolidation
Cordectomy	Surgical removal of vocal cord(s)	Pneumonolysis/ pneumolysis	Surgical separation of lung from chest wall to allow lung to collapse
Crackle	Abnormal sound when breathing (heard on auscultation)		
Croup	Acute viral infection (obstruction of larynx), stridor	Pneumonotomy/ pneumotomy	Incision of lung
Cyanosis	Bluish discoloration		
Drainage	Free flow or withdrawal of fluids from a wound or cavity	Pulmonary edema	Accumulation of fluid in pulmonary tissues and air spaces
Dysphonia	Speech impairment	Pulmonary embolism	Thrombus or other foreign material lodged in pulmonary artery or one of its branches
Dyspnea	Shortage of breath, difficult breathing		
Emphysema	Air accumulated in organ or tissue	Rales	An abnormal respiratory sound heard in auscultation, indicating some pathologic condition
Epiglottidectomy	Excision of covering of larynx		
Epistaxis	Nose bleed		
Glottis	True vocal cords	Rhinoplasty	Surgical repair of nose
Hemoptysis	Bloody sputum	Rhinorrhea	Free discharge of a thin nasal mucus
Intramural	Within organ wall		
Intubation	Insertion of a tube	Sarcoidosis	Chronic inflammatory disease with nodules developing in lungs, lymph nodes, other organs
Laryngeal web	Congenital abnormality of connective tissue between vocal cords		
Laryngectomy	Surgical removal of larynx		
Laryngoplasty	Surgical repair of larynx	Segmentectomy	Surgical removal of the smaller subdivisions (segment) of lobes of a lung
Laryngoscope	Fiberoptic scope used to view inside of larynx		

TABLE 3-5

Medical Terms—cont'd

Term	Meaning	Term	Meaning
Septoplasty	Surgical repair of nasal septum	Thoracostomy	Surgical incision into chest wall and insertion of a chest tube
Sinusotomy	Surgical incision into a sinus	Thoracotomy	Surgical incision into chest wall
Spirometry	Measuring breathing capacity	Total pneumonectomy	Surgical removal of an entire lung
Tachypnea	Quick, shallow breathing	Tracheostomy	Creation of an opening into trachea
Thoracentesis/ thoracocentesis (pleuracentesis/ pleurocentesis)	Surgical puncture of thoracic cavity, usually using a needle, to remove fluids	Tracheotomy	Incision into trachea
		Transtracheal	Across trachea
Thoracoplasty	Surgical procedure that removes rib(s) and thereby allows collapse of a lung	Tuberculosis	Infection of the lungs caused by bacteria (tubercle bacillus)
Thoracoscopy	Use of a lighted endoscope to view pleural spaces and thoracic cavity or to perform surgical procedures		

Chapter 3: Anatomy and Terminology Quiz

(Quiz Answers Are Located in Appendix B)

1. This is NOT a part of lower respiratory tract:
   a. trachea
   b. larynx
   c. bronchi
   d. lungs
2. Another name for voice box is:
   a. oropharynx
   b. pharynx
   c. laryngopharynx
   d. larynx
3. This is the windpipe:
   a. pharynx
   b. larynx
   c. trachea
   d. sphenoid
4. Interior of nose is divided by the:
   a. septum
   b. sphenoid
   c. oropharynx
   d. apical
5. This combining form means "incomplete":
   a. atel/o
   b. alveol/o
   c. ox/i
   d. pneumat/o
6. This combining form means "breath":
   a. py/o
   b. lob/o
   c. spir/o
   d. pleur/o
7. This prefix means "all":
   a. a-
   b. an-
   c. pan-
   d. poly-
8. This abbreviation refers to a syndrome that involves difficulty in breathing:
   a. ABG
   b. ARDS
   c. BiPAP
   d. FEF
9. This abbreviation refers to amount of air patient can expel from the lungs in 1 second:
   a. PFT
   b. PND
   c. RDS
   d. FEV_1
10. This suffix means "breathing":
    a. -stenosis
    b. -spasm
    c. -pexy
    d. -pnea

PATHOPHYSIOLOGY

Signs and Symptoms of Pulmonary Disorders

Dyspnea

Difficult breathing (sense of air hunger)
Increased respiratory effort

Hypoventilation

Decreased alveolar ventilation

Hyperventilation

Increased alveolar ventilation

Hemoptysis

Bloody sputum

Hypoxia

Reduced oxygenation of tissue cells

Cough

Caused by irritant
Protective reflex
Acute cough is up to 3 weeks
Chronic cough is over 3 weeks

Tachypnea

Rapid breathing

Apnea

Lack of breathing

Orthopnea

Requiring sitting upright to facilitate breathing

Pulmonary Diseases and Disorders

Hypercapnia

Increased carbon dioxide in arterial blood
Caused by inadequate ventilation of alveoli
Can result in respiratory acidosis

Hypoxemia

Reduced oxygenation of arterial blood

Acute Respiratory Failure

Inadequate gas exchange
Hypoxemia
Can result from trauma or disease

Adult Respiratory Distress Syndrome (ARDS)

Acute injury to alveolocapillary membrane
Results in edema and atelectasis
In infants, infant respiratory distress syndrome (IRDS)

Pulmonary Edema

Accumulation of fluid in lung tissue
Most common cause is left ventricular failure

Aspiration

Passage of fluid and solid particles into lung
Can cause severe pneumonitis
* Localized inflammation of lung

Atelectasis

Collapse of lung
Three most common types are:
* Adhesive
* Compression
* Obstruction
May be chronic or acute
* Acute, such as compression as a result of an automobile accident
* Chronic from structural defect

Absorption Atelectasis

Results from absence of air in alveoli

Caused by
Foreign body
Tumor
Abnormal external pressure

Bronchiectasis

Chronic, irreversible dilation of bronchi

Common Types That Describe Severity of Condition
* Cylindrical
* Varicose
* Saccular or cystic

Respiratory Acidosis

Decreased level of pH
Due to excess retention of carbon dioxide

Bronchiolitis

Inflammation and obstruction of bronchioles
Usually in children younger than 2 years old—preceded by URI
Viral infection (respiratory syncytial virus, or RSV)

Common Types
* Constrictive
* Proliferative
* Obliterative

Pneumothorax

Air collected in pleural cavity
* Leads to lung collapse
* Communicating pneumothorax is barometric air pressure in pleural space

- Spontaneous pneumothorax is spontaneous rupture of visceral pleura
- Secondary pneumothorax is a result of trauma to chest

Pneumoconiosis

Dust particles or other particulate matter in lung

Common Types
- Coal
- Asbestos
- Fiberglass

Pleural Effusion–Fluid in Pleural Space

Common Types
- Hemothorax—hemorrhage into pleural cavity
- Empyema—Infectious materials in pleural space
- Exudate—Fluid remaining after infection, inflammation, malignancy

Empyema

Infectious Pleural Effusion

Pus in pleural space
    Complication of respiratory infection
    Commonly follows pneumonia and is treated like pneumonia

Pulmonary Embolism

Air, tissue, or clot occlusion
    Lodges in pulmonary artery or branch of artery
    Risk with congestive heart failure
    Most clots originate in leg veins

Cor Pulmonale

Hypertrophy or failure of right ventricle
    Result of lung, pulmonary vessels, or chest wall disorders
    Acute is secondary to pulmonary embolus
    Chronic is secondary to obstructive lung disease

Pleurisy (Pleuritis)

Inflammation of pleura
    Often preceded by an upper respiratory infection

Infectious Disease

Upper Respiratory Infection (URI)

Acute inflammatory process of mucous membranes in trachea and above

Common Types
- Common cold
- Croup
- Sinusitis
- Laryngitis

Lower Respiratory Infection (LRI)

Pneumonia

Inflammation of lungs with consolidation

Categorized according to causative organism
Can be caused by
    Aspiration
    Bacteria
    Protozoa
    Fungi
    Chlamydia
    Virus

Common Types
Aspiration pneumonia
Bacterial
Chlamydial
Drug resistant
Eosinophil
Fungal
Hospital acquired (nosocomial)
Legionnaires' disease
Mycoplasma
Pneumococcal
Viral

Tuberculosis

Communicable lung disease—airborne droplet
    Caused by *Mycobacterium tuberculosis* (bacilli)

Chronic Obstructive Pulmonary Disease (COPD)

Irreversible airway obstruction that decreases expiration

Includes
Chronic bronchitis
- Bronchial spasms
- Dyspnea
- Wheezing
- Productive cough
- Cyanosis
- Chronic hypoventilation
- Polycythemia
- Cor pulmonale
- Prolonged expiration

Emphysema
- Loss of elasticity and enlargement of alveoli
- Mimics symptoms of chronic bronchitis but more exaggerated

Chapter 3: Pathophysiology Quiz

(Quiz Answers Are Located in Appendix B)

1. Acute injury to alveolocapillary membrane that results in edema and atelectasis:
   a. hypoxemia
   b. adult respiratory distress syndrome
   c. bronchiolitis
   d. pneumoconiosis

2. Condition in which pus is in pleural space and is often a complication of pneumonia:
   a. empyema
   b. cor pulmonale
   c. pneumothorax
   d. atelectasis

3. Which of the following is NOT one of the most common types of atelectasis?
   a. adhesive
   b. compression
   c. obstruction
   d. expansion

4. This condition is a result of accumulation of dust particles in lung:
   a. pleurisy
   b. tuberculosis
   c. chronic obstructive pulmonary disease
   d. pneumoconiosis

5. An irreversible airway obstructive disease in which symptoms are bronchial spasm, dyspnea, and wheezing:
   a. pleurisy
   b. empyema
   c. bronchiolitis
   d. COPD

6. Cylindrical, varicose, and secular/cystic are examples of:
   a. bronchiectasis
   b. cor pulmonale
   c. pneumothorax
   d. atelectasis

7. Condition in which there is a loss of elasticity and enlargement of alveoli:
   a. chronic bronchitis
   b. asthma
   c. emphysema
   d. empyema

8. Definition of a chronic cough is one that lasts for more than this number of weeks:
   a. 2
   b. 3
   c. 4
   d. 5

9. A condition marked by an increase in carbon dioxide in arterial blood and decreased ability to breathe that can result in respiratory acidosis:
   a. hypercapnia
   b. hypoxemia
   c. acute respiratory failure
   d. pulmonary edema

10. This condition often follows a viral infection and occurs in children under 2 years of age. Examples of various types of this condition are constrictive, proliferating, and obliterative.
    a. pneumoconiosis
    b. pulmonary edema
    c. bronchiolitis
    d. bronchiectasis

4

Cardiovascular System

Consists of blood, blood vessels, and heart

Blood (Function Is to Maintain a Constant Environment)

Composed of cells suspended in plasma (clear, straw-colored liquid)

Carries

Oxygen and nutrients to cells
Waste and carbon dioxide to kidneys, liver, and lungs
Hormones from endocrine system

Regulates

Temperature by circulating blood

Protection

White cells (leukocytes) produce antibodies

Composed of Two Parts

Liquid Part (Extracellular) Is Plasma
Water 91%
Protein 1%, albumin, globulins, fibrinogen, ferritin, transferrin
2% ions, nutrients, waste products, gases, regulating substances

Cellular Structures
Leukocytes (WBCs)—granular and agranular—fight infections
- Neutrophils
- Lymphocytes
- Monocytes
- Eosinophils
- Basophils

Erythrocytes (red blood cells)—hemoglobin carries oxygen
Thrombocytes (platelets)—important for hemostasis
Blood types: A, B, AB, and O are genetically endowed
- Blood type O negative is known as universal donor (no Rh and no red cell antigens present)

Vessels—Circulatory System

Function

To carry blood delivering nutrients and oxygen (arterial system) and carry away cell waste and carbon dioxide (venous system)

Types

Arteries (Fig. 4.1) **Carrying Oxygenated Blood**
Inner layer, endothelium
Lead away from heart
Branches are arterioles

Capillaries
Connection between arterioles and venules
Exchange structure (oxygen and carbon dioxide, nutrients, and waste)

Veins (Fig. 4.2) **Carrying Deoxygenated Blood**
Carry blood to heart
Venules are small branches

Heart

Circulates blood

Four Chambers (Fig. 4.3)

Two Upper
Right and left atria (singular: atrium) receive blood

Two Lower
Right and left ventricles discharge blood (pump)

Chamber Walls

Composed of three layers
- Endocardium: smooth inner layer
- Myocardium: middle muscular layer
- Epicardium: outer layer

Septa (Singular: Septum)

Divide chambers
- Interatrial septum
  Separates two upper chambers

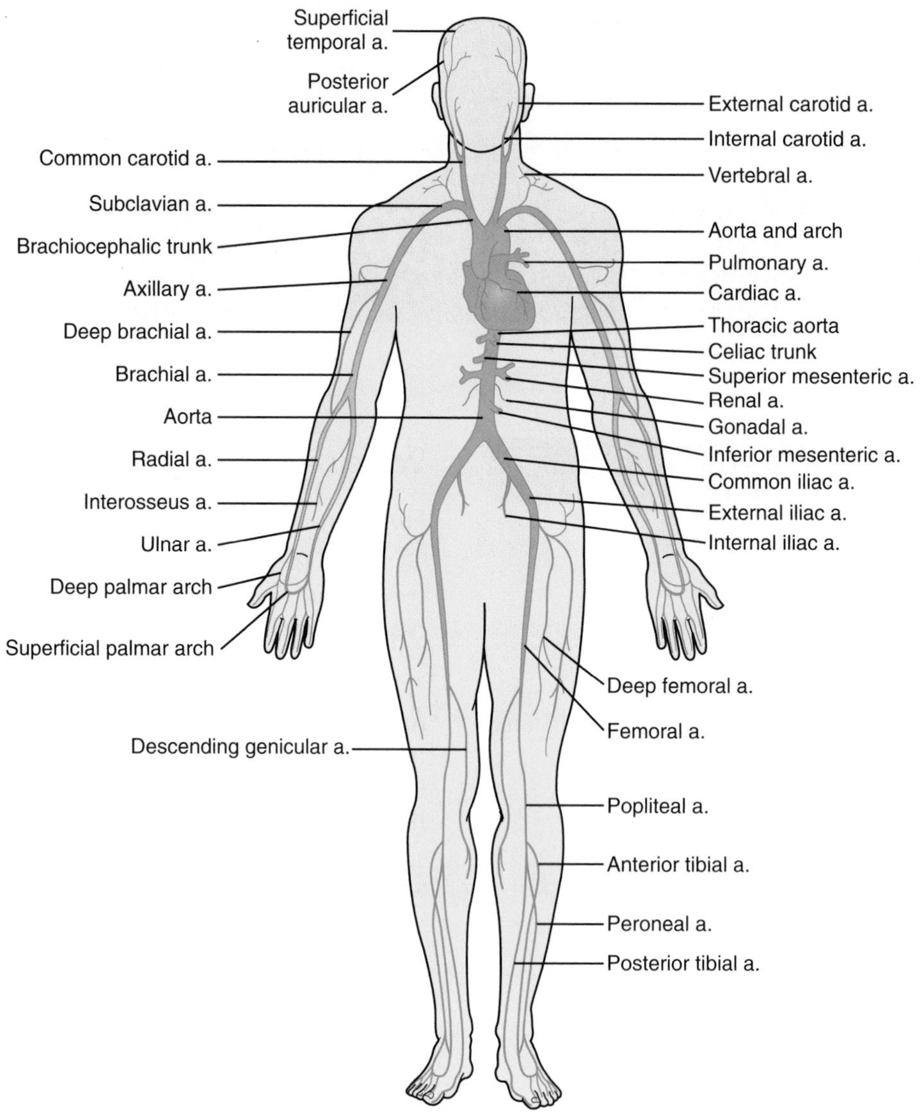

• **Figure 4.1** Arteries of circulatory system.

- Interventricular septum
  Separates two lower chambers

Major Blood Vessels

Inferior vena cava—carries deoxygenated blood from lower extremities, pelvic, and abdominal viscera to right atrium

Superior vena cava—drains deoxygenated blood from head, neck, upper extremities, and chest to right atrium

Pulmonary artery bifurcates and becomes right and left pulmonary artery—carries deoxygenated blood from right ventricle to lungs

Right and left pulmonary veins (4)—carry oxygenated blood from lungs to left atrium

Aorta—carries oxygenated blood from left side of heart to body

Pericardium

Sac comprising two layers that covers heart

- Parietal pericardium: outermost covering

- Visceral pericardium: innermost (epicardium)
- Pericardial cavity: contains about 30 cc of fluid

Valves (4 in Heart)

Tricuspid: between right atrium and right ventricle

Pulmonary: at entrance of pulmonary artery leading from right ventricle

Aortic: at entrance of aorta leading from left ventricle

Bicuspid (mitral): between left atrium and left ventricle

Conduction System (Fig. 4.4)

Sinoatrial node: SAN, nature's pacemaker, sends impulses to atrioventricular node

Atrioventricular node (AVN): located on interatrial septum and sends impulses to bundle of His

Bundle of His: divides into right bundle branch (RBB) and left bundle branch (LBB) in septum

Purkinje fibers: merge from bundle branches into specialized cells of myocardium, located in ventricular endocardium

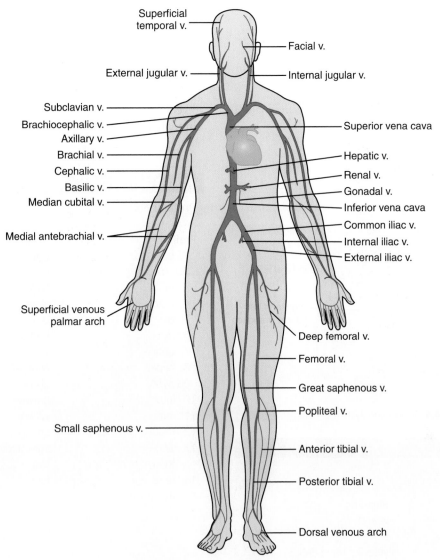

Superficial temporal v.
Facial v.
External jugular v.
Internal jugular v.
Subclavian v.
Brachiocephalic v.
Axillary v.
Brachial v.
Cephalic v.
Basilic v.
Median cubital v.
Medial antebrachial v.
Superior vena cava
Hepatic v.
Renal v.
Gonadal v.
Inferior vena cava
Common iliac v.
Internal iliac v.
External iliac v.
Superficial venous palmar arch
Deep femoral v.
Femoral v.
Great saphenous v.
Popliteal v.
Small saphenous v.
Anterior tibial v.
Posterior tibial v.
Dorsal venous arch

• **Figure 4.2** Veins of circulatory system.

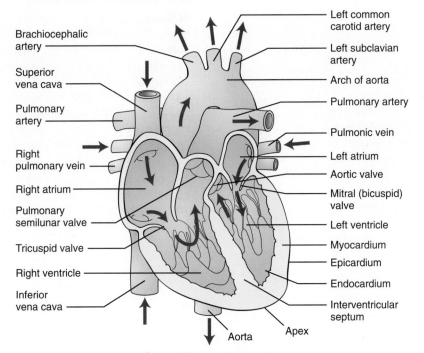

Brachiocephalic artery
Superior vena cava
Pulmonary artery
Right pulmonary vein
Right atrium
Pulmonary semilunar valve
Tricuspid valve
Right ventricle
Inferior vena cava
Left common carotid artery
Left subclavian artery
Arch of aorta
Pulmonary artery
Pulmonic vein
Left atrium
Aortic valve
Mitral (bicuspid) valve
Left ventricle
Myocardium
Epicardium
Endocardium
Interventricular septum
Aorta
Apex

• **Figure 4.3** Internal view of heart.

Heartbeat

Two Phases—Correspond to Blood Pressure Readouts

Systole: contraction—top number reading
Diastole: relaxation—lower number reading
Trace a drop of blood from trunk of body (deoxygenated) to trunk of body (oxygenated)

Inferior vena cava to right atrium
Through tricuspid valve to right ventricle
From right ventricle to pulmonary artery to lung capillaries
From lung capillaries to pulmonary veins
To left atrium through mitral (bicuspid) valve to left ventricle
Through aortic valve to aorta

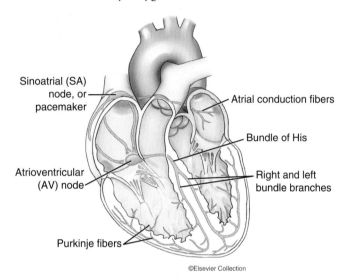

Sinoatrial (SA) node, or pacemaker

Atrial conduction fibers

Bundle of His

Atrioventricular (AV) node

Right and left bundle branches

Purkinje fibers

©Elsevier Collection

• **Figure 4.4** Conduction system of heart.

TABLE 4-1	
Combining Forms	
Combining Form	**Meaning**
1. angi/o	vessel
2. aort/o	aorta
3. ather/o	yellow plaque (fat)
4. arter/o	artery
5. arteri/o	artery
6. atri/o	atrium
7. brachi/o	arm
8. cardi/o	heart
9. cholesterol/o	cholesterol
10. coron/o	heart
11. cyan/o	blue
12. my/o, muscul/o	muscle
13. myx/o	mucus
14. ox/o	oxygen
15. pericardi/o	pericardium
16. phleb/o	vein
17. sphygm/o	pulse
18. steth/o	chest
19. thromb/o	clot
20. valv/o	valve
21. valvul/o	valve
22. vascul/o	vessel
23. vas/o	vessel
24. ven/o	vein
25. ventricul/o	ventricle

TABLE 4-2	
Prefixes	
Prefix	**Meaning**
1. a-	not
2. an-	not
3. bi-	two
4. brady-	slow
5. de-	lack of
6. dys-	bad, difficult, painful
7. endo-	in
8. hyper-	over
9. hypo-	under
10. inter-	between
11. intra-	within
12. meta-	change, after
13. peri-	surrounding
14. tachy-	fast
15. tetra-	four
16. tri-	three

TABLE 4-3	
Suffixes	
Suffix	**Meaning**
1. -dilation	widening, expanding
2. -emia	blood
3. -graphy	recording process
4. -lysis	separation
5. -megaly	enlargement
6. -oma	tumor
7. -osis	condition
8. -plasty	repair
9. -sclerosis	hardening
10. -stenosis	blockage, narrowing
11. -tomy	cutting, incision

TABLE 4-4

Medical Abbreviations

Abbreviation	Meaning	Abbreviation	Meaning
1. ASCVD	arteriosclerotic cardiovascular disease	15. MI	myocardial infarction
2. ASD	atrial septal defect	16. NSR	normal sinus rhythm
3. ASHD	arteriosclerotic heart disease	17. PAC	premature atrial contraction
4. AV	atrioventricular	18. PAT	paroxysmal atrial tachycardia
5. CABG	coronary artery bypass graft	19. PST/PSVT	paroxysmal supraventricular tachycardia
6. CHF	congestive heart failure	20. PTCA	percutaneous transluminal coronary angioplasty
7. CK	creatine kinase		
8. CPK	creatine phosphokinase	21. PVC	premature ventricular contraction
9. CVI	cerebrovascular insufficiency	22. RBBB	right bundle branch block
10. DSE	dobutamine stress echocardiography	23. RSR	regular sinus rhythm
11. HCVD	hypertensive cardiovascular disease	24. RVH	right ventricular hypertrophy
12. LBBB	left bundle branch block	25. SVT	supraventricular tachycardia
13. LVH	left ventricular hypertrophy	26. TEE	transesophageal echocardiography
14. MAT	multifocal atrial tachycardia	27. TST	treadmill stress test

TABLE 4-5

Medical Terms

Term	Meaning	Term	Meaning
Acute coronary syndrome (ACS)	An umbrella term used to cover clinical symptoms compatible with acute myocardial ischemia	Edema	Swelling due to abnormal fluid collection in tissue spaces
Anastomosis	Surgical connection of two tubular structures, such as two pieces of the intestine	Electrode	Lead attached to a generator that carries electric current from the generator to atria or ventricles
Aneurysm	Abnormal dilation of vessels, usually an artery	Electrophysiology	Study of electrical system of heart, including study of arrhythmias
Angina	Spasmotic, choking, or suffocative pain	Embolectomy	Removal of blockage (embolism) from vessel
Angiography	Radiography of blood vessels	Endarterectomy	Incision into an artery to remove inner lining
Angioplasty	Procedure in a vessel to dilate vessel opening	Epicardial	Over heart
Atherectomy	Removal of plaque from an artery (can be done by a percutaneous or open procedure)	False aneurysm	Sac of clotted blood that has completely destroyed vessel and is being contained by tissue that surrounds vessel
Auscultation	Listening for sounds within body	Fistula	Abnormal opening from one area to another area or to outside of the body
Bundle of His	Muscular cardiac fibers that provide heart rhythm to ventricles	Hematoma	Mass of blood that forms outside vessel
Bypass	To go around	Hemolysis	Breakdown of red blood cells
Cardiopulmonary	Refers to heart and lungs	Hypoxemia	Low level of oxygen in blood
Cardiopulmonary bypass	Blood bypasses heart through a heart-lung machine	Hypoxia	Low level of oxygen in tissue
Circumflex	A coronary artery that circles heart	Implantable defibrillator	Surgically placed or wearable device that directs an electric shock to the heart to restore rhythm
Cutdown	Incision into a vessel for placement of a catheter	Intracardiac	Inside heart

Continued

TABLE 4-5

Medical Terms—cont'd

Term	Meaning	Term	Meaning
Invasive	Entering body, breaking skin	Pericardium	Membranous sac enclosing heart and ends of great vessels
Noninvasive	Not entering body, not breaking skin		
Nuclear cardiology	Diagnostic specialty that uses radiologic procedures to aid in diagnosis of cardiologic conditions	Swan-Ganz catheter	A catheter that measures pressure in right side of heart and in pulmonary artery
Order	Shows subordination of one thing to another; family or class	Thoracostomy	Incision into chest wall and insertion of a chest tube
		Thromboendarterectomy	Removal of thrombus and atherosclerotic lining from an artery (percutaneous or open procedure)
Pericardiocentesis	Procedure in which a surgeon withdraws fluid from pericardial space by means of a needle inserted percutaneously	Transvenous	Through a vein

Chapter 4: Anatomy and Terminology Quiz

(Quiz Answers Are Located in Appendix B)

1. These carry blood to the heart:
   a. capillaries
   b. arteries
   c. arterioles
   d. veins
2. Relaxation phase of heartbeat:
   a. diastole
   b. systole
3. Nature's pacemaker is this node:
   a. atrioventricular
   b. Bundle of His
   c. sinoatrial
   d. mitral
4. Node located on interatrial septum:
   a. atrioventricular
   b. Bundle of His
   c. sinoatrial
   d. Purkinje
5. Which of the following is NOT one of the three layers of chamber walls of the heart?
   a. endocardium
   b. myocardium
   c. epicardium
   d. parietal

6. Septum that divides upper two chambers of heart:
   a. intraventricular
   b. interatrial
   c. tricuspid
   d. myocardium
7. Valve between right atrium and right ventricle:
   a. pulmonary
   b. aortic
   c. bicuspid
   d. tricuspid
8. Outer two-layer covering of heart:
   a. pericardium
   b. mitral
   c. myocardium
   d. epicardium
9. These are chambers that receive blood:
   a. right and left ventricle
   b. left ventricle and right atrium
   c. right atrium and right ventricle
   d. right and left atria
10. This combining form means "plaque":
    a. atri/o
    b. brachi/o
    c. cyan/o
    d. ather/o

PATHOPHYSIOLOGY

Vascular Disorders

Coronary Artery Disease (CAD)/Ischemic Heart Disease (IHD)

Thickening and hardening of arterial intima (innermost layer) with lipid and fibrous plaque (atherosclerosis)

- Produces narrowing and stiffening of vessel
  Location of lesions leads to various vascular diseases
- Femoral and popliteal arteries = peripheral vascular disease
- Carotid arteries = stroke
- Aorta = aneurysms (dilation/weakening of vessel walls)
- Coronary arteries = ischemic heart disease or myocardial infarction
- Resulting in decreased oxygen supply

Risk factors increased by:

- Age
- Family history of CAD
- Hyperlipidemia
- Low HDL-C (good cholesterol)
- Hypertension
- Cigarette smoking
- Diabetes mellitus
- Obesity, particularly abdominal

Ischemia

Deficiency of oxygenated blood

- Often due to constriction or obstruction of blood vessel

Localized Myocardial Ischemia—Most Common Cause: Atherosclerosis of Vessels

Oxygen demand of tissues greater than supply
Presenting symptoms

- Chest pain (angina pectoris)
- Hypotension
- Changes in ECG

Transient Ischemia

Heart muscle begins to perform at a low level due to lack of oxygen (reversible ischemia)

Irreversible Ischemia—Is Cause of an MI (Myocardial Infarction)

Heart muscle dies—necrosis (myocardial infarction)

- Prolonged ischemia of 30 minutes or more
- Reestablishment of blood flow reduces residual necrosis
- Thrombolytic agents to dissolve or split up thrombus
- Primary percutaneous transluminal coronary angioplasty (PTCA)

Cardiac enzymes are released from damaged cells

- Blood test reveals elevation of enzymes, confirming myocardial infarction

Classification of blood pressure for adults aged 18 years or older[1]

Category	Systolic (mm Hg)	Diastolic (mm Hg)
Normal	<120	<80
Prehypertension (stays between)	120–139	80–89
Hypertension[2]		
Stage 1 (mild)	140–159	90–99
Stage 2 (moderate)	160–179	100–109
Stage 3 (severe)	≥180	≥110

[1] Not taking antihypertensive drugs and not acutely ill. When systolic and diastolic pressures fall into different categories, the higher category should be selected.

[2] Based on the average of two or more readings taken at each of two or more visits after an initial screening.

• **Figure 4.5** Classification of blood pressure.

Hypertension (HTN)

Normal is less than 120/80 for adults

- Fig. 4.5 illustrates new hypertension classifications

Leading cause of death in United States due to damage to brain, heart, kidneys, eyes, and arteries of the lower extremities

Cause is unknown in 95% of cases

- Known as
  - Primary hypertension
  - Essential hypertension

5% of cases are secondary to underlying disease
Increased resistance damages heart and blood vessels

- Retinal vascular changes are monitored to assess therapy and disease progression

Chronic hypertension often leads to end-stage renal disease

- Result of progressive sclerosis of renal vessels

Treatment

Medications

- ACE (angiotensin-converting enzyme) inhibitor
- Alpha-adrenergic or beta-adrenergic receptor blocker
- Diuretic
- Calcium channel blocker

Lifestyle changes

Hypotension

Abnormally Low Blood Pressure

Types

Orthostatic (postural) hypotension

- Fall in both systolic and diastolic arterial blood pressure on standing
- Associated with
  - Dizziness
  - Blurred vision
  - Fainting (syncope)

- Caused by insufficient oxygenated blood flow through brain
- Can be acute (temporary) or chronic

Chronic orthostatic hypotension—types

- Primary of unknown cause
- Secondary to certain disease processes such as:
  - Endocrine
  - Metabolic
  - Central nervous system disorders
- Treatment for secondary hypotension is correction of underlying disease

Aneurysm

Dilation of an arterial blood vessel wall or cardiac chamber

- Danger is rupture of aneurysm

Atherosclerosis is common cause

Arteriosclerosis and hypertension also common in persons with aneurysms

True Aneurysm

Involves all three layers of arterial wall

Causes weakening and ballooning of arterial wall

False or Pseudoaneurysm

Usually result of trauma

Also known as saccular

Separation of arterial wall layers (dissecting) in artery wall (crisis situation—a medical emergency)

Bleeds into dissected space and is contained by arterial connective tissue wall

Thrombus

Blood clot that remains attached to vessel wall and occludes vessel

Dislodged thrombus is a thromboembolus

Causes

Trauma

Interior wall lining irritation/roughening

Infection

Inflammation

Low blood pressure/blood stagnation

Obstruction

Atherosclerosis

Risks Related to Thrombus

Dislodges and moves to lungs, brain, heart

Grows to occlude blood flow

Treatment

Pharmacologic, anticoagulants

Heparin

Warfarin derivatives

Noninvasive Intervention

Balloon-tipped catheter to remove or compress thrombus

Thrombophlebitis Caused by Inflammation (Phlebitis)

Causes

Trauma

Infection

Immobility

Commonly Associated With

Endocarditis

Rheumatic heart disease

Embolism

Mass that is present and circulating in blood

Common Types

Air bubble

Fat

Bacterial mass

Cancer cells

Foreign substances

Dislodged thrombus

Amniotic fluid

Obstructs Vessel

Pulmonary emboli travel through venous side or right side of the heart to the pulmonary artery

Systemic or arterial emboli originate in left side of the heart

Associated with

- Myocardial infarction
- Left-sided heart failure
- Endocarditis
- Valvular conditions
- Dysrhythmias

Peripheral Arterial Disease

Thromboangiitis Obliterans (Buerger's Disease)

Occurs most often in young men who are heavy smokers

Inflammatory disease of peripheral arteries creating thrombi and vasospasms

Involves small or medium arteries of feet and often hands

- May necessitate amputation

Raynaud's Disease

Vasospasms and constriction of small arterioles of fingers and toes

Affects young women as a secondary condition

Triggered by cold temperatures, emotional stress, cigarette smoking

Fingertips thicken and nails become brittle

Raynaud's phenomenon is secondary to primary disease, such as

- Scleroderma
- Pulmonary hypertension

Treatment of Underlying Condition

No known origin or treatment

Varicose Veins

Blood pools in veins, distending them
Tends to be progressive/vein valve failure
Occurs most commonly in saphenous veins
Hemorrhoids are varicose veins of anus

Leads to
Swelling and discomfort
Fatigue when in legs
Possible ulcerations

Heart Disorders

Congestive Heart Failure (CHF)—Heart Cannot Pump Required Amounts of Blood

Can be left-sided or right-sided heart failure
Left-sided heart failure (systolic); cannot generate adequate output, causing pulmonary edema
Common causes:
    Myocardial infarction
    Myocarditis
    Cardiomyopathies leading to ischemia
Symptoms of left-sided congestive heart failure include:
    Shortness of breath
    Fatigue
    Exercise intolerance
Right-sided heart failure (diastolic) results in right ventricle stasis, inadequate pulmonary circulation, and peripheral edema/hepatosplenomegaly

Abnormal Heart Rhythms (Conduction Irregularities)

Bradycardia and heart block (atrioventricular block)
    Inadequate conduction impulses from SA node though AV node to AV bundle
    Treatment
        Cardiac pacemaker to maintain proper heart rate
Flutter—rapid regular contractions (most commonly of atria)
    Symptoms—palpitations
    Treatment
        Cardioversion (electronic shock to heart)
        Ablation (radiofrequency catheter destroying tissue causing arrhythmia)
Fibrillation—rapid, erratic, inefficient contractions of atria and ventricles
Atrial fibrillation—most common (electrical impulses move randomly in atria)
    Symptoms—palpitation, risk of stroke due to clot formations from poor atrial outputs
    Treatment
        Cardioversion
        Ablation
Ventricular fibrillation—life-threatening, random electrical impulses throughout ventricles
    Symptoms—cardiac death or arrest without immediate treatment

Treatment
    Cardioversion
    Digoxin—drug used to slow heart rate
    Implantable defibrillator
    Emergency treatment—automatic external defibrillators (AEDs)
    Radiofrequency catheter ablation (RFA) is a minimally invasive technique used to treat cardiac arrhythmias

Infective Endocarditis

Inflammation of interior-most lining of heart
Leads to destruction and permanent damage to heart valves
Caused by
    Bacteria (most commonly streptococci and staphylococci)
    Virus
    Fungi
    Parasites
Patients with heart defects or damage usually take antibiotics prior to invasive procedures

Pericarditis

Inflammation of pericardium of heart

Common Types
- Acute
- Pericardial effusion
- Constrictive

Rheumatic Fever/Rheumatic Heart Disease

Results in formation of scar tissue of the endocardium and heart valves
In 10% of cases leads to rheumatic heart disease
Family tendency to develop
Begins as carditis (inflammation of all layers of heart wall)
Long-term effects:
    Mitral and/or aortic valve disease
    Stenosis
    Regurgitation
    Insufficiency
Tricuspid valve
    Affected in about 10% of cases
Pulmonary valve
    Rarely affected

Valvular Heart Disease

Valves are extensions of endocardial tissue
    Endocardial damage can be congenital or acquired
    Damage leads to stenosis and/or incompetent valve
    Includes
    - Valvular stenosis is narrowing, stiffness, thickening, fusion, or blockage of valve, creating resistance, resulting in increased pressure in cardiac chamber behind valve

- Valvular regurgitation is failure of valve leaflet to close tightly, allowing backflow of blood
- Result of lesions causing valve leaflets to shrink
- Functional valvular regurgitation results in increased chamber size (cardiomegaly)

Stenosis

Aortic Valve Stenosis

Caused by
  Congenital malformation
  Degeneration
  Infection
Results in slowing blood circulatory rate
Symptoms
  Bradycardia
  Faint pulse
  May lead to heart murmur and hypertrophy

Mitral Valve Stenosis

Impaired flow from left atrium to left ventricle
Caused by
  Rheumatic fever
  Bacterial infections
Symptom
  Decreased cardiac output
May lead to
- Pulmonary hypertension
- Right ventricular heart failure
- And/or edema

Valvular Regurgitation

Flow in opposite direction from normal
Mitral regurgitation (MR)
  Backflow of blood from left ventricle into left atrium
Aortic regurgitation (AR)
  Backflow of blood from aorta into left ventricle
Pulmonic regurgitation (PR)
  Backflow of blood from pulmonary artery into right ventricle
Tricuspid regurgitation (TR)
  Backflow of blood from right ventricle into right atrium

Heart Wall Disorders

Acute Pericarditis

Roughening and inflammation of pericardium (sac around heart)

Treatment
  Anti-inflammatory drugs and pain medication

Constrictive Pericarditis (Restrictive Pericarditis)

Forms Fibrous Lesions That Encase Heart

Compresses heart—thickened pericardial sac prevents heart from expanding when blood enters it
  Tamponade occurs when fluid builds up in pericardial space

Pressure stops heart from beating—pericardial effusion or bleeding after heart surgery
Reduces output

Pericardial Effusion

Accumulation of fluid in pericardial cavity
Results in pressure on heart
- Sudden development of pressure on heart is tamponade

Cardiomyopathies

Myocardium: muscular wall (middle layer) of heart musculature
Group of diseases that affect myocardium
Cause
  Idiopathic (most common)
  Underlying condition

Types of Cardiomyopathy

Dilated cardiomyopathy (congestive cardiomyopathy)
- Ventricular distention and impaired systolic function
Hypertrophic cardiomyopathy
- Cause is often hypertensive or valvular heart disease
- Results in thickened interventricular septum (septum between the ventricle chambers)
Restrictive cardiomyopathy
- Myocardium becomes stiffened
- Heart enlarges (cardiomegaly)
- Dysrhythmias common
- Caused by infiltrative diseases such as amyloidosis

Congenital Heart Defects

Coarctation of aorta (CoA)—narrowing of the aorta
- Treatment
    Surgical removal of narrow segment/end-to-end anastomosis
Patent ductus arteriosus (PDA)—opening between aorta and pulmonary artery
- Treatment
    Drugs to close/embolize or plug ductus or tying off surgically
Tetralogy of Fallot—malformation of heart includes four defects
1. Pulmonary artery stenosis—
   - Narrowing/obstruction
2. Ventricular septal defect
   - Hole between two bottom chambers (ventricles) of heart
3. Overriding aorta
   - Shift of aorta to right—aorta overrides the interventricular septum
4. Hypertrophy of right ventricle
   - Myocardium enlarges to pump blood through narrowed pulmonary artery
   Treatment
   - Open-heart technique with heart-lung machine support to relieve right ventricular outflow tract stenosis and repair of ventriculoseptal defect

Chapter 4: Pathophysiology Quiz

(Quiz Answers Are Located in Appendix B)

1. Lesion of carotid artery may lead to:
   a. heart attack
   b. stroke
   c. peripheral vascular disease
   d. ischemic heart disease

2. This blood pressure is hypertension:
   a. 120/80
   b. 130/70
   c. 140/90
   d. 110/70

3. Infective endocarditis is inflammation of the interior of the lining of the heart, and when caused by streptococci or staphylococci, the infection is:
   a. viral
   b. fungal
   c. bacterial
   d. parasitic

4. Angina pectoris is:
   a. heart block
   b. heart murmur
   c. chest pain
   d. barrel chest

5. In this type of regurgitation, there is a backflow of blood from left ventricle into left atrium:
   a. aortic
   b. pulmonic
   c. tricuspid
   d. mitral

6. In this type of heart wall disorder, fibrous lesions form and encase the heart:
   a. constrictive pericarditis
   b. acute pericarditis
   c. pericardial effusion
   d. cardiomyopathy

7. Which of the following terms means "of unknown cause"?
   a. etiology
   b. manifestation
   c. idiopathic
   d. late effect

8. This condition is also known as congestive cardiomyopathy:
   a. hypertrophic
   b. valvular
   c. dilated
   d. restrictive

9. This peripheral arterial disease most often occurs in young men who are heavy smokers:
   a. Buerger's
   b. Pick's
   c. Addison's
   d. Glasser's

10. This cardiomyopathy results in a thickened interventricular septum:
    a. restrictive
    b. congestive
    c. dilated
    d. hypertrophic

5

Female Genital System and Pregnancy

Terminology

Ovaries (Pair)

Produce ova (single female gamete) and hormones; ova: plural; ovum: singular (Fig. 5.1). Each ovum/gamete contains 23 chromosomes.

Fallopian Tubes (Uterine Tubes or Oviducts)

Ducts from ovary to uterus

Uterus (Womb)

Muscular organ that holds embryo
Three layers
- Endometrium: inner mucosa
- Myometrium: middle layer/muscle
- Perimetrium/Uterine serosa: outer layer
  - Cervix: lower narrow portion of uterus
  - Fundus: the upper rounded part of the uterus

Vagina

Tube from uterus to outside of body

Vulva

External genitalia
- Clitoris: erectile tissue
- Labia majora: outer lips of vagina
- Labia minora: inner lips of vagina
- Urinary meatus: opening to urethra
- Bartholin's gland: glands on either side of vagina
- Hymen: membrane partially or wholly occludes entrance to vagina

Perineum

Area between anus and vaginal orifice

Accessory Organs (Fig. 5.2)

Breasts

Mammary glands
  Composed of glandular tissue containing milk glands/lactiferous ducts
  In response to hormones from pituitary gland, milk is produced in acini (also known as alveoli) (lactation)
  Lactiferous ducts transfer milk to nipple
  Nipple, surrounded by areola

Menstruation and Pregnancy

Proliferation Phase

Menstruation (Days 1-5): discharge of blood fluid containing endometrial cells, blood cells, and glandular secretions from endometrium
Endometrium repair (Days 6-12): maturing follicle in ovary produces estrogen (hormone), which causes endometrium to thicken and ovum (egg) to mature in graafian follicle

Secretory Phase

Ovulation (Days 13-14): occurs when graafian follicle ruptures and ovum travels down fallopian tube
  Usually only one graafian follicle develops each month
Premenstruation (Days 15-28): a period of time in which graafian follicle converts to corpus luteum secreting progesterone to stimulate build-up of uterine lining. If after 5 days no fertilization occurs, cycle repeats.

Pregnancy

Prenatal stage of development from fertilization to birth (39 weeks)
  Fertilized ovum or zygote develops in a double cavity: yolk sac (produces blood cells) and amniotic cavity (contains amniotic fluid)

Embryo, stage of development from 4th to 8th week
Fetus, unborn offspring, 9 weeks until birth

Placenta Forms Within Uterine Wall and Produces Hormone—Human Chorionic Gonadotropin (HCG)

HCG is hormone tested in urine pregnancy tests
    HCG stimulates corpus luteum to produce estrogen and progesterone until the third month of pregnancy
    Placenta then produces hormones
    Expelled after delivery (afterbirth)

Gestation, Approximately 266 Days

280 days used when calculating estimated date of delivery (EDD) or time from last menstrual period (LMP)
    Three trimesters

- First   LMP-12 weeks
- Second   13-27 weeks
- Third   28 weeks-EDD

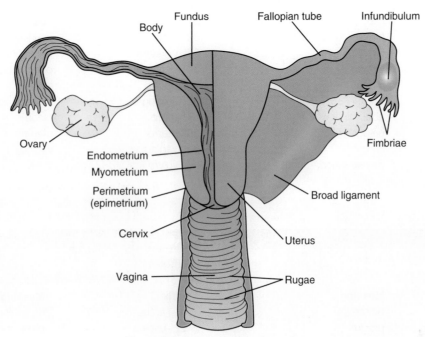

• **Figure 5.1** Female reproductive system.

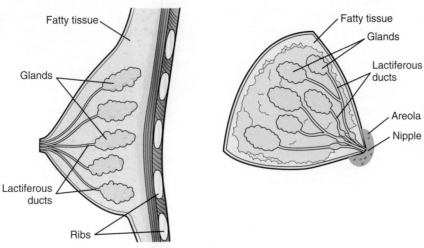

• **Figure 5.2** Breast structure.

TABLE 5-1

Combining Forms

Combining Form	Meaning	Combining Form	Meaning
1. amni/o	amnion	21. metr/o	uterus, measure
2. arche/o	first	22. metr/i	uterus
3. cephal/o	head	23. my/o, muscul/o	muscle
4. cervic/o	cervix	24. nat/a	birth
5. chori/o	chorion	25. nat/i	birth
6. colp/o	vagina	26. obstetr/o	pregnancy/childbirth
7. crypt/o	hidden	27. olig/o	few
8. culd/o	cul-de-sac	28. oo/o	egg
9. episi/o	vulva	29. oophor/o	ovary
10. fet/o	fetus	30. ov/o	egg
11. galact/o	milk	31. ovari/o	ovary
12. gynec/o	female	32. ovul/o	ovulation
13. gyn/o	female	33. perine/o	perineum
14. hymen/o	hymen	34. peritone/o	peritoneum
15. hyster/o	uterus	35. phor/o	to bear
16. lact/o	milk	36. salping/o	uterine tube, fallopian tube
17. lapar/o	abdominal wall	37. top/o	place
18. mamm/o	breast	38. uter/o	uterus
19. mast/o	breast	39. vagin/o	vagina
20. men/o	menstruation, month	40. vulv/o	vulva

TABLE 5-2

Prefixes

Prefix	Meaning
1. ante-	before
2. dys-	painful
3. ecto-	outside
4. endo-	in
5. extra-	outside
6. in-	into
7. intra-	within
8. multi-	many
9. neo-	new
10. nulli-	none
11. nulti-	none
12. post-	after
13. primi-	first
14. pseudo-	false
15. retro-	backwards
16. uni-	one

TABLE 5-3

Suffixes

Suffix	Meaning
1. -arche	beginning
2. -cyesis	pregnancy
3. -gravida	pregnancy
4. -rrhexis	rupture
5. -para	woman who has given birth
6. -parous	to bear
7. -rrhea	discharge
8. -salpinx	uterine tube
9. -tocia	labor
10. -version	turning

TABLE 5-4

Medical Abbreviations

Abbreviation	Meaning	Abbreviation	Meaning
1. AFI	amniotic fluid index	20. EMC	endometrial curettage
2. AGA	appropriate for gestational age	21. ERT	estrogen replacement therapy
3. ARM	artificial rupture of membrane	22. FAS	fetal alcohol syndrome
4. BPD	biparietal diameter	23. FHR	fetal heart rate
5. BPP	biophysical profile	24. FSH	follicle-stimulating hormone
6. BV	bacterial vaginosis	25. HPV	human papillomavirus
7. CHL	crown-to-heel length	26. HSG	hysterosalpingogram
8. CNM	certified nurse midwife	27. HSV	herpes simplex virus
9. CPD	cephalopelvic disproportion	28. IVF	in vitro fertilization
10. CPP	chronic pelvic pain	29. LEEP	loop electrosurgical excision procedure
11. D&C	dilation and curettage	30. LGA	large for gestational age
12. D&E	dilation and evacuation	31. PID	pelvic inflammatory disease
13. DUB	dysfunctional uterine bleeding	32. PROM	premature rupture of membranes
14. ECC	endocervical curettage	33. SHG	sonohysterogram
15. EDC	estimated date of confinement	34. SROM	spontaneous rupture of membranes
16. EDD	estimated date of delivery	35. SUI	stress urinary incontinence
17. EFM	electronic fetal monitoring	36. TAH	total abdominal hysterectomy
18. EFW	estimated fetal weight	37. VBAC	vaginal birth after cesarean
19. EGA	estimated gestational age		

TABLE 5-5

Medical Terms

Term	Meaning	Term	Meaning
Abortion	Termination of pregnancy	Introitus	Opening or entrance to vagina
Amniocentesis	Percutaneous aspiration of amniotic fluid	Ligation	Binding or tying off, as in constricting blood flow of a vessel or binding fallopian tubes for sterilization
Amniotic sac	Sac containing fetus and amniotic fluid		
Antepartum	Before childbirth		
Cesarean	Surgical opening through abdominal wall for delivery	Multipara	More than one pregnancy
		Oophorectomy	Surgical removal of ovary(ies)
Chorionic villus sampling	CVS, biopsy of outermost part of placenta	Perineum	Area between vulva and anus; also known as pelvic floor
Cordocentesis	Procedure to obtain a fetal blood sample; also called a percutaneous umbilical blood sampling	Placenta	A structure that connects fetus and mother during pregnancy
		Postpartum	After childbirth
Curettage	Scraping of a cavity using a spoon-shaped instrument	Primigravida	First pregnancy
		Primipara	First delivered infant/given birth to only one child
Cystocele	Herniation of bladder into vagina		
Delivery	Childbirth	Salpingectomy	Surgical removal of uterine tube
Dilation	Expansion (of cervix)	Salpingostomy	Creation of a fistula into uterine tube
Ectopic	Pregnancy outside uterus (i.e., in fallopian tube)	Tocolysis	Repression of uterine contractions
		Vesicovaginal fistula	Abnormal opening/channel between vagina and bladder
Hysterectomy	Surgical removal of uterus		
Hysterorrhaphy	Suturing of uterus		
Hysteroscopy	Visualization of canal and cavity of uterus using a scope placed through vagina		

Chapter 5: Anatomy and Terminology Quiz

(Quiz Answers Are Located in Appendix B)

1. This is NOT one of the three layers of uterus:
   a. perimetrium
   b. endometrium
   c. myometrium
   d. barametrium
2. Located at the lower end of uterus is the:
   a. cervix
   b. vagina
   c. perineum
   d. labia majora
3. Approximate gestation of a human fetus is:
   a. 266 days
   b. 276 days
   c. 290 days
   d. 292 days
4. LMP is the:
   a. later maternity phase
   b. last menstrual period
   c. low metabolic pregnancy
   d. late menstruation phase
5. Name of stage that describes development of fetus from fertilization to birth is:
   a. postpartum
   b. antepartum
   c. prenatal
   d. natal
6. Which of the following correctly identifies three trimesters of gestation?
   a. LMP to less than 14 weeks 0 days, 14 weeks 0 days to less than 28 weeks 0 days, 28 weeks 0 days until delivery
   b. LMP to less than 16 weeks 0 days, 16 weeks 0 days to less than 28 weeks 0 days, 28 weeks 0 days until delivery
   c. LMP to less than 16 weeks 0 days, 16 weeks 0 days to less than 29 weeks 0 days, 29 weeks 0 days until delivery
   d. LMP to less than 13 weeks 0 days, 13 weeks 0 days to less than 27 weeks 0 days, 27 weeks 0 days until delivery
7. Combining form meaning "few":
   a. oopho/o
   b. olig/o
   c. nati/i
   d. top/o
8. Combining form meaning "hidden":
   a. amni/o
   b. crypt/o
   c. chori/o
   d. fet/o
9. Suffix meaning "beginning":
   a. -cyesis
   b. -rrhea
   c. -arche
   d. -orrhexis
10. Prefix meaning "within":
    a. ante-
    b. dys-
    c. ecto-
    d. endo-

PATHOPHYSIOLOGY

Menstrual and Hormonal Disorders

Dysmenorrhea

Painful menstruation

Common Types
- Primary and secondary

Primary Dysmenorrhea

No underlying condition but begins with commencement of ovulation

Cramping is caused by excess of prostaglandin
- Causes contractions and uterine ischemia
- Develops 24 to 48 hours prior to menstruation

Treatment
- Nonsteroidal anti-inflammatory agents
- Progesterone

Secondary Dysmenorrhea

Caused by an underlying disorder, such as
- Polyps
- Tumors
- Endometriosis
- Pelvic inflammatory disease

Treatment

Directed at underlying disorder

Amenorrhea

Amenorrhea is absence of menstruation

Common Types
- Primary and secondary

Primary Amenorrhea

Menstruation has never occurred
May be genetic disorder
- Turner's syndrome (ovaries do not function)

Secondary Amenorrhea

Cessation of menstruation for 3 cycles or 6 months
- Individual has previously menstruated

Various causes of anovulation/amenorrhea

Examples:
- Tumors
- Stress
- Eating disorders
- Competitive sports participation

Dysfunctional Uterine Bleeding (DUB)

Abnormal bleeding patterns

Occurs when no organic cause can be identified

Abnormal Menstruation Types

Oligomenorrhea: in excess of 6 weeks between periods
  Polymenorrhea: less than 3 weeks between periods
  Metrorrhagia: bleeding between cycles
  Menorrhagia: increase in amount and duration of flow
  Hypomenorrhea: light or spotty flow
  Menometrorrhagia: irregular cycle with varying amounts and duration of flow
  Menorrhea: lengthy menstrual flow
  Dysmenorrhea: painful menstruation

Premenstrual Syndrome (PMS)

Also known as premenstrual tension (PMT)

Occurs before onset of menses (luteal phase) and ends at onset of menses

Cluster of Common Symptoms

Weight gain
Breast tenderness
Sleep disturbances
Headache
Irritability
Cause is unknown

Treatment

Varies depending on individual symptoms

Endometriosis

Endometrial tissue (uterine lining) develops outside the uterus (on ovaries, fallopian tubes, small intestine, etc.)

Responses to Hormone Cycle

Ectopic (out of place) endometrial tissue degenerates, sheds, and bleeds

Causes

- Irritation
- Inflammation
- Pain

Continued cycles produce fibrous tissue
- Adhesions and obstructions can then form
- Interferes with normal bodily function

- For example, fallopian tube endometriosis may lead to obstructed tubes

Primary symptom is dysmenorrhea
- May also cause painful intercourse (dyspareunia)

Risks

Increased risk for cancers
- Breast
- Ovaries
- Non-Hodgkin lymphoma

Treatment Includes

Hormonal suppression

Surgical removal of endometrial tissue
- May require hysterectomy and BSO (bilateral salpingo-oophorectomy)

Infection, Inflammation, and Sexually Transmitted Diseases

Pelvic Inflammatory Disease (PID)

Infection and inflammation of reproductive tract
- Primarily ovaries and fallopian tubes
- Usually originates in cervix or vagina
- Migrates up through reproductive tract

Types

Acute
Chronic
- Commonly forms adhesions and strictures
- May lead to infertility

Candidiasis

Yeast infection
- *Candida albicans (Monilia)*

Not sexually transmitted

Opportunistic infection may follow
- Infection treated with antibiotics
- Period of reduced resistance
- Increased glucose or glycogen levels (often associated with diabetes mellitus)

Affects mucous membranes
- Produces a white, thick, curdlike discharge

Result may be dyspareunia and dysuria

Treatment

Antifungal substances such as nystatin

Identification and treatment of underlying condition

Chlamydia

Most common sexually transmitted disease (STD)

Cause

Bacteria, *Chlamydia trachomatis*

Symptoms
Asymptomatic or mild discharge and dysuria

Treatment
Antimicrobial

Genital Herpes

Cause
Virus, herpes simplex 2 (HSV-2)

Symptoms
Ulcers and vesicles

Treatment
Antiviral, manage outbreaks
There is no cure for genital herpes

Genital Warts

Cause
Virus, human papillomavirus

Symptoms
Polyps or grey lesions

Treatment
Excision

Prevention
Vaccine
There is no cure for genital warts

Gonorrhea

Cause
Bacteria, *Neisseria gonorrhoeae*

Symptoms
Dysuria
Discharge

Treatment
Antibacterial drugs
Some strains are drug-resistant

Syphilis

Cause
Bacteria, *Treponema pallidum*

Symptoms
Primary syphilis
  • Ulcer or chancre at site of entry
Secondary syphilis
  • Headache
  • Fever
  • Rash
  • Tertiary
  • Affects cardiovascular and nervous systems

Treatment
Penicillin

Trichomoniasis

Cause
Protozoan, *Trichomonas vaginalis*

Symptoms
Usually asymptomatic

Treatment
Antimicrobial drugs

Benign Lesions

Leiomyomas—Uterine Fibroids

Well-defined, solid uterine tumor

Also known as
  • Uterine fibroids
  • Fibromyoma
  • Fibroma
  • Myoma
  • Fibroid
Classification is based on location of tumor within uterine wall
  Submucous: beneath endometrium
  Subserous: beneath serosa
  Intramural: in muscle wall

Symptoms
May be asymptomatic
Abnormal uterine bleeding
Pressure on nearby structures, such as bladder and rectum
Constipation
Pain
Sensation of heaviness

Treatment
Surgical excision of lesions
Hysterectomy may be necessary

Adenomyosis

Within uterine myometrium

Symptoms
Usually asymptomatic
Abnormal menstrual bleeding
Enlarged uterus
  Commonly develops in late reproductive years
  Common in those taking tamoxifen

Treatment
Symptomatic in mild cases
Surgical in severe cases
  • Excision of adenomyosis or hysterectomy

Malignant Lesions

Carcinoma of Breast

Accessory of reproductive system
  Most often develops in upper outer quadrant
  - Due to location, often spreads to lymph nodes
  - May metastasize to lungs, brain, bone, liver, etc.
  Majority arise from epithelial cells of ducts and lobules
  Second most common cancer of women
  Most are adenocarcinoma
  - Invasive ductal carcinoma most common type
  - Invasive lobular carcinoma second most common type
  - Lymph node spread is determined by sentinel node biopsy (SNB)
  - Small primary tumors are excised in a lumpectomy (tumor and immediate surrounding tissue only)
  - Mastectomy is alternative surgical procedure removing entire breast
  - Chemotherapy and radiation may be indicated to prevent recurrence
If neoplasm is responsive to hormone, hormone-blocking agents are administered

Increased Risks

- Heredity
  - Especially history of mother or sister who developed breast cancer
  - Mutated breast cancer gene (BRCA-1)
  - Familial breast cancer syndrome associated with BRCA-2
- Lower socioeconomic status
- Radiation exposure

Carcinoma of Uterus (Endometrial Cancer)

Most frequent pelvic cancer
  Usually postmenopausal
  Associated with higher levels of estrogen

Increases Risk

Obesity (estrogen produced by fat tissue)
Early menarche
Delayed menopause
Hypertension
Diabetes mellitus
Nulliparity (no viable births)
Some types of colorectal cancer
Oral contraceptives (estrogen)
Estrogen-producing tumors

Symptoms

Abnormal, excessive uterine bleeding
Postmenopausal bleeding
No simple screening test available
- Uterine cells may be aspirated for evaluation

Staging of Endometrial, Cervical, and Ovarian Malignancies

I—Confined to corpus
II—Involves corpus and cervix
III—Extends outside uterus but not outside true pelvis
IV—Extends outside true pelvis or involves rectum or bladder

Treatment

Pharmaceutical
Surgical
Irradiation
Chemotherapy
Combination of above

Carcinoma of Cervix

Routinely found on Papanicolaou (Pap) smear
  Dysplasia is an early change in cervical epithelium

Increases Risks

Herpes simplex virus type 2 (HSV-2)
Human papillomavirus (HPV)
Young age of sexual activity
Smoking
Lower socioeconomic status

Stages of cervical cancer

Stage 1—Carcinoma of cervix
Stage 2—Carcinoma spread from cervix to upper vagina
Stage 3—Carcinoma spread to lower portion of vagina/pelvic wall
Stage 4—Most invasive stage spreading to other body parts

Symptoms

Early stages asymptomatic
Later stages
- Bleeding
- Discharge
Biopsy is used to confirm

Treatment

Pharmaceutical
Surgical
Irradiation
Chemotherapy
Combination of above

Carcinoma of Ovary

Cause is unknown—considered silent killer

Increased Risks

Genetic factors (BRCA-1)
Endocrine
- Nulliparous
- Early menarche

- Late menopause
- Non–breast feeding
- Late first pregnancy
- Postmenopausal estrogen replacement therapy (ERT)

Tumor Categories

Germ Cell Tumors

Arise from primitive germ cells, usually the testis and ovum

Types

- Germinoma
- Yolk sac
- Endodermal sinus tumor
- Teratoma
- Embryonal carcinoma
- Polyembryoma
- Gonadoblastoma
- Some types of choriocarcinoma

Categories

- Dermoid cysts (benign)
- Malignant tumors
- Primitive malignant
  - Embryonic
  - Extraembryonic cells

Epithelial Tumors

Most common gynecologic cancer

Gonadal Stromal Tumors

Symptoms

Pelvic heaviness
Dysuria
Increased urinary frequency
Sometimes vaginal bleeding

Treatment

Excision
   Hysterectomy, including bilateral salpingo-oophorectomy with omentectomy (fold of peritoneum)
Chemotherapy
Radiation therapy
Combination of above

Carcinoma of Fallopian Tubes

Primary Fallopian Tube Tumors

Rare
Must be located within tube to be considered primary
- Adenocarcinoma most common primary tumor
Most tumors are secondary

Symptoms

Often asymptomatic
Bleeding or discharge
Irregular menstruation
Pain

Treatment

Hysterectomy, including bilateral salpingo-oophorectomy with any necessary omentectomy (fold of peritoneum)
Chemotherapy
Radiation therapy
Combination of above

Carcinoma of Vulva

Usually squamous cell carcinoma (90%)
Increased risk with STDs

Symptoms

Can be asymptomatic
Pruritic vulvular lesion

Treatment

Radical vulvectomy with node dissection
Wide local excision

Carcinoma of Vagina

Usually squamous cell carcinoma

Increased Risk

Human papillomavirus (HPV)
Postmenopausal hysterectomy
History of abnormal Pap
History of other carcinomas

Symptoms

Often asymptomatic
Vaginal pain, discharge, or bleeding

Treatment

Squamous cell—radiation
Early tumors may be excised
Vaginectomy
Hysterectomy
Lymph node dissection

Pregnancy

Placenta Previa

Opening of cervix is obstructed by displaced placenta

Types (Fig. 5.3)
Marginal
Partial
Total

Abruptio Placentae (Fig. 5.4)

Premature separation of placenta from uterine wall

Eclampsia

Serious condition of pregnancy characterized by
- Hypertension
- Edema
- Proteinuria

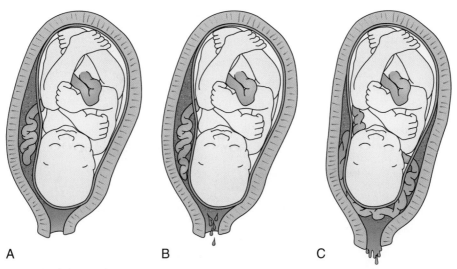

• **Figure 5.3** **A.** Marginal placenta previa. **B.** Partial placenta previa. **C.** Total placenta previa.

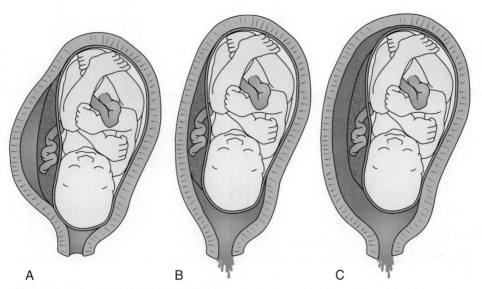

• **Figure 5.4** Abruptio placentae is classified according to the grade of separation of the placenta from uterine wall. **A.** Mild separation in which hemorrhage is internal. **B.** Moderate separation in which there is external hemorrhage. **C.** Severe separation in which there is external hemorrhage and extreme separation.

Ectopic Pregnancy (Extrauterine)
(Fig. 5.5)

Implantation of fertilized ovum outside uterus
- Often fallopian tubes (tubal pregnancy)

Hydatidiform Mole

Benign tumor of placenta
Secretes hormone (chorionic gonadotropic hormone, CGH)
Indicates positive pregnancy test

Malpositions and Malpresentations
(Fig. 5.6)

Vaginal Delivery

Breech
    Vertex
    Face
    Brow
    Shoulder

Abortion

Types
Spontaneous
- Miscarriage
- Happens naturally
- Uterus completely empties

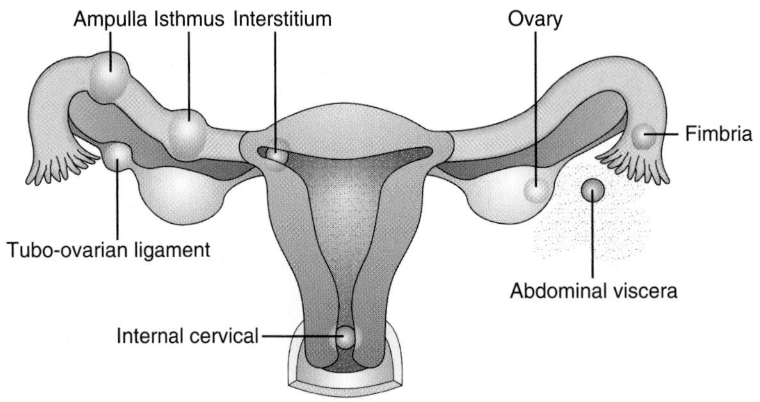

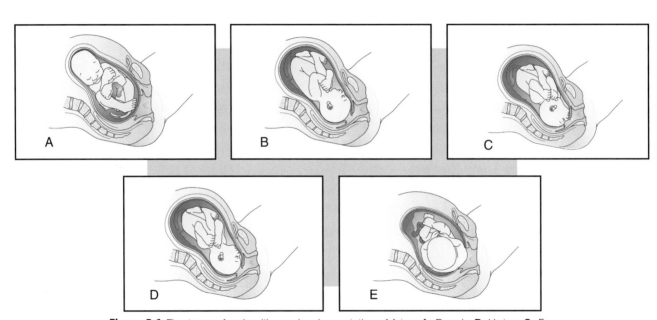

• Figure 5.5 Ectopic pregnancy most often occurs in fallopian tube. Pregnancy outside the uterus may end in life-threatening rupture.

• Figure 5.6 Five types of malposition and malpresentation of fetus: **A.** Breech. **B.** Vertex. **C.** Face. **D.** Brow. **E.** Shoulder.

Incomplete
- Uterus does not completely empty
- Requires intervention to remove remaining fetal material

Missed
- Fetus dies naturally
- Requires intervention to remove fetal material

Septic
- Similar to missed
- Has added complication of infection
- Requires intervention to remove fetal material
- Vigorous treatment of infection

Methods

D&C
- Dilation and curettage (scraping)

Evacuation (suction)

Intra-amniotic injections
- Saline (salt) solution

Vaginal suppositories
- Such as prostaglandin

Chapter 5: Pathophysiology Quiz

(Quiz Answers Are Located in Appendix B)

1. Most common solution used for intra-amniotic injections is:
   a. prostaglandin
   b. saline
   c. estrogen
   d. chorionic gonadotropic hormone
2. This type of dysmenorrhea is treated with nonsteroidal anti-inflammatory agents and progesterone:
   a. secondary
   b. constrictive
   c. periodic
   d. primary
3. In this type of amenorrhea there is a cessation of menstruation:
   a. secondary
   b. constrictive
   c. periodic
   d. primary

For questions 4 to 6, match the abnormal menstruation type with correct definition from items a-c below.
   a. increased amount and duration of flow
   b. bleeding between cycles
   c. in excess of 6 weeks

4. oligomenorrhea
5. metrorrhagia
6. menorrhagia
7. Increased risks of breast cancer, ovarian cancer, and non-Hodgkin lymphoma exist with this condition:
   a. endometriosis
   b. pelvic inflammatory disease
   c. sexually transmitted disease
   d. dysfunctional uterine bleeding
8. This benign lesion is also known as uterine fibroids:
   a. adenomyosis
   b. squamous cell
   c. leiomyoma
   d. extraembryonic cell primitive
9. Marginal, partial, and total are types of this condition:
   a. abruptio placentae
   b. placenta previa
   c. ectopic pregnancy
   d. hydatidiform mole
10. Which of the following is NOT a malposition of fetus?
    a. breech
    b. shoulder
    c. back
    d. brow

6

Male Genital System

ANATOMY AND TERMINOLOGY

Function, reproduction
  Structure, essential organs, and accessory organs (Fig. 6.1)

Essential Organs

Testes (Gonads)

Produce sperm (male gamete with 23 chromosomes) in seminiferous tubules
  Covered by tunica albuginea, located in scrotum
  Produce testosterone in Leydig cells

Vas Deferens

Is a tube
End of epididymis

Accessory Organs

Ducts (carry sperm from testes to exterior), sex glands (produce solutions that mix with sperm), and external genitalia

Seminal vesicles produce most seminal fluid
Prostate gland produces some seminal fluid and activates sperm
Bulbourethral gland (Cowper's gland) secretes a very small amount of seminal fluid
External genitalia: penis and scrotum
- Penis contains three columns of erectile tissue: two corpora cavernosa and one spongiosum
- Urethra passes through corpora spongiosum
- Scrotum encloses testes
Passage of sperm from production to exterior

Sperm are produced in seminiferous tubules (testes) and pass into:
- Epididymis then to vas deferens (within seminal vesicles) to ejaculatory duct then through urethra (prostate gland and Cowper's [bulbourethral] gland)
- Pass though penis to outside of body

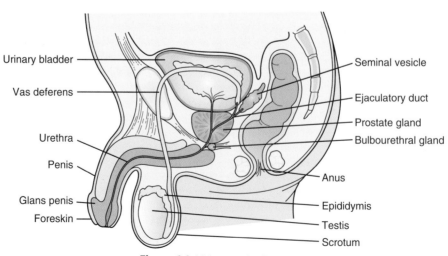

• **Figure 6.1** Male reproductive system.

TABLE 6-1
Combining Forms

Combining Form	Meaning
1. andr/o	male
2. balan/o	glans penis
3. cry/o	cold
4. crypt/o	hidden
5. epididym/o	epididymis
6. gon/o	seed
7. hydr/o	water, fluid
8. orch/i	testicle
9. orch/o	testicle
10. orchi/o	testicle
11. orchid/o	testicle
12. prostat/o	prostate gland
13. semin/i	semen
14. sperm/o	sperm
15. spermat/o	sperm
16. test/o	testicle
17. varic/o	varicose veins
18. vas/o	vessel, vas deferens
19. vesicul/o	seminal vesicles

TABLE 6-2
Suffixes

Suffix	Meaning
1. -one	hormone
2. -pexy	fixation
3. -ectomy	removal
4. -stomy	new opening

TABLE 6-3
Medical Abbreviations

Abbreviation	Meaning
1. BPH	benign prostatic hypertrophy
2. PSA	prostate-specific antigen
3. TURBT	transurethral resection of bladder tumor
4. TURP	transurethral resection of prostate

TABLE 6-4
Medical Terms

Term	Meaning
Cavernosa	Connection between cavity of penis and a vein
Cavernosography	Radiographic recording of a cavity, e.g., pulmonary cavity or main part of penis
Cavernosometry	Measurement of pressure in a cavity, e.g., penis
Chordee	Condition resulting in penis being bent downward
Corpora cavernosa	The two cavities of penis
Epididymectomy	Surgical removal of epididymis
Epididymis	Tube located at the top of testes that stores sperm
Epididymovasostomy	Creation of a new connection between vas deferens and epididymis
Meatotomy	Surgical enlargement of opening of urinary meatus
Orchiectomy	Castration, removal of testes
Orchiopexy	Surgical procedure to release undescended testis and fixate within scrotum
Penoscrotal	Referring to penis and scrotum
Plethysmography	Determining changes in volume of an organ part or body
Priapism	Painful condition in which penis is constantly erect
Prostatotomy	Incision into prostate
Transurethral resection, prostate	Procedure performed through urethra by means of a cystoscopy to remove part or all of prostate
Tumescence	State of being swollen
Tunica vaginalis	Covering of testes
Varicocele	Swelling of a scrotal vein
Vas deferens	Tube that carries sperm from epididymis to ejaculatory duct and seminal vesicles
Vasectomy	Removal of segment of vas deferens
Vasogram	Recording of the flow in vas deferens
Vasotomy	Incision in vas deferens
Vasorrhaphy	Suturing of vas deferens
Vasovasostomy	Reversal of a vasectomy
Vesiculectomy	Excision of seminal vesicle
Vesiculotomy	Incision into seminal vesicle

Chapter 6: Anatomy and Terminology Quiz

(Quiz Answers Are Located in Appendix B)

1. This gland activates sperm and produces some seminal fluid:
   a. seminal vesicle
   b. bulbourethral gland
   c. prostate gland
   d. scrotum
2. Carries sperm from testes to ejaculatory duct:
   a. vas deferens
   b. sex gland
   c. tunica
   d. seminal
3. Penis contains these erectile tissues:
   a. one corpora cavernosa and two spongiosa
   b. two corpora cavernosa and two spongiosa
   c. one corpora cavernosa and one spongiosum
   d. two corpora cavernosa and one spongiosum
4. Also known as Cowper's gland:
   a. seminal vesicles
   b. bulbourethral gland
   c. prostate gland
   d. scrotum
5. Which of the following is NOT an accessory organ?
   a. gonads
   b. seminal vesicles
   c. prostate
   d. penis
6. Combining form meaning "male":
   a. andr/o
   b. balan/o
   c. orchi/o
   d. test/o
7. Combining form meaning "glans penis":
   a. balan/o
   b. vas/o
   c. vesicul/o
   d. orch/o
8. Testes are covered by the:
   a. seminal vesicles
   b. androgen
   c. chancre
   d. tunica albuginea
9. This abbreviation describes a surgical resection of prostate that is accomplished by means of an endoscope inserted into the urethra:
   a. TURBT
   b. BPH
   c. UPJ
   d. TURP
10. This abbreviation describes a condition of prostate in which there is an enlargement that is benign:
    a. TURBT
    b. BPH
    c. UPJ
    d. TURP

PATHOPHYSIOLOGY

Male Genital System Disorders

Disorders of Scrotum, Testes, and Epididymis

Cryptorchidism

Undescended testes—condition at birth
- Unilateral or bilateral
- Primarily result from obstruction
- Risk neoplastic processes

Treatment
- May descend spontaneously
- Administration of hormone to stimulate testosterone production
- Surgical intervention (orchiopexy) near age 1 to avoid risk of infertility

Orchitis

Inflammation of testes
Most common cause is virus
- Such as mumps orchitis
- Atrophy with irreversible loss of sperm production at risk

May be associated with
- Mumps or epidemic parotitis
- Gonorrhea
- Syphilis
- Tuberculosis

Symptoms
- Mild to severe pain in testes
- Mild to severe edema
- Feeling of weight in testicular area

Treatment
- Depends on presence of underlying condition

Epididymitis

Inflammation of epididymis
Inflammatory response to trauma or infection
Abscess may form

Types

Sexually transmitted epididymitis
- Gonorrhea
- *T. pallidum*
- *T. vaginalis*

Nonspecific bacterial epididymitis
- *E. coli*
- Streptococci

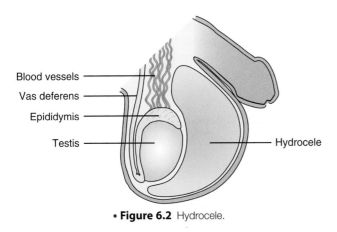

• **Figure 6.2** Hydrocele.

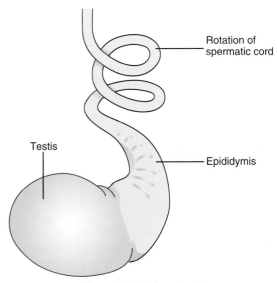

• **Figure 6.3** Torsion of testis.

- Staphylococci
- Associated with underlying urological disorder

Symptoms
Scrotal pain
Swelling
Erythema
Perhaps hydrocele formation

Treatment
Antibiotic
Bed rest
Ice packs
Scrotal support
Analgesics

Hydrocele (Fig. 6.2)
Collection of fluid in membranes of tunica vaginalis
May be congenital or acquired (response to infection or tumors)
Congenital hydrocele may reabsorb due to a communication between the scrotal sac and peritoneal cavity and require no intervention

Symptoms
Scrotal enlargement

Usually painless
- Unless infection is present

Varicocele
Abnormal dilation of plexus of veins
Decreases sperm production and motility

Symptoms
Usually painless
In elderly, may signal renal tumor

Treatment
Surgical intervention

Torsion of Testes (Fig. 6.3)
Twisting of testes
Congenital abnormal development of tunica vaginalis and spermatic cord
Trauma may precipitate

Symptoms
Sudden onset of severe pain
Nausea
Vomiting
Scrotal edema and tenderness
Fever

Treatment
Immediate surgical intervention

Cancer of Testes
Rare form of cancer

Cure rate high (95%)
Cause unknown
Usually occurs in younger men
Two main groups
- Germ cell tumors (GCT)—90% of testicular tumors
- Sex cord–stromal tumors

Cancer of Scrotum
Rare form of cancer
- Squamous cell carcinoma

Symptoms
Asymptomatic in early stages
Ulcerations in later stages

Treatment
Wide local excision
Mohs micrographic surgery

- Precise removal of tumor
- Layers are removed until no further microscopic evidence of abnormal cells is seen

Laser therapy

Lymph nodes are examined for metastasis

Disorders of Urethra

Epispadias

Congenital anomaly

Urethral meatus is located on dorsal side of penis

Usually occurs in conjunction with other abnormalities

Treatment

Surgical reconstruction

Hypospadias

Most common abnormality of penis

Urethral opening on ventral side of penis

Results in curvature of penis

- Due to chordee

Treatment

Surgical reconstruction

Urethritis

Inflammation of urethra

Infectious urethritis can be gonococcal or nongonococcal

Nongonococcal organisms

- C. trachomatis
- *U. urealyticum*

Symptoms

Discharge

Inflammation of meatus

Burning

Itching

Urgent and frequent urination

In nongonococcal, symptoms are fewer

Treatment

Antibiotics based on organism

Disorders of Penis

Balanitis

Inflammation of glans

Causes

Syphilis

Trichomoniasis

Gonorrhea

Candida albicans

Tinea

Underlying disease—diabetes mellitus and candidiasis

No circumcision

Symptoms

Irritation

Tenderness

Discharge

Edema

Ulceration

Swelling of lymph nodes

Treatment

Culture of discharge

Saline irrigation

Antibiotics

Phimosis and Paraphimosis, Phimosis

Condition in which prepuce (foreskin) is constricted

- Prepuce cannot be retracted over glans penis

Can occur at any age

Associated with poor hygiene and chronic infection in uncircumcised males

Symptoms

Erythema

Edema

Tenderness

Purulent discharge

Treatment

Surgical circumcision

Paraphimosis

Condition in which prepuce (foreskin) is constricted

Prepuce is retracted over glans penis and cannot be moved forward

Symptom

Edema

Treatment

Surgical

Peyronie's Disease

Also known as bent nail syndrome

Fibrotic condition

- Results in lateral curvature of penis during erection

Occurs most often in middle-aged men

Cause is unknown but associated with

- Diabetes
- Keloid development
- Dupuytren's contracture (flexion deformity of toes and fingers)

Treatment

Sometimes spontaneous remission

Pharmacologic, oxygen-increasing therapies

Surgical resection of fibrous bands

Cancer of Penis

Rare form of cancer

Occurs most often in men over age 60
Squamous cell carcinoma
Increased risks
- More common in uncircumcised men
- Sexual partner with cervical carcinoma
- Human papillomavirus

Usually begins with small lesion beneath prepuce
Intraepithelial neoplasia is also known as
- Bowen's disease
- Erythroplasia of Queyrat

Begins as noninvasive
Progresses to invasive if untreated
Metastasis to lymph nodes

Treatment
Excision
Mohs micrographic surgery
Radiation therapy
Laser therapy
Cryosurgery

Advanced tumors are treated with partial or total penectomy and chemotherapy

Disorders of Prostate Gland

Benign Prostatic Hyperplasia/Hypertrophy (BPH)
Multiple fibroadenomatous nodules; usually located on outside of gland, so easily palpable on digital exam
- Related to aging; common in men over 60 years of age
- Enlarging prostate obstructs bladder neck and urethra
- Decreases urine flow

It is thought that increased levels of estrogen/androgen cause BPH

Symptoms
Increased frequency and urgency of urination
Nocturia
Incontinence
Hesitancy
Diminished force
Postvoiding dribble

Screening
Prostate-specific antigen (PSA)
Digital rectal examination (DRE)

Treatment
Partial prostatectomy
Transurethral resection of prostate (TURP)
Excision of nodules
Hormone therapy
Placement of urethral stents

Pharmaceuticals—those that inhibit production of testosterone and those that relax smooth muscle of gland and neck of bladder

Prostatitis
Inflammation of prostate
- Acute or chronic bacterial prostatitis

Bacterial Causes
Escherichia coli
Enterococci
Staphylococci
Streptococci
Chlamydia trachomatis
Ureaplasma urealyticum
Neisseria gonorrhea

Nonbacterial Causes
Spontaneous
Prostatodynia

Symptoms
Acute Prostatitis
Fever and chills
Lower back pain
Perineal pain
Dysuria
Tenderness, suprapubic
Urinary tract infection

Chronic Prostatitis
Recurring
Same as acute only with no infection in urinary tract

Treatment
Acute. Antibiotic based on culture
Chronic. No treatment available

Cancer of Prostate
Most common malignancy diagnosed in men, occurring in men over age 60
Indications are that the cause is related to androgens
Predominately adenocarcinoma (95%)
No relationship between BPH and cancer of prostate

Symptoms
Asymptomatic in early stages

Later symptoms include
- Dysuria
- Back pain
- Hematuria
- Frequent urination
- Urinary retention
- Increased incidence of uremia

Stages

Two systems used to stage prostate cancer
- Whitmore-Jewett stages as indicated in Fig. 6.4
- Tumor-node-metastasis (TNM) as indicated in Fig. 6.5

Treatment

Dependent on stage

WHITMORE-JEWETT STAGES:

Stage A is clinically undetectable tumor confined to the gland and is an incidental finding at prostate surgery.
A1: well-differentiated with focal involvement
A2: moderately or poorly differentiated or involves multiple foci in the gland
Stage B is tumor confined to the prostate gland.
B0: nonpalpable, PSA-detected
B1: single nodule in one lobe of the prostate
B2: more extensive involvement of one lobe or involvement of both lobes
Stage C is a tumor clinically localized to the periprostatic area but extending through the prostatic capsule; seminal vesicles may be involved.
C1: clinical extracapsular extension
C2: extracapsular tumor producing bladder outlet or ureteral obstruction
Stage D is metastatic disease.
D0: clinically localized disease (prostate only) but persistently elevated enzymatic serum acid phosphatase
D1: regional lymph nodes only
D2: distant lymph nodes, metastases to bone or visceral organs
D3: D2 prostate cancer patients who relapse after adequate endocrine therapy

• **Figure 6.4** Whitmore-Jewett stages.

TNM STAGES:

Primary Tumor (T)
TX: Primary tumor cannot be assessed
T0: No evidence of primary tumor
T1: Clinically inapparent tumor not palpable or visible by imaging
    T1a: Tumor incidental histologic finding in 5% or less of tissue resected
    T1b: Tumor incidental histologic finding in more than 5% of tissue resected
    T1c: Tumor identified by needle biopsy (e.g., because of elevated PSA)
T2: Tumor confined within the prostate
    T2a: Tumor involves half a lobe or less
    T2b: Tumor involves more than half of a lobe, but not both lobes
    T2c: Tumor involves both lobes; extends through the prostatic capsule
T3a: Unilateral extracapsular extension
T3b: Bilateral extracapsular extension
T3c: Tumor invades the seminal vesicle(s)
T4: Tumor is fixed or invades adjacent structures other than the seminal vesicle(s)
    T4a: Tumor invades any of bladder neck, external sphincter, or rectum
    T4b: Tumor invades levator muscles and/or is fixed to the pelvic wall
Regional lymph nodes (N)
NX: Regional lymph nodes cannot be assessed
N0: No regional lymph node metastasis
N1: Metastasis in a single lymph node, 2 cm or less in greatest dimension
N2: Metastasis in a single lymph node, more than 2 cm but not more than 5 cm in greatest dimension; or multiple lymph node metastases, none more than 5 cm in greatest dimension
N3: Metastasis in a single lymph node more than 5 cm in greatest dimension
Distant metastases (M)
MX: Presence of distant metastasis cannot be assessed
M0: No distant metastasis
M1: Distant metastasis
    M1a: Nonregional lymph node(s)
    M1b: Bone(s)
    M1c: Other site(s)

• **Figure 6.5** TNM stages.

Chapter 6: Pathophysiology Quiz

(Quiz Answers Are Located in Appendix B)

1. What is the condition in which testes do not descend?
   a. cryptorchidism
   b. Bowen's disease
   c. torsion
   d. hypospadias
2. Orchitis is most often caused by a:
   a. bacteria
   b. virus
   c. parasite
   d. fungus
3. A condition that can be either congenital or acquired through trauma and that involves twisting of testes is:
   a. hydrocele
   b. hypospadias
   c. cryptorchidism
   d. torsion
4. Cancer of the _____ is divided into two main groups of germ cell tumors and sex stromal cord tumors.
   a. testes
   b. penis
   c. scrotum
   d. prostate
5. This type of surgical technique involves excision of a lesion in layers until no further evidence of abnormality is seen:
   a. Bowen's
   b. Addison's
   c. Mohs
   d. laser

6. Epispadias is a disorder of the urethra in which urethral meatus is located on the _____ side of penis:
   a. ventral
   b. dorsal
   c. lateral
   d. medial

7. Inflammation of glans is:
   a. phimosis
   b. paraphimosis
   c. urethritis
   d. balanitis

8. This disease is also known as bent nail syndrome:
   a. Bowen's
   b. Peyronie's
   c. Addison's
   d. Whitmore-Jewett

9. Condition in which multiple fibroadenomatous nodules form and lead to decreased urine flow. Condition is thought to be related to increased levels of estrogen/androgen.
   a. BPH
   b. DRE
   c. GCT
   d. TNM

10. Cancer of prostate is predominately this type of cancer:
   a. sex cord
   b. adenocarcinoma
   c. squamous cell
   d. seminoma

7

Urinary System

ANATOMY AND TERMINOLOGY

Removes metabolic waste materials (nitrogenous waste: urea, creatinine, and uric acid)

Conserves nutrients and water
Balances: electrolytes (acids/bases balance)
  Electrolytes are electrically charged molecules required for nerve and muscle function
Assists liver in detoxification

Organs (Fig. 7.1)

Kidneys
Ureters
Urinary bladder
Urethra

Kidneys (Fig. 7.2)

Electrolytes and fluid balance
Control pH balance (acid/base)
Secrete renin (which affects blood pressure) and erythropoietin (which stimulates red blood cell production in bone marrow)
Secrete active vitamin D required for calcium absorption from intestines
Two organs located behind peritoneum (retroperitoneal space)

Kidney Structure
Cortex (outer layer)
Medulla (inner portion)
Hilum (depression on medial border through which blood vessels and nerves pass)
Pyramids (divisions of medulla)
Papilla (inner part of pyramids)
Pelvis (receptacle for urine within kidney)
Calyces surround top of renal pelvis
Nephrons (3 types) are operational units of kidney

Ureters

Narrow tubes transporting urine from kidneys to bladder

Urinary Bladder
Reservoir for urine

Shaped like an upside-down pear with three surfaces
  • Posterior (base)
  • Anterior (neck)
  • Superior (peritoneum)
Trigone
  • Smooth triangular area inside bladder—size never changes
  • Formed by openings of ureters and urethra

Urethra

Canal from bladder to exterior of body
Urinary meatus, outside opening of urethra

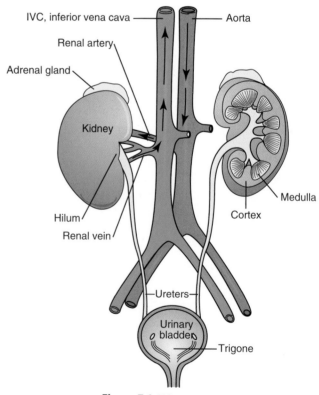

• **Figure 7.1** Urinary system.

TABLE 7-1

Combining Forms

Combining Form	Meaning
1. albumin/o	albumin
2. azot/o	urea
3. bacteri/o	bacteria
4. cali/o	calyx
5. cyst/o	urinary
6. dips/o	thirst
7. glomerul/o	glomerulus
8. glyc/o	sugar
9. glycos/o	sugar
10. hydr/o	water
11. ket/o	ketone bodies/ketoacidosis
12. lith/o	stone
13. meat/o	meatus
14. nephr/o	kidney
15. noct/i	night
16. olig/o	scant, few
17. pyel/o	renal pelvis
18. ren/o	kidney
19. son/o	sound
20. tripsy	to crush
21. tryg/o	trigone region/kidney
22. ur/o	urine
23. ureter/o	ureter
24. urethr/o	urethra
25. uria	urination/urinary condition
26. urin/o	urine
27. vesic/o	bladder

TABLE 7-2

Prefixes

Prefix	Meaning
1. dys-	painful
2. peri-	surrounding
3. poly-	many
4. retro-	behind

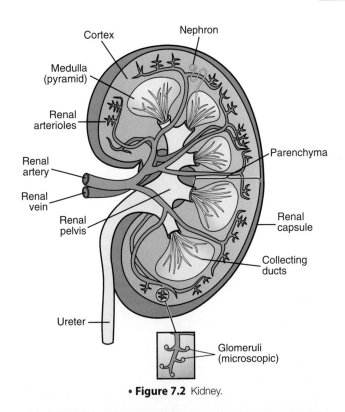

• **Figure 7.2** Kidney.

TABLE 7-3

Suffixes

Suffix	Meaning
1. -eal	pertaining to
2. -lithiasis	condition of stones
3. -lysis	separation
4. -plasty	repair
5. -rrhaphy	suture
6. -tripsy	crush

TABLE 7-4

Medical Abbreviations

Abbreviation	Meaning
1. ARF	acute renal failure
2. BUN	blood urea nitrogen
3. ESRD	end-stage renal disease
4. HD	hemodialysis
5. IVP	intravenous pyelogram
6. KUB	kidney, ureter, bladder
7. pH	symbol for acid/base level
8. PKU	phenylketonuria
9. sp gr	specific gravity
10. UA	urinalysis
11. UPJ	ureteropelvic junction
12. UTI	urinary tract infection

TABLE 7-5

Medical Terms

Term	Meaning	Term	Meaning
Bulbocavernosus	Muscle that constricts vagina in a female and urethra in a male	Nephrocutaneous fistula	An abnormal channel from kidney to skin
Bulbourethral	Gland with duct leading to urethra	Nephrolithotomy	Removal of a kidney stone through an incision made into the kidney
Calculus	Concretion of mineral salts, also called a stone	Nephrorrhaphy	Suturing of kidney
Calycoplasty	Surgical reconstruction of recess of renal pelvis	Nephrostomy	Creation of a channel into renal pelvis of kidney
Calyx	Recess of renal pelvis	Transureteroureterostomy	Surgical connection of one ureter to other ureter
Cystolithectomy	Removal of a calculus (stone) from urinary bladder	Transvesical ureterolithotomy	Removal of a ureter stone (calculus) through bladder
Cystometrogram	CMG, measurement of pressures and capacity of urinary bladder	Ureterectomy	Surgical removal of a ureter, either totally or partially
Cystoplasty	Surgical reconstruction of bladder	Ureterocutaneous fistula	Channel from ureter to exterior skin
Cystorrhaphy	Suture of bladder	Ureteroenterostomy	Creation of a connection between intestine and ureter
Cystoscopy	Use of a scope to view bladder	Ureterolithotomy	Removal of a stone from ureter
Cystostomy	Surgical creation of an opening into bladder	Ureterolysis	Freeing of adhesions of ureter
Cystotomy	Incision into bladder	Ureteroneocystostomy	Surgical connection of ureter to a new site on bladder
Cystourethroplasty	Surgical reconstruction of bladder and urethra	Ureteropyelography	Ureter and renal pelvis radiography
Cystourethroscopy	Use of a scope to view bladder and urethra	Ureterotomy	Incision into ureter
Dilation	Stretching or expansion	Urethrocystography	Radiography of bladder and urethra
Dysuria	Painful urination	Urethromeatoplasty	Surgical repair of urethra and meatus
Endopyelotomy	Procedure involving bladder and ureters, including insertion of a stent into renal pelvis	Urethropexy	Fixation of urethra by means of surgery
Extracorporeal	Occurring outside of body	Urethroplasty	Surgical repair of urethra
Fundoplasty	Repair of the bottom of bladder	Urethrorrhaphy	Suturing of urethra
Hydrocele	Sac of fluid	Urethroscopy	Use of a scope to view urethra
Kock pouch	Surgical creation of a urinary bladder from a segment of the ileum	Vesicostomy	Surgical creation of a connection of viscera of bladder to skin

Chapter 7: Anatomy and Terminology Quiz

(Quiz Answers Are Located in Appendix B)

1. The outer covering of kidney:
   a. medulla
   b. pyramids
   c. cortex
   d. papilla
2. Which is not a division of kidneys?
   a. pelvis
   b. pyramids
   c. cortex
   d. trigone
3. The inner portion of kidneys:
   a. medulla
   b. pyramids
   c. cortex
   d. papilla
4. The smooth area inside bladder:
   a. pyramids
   b. calyces
   c. trigone
   d. cystocele
5. The narrow tube connecting kidney and bladder:
   a. urethra
   b. ureter
   c. meatus
   d. trigone
6. Which of the following is NOT a surface of urinary bladder?
   a. posterior
   b. anterior
   c. superior
   d. inferior
7. Combining form that means "stone":
   a. azot/o
   b. cyst/o
   c. lith/o
   d. olig/o
8. Term meaning "painful urination":
   a. pyuria
   b. dysuria
   c. diuresis
   d. hyperemia
9. Combining form meaning "scant":
   a. glyc/o
   b. hydr/o
   c. meat/o
   d. olig/o
10. Term that describes renal failure that is acute:
    a. ARF
    b. ESRD
    c. HD
    d. BPH

PATHOPHYSIOLOGY

Renal Failure

Acute Renal Failure

Sudden onset of renal failure

Causes
Extreme hypotension
Trauma
Infection
Inflammation
Toxicity
Obstructed vascular supply

Symptoms
Uremia
Oliguria (decreased output) or anuria (no output)
Hyperkalemia (high potassium in blood)
Pulmonary edema

Types
Prerenal
 • Associated with poor systemic perfusion
 • Decreased renal blood flow
   • Such as with congestive heart failure

Intrarenal
 • Associated with renal parenchyma disease (functional tissue of kidney)
   • Such as acute interstitial nephritis, glomerulopathies, and malignant hypertension
Postrenal
 • Resulting from urine flow obstruction outside kidney (ureters or bladder neck)

Treatment
Underlying condition
Dialysis
Monitoring of fluid and electrolyte balance

Chronic Renal Failure

Gradual loss of function
 • Progressively more severe renal insufficiency until end stage of
   • Renal disease
   • Irreversible kidney failure

Stages—Based on Level of Creatinine Clearance
Stage 1: Blood flow through kidney increases, kidney enlarges
Stage 2 (mild): Small amounts of blood protein (albumin) leak into urine (microalbuminuria)

Stage 3 (moderate): Albumin and other protein losses increase; patient may develop high blood pressure and kidney loses ability to filter waste

Stage 4 (severe): Large amounts of urine pass through kidney; blood pressure increases

Stage 5: End-stage renal failure. Ability to filter waste nearly stops; dialysis or transplant only option

Causes
Long-term exposure to nephrotoxins
Diabetes
Hypertension

Symptoms
No symptoms until well advanced
Polyuria
Nausea or anorexia
Dehydration
Neurologic manifestations

Stages of Nephron Loss
Decreased reserve
- 60% loss

Renal insufficiency
- 75% loss

End-stage renal failure
- 90% loss

Treatment
No cure
Dialysis
Kidney transplant

Urinary Tract Infections (UTI)

Cystitis—Bacterial

Cause
Bacteria, usually *E. coli*

Symptoms
Lower abdominal pain
Dysuria
Lower back pain
Urinary frequency and urgency
Cloudy, foul-smelling urine

Systemic Signs
Fever
Malaise
Nausea

Treatment
Antibiotics
Increased fluid intake

Cystitis—Noninfectious, Nonbacterial

Cause
Radiation, chemotherapy, autoimmune disorder, etc.
May later produce bacterial infection

Symptoms
Urinary frequency and urgency
Dysuria
Negative urine culture

Treatment
No known treatment

Acute Pyelonephritis (Fig. 7.3)

Bacterial infection with multiple abscesses of renal pelvis and medullary tissue
- May involve one or both kidneys

Causes
E. coli
Proteus
Pseudomonas
Obstruction and reflux of urine from bladder

Symptoms
Fever
Chills
Groin or flank pain
Dysuria
Pyuria
Nocturia

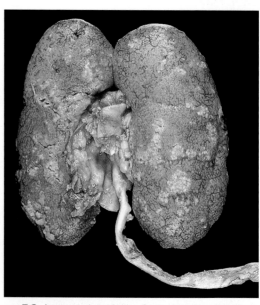

• **Figure 7.3** Acute pyelonephritis. Cortical surface exhibits grayish white areas of inflammation and abscess formation.

Treatment
Antibiotics
Surgical correction of obstruction

Chronic Pyelonephritis

Recurrent infection that causes scarring of kidney
Cause is difficult to determine
- Repeated infections
- Obstructive conditions

Symptoms
Hypertension
Dysuria
Flank pain
Increased frequency of urination

Treatment
Antibiotics for extended periods when recurring
Surgical reduction of obstruction

Glomerular Disorders

May be acute or chronic
Function of glomerulus is blood filtration

Glomerulonephritis

Inflammation of glomerulus

Causes
Drugs or toxins
Systemic disorder affecting many organs or idiopathic
May follow acute infections—most commonly streptococcal infections
Vascular pathology
Immune disorders

Treatment
Follows cause

Nephrotic Syndrome (Nephrosis)

Disease of kidneys that includes damage to membrane of the glomerulus causing excessive protein loss to urine

Accompanied by
- Hypoalbuminemia
- Hypercholesterolemia
- Hypercoagulability (excessive clotting)
- Prone to infections
- Edema
- Protein loss of >3.5 g

Damage to glomerulus results from
- Infection
- Immune response
  - Most predominant cause of dysfunction is exposure to toxins

May be a manifestation of an underlying condition, such as diabetes

Symptoms
Edema
Weight gain
Pallor
Proteinuria
Lipiduria

Treatment
Glucocorticoids, such as prednisone
- Reduces inflammation

Sodium- and fat-reduced diet
Protein supplements
Careful monitoring for continued inflammation

Acute Poststreptococcal Glomerulonephritis (APSGN)

Cause
Streptococcus infection
- With certain types of group A beta-hemolytic *Streptococcus* Creates an antigen-antibody complex
- Infiltrates glomerular capillaries
- Results in inflammation in kidneys
- Inflammation interferes with normal kidney function
- Fluid and waste build-up
- Can lead to acute renal failure and scarring Usually occurs in children 3 to 7 years of age
- Most often in boys

Symptoms
Back and flank pain
Cloudy, dark urine
Oliguria (decreased output)
Edema
Elevated blood pressure
Fatigue
Malaise
Headache
Nausea

Treatment
Sodium reduction
Antibiotics
Careful monitoring for continued inflammation

Urinary Tract Obstructions

Interference with urine flow

Causes urine backup behind obstruction of urinary system
Damage occurs to structures behind blockages
Increased urinary tract infection
Obstruction can be

- Functional
- Anatomic
  - Also known as obstructive uropathy

Kidney Stones (Nephrolithiasis—Renal Calculi)

Formed of mineral salts (uric and calcium)

Develop anywhere in urinary tract
Tend to form in presence of excess salt and decreased fluid intake
Most stones are formed of calcium salts
Staghorn calculus forms in renal pelvis

Symptoms
Asymptomatic until obstruction occurs

Obstruction results in renal colic
- Extremely intense pain in flank
- Nausea
- Vomiting
- Cold, clammy skin
- Increased pulse rate

Treatment
Stone usually passes spontaneously
May use extracorporeal ultrasound or laser lithotripsy to break up stone (also known as extracorporeal shock wave lithotripsy, or ESWL)
Drugs may be used to dissolve stone
Preventative treatment to adjust pH level
- Increased fluid intake

Bladder Carcinoma

Malignant Tumor
Most common site of malignancy in urinary system
Tumors originate in transitional epithelial lining
Tends to recur
Often metastatic to liver and bone

Tumor Staging for Renal Cancer
Stage 1—Tumor of kidney capsule only
Stage 2—Tumor invading renal capsule/vein but within fascia
Stage 3—Tumor extending to regional lymph nodes/vena cava
Stage 4—Other organ metastasis

Symptoms
Often asymptomatic in early stage
Hematuria
Dysuria
Frequent urination
Infections common

Increased Risks
Cigarette smoking
Males age 50+
Working with industrial chemicals
Analgesics used in large amounts
Recurrent bladder infections

Treatment
Immunotherapy (Bacillus Calmette-Guérin [BCG] vaccine)
Excision
Chemotherapy
Radiation therapy

Hydronephrosis

Distention of kidney with urine
- Due to an obstruction
- Usually as a result of a kidney stone
- May also be due to scarring, tumor, edema from infection, or other obstruction

Symptoms
Usually asymptomatic
Mild flank pain
Infection may develop
May lead to chronic renal failure

Treatment
Treat underlying condition, such as removal of stone or antibiotics for infection
Dilation of stricture

Vascular Disorders

Nephrosclerosis

Excessive hardening and thickening of vascular structure of kidney
- Reduces blood supply
  - Increases blood pressure
  - Results in atrophy and ischemia of structures
  - May lead to chronic renal failure

Symptoms
Asymptomatic in early stages

Treatment
Diuretics
ACE (angiotensin-converting enzyme) inhibitors
Beta blockers that block release of resin
Antihypertensive drugs
Sodium intake reduction

Congenital Disorders

Polycystic Kidney Disease (PKD)

Numerous kidney cysts
  Genetic disease

Symptoms
Asymptomatic until 40s
Cysts progressive in development (both kidneys)

Nephromegaly, hematuria, UTI, hypertension, uremia
Develops chronic renal failure
Cysts may spread to other organs, such as liver

Treatment
As for chronic renal failure

Wilms' Tumor—Nephroblastoma
Usually unilateral kidney tumors

Most common tumor in children
Usually advanced at time of diagnosis
- Metastasis to lungs at time of diagnosis is common

Symptoms
Asymptomatic until abdominal mass becomes apparent at age 1 to 5

Treatment
Excision
Radiation therapy
Chemotherapy
Usually a combination of above

Chapter 7: Pathophysiology Quiz

(Quiz Answers Are Located in Appendix B)

1. Which of the following is NOT a type of acute renal failure?
   a. prerenal
   b. intrarenal
   c. interrenal
   d. postrenal
2. The loss of nephron function in end-stage renal disease is:
   a. 60%
   b. 70%
   c. 80%
   d. 90%
3. The cause of bacterial cystitis is usually:
   a. Proteus
   b. Pseudomonas
   c. Staphylococcus
   d. *E. coli*
4. The primary treatment for acute pyelonephritis would be:
   a. prednisone
   b. sodium reduction
   c. antibiotics
   d. BCG
5. APSGN stands for:
   a. advanced poststaphylococcal glomerulonephritis
   b. acute poststreptococcal glomerulonephritis
   c. acute poststaphylococcal glomerulonephritis
   d. advanced poststreptococcal glomerulonephritis
6. Obstructive uropathy is also known as:
   a. pyelonephritis
   b. renal failure
   c. urinary tract obstruction
   d. nephrotic syndrome
7. A treatment for kidney stone may be:
   a. ESWL
   b. prednisone
   c. open surgical procedure
   d. diuretics
8. The treatment for hydronephrosis involves:
   a. an open surgical procedure
   b. use of diuretics
   c. treatment of the underlying condition
   d. BCG
9. This is a congenital condition in which numerous cysts form in the kidney:
   a. Wilms' tumor
   b. polycystic kidney
   c. nephrosclerosis
   d. nephrotic syndrome
10. The treatment of Wilms' tumor would NOT include which of the following?
    a. excision
    b. chemotherapy
    c. diuretic
    d. radiation therapy

8

Digestive System

ANATOMY AND TERMINOLOGY

Function: digestion, absorption, and elimination
Includes gastrointestinal tract (alimentary canal) and accessory organs

Mouth (Fig. 8.1)

Roof: hard palate, soft palate, uvula (projection at back of mouth)
Floor: contains tongue (Fig. 8.2), muscles, taste buds, and lingual frenulum, which anchors tongue to floor of mouth

Teeth

Thirty-two teeth (permanent)

Names of teeth: incisor, cuspid, bicuspid, and tricuspid
Tooth has crown (outer portion), neck (narrow part below gum line), root (end section), and pulp cavity (core)

Salivary Glands (Fig. 8.3)

Surround mouth and produce saliva—1.5 liters daily

Parotid
Submandibular
Sublingual

Pharynx or Throat (Fig. 8.4)

Muscular tube (5 inches long) lined with mucous membrane through which air and food/water travel

Epiglottis covers larynx/esophagus when swallowing

Esophagus

Muscular tube (9-10 inches long) that carries food from pharynx to stomach by means of peristalsis (rhythmic contractions)

Stomach

Sphincter (ring of muscles) at entry into stomach (gastro-esophageal or cardiac)

Three parts of stomach:
Fundus (upper part)
Body (middle part)
Antrum/pylorus (lower part)
Lined with rugae (folds of mucosal membrane)
Pyloric sphincter opens to allow chyme (thick liquid) to leave stomach and enter small intestine

Small Intestine

Duodenum (2 inches long): first portion beyond stomach—bile and pancreatic juice delivered here
Jejunum (96 inches long): connects duodenum to ileum
Ileum (132 inches long): attaches to large intestine

Large Intestine

Extends from ileum to anus
Cecum, from which appendix extends, connects ileum and colon
Colon (60 inches long), divided into:
Ascending
Transverse
Descending
Sigmoid
Sigmoid colon connected to rectum, which terminates at anus

Accessory Organs

Liver produces bile, sent to gallbladder via hepatic duct and cystic duct

Gallbladder stores bile, sent to duodenum from cystic duct into common bile duct
Bile emulsifies fat (breaks up large globules)

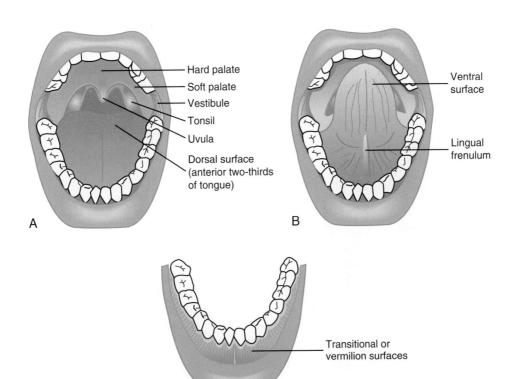

A

- Hard palate
- Soft palate
- Vestibule
- Tonsil
- Uvula
- Dorsal surface (anterior two-thirds of tongue)

B

- Ventral surface
- Lingual frenulum

C

- Transitional or vermilion surfaces

Lips are connected to the gums by frenulum

• **Figure 8.1** Anatomic structures of the mouth.

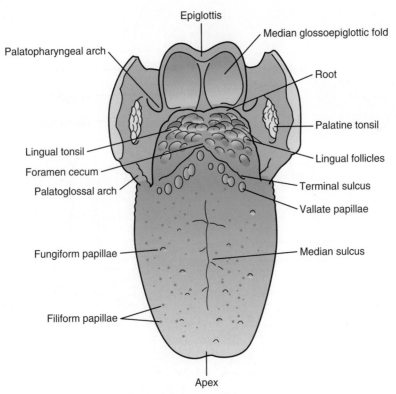

- Epiglottis
- Median glossoepiglottic fold
- Palatopharyngeal arch
- Root
- Palatine tonsil
- Lingual tonsil
- Lingual follicles
- Foramen cecum
- Terminal sulcus
- Palatoglossal arch
- Vallate papillae
- Fungiform papillae
- Median sulcus
- Filiform papillae
- Apex

• **Figure 8.2** Dorsum of the tongue.

Pancreas produces enzymes sent through pancreatic duct to hepatopancreatic ampulla (ampulla of Vater) then to duodenum

Pancreatic cells—islets of Langerhans produce insulin and glucagon

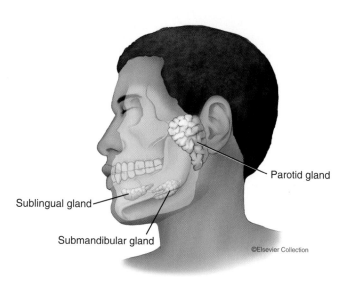

©Elsevier Collection

• **Figure 8.3** Major salivary glands.

Peritoneum

Serous membrane lines abdominal cavity and maintains organs in correct anatomic position

Food passes through digestive tract via:
Mouth—including salivary glands
Pharynx
Esophagus
Stomach
Duodenum—pancreatic enzymes and bile produced in liver and stored in gallbladder enter
Jejunum
Ileum
Cecum
Ascending colon
Transverse colon
Descending colon
Sigmoid colon
Rectum
Anus

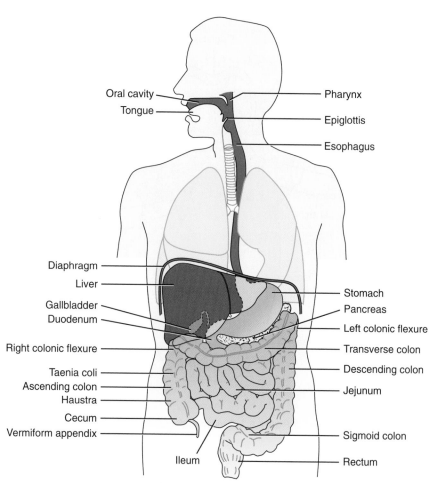

• **Figure 8.4** Digestive system.

TABLE 8-1

Combining Forms

Combining Form	Meaning	Combining Form	Meaning
1. abdomin/o	abdomen	25. herni/o	hernia
2. an/o	anus	26. ile/o	ileum
3. appendic/o	appendix	27. jejun/o	jejunum
4. bil/i	bile	28. labi/o	lip
5. bilirubin/o	bile pigment	29. lapar/o	abdomen
6. bucc/o	cheek	30. lingu/o	tongue
7. cec/o	cecum	31. lip/o	fat
8. celi/o	abdomen	32. lith/o	stone
9. cheil/o	lip	33. or/o	mouth
10. chol/e	gall/bile	34. ordont/o	tooth
11. cholangio/o	bile duct	35. palat/o	palate
12. cholecyst/o	gallbladder	36. pancreat/o	pancreas
13. choledoch/o	common bile duct	37. peritone/o	peritoneum
14. col/o	colon	38. pharyng/o	throat
15. dent/i	tooth	39. polyp/o	polyp
16. diverticul/o	diverticulum	40. proct/o	rectum
17. duoden/o	duodenum	41. pylor/o	pylorus
18. enter/o	small intestine	42. rect/o	rectum
19. esophag/o	esophagus	43. sial/o	saliva
20. faci/o	face	44. sialaden/o	salivary gland
21. gastr/o	stomach	45. sigmoid/o	sigmoid colon
22. gingiv/o	gum	46. steat/o	fat
23. gloss/o	tongue	47. stomat/o	mouth
24. hepat/o	liver	48. uvul/o	uvula

TABLE 8-2

Suffixes

Suffix	Meaning
1. -ase	enzyme
2. -cele	hernia
3. -chezia	defecation
4. -iasis	abnormal condition
5. -phagia	eating
6. -prandial	meal

TABLE 8-3

Medical Abbreviations

Abbreviation	Meaning
1. EGD	esophagogastroduodenoscopy
2. EGJ	esophagogastric junction
3. ERCP	endoscopic retrograde cholangiopancreatography
4. GERD	gastroesophageal reflux disease
5. GI	gastrointestinal
6. HJR	hepatojugular reflux
7. LLQ	left lower quadrant
8. LUQ	left upper quadrant
9. PEG	percutaneous endoscopic gastrostomy
10. RLQ	right lower quadrant
11. RUQ	right upper quadrant

TABLE 8-4

Medical Terms

Term	Meaning	Term	Meaning
Anastomosis	Surgical connection of two tubular structures, such as two pieces of intestine	Hernia	Organ or tissue protruding through wall or cavity that usually contains it
Biliary	Refers to gallbladder, bile, or bile duct	Ileostomy	Artificial opening between ileum and abdominal wall
Cholangiography	Radiographic recording of bile ducts	Imbrication	Overlapping
Cholecystectomy	Surgical removal of gallbladder	Incarcerated	Regarding hernias, a constricted, irreducible hernia that may cause obstruction of an intestine
Cholecystoenterostomy	Creation of a connection between gallbladder and intestine	Intussusception	Slipping of one part of intestine into another part
Colonoscopy	Fiberscopic examination of entire colon that may include part of terminal ileum	Jejunostomy	Artificial opening between jejunum and abdominal wall
Colostomy	Artificial opening between colon and abdominal wall	Laparoscopy	Exploration of the abdomen and pelvic cavities using a scope placed through a small incision in abdominal wall
Diverticulum	Protrusion in wall of an organ		
Dysphagia	Difficulty swallowing		
Enterolysis	Releasing of adhesions of intestine	Lithotomy	Incision into an organ or a duct for the purpose of removing a stone
Eventration	Protrusion of bowel through an opening in abdomen	Lithotripsy	Crushing of a stone by sound wave or force
Evisceration	Pulling viscera outside of the body through an incision	Paraesophageal or hiatal hernia	Protrusion of any structure through esophageal hiatus of diaphragm
Exstrophy	Condition in which an organ is turned inside out		
Fulguration	Use of electric current to destroy tissue	Proctosigmoidoscopy	Fiberscopic examination of sigmoid colon and rectum
Gastrointestinal	Pertaining to stomach and intestine	Sialolithotomy	Surgical removal of a stone of salivary gland or duct
Gastroplasty	Operation on stomach for repair or reconfiguration	Varices	Varicose veins
Gastrostomy	Artificial opening between stomach and abdominal wall	Volvulus	Twisted section of intestine

Chapter 8: Anatomy and Terminology Quiz

(Quiz Answers Are Located in Appendix B)

1. This is NOT a part of the small intestine:
   a. ileum
   b. cecum
   c. duodenum
   d. jejunum

2. Term meaning "ring of muscles":
   a. pyloric
   b. parotid
   c. epiglottis
   d. sphincter

3. The throat is also known as the:
   a. larynx
   b. epiglottis
   c. esophagus
   d. pharynx

4. The three parts of the stomach:
   a. pyloric, rugae, fundus
   b. fundus, body, antrum
   c. antrum, pyloric, rugae
   d. ilium, fundus, pyloric

5. The projection at the back of the mouth:
   a. palate
   b. sublingual
   c. uvula
   d. parotid

6. Mucosal membrane that lines the stomach:
   a. cecum
   b. rugae
   c. frenulum
   d. fundus

7. The parts of the colon are:
   a. ascending, transverse, descending, sigmoid
   b. ascending, descending, sigmoid
   c. transverse, descending, sigmoid
   d. descending, sigmoid

8. Combining form meaning "abdomen":
   a. an/o
   b. cec/o
   c. celi/o
   d. col/o

9. Term that means connecting two ends of a tube:
   a. anastomosis
   b. amylase
   c. aphthous stomatitis
   d. atresia

10. Abbreviation that means a scope placed through the esophagus, into the stomach, and to the duodenum:
    a. ERCP
    b. EGD
    c. GERD
    d. PEG

PATHOPHYSIOLOGY

Disorders of Oral Cavity

Cleft Lip and Cleft Palate (Orofacial Cleft) (Fig. 8.5)

Congenital defect
Cleft lip and palate
  Lip and palate do not properly join together
Causes feeding problems
- Infants cannot create sufficient suction for feeding
- Danger of aspirating food
- Results in speech defects

Treatment
Surgical repair of defects

Ulceration

Canker sore—caused by herpes simplex virus
- Ulceration of oral mucosa
  Also known as
- Aphthous ulcer (aphtha: small ulcer)
- Aphthous stomatitis
  Heals spontaneously

Infections

Candidiasis
Candida albicans is naturally found in mouth

Thrush (oral candidiasis) is overarching infection

Causes
Antibiotic regimen
Chemotherapy
Glucocorticoids
Common in patients with diabetes and AIDS patients

Treatment
Nystatin (topical fungal agent)

Herpes Simplex Type 1
Herpetic stomatitis
- Viral cold sores and blisters
- Associated with herpes simplex virus type 1 (HSV-1)

Treatment
No cure
  May be alleviated somewhat by antiviral medications

Cancer of Oral Cavity

Most common type is squamous cell carcinoma
  Kaposi's sarcoma is type seen in AIDS patients
  Increased in smokers
  Lip cancer also increased in smokers, particularly pipe
    smokers
  Poor prognosis
  Usually asymptomatic until later stages
  Metastasis through lymph nodes

Esophageal Disorders

Scleroderma

Also known as progressive systemic sclerosis

Atrophy of smooth muscles of lower esophagus
Lower esophageal sphincter (LES) does not close properly

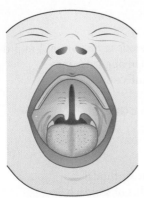

• **Figure 8.5** Cleft palate.

- Leads to esophageal reflux
- Strictures form

Symptom
Predominantly dysphagia

Esophagitis
Inflammation of esophagus

Types
Acute
Most common type is that caused by hiatal hernia
Infectious esophagitis is common in patients with AIDS
Ingestion of strong alkaline or acid substances
- Such as those in household cleaners
Inflammation leads to scarring
Chronic
Most common type is that caused by LES reflux

Cancer of Esophagus
Most common type is squamous cell or secondary adenocarcinoma

Usually caused by continued irritation
- Smoking
- Alcohol
- Hiatal hernia
- Chronic esophagitis/GERD
Poor prognosis

Hiatal Hernia (Diaphragmatic Hernia)
Diaphragm goes over stomach
- Esophagus passes through diaphragm at natural opening (hiatus)
- Part of the stomach protrudes (herniates) through opening in diaphragm into thorax

Types (Fig. 8.6)
Sliding
- Stomach and gastroesophageal junction protrude through the hiatus
Paraesophageal/rolling hiatal
- Part of fundus protrudes

HIATAL HERNIAS

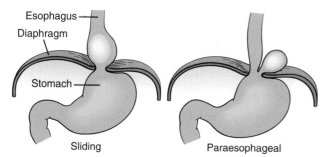

Esophagus
Diaphragm
Stomach
Sliding   Paraesophageal

• **Figure 8.6** Sliding and paraesophageal hernias (hiatal hernias).

Symptoms
Heartburn
Reflux
Belching
Lying down causes discomfort
Dysphagia
Substernal pain after eating

Gastroesophageal Reflux Disease (GERD)
Associated with hiatal hernias
Reflux of gastric contents
Lower esophageal sphincter does not constrict properly

Treatment
Reduce irritants, such as
- Smoking
- Spicy foods
- Alcohol
Antacids
Elevate head of bed
Avoid tight clothing

Stomach and Duodenum Disorders

Gastritis
Inflammation of stomach mucosa

Acute Superficial Gastritis
Mild, transient irritation

Causes
Excessive alcohol
Infection
Food allergies
Spicy foods
Aspirin
H. pylori (Helicobacter pylori)

Symptoms
Nausea
Vomiting
Anorexia
Bleeding in more severe cases
Epigastric pain

Treatment
Usually spontaneous remission in 2 to 3 days
Removal of underlying irritation
Antibiotics for infection

Chronic Atrophic Gastritis
Progressive atrophy of epithelium

Types
Type A, atrophic or fundal
- Involves fundus of stomach
- Autoimmune disease

- Decreases acid secretion
- Results in high gastrin levels

Type B, antral
- Involves antrum region of stomach
- Often associated with elderly
  - May be associated with pernicious anemia
- Low gastrin levels
- Usually caused by infection
- Irritated by alcohol, drugs, and tobacco
Symptom abatement
- Bland diet
- Alcohol avoidance
- ASA avoidance
- Antibiotics for *H. pylori*

Peptic Ulcers

Erosive area on mucosa
Extends below epithelium
Chronic ulcers have scar tissue at base of erosive area
Ulcers can occur anywhere on gastrointestinal tract but typically are found on the
- Lower esophagus
- Stomach
- Proximal duodenum

Some Causes

Alcohol
Smoking
Aspirin
Severe stress
Bacterial infection caused by *Helicobacter pylori (H. pylori)*, 90% of the time
Genetic factor
Constant use of anti-inflammatory drugs

Symptoms

Epigastric pain when stomach is empty
- Relieved by food or antacid
- Burning
May include
- Vomiting blood
- Nausea
- Weight loss
- Anorexia
Severe cases may include
- Obstruction
- Hemorrhage
- Perforation

Treatment

Surgical intervention
Antacids
Dietary restrictions
Rest
Antibiotics

Gastric Cancer (Malignant Tumor of Stomach)

Most often occurs in men over 40
Cause is unknown, but often associated with *Helicobacter pylori* (bacterial infection)

Predisposing Factors

Atrophic gastritis
Pernicious anemia
History of nonhealing gastric ulcer
Blood type A
Geographic factors
Environmental factors
Carcinogenic foods
- Smoked meats
- Nitrates
- Pickled foods

Symptoms

Usually asymptomatic in early stages

Treatment

Excision
Chemotherapy
Radiation (poor response)
Prognosis is poor

Pyloric Stenosis

Narrowing of the pyloric sphincter
Signs appear soon after birth
- Failure to thrive
- Projectile vomiting

Treatment

Surgery to relieve stenosis (pyloromyotomy)

Intestinal Disorders

Small Intestine

Malabsorption Conditions

Celiac Disease

Most important malabsorption condition
Villi atrophy in response to food containing gluten and lose ability to absorb
- Gluten is a protein found in wheat, rye, oats, and barley

Symptoms

Malnutrition
Muscle wasting
Distended abdomen
Diarrhea
Fatigue
Weakness
Steatorrhea (excess fat in feces)

Treatment

Gluten-free diet

Steroids when necessary

Lactase Deficiency

Enzyme deficiency

- Secondary to gastrointestinal damage, such as
  - Regional enteritis
  - Infection
- Common in African Americans, occurring in adulthood

Symptoms

Intolerance to milk

Intestinal cramping

Diarrhea

Flatulence

Treatment

Elimination of milk products

Inflammatory Bowel Disease (IBD)

Affects terminal ileum and colon

For example, Crohn's Disease (regional enteritis)

Cause

Unknown

Symptoms

Vary greatly

Inflammatory disease of GI tract

Diarrhea

Gas

Fever

Abdominal pain

Malaise

Anorexia

Weight loss

Treatment

No specific treatment

Palliative medications to control symptoms

Resection of affected section of intestine with anastomosis

Diet modifications

Duodenal Ulcers

Most common ulcer

Develop in younger population

Common in type O blood types

Appendicitis

Inflammation of vermiform appendix that projects from cecum

Obstruction of lumen leads to infection

- Appendix becomes hypoxic (decreased oxygen levels)
- May cause gangrene
- May rupture, causing peritonitis

Symptoms

Periumbilical (around umbilicus) pain, initially

Right lower quadrant (RLQ) pain as inflammation progresses

Nausea

Vomiting

Possible diarrhea

Treatment

Appendectomy

Management of any perforation or abscess

Meckel's Diverticulum

- Appendage of ileum near cecum derived from an unobliterated yolk stalk in fetal development
- Symptoms can mimic appendicitis

Peritonitis

Inflammation of peritoneum (membrane that lines abdominal cavity)

Usually a result of

- Spread of infection from abdominal organ
- Puncture wound to abdomen
- Rupture of gastrointestinal tract—appendicitis or Meckel's diverticulum

Abscesses form, resulting in adhesions

- May result in obstruction

Types

Acute, chronic

Symptoms

Abdominal pain

Vomiting

Rigid abdomen

Fever

Leukocytosis (increased white cells in blood)

Treatment

Antibiotics

Suction of stomach and intestines

If possible, surgical removal of origin of infection, such as appendix

Fluid replacement

Bed rest

Obstruction

Any interference with passage of intestinal contents

May be

- Acute
- Chronic
- Partial
- Total

Types

Nonmechanical

- Paralytic ileus
- Result of trauma or toxin

Mechanical
- Result of tumors, adhesions, hernias
- Simple mechanical obstruction
  - One point of obstruction
- Closed-loop obstruction
  - At least two points of obstruction
- Diverticulosis
- Twisted bowel (volvulus)
- Telescoping bowel (intussusception)

Symptoms
Abdominal distention
Pain
Vomiting
Total constipation

Treatment
Surgical intervention
Symptomatic treatment

Large Intestine

Diverticulosis
Herniation of intestinal mucosa
- Forms sacs in lining, called diverticula

Diverticulitis
Sacs fill and become inflamed
- Common in aged persons

Symptoms
Diarrhea or constipation
Gas
Abdominal discomfort

Complications
Perforation
Bleeding
Peritonitis
Abscess
Obstruction

Treatment
Antimicrobials as necessary
High-fiber diet (greater than 20 g daily)
Stool softeners
Dietary restrictions of solid foods
Surgical intervention if necessary

Ulcerative Colitis (Fig. 8.7)
Inflammation of rectum that progresses to sigmoid colon
Intermittent exacerbations and remissions
May develop into toxic megacolon
- Leads to obstruction and dilation of colon
Increased risk for colorectal cancer

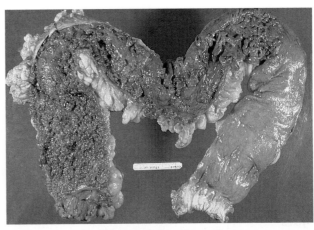

• **Figure 8.7** Ulcerative colitis.

Symptoms
Diarrhea
- Blood and mucus may be present
Cramping
Fever
Weight loss

Treatment
Remove physical or emotional stressors
Anti-inflammatory medications
Antimotility agents
Nutritional supplementation
Surgical intervention, if necessary

Colorectal Cancer
Usually develop from polyp
- In those 55 and older

Increased Risks
Genetic factors
40 years of age and older
Diets high in
- Fat
- Sugar
- Red meat
Low-fiber diets

Symptoms
Asymptomatic until advanced
Some may experience
- Cramping
- Ribbon stools
- Feeling of incomplete evacuation
- Fatigue
- Weight loss
- Change in bowel habits
- Blood in stool

Treatment
Surgical excision

Radiation
Chemotherapy
Combination of above

Disorders of Liver, Gallbladder, and Pancreas

Disorders of Liver

Jaundice (Hyperbilirubinemia)

A sign of biliary disease, not a disease itself
• Results in yellow eyes (sclera) and skin

Types
Prehepatic
• Excess destruction of red blood cells
• Result of hemolytic anemia or reaction to transfusion
Intrahepatic
• Impaired uptake of bilirubin and decreased blending of bilirubin by hepatic cells
• Result of liver disease, such as cirrhosis or hepatitis
Posthepatic
• Excess bile flows into blood
• Result of obstruction
   • Due to conditions such as inflammation of liver, tumors, cholelithiasis

Treatment
Removal of cause

Cancer of Liver

Most commonly a metastasis; primary CA rare
Risk for primary liver CA
• Hepatitis B, C, and D
• Cirrhosis
• Myotoxins
• Heavy smoking/alcohol use

Treatment
Surgical resection if localized
   Survival typically 3 or 4 months

Viral Hepatitis

Liver cells are damaged
   Results in inflammation and necrosis
   Damage can be mild or severe
   Scar tissue forms in liver
   • Leads to ischemia

Hepatitis A (HAV)
Infectious hepatitis—caused by hepatitis A virus

Transmission
   • Most commonly fecal-oral route—contaminated food or water
Does not have a chronic state
Slow onset—complete recovery characteristic

Vaccine available for those who are traveling
Gamma globulin may be administered to those just exposed

Hepatitis B (HBV)
Serum hepatitis

Carrier state is common
Caused by hepatitis B virus
   • Asymptomatic but contagious
Long incubation period
Transmission
   • Intravenous drug users
   • Transfusion
   • Exposure to blood and bodily fluids
   • Sexual transmission
   • Mother-to-fetus transmission
   • Immune globulin is temporary prophylactic
   • Vaccine is now routine for children and is given to those at risk
Severe forms cause liver cell destruction, cirrhosis, death

Hepatitis C (HCV)
Transmission of virus
• Most commonly by transfusion
• IV drug users
   Half of cases develop into chronic hepatitis
   Increases risk of hepatocellular cancer
   Carrier state may develop

Hepatitis D (HDV)
Transmission of hepatitis D virus
• Blood
• Intravenous drug users
   Hepatitis B is present for this type to develop

Hepatitis E (HEV)
Transmission of hepatitis E virus
• Fecal-oral route
   Does not develop into chronic or carrier

Hepatitis G
Transmission of hepatitis G virus
• IV drug use
• Sexual transmission

Symptoms of Hepatitis
   Stages
Preicteric
   • Anorexia
   • Nausea and vomiting
Liver enzymes may be elevated—indication of liver cell damage
   • Fatigue
   • Malaise
   • Generalized pain with low-grade fever
   • Cough

Icteric
- Jaundice
- Hepatomegaly (enlarged liver)
- Biliary obstruction
- Light-colored stools and dark urine
- Pruritus
- Abdominal pain

Posticteric (recovery)
- Reduction of symptoms

Treatment
None
In early stages gamma globulins may be used
Interferon may be used for cases of chronic hepatitis B and C

Nonviral Hepatitis
Hepatitis that results from hepatotoxins

Symptoms
- Similar to viral hepatitis

Treatment
- Removal of hepatotoxin

Cirrhosis
Profuse liver damage
- Extensive fibrosis
  - Results in inflammation
  - Progressive disorder
  - Leads to liver failure

Types
Alcoholic liver
- Known as Laënnec's cirrhosis or portal cirrhosis
- Largest group
- Biliary
- Associated with immune disorders
- Obstructions (intrahepatic or extrahepatic blood vessels) occur and disrupt normal function
- Postnecrotic
- Associated with chronic hepatitis (A or C) and exposure to toxins

Symptoms
Asymptomatic in early stages
Nausea
Vomiting
Fatigue
Weight loss
Pruritus
Jaundice
Edema

Treatment
Symptomatic
Dietary restrictions
- Reduced protein and sodium

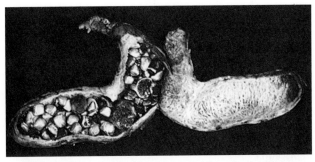

• **Figure 8.8** Resected gallbladder containing mixed gallstones.

- Increased vitamins and carbohydrates
Diuretics
Antibiotics
Liver transplant

Disorders of Gallbladder
Cholecystitis
Inflammation of gallbladder and cystic duct

Cholangitis
Inflammation of bile duct

Cholelithiasis
Formation of gallstones (Fig. 8.8)
- Consists of cholesterol or bilirubin
- Occurs most often in those with high levels of cholesterol, calcium, or bile salts

Stones cause irritation and inflammation
- May lead to infection
- Obstruction
  - May result in pancreatitis
  - Rupture is possible

Symptoms
Often asymptomatic
Dietary intolerance particularly to fat
Right upper quadrant (RUQ) pain
Pain in back and/or shoulder
Epigastric discomfort
Bloating heartburn, flatulence

Treatment
Surgical intervention (laparoscopic cholecystectomy)
Lithotripsy
Medical management by use of drugs that break down stone

Disorders of Pancreas
Pancreatitis
Inflammation of pancreas resulting from digestive enzyme attack to pancreas

Acute and chronic forms

Commonly associated with alcoholism, biliary tract obstruction, drug toxicity, gallstone obstruction of common bile duct, and viral infections

Symptoms
Severe pain
Fever
Acute form is a medical emergency
Neurogenic shock
Septicemia
General sepsis

Complications
Adult respiratory distress syndrome (ARDS)

Renal failure

Treatment
No oral intake
• IV fluids given and carefully monitored

Analgesics
Stop process of autodigestion
Prevent systemic shutdown

Pancreatic Cancer

Increased Risk
Cigarette smoking
Diet high in fat and protein

Symptoms
Weight loss
Jaundice
Anorexia
Most types of pancreatic cancer are asymptomatic until well advanced

Treatment
Surgery
Chemotherapy and radiation therapy

Chapter 8: Pathophysiology Quiz

(Quiz Answers Are Located in Appendix B)

1. This type of hyperbilirubinemia is characterized by excess bile flow into the blood:
   a. intrahepatic
   b. prehepatic
   c. posthepatic
   d. jaundice

2. This type of hepatitis is transmitted by the fecal-oral route:
   a. A
   b. B
   c. C
   d. D

3. Which of the following is the recovery stage of hepatitis?
   a. prehepatic
   b. posthepatic
   c. preicteric
   d. posticteric

4. This type of cirrhosis is also known as portal cirrhosis:
   a. biliary
   b. alcoholic liver
   c. postnecrotic
   d. traumatic

5. This condition is the inflammation of the bile ducts:
   a. cholangitis
   b. cholecystitis
   c. cholelithiasis
   d. cholangioma

6. Formation of gallstones most often occurs with high levels of the following:
   a. bile salts and toxins
   b. cholesterol and toxins
   c. cholesterol and bile salts
   d. toxins

7. The primary factor that increases the risk of pancreatic cancer is:
   a. smoking
   b. alcohol
   c. intravenous drug use
   d. hepatitis

8. A potential complication of this condition is ARDS:
   a. hyperbilirubinemia
   b. hepatitis
   c. pancreatitis
   d. pancreatic cancer

9. The primary treatment for jaundice is:
   a. removal of cause
   b. antibiotics
   c. dialysis
   d. vaccine

10. This condition has the largest group of those who abuse alcohol:
   a. cirrhosis
   b. hepatitis
   c. pancreatitis
   d. pancreatic cancer

9
Mediastinum and Diaphragm

ANATOMY AND TERMINOLOGY

Not an organ system

Mediastinum

The area between lungs that a median (partition) divides (Fig. 9.1) into
- Superior
- Anterior
- Posterior
- Middle
  Space that houses heart, thymus gland, trachea, esophagus, nerves, lymph and blood vessels, and major blood vessels
- Aorta
- Inferior vena cava

Diaphragm

A dome-shaped muscular partition that separates abdominal cavity from thoracic cavity
- Assists in breathing

- Expands to assist lungs in exhalation/relaxation of diaphragm
- Flattens out during inspiration/contraction of diaphragm
- Diaphragmatic hernia: esophageal hernia

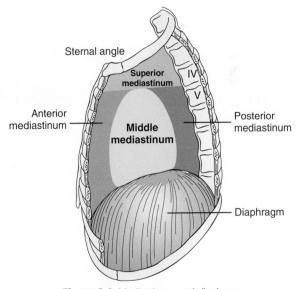

• **Figure 9.1** Mediastinum and diaphragm.

Chapter 9: Anatomy and Terminology Quiz

1. The mediastinum is NOT an organ system.
   a. true
   b. false
2. The mediastinum is divided into:
   a. superior, anterior, posterior
   b. superior, anterior, posterior, middle
   c. anterior, posterior, middle
   d. middle, anterior, superior
3. During inspiration, the diaphragm:
   a. expands
   b. moves upward
   c. collapses
   d. flattens out
4. Term meaning "partition":
   a. middle
   b. aspect
   c. median
   d. diaphragm

5. The diaphragm is said to be this shape:
   a. square
   b. flat
   c. dome
   d. round

6. This separates the abdominal cavity from the thoracic cavity:
   a. mediastinum
   b. diaphragm
   c. superior
   d. inferior

7. This is the area between the lungs:
   a. mediastinum
   b. diaphragm
   c. superior
   d. inferior

8. This is an esophageal hernia:
   a. mediastinal
   b. diaphragmatic
   c. paraesophageal
   d. hiatal

9. A diaphragmatic hernia is also known as:
   a. esophageal
   b. epiglottis
   c. partitional
   d. medial

10. The diaphragm assists in:
    a. percussion
    b. auscultation
    c. contraction
    d. breathing

10
Hemic and Lymphatic System

ANATOMY AND TERMINOLOGY

Hemic refers to blood

Lymphatic system removes excess tissue fluid
- Lymph tissue is scattered throughout body
- Composed of lymph nodes, vessels, and organs

Lymph

Colorless fluid containing lymphocytes and monocytes
Originates from blood and after filtering, returns to blood
Transports interstitial fluids and proteins that have leaked from blood system into venous system
Absorbs and transports fats from villi of small intestine to venous system
Assists in immune function

Lymph Vessels

Similar to veins
  Organized circulatory system throughout body

Lymph Organs

Lymph nodes, spleen, bone marrow, thymus, tonsils, and Peyer's patches (lymphoid tissue on mucosa of small intestine)

Lymph nodes, areas of concentrated tissue (Fig. 10.1)
Spleen, located in left upper quadrant (LUQ) of abdomen
- Composed of lymph tissue
  - Function is to filter blood; activates lymphocytes and B cells to filter antigens
  - Stores blood
Thymus secretes thymosin, causing T cells to mature
- Larger in infants and shrinks with age
Tonsils
- Palatine tonsils
- Pharyngeal tonsils/adenoids

Hematopoietic Organ

Bone marrow, contains tissue that produces RBCs, WBCs, and platelets
- Produces stem cells

TABLE 10-1

Combining Forms

Combining Form	Meaning
1. aden/o	gland
2. adenoid/o	adenoids
3. axill/o	armpit
4. cervic/o	neck/cervix
5. immune/o	immune
6. inguin/o	groin
7. lymph/o	lymph
8. lymphaden/o	lymph gland
9. splen/o	spleen
10. thym/o	thymus gland
11. tonsill/o	tonsil
12. tox/o	poison

TABLE 10-2

Prefixes

Prefix	Meaning
1. hyper-	excess
2. inter-	between
3. retro-	behind

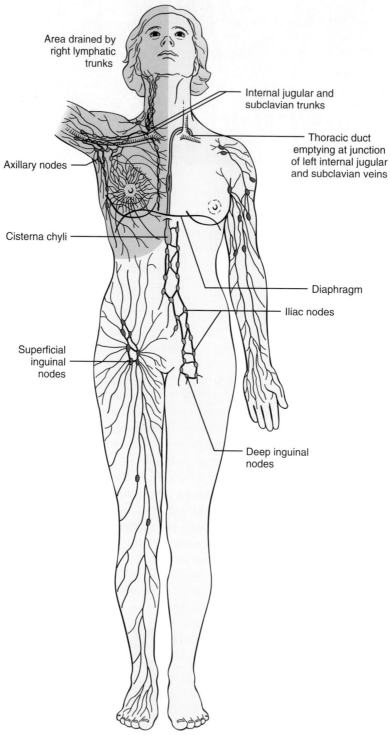

Area drained by right lymphatic trunks

Internal jugular and subclavian trunks

Thoracic duct emptying at junction of left internal jugular and subclavian veins

Axillary nodes

Cisterna chyli

Diaphragm

Iliac nodes

Superficial inguinal nodes

Deep inguinal nodes

• **Figure 10.1** Lymphatic system.

TABLE 10-3

Suffixes

Suffix	Meaning	Suffix	Meaning
1. -ectomy	removal	6. -oma	tumor
2. -edema	swelling	7. -penia	deficient
3. -itis	inflammation	8. -pexy	fixation
4. -megaly	enlargement	9. -phylaxis	protection
5. -oid	resembling	10. -poiesis	production

TABLE 10-4

Medical Terms

Term	Meaning	Term	Meaning
Axillary nodes	Lymph nodes located in armpit	Parathyroid	Produces a hormone to mobilize calcium from bones to blood
Cloquet's node	Also called a gland; it is highest of deep groin lymph nodes	Splenectomy	Excision of spleen
Inguinofemoral	Referring to groin and thigh	Splenography	Radiographic recording of spleen
Jugular nodes	Lymph nodes located next to large vein in neck	Splenoportography	Radiographic procedure to allow visualization of splenic and portal veins of spleen
Lymph node	Station along lymphatic system		
Lymphadenectomy	Excision of a lymph node or nodes	Stem cell	Immature blood cell
Lymphadenitis	Inflammation of a lymph node	Thoracic duct	Largest lymph vessel; it collects lymph from portions of body below diaphragm and from left side of body above diaphragm
Lymphangiography	Radiographic recording of lymphatic vessels and nodes		
Lymphangiotomy	Incision into a lymphatic vessel		
Lymphangitis	Inflammation of lymphatic vessel or vessels	Transplantation	Grafting of tissue from one source to another

Chapter 10: Anatomy and Terminology Quiz

(Quiz Answers Are Located in Appendix B)

1. The spleen is located in this quadrant of the abdomen:
   a. RUQ
   b. LUQ
   c. LLQ
   d. LRQ

2. Produces RBCs and platelets:
   a. thymus
   b. tonsils
   c. lymph node
   d. bone marrow

3. Which of the following is NOT a lymph organ?
   a. adrenal
   b. spleen
   c. thymus
   d. tonsil

4. Lymph transports fluids and _____ that have leaked from the blood system back to veins.
   a. stem cells
   b. lymphocytes
   c. B cells
   d. proteins

5. This is largest in infants and shrinks with age:
   a. tonsils
   b. spleen
   c. thymus
   d. bone marrow

6. Combining form meaning "gland":
   a. axill/o
   b. thym/o
   c. aden/o
   d. tox/o

7. Prefix meaning "excess":
   a. hyper-
   b. hypo-
   c. inter-
   d. retro-
8. Suffix meaning "enlargement":
   a. -edema
   b. -poiesis
   c. -penia
   d. -megaly

9. Lymph node located on neck:
   a. thoracic
   b. jugular
   c. Cloquet's
   d. axillary
10. These cells originate in the bone marrow:
    a. B cells
    b. antigens
    c. erythrocytes
    d. stem cells

PATHOPHYSIOLOGY

Anemia

Reduction in number of erythrocytes or decrease in quality of hemoglobin
- Less oxygen is transported in the blood

Aplastic Anemia

Diverse group of anemias
Characterized by bone marrow failure with reduced numbers of red and white blood cells and platelets

Causes

Genetic or acquired (primary or secondary)

Toxins/chemical agents
   - Benzene and antibiotics such as chloramphenicol
Irradiation
Immunologic
Idiopathic (unknown)

Treatment

Blood transfusion
Bone marrow transplant

Iron Deficiency Anemia

Characterized by small erythrocytes and a reduced amount of hemoglobin
Caused by low or absent iron stores or serum iron concentrations
   - Blood loss
   - Decreased intake of iron
   - Malabsorption of iron

Symptoms

Pallor
Headache
Stomatitis
Oral lesions
Gastrointestinal complaints
Retinal hemorrhages
Thinning, brittle nails and hair

Treatment

Iron supplement

Pernicious Anemia

Megaloblastic anemia (large stem cells)
Inability to absorb vitamin B_{12} due to a lack of intrinsic factor (found in gastric juices)
Usually in older adults
Caused by impaired intestinal absorption of vitamin B_{12}

Symptoms

Pallor
Weakness
Neurologic manifestations
Gastric discomfort

Treatment

Injections of vitamin B_{12}
Transfusions

Hemolytic Anemia

May be acute or chronic

Shortened survival of mature erythrocytes—excessive destruction of RBCs
   - Inability of bone marrow to compensate for decreased survival of erythrocytes

Treatment

Treat cause

Sickle Cell Anemia

Occurs primarily in those of West African descent
Abnormal sickle-shaped erythrocytes (sickle cell) caused by an abnormal type of hemoglobin (Hemoglobin S)

Symptoms

Abdominal pain
Arthralgia
Ulceration of lower extremities
Fatigue
Dyspnea
Increased heart rate

Treatment
Symptomatic

Granulocytosis

Increase in granulocytes
- Neutrophils
- Eosinophils
- Basophils

Eosinophilia

Increase in number of eosinophilic granulocytes

Cause
Allergic disorders
Dermatologic disorders
Parasitic invasion
Drugs
Malignancies

Basophilia

Increase in basophilic granulocytes seen in leukemia

Monocytosis

Increased number of monocytes

Cause
Infection
Hematologic factors

Leukocytosis

Increased number of leukocytes

Cause
Acute viral infections, such as hepatitis
Chronic infections, such as syphilis

Leukocytopenia

Decreased number of leukocytes

Cause
Neoplasias
Immune deficiencies
Drugs
Virus
Radiation

Infectious Mononucleosis

Acute Infection of B Cells

Epstein-Barr virus most common cause

Symptoms
Fatigue
Fever
Weakness (asthenia)
Pharyngitis
Atypical lymphocytes in blood
Lymph node enlargement
Splenomegaly
Hepatomegaly

Transmission
Saliva
- Known as kissing disease

Treatment
Rest
Treatment of symptoms

Leukemia

Malignant disorder of blood and blood-forming organs

Leads to dysfunction of cells
- Primarily leads to proliferation of abnormal leukocytes—filling bone marrow and bloodstream

Acute Myelogenous Leukemia (AML)

Rapid onset
Short survival time

Symptoms
Abrupt onset
Fatigue
Lymphadenopathy
Bone pain and tenderness
Anemia
Bleeding
Fever
Infection
Anorexia
Splenomegaly
Hepatomegaly
Headache, vomiting, paralysis

Treatment
Chemotherapy
Bone marrow transplant following high-dose chemotherapy to eradicate leukemic cells

Acute Lymphocytic Leukemia (ALL)

Immature lymphocytes (lymphoblasts)
Most cases occur in children and adolescents
Sudden onset

Treatment
Chemotherapy with drugs that suppress cell division and destroy rapidly dividing cells

Remission
Relapse—leukemia cells in bone marrow and blood requiring treatment

Chronic Myelogenous Leukemia (CML)

Mature and immature granulocytes in bone marrow and blood

Slow, progressive disease (those over 55 years live many years without life threat)
Cells are more differentiated
Gradual onset with milder symptoms
- Majority of cases are in adults

Symptoms
Extreme fatigue
Weight loss
Splenomegaly
Night sweats
Fever
Infections

Treatment
Chemotherapy—target abnormal proteins
Bone marrow transplant following high-dose chemotherapy

Chronic Lymphocytic Leukemia (CLL)

Increased numbers of mature lymphocytes in marrow, lymph nodes, spleen

Most common form seen in elderly
Slowly progressive

Treatment
Chemotherapy

Lymphadenopathy

Any abnormality of lymph node
Enlargement of lymph node

Lymphangitis

Inflammation of lymphatic vessel

Lymphadenitis

Inflammation of lymph node
Localized inflammation associated with inflamed lesion
Generalized inflammation associated with disease
Inflammation can occur as result of
- Trauma
- Infection
- Drug reaction
- Autoimmune disease
- Immunologic disease

Malignant Lymphoma

Hodgkin Disease

Initial sign is a painless mass commonly located on neck
Giant Reed-Sternberg cells are present in lymphatic tissue

Presentation
Enlarged spleen (splenomegaly)
Abdominal mass
Mediastinal mass
Localized node involvement
- Orderly spreading of node involvement
- Cervical, axillary, inguinal, and retroperitoneal lymph node involvement

Symptoms
Night sweats
Fever
Weight loss
Itching (pruritus)
Anorexia
Weakness

Treatment
If localized: radiation therapy and chemotherapy
If systemic: chemotherapy alone
High probability of cure with new treatments

Non-Hodgkin Lymphoma

No giant Reed-Sternberg cells present
Involves multiple nodes scattered throughout body (follicular lymphoma)
Large cell lymphoma (large lymphocytes in diffuse nodes and lymph tissue)
- Noncontiguous spread of node involvement
- Not localized
Usually begins as a painless enlargement of node

Symptoms
Presents similar to Hodgkin disease

Treatment
Chemotherapy cures or stops disease progression

Burkitt's Lymphoma

Type of non-Hodgkin lymphoma
Usually found in Africa and New Guinea
Characterized by lesions in jaw and face
Epstein-Barr (herpes virus) has been found in Burkitt's lymphoma

Treatment
Radiation and chemotherapy for African type

Myeloma

Multiple Myeloma

B-cell cancer—lymphocytes that produce antibodies destroying bone tissue
- Also known as plasma cell myeloma
- Increased plasma cells replace bone marrow
- Overproduction of immunoglobulins—Bence Jones protein (found in urine)
- Multiple tumor sites cause bone destruction
- Results in weakened bone
- Hypercalcemia
- Anemia
- Renal damage
- Increased susceptibility to infections

Cause
Unknown

Treatment
Chemotherapy
Radiotherapy
Autologous bone marrow transplant (ABMT) prolongs remission—may be a cure
Palliative treatments

Chapter 10: Pathophysiology Quiz

(Quiz Answers Are Located in Appendix B)

1. This condition involves a reduced number of erythrocytes and decreased quality of hemoglobin:
   a. monocytosis
   b. eosinophilia
   c. anemia
   d. leukocytosis

2. This condition is characterized by a shortened survival of mature erythrocytes and inability of bone marrow to compensate for decreased survival:
   a. hemolytic anemia
   b. granulocytosis
   c. eosinophilia
   d. monocytosis

3. The most common cause of this disease is Epstein-Barr virus:
   a. leukocytopenia
   b. infectious mononucleosis
   c. leukocytosis
   d. hemolytic anemia

4. Inflammation of the lymphatic vessels is:
   a. lymphadenitis
   b. lymphoma
   c. lymphadenopathy
   d. lymphangitis

5. What giant cell is present in Hodgkin disease?
   a. B cell
   b. Reed-Sternberg
   c. T cell
   d. C cell

6. This condition increases plasma cells, which replace bone marrow:
   a. Burkitt's lymphoma
   b. multiple myeloma
   c. Hodgkin disease
   d. leukemia

7. Injection of vitamin B may be prescribed for this type of anemia:
   a. pernicious
   b. aplastic
   c. sideroblastic
   d. sickle cell

8. These are large stem cells:
   a. megaloblasts
   b. leukocytes
   c. erythrocytes
   d. granulocytes

9. This is known as the kissing disease:
   a. monocytosis
   b. leukocytopenia
   c. infectious mononucleosis
   d. granulocytosis

10. This lymphoma is usually found in Africa:
    a. multiple
    b. Burkitt's
    c. B-cell
    d. T-cell

11

Endocrine System

ANATOMY AND TERMINOLOGY

Regulates body through hormones (chemical messengers)
Ductless endocrine glands secrete hormones directly to bloodstream
Affects growth, development, and metabolism

Endocrine Glands (Fig. 11.1)

Pituitary (Hypophysis): Master Gland

Located at base of brain in a depression in skull (sella turcica)

Anterior pituitary (adenohypophysis)
- Adrenocorticotropic hormone (ACTH)—stimulates adrenal cortex and increases production of cortisol
- Follicle-stimulating hormone (FSH)—males, stimulates sperm and testosterone production; females, with luteinizing hormone (LH) stimulates secretion of estrogen and follicle development and ovulation
- Growth hormone (GH or somatotropin STH)—stimulates protein processing resulting in growth of bones, muscle, and fat metabolism, and maintains blood glucose levels
- Luteinizing hormone (LH)—males, stimulates testosterone production; females, stimulates secretion of progesterone and estrogen
- Melanocyte-stimulating hormone (MSH)—increases skin pigmentation
- Prolactin (PRL)—secreted by anterior pituitary, stimulates milk production and breast development
- Thyroid-stimulating hormone (TSH or thyrotropin)—stimulates thyroid gland

Posterior pituitary (neurohypophysis)—stores and releases hormones
- Antidiuretic hormone (ADH) or vasopressin—stimulates reabsorption of water by kidney tubules and increases blood pressure by constricting arterioles

- Oxytocin (OT)—stimulates contractions during childbirth, production and release of milk

Thyroid

Two lobes overlying trachea
Secretes two hormones that increase cell metabolism—thyroxine (T_4) and triiodothyronine (T_3)—synthesized from iodine
Secretes one hormone that decreases blood calcium—thyrocalcitonin (nasal spray used to treat osteoporosis)

Parathyroid Glands (4)

Located on posterior side of thyroid
Secretes PTH (parathyroid hormone) or parathormone
Promotes calcium homeostasis in bloodstream

Adrenal Gland (Pair)

Located on top of each kidney
Adrenal cortex—outer region that secretes corticosteroids
- Cortisol—increases blood glucose
- Aldosterone—increases reabsorption of sodium (salt)
- Androgen, estrogen, progestin—sexual characteristics
Adrenal medulla—inner region that secretes catecholamines (epinephrine to dilate blood vessels to lower blood pressure, increase heart rate, dilate bronchial tubes, and release glycogen for energy and norepinephrine to constrict blood vessels to raise blood pressure)

Pancreas

Located behind stomach
Contains specialized cells (islets of Langerhans) that produce insulin and glycogen hormones
Insulin (decreases blood glucose), glucagon (converts glycogen to glucose, raising blood sugar), and somatostatin (regulates other cells of pancreas)

Thymus

Located behind sternum
Atrophies during adolescence

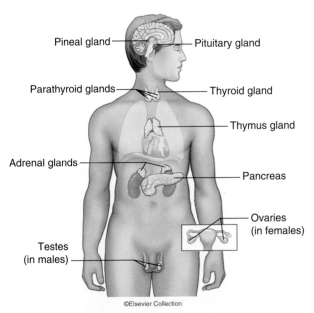

Pineal gland — Pituitary gland

Parathyroid glands — Thyroid gland

— Thymus gland

Adrenal glands — Pancreas

— Ovaries (in females)

Testes (in males)

©Elsevier Collection

• **Figure 11.1** Endocrine system.

Produces thymosin—stimulates T-lymphocytes, effecting a positive immune response

Hypothalamus (Part of Brain)

Located below thalamus and above pituitary gland

Stimulates anterior pituitary to release hormones and posterior hypothalamus to store and release hormones

Pineal

Located between two cerebral hemispheres and above third ventricle

Secretes melatonin—more so at night, which affects sleep cycle

Also responsible for delaying sexual maturation in children

Also has neurotransmitters such as somatostatin, norepinephrine, serotonin, and histamine

Ovaries (Pair, Females)

Estrogen production stimulates ova production and secondary female sex characteristics

Progesterone—prepares the uterus for and maintains pregnancy

Placenta

Produces HCG (human chorionic gonadotropin) to sustain a pregnancy

Testes (Pair, Males)

Testosterone—male sex characteristics

TABLE 11-1			
Combining Forms			
Combining Form	**Meaning**	**Combining Form**	**Meaning**
1. aden/o	in relationship to a gland	16. lact/o	milk
2. adren/o	adrenal gland	17. myx/o	mucus
3. adrenal/o	adrenal gland	18. natr/o	sodium
4. andr/o	male	19. pancreat/o	pancreas
5. calc/o, calc/i	calcium	20. parathyroid/o	parathyroid gland
6. cortic/o	cortex	21. phys/o	growing
7. crin/o	secrete	22. pituitar/o	pituitary gland
8. dips/o	thirst	23. somat/o	body
9. estr/o	female	24. ster/o, stere/o	solid, having three dimensions
10. gluc/o	sugar	25. thry/o	thyroid gland
11. glyc/o	sugar	26. thyroid/o	thyroid gland
12. gonad/o	ovaries and testes	27. toc/o	childbirth
13. home/o	same	28. toxic/o	poison
14. hormon/o	hormone	29. ur/o	urine
15. kal/i	potassium		

TABLE 11-2

Prefixes

Prefix	Meaning
1. eu-	good/normal
2. oxy-	sharp, oxygen
3. pan-	all
4. tetra-	four
5. tri-	three
6. tropin-	act upon

TABLE 11-3

Suffixes

Suffix	Meaning
1. -agon	assemble
2. -drome	run, relationship to conducting, to speed
3. -emia	blood condition
4. -in	a substance
5. -ine	a substance
6. -tropin	act upon
7. -uria	urine

TABLE 11-4

Medical Terms

Term	Meaning
Adrenals	Glands, located at top of kidneys, that produce steroid hormones (cortex) and catecholamines (medulla)
Contralateral	Opposite side
Hormone	Chemical substance produced by body's endocrine glands
Isthmus	Connection of two regions or structures
Isthmus, thyroid	Tissue connection between right and left thyroid lobes
Isthmusectomy	Surgical removal of isthmus
Lobectomy	Removal of a lobe
Thymectomy	Surgical removal of thymus
Thymus	Gland that produces hormones important to immune response
Thyroglossal duct	A duct in embryo between thyroid and posterior tongue that occasionally persists into adult life and causes cysts, fistulas, or sinuses
Thyroid	Part of endocrine system that produces hormones that regulate metabolism
Thyroidectomy	Surgical removal of thyroid

Chapter 11: Anatomy and Terminology Quiz

(Quiz Answers Are Located in Appendix B)

1. Which of the following is NOT affected by the endocrine system?
   a. digestion
   b. development
   c. progesterone
   d. metabolism

2. Gland that overlies the trachea:
   a. parathyroid
   b. adrenal
   c. pancreas
   d. thyroid

3. Gland that is located on the top of each kidney:
   a. parathyroid
   b. adrenal
   c. pancreas
   d. thyroid

4. The outer region of the adrenal gland that secretes corticosteroids:
   a. cortex
   b. medulla
   c. sternum
   d. medullary

5. Located on the thyroid:
   a. hypophysis
   b. thymus
   c. pineal
   d. parathyroid

6. Located at the base of the brain in a depression in the skull:
   a. pituitary
   b. thymus
   c. adrenal
   d. pineal

7. Stimulates contractions during childbirth:
   a. cortisol
   b. PTH
   c. ADH
   d. oxytocin

8. Produced only during pregnancy by the placenta:
   a. estrogen and progesterone
   b. melatonin
   c. thymosin
   d. adrenocorticotropic hormone

9. Combining form meaning "secrete":
   a. dips/o
   b. crin/o
   c. gluc/o
   d. kal/i

10. Prefix meaning "good":
   a. tri-
   b. tropin-
   c. pan-
   d. eu-

PATHOPHYSIOLOGY

Diabetes Mellitus

Caused by a deficiency in insulin production or poor use of insulin by body cells

Islets of Langerhans (pancreatic cells) secrete glucagon and insulin to regulate fat, carbohydrate, and protein metabolism

Types of Diabetes Mellitus

Type 1, IDDM (Insulin-Dependent Diabetes Mellitus), Immune Mediated

Onset before age 30—peak onset age 12
Includes beta islet cell destruction, insulin deficiency
Acute onset
Positive family history
Requires insulin
Ketoacidosis (fats improperly burned leads to ketones and acids circulating)

Type 2, NIDDM (Non–Insulin-Dependent Diabetes Mellitus)

Adult onset, after age 30, but it is now occurring earlier
Insidious onset/asymptomatic
Positive in immediate family
Dietary management and/or oral hypoglycemics and/or insulin
Most common type—85% are obese at onset
Insulin is present
Ketoacidosis does not occur

Symptoms

Polyuria
Polydipsia
Glycosuria
Hyperglycemia
Polyphagia
Unexplained weight loss

Acute Complications

Hypoglycemia
Hyperglycemia with coma
Diabetic ketoacidosis

Chronic Complications

Diabetic neuropathy (Fig. 11.2)
Retinopathy
Coronary artery disease (atherosclerosis)

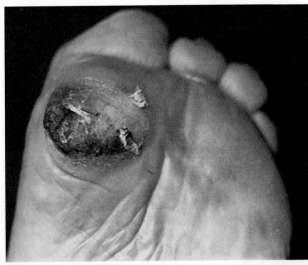

• **Figure 11.2** Patient with diabetes mellitus and neuropathy had severe claw toes, and shear forces across plantar surface of first metatarsal head caused recurrent ulceration.

Stroke
Peripheral vascular disease
Infection

Gestational Diabetes Mellitus— Predisposition to Diabetes

Most often recognized in second trimester
Glucose intolerance may be temporary, occurring only during pregnancy
Many will develop diabetes mellitus within 15 years

Pituitary Disorders

Tumors
Most common cause of pituitary disorders
May secrete hormone
   Such as prolactin or ACTH

Anterior Pituitary

Dwarfism (Hypopituitarism)

Can be caused by deficiency of somatotropin (growth hormone)

Gigantism (Fig. 11.3) (Hyperpituitarism)

Can be caused by excess of somatotrophin (growth hormone) in childhood

Treatment

Resection of tumor or irradiation of pituitary

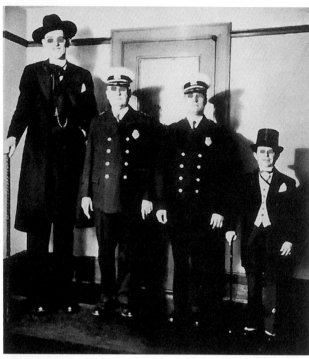

• **Figure 11.3** Gigantism. A pituitary giant and dwarf contrasted with normal-size men.

Acromegaly (Hyperpituitarism)

Increased GH in adulthood
Enlargement of facial bones, feet, and hands

Treatment

Pituitary adenoma is irradiated or removed

Posterior Pituitary

Diabetes Insipidus

Insufficient antidiuretic hormone—kidney tubules fail to retain needed water and salts
Causes polyuria, polydipsia, and dehydration
ADH or SIADH—syndrome of inadequate antidiuretic hormone
Excessive secretion of antidiuretic hormone
Causes excessive water retention

Treatment

Some types have no treatment
Others can be controlled with vasopressin (drug)

Thyroid Disorders

Goiter (Fig. 11.4)

Enlargement of thyroid gland in the neck

Cause

Hypothyroid disorders
Hyperthyroid disorders

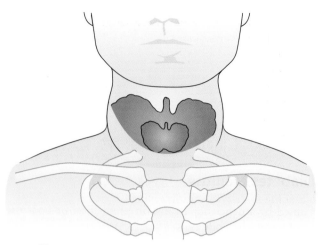

• **Figure 11.4** Goiter is an enlargement of thyroid gland.

Hyperthyroidism—Thyrotoxicosis

Excessive thyroid hormone production
Most common form: Graves' disease (familial)—results of autoimmune process

Characterized by

Goiter
Tachycardia
Atrial fibrillation
Dyspnea
Palpitations
Fatigue
Tremor
Nervousness
Weight loss
Exophthalmos (protruding eyes)
  • Decreased blinking

Treatment

Medication (antithyroid drugs)
Radioactive iodine
Surgical excision

Thyrotoxicosis Storm/Crisis

Thyroid storm/crisis is an acute, life-threatening hypermetabolic state induced by excessive release of thyroid hormones
  • Most extreme state of thyrotoxicosis

Hypothyroidism

Primary: inadequate thyroid hormone production
  Resulting in increasing levels of thyroid-stimulating hormone (TSH) production
Secondary: inadequate amounts of thyroid-stimulating hormone synthesized

Types

Cretinism
  • Congenital
  • Occurs in children

- If not treated, it will cause a severe delay in physical and mental development

Myxedema
- Severe form
- Occurs in adults
  - Atherosclerosis
- Symptoms
  - Cold intolerance
  - Weight gain
  - Mental sluggishness
  - Fatigue

Hashimoto's thyroiditis
- Autoimmune disorder

Treatment
Medication (levothyroxine synthetic hormone replacement)

Parathyroid Disorders

Hyperparathyroidism—Excessive Parathyroid Hormone (PTH)

Leads to hypercalcemia
Affects heart and bones and damages kidneys

Symptoms
Brittle bones
Kidney stones
Cardiac disturbances

Treatment
Surgical excision

Hypoparathyroidism—Abnormally Low PTH

Leads to hypocalcemia

Symptoms
Nerve irritability—twitching or spasms
Muscle cramps
Tingling and burning (paresthesias) of fingertips, toes, and lips
Anxiety, nervousness
Tetany (constant muscle contraction)

Treatment
Calcium and vitamin D

Adrenal Gland Disorders

Cushing Syndrome—Hypercortisolism
Excess levels of adrenocorticotropic hormone (ACTH)

Cause
Hyperfunction of adrenal cortex
Long-term use of steroid medications

Symptoms
Weight gain

- Fat deposits on face (moonface) and trunk (buffalo hump)

Glucose intolerance
- Diabetes may develop (20%)

Hypernatremia
Hypokalemia
Virilization
Hypertension
Muscle wasting
Osteoporosis
Change in mental status
Delayed healing

Treatment
Medication
Radiation therapy
Surgical intervention

Addison's Disease—Primary Adrenal Insufficiency

Deficiency of adrenocortical hormones resulting from destruction of adrenal glands
- Glucocorticoids
- Mineralocorticoids

Cause
Tumors
Autoimmune disorders
Viral
Tuberculosis
Infection

Symptoms
Decreased blood glucose levels
Elevated serum ACTH
Fatigue
Lack of ability to handle stress
Weight loss
Infections
Hypotension
Decreased body hair
Hyperpigmentation

Treatment
Hormone (glucocorticoid) replacement

Hyperaldosteronism

Excess aldosterone secreted by adrenal cortex

Types
Primary hyperaldosteronism (Conn's syndrome)
- Caused by an abnormality of adrenal cortex
  - Usually an adrenal adenoma
Secondary hyperaldosteronism
- Caused by other than adrenal stimuli

Symptoms
Hypertension

Hypokalemia
Neuromuscular disorders

Treatment
Treat the underlying condition that caused hyperaldosteronism
* Such as adrenal adenoma

Adrenal Medulla

Hypersecretion
    Pheochromocytoma—benign tumor of medulla
    Excessive production of epinephrine and norepinephrine

Symptoms
Severe headaches
Sweating
Flushing
Hypertension
Muscle spasms

Treatment
Antihypertensive drugs
Remove tumor

Androgen and Estrogen Hypersecretion

Androgen, male characteristic hormone
    * Virilization, development of male characteristics
Hypersecretion of estrogen, female characteristic hormone
    * Feminization

Cause
Underlying condition
* Adrenal tumor
* Cushing syndrome
* Adenomas or carcinomas
* Defects in steroid metabolism

Treatment
Surgical intervention for tumor
    Underlying condition

Chapter 11: Pathophysiology Quiz

(Quiz Answers Are Located in Appendix B)

1. This type of diabetes typically occurs before age 30:
   a. type 1
   b. type 2
2. The acronym that indicates that insulin is not required is:
   a. IDDM
   b. NIDDM
   c. PIDDM
   d. NDDMI
3. The most common cause of pituitary disorders is:
   a. hypersecretion
   b. hyposecretion
   c. tumor
   d. infection
4. In excess, this hormone can cause gigantism:
   a. somatotrophin
   b. thyroid
   c. mineralocorticoids
   d. adrenocortical
5. Goiter can be caused by which of the following:
   a. hypothyroidism
   b. parathyroidism
   c. hyperthyroidism
   d. both a and c
6. This type of hypothyroidism is an autoimmune disorder:
   a. myxedema
   b. Hashimoto's
   c. cretinism
   d. hypokalemia
7. Tetany can be caused by:
   a. hypoparathyroidism
   b. hyperthyroidism
   c. hyperparathyroidism
   d. hyperaldosteronism
8. Conn's syndrome is also known as:
   a. primary hypoparathyroidism
   b. primary hyperthyroidism
   c. primary hyperparathyroidism
   d. primary hyperaldosteronism
9. Development of male characteristics is known as:
   a. virilization
   b. feminization
   c. hypertrophy
   d. hyperaldosteronism
10. The treatment for Addison's disease is often:
    a. chemotherapy
    b. radiation
    c. hormone replacement
    d. all of the above

12

Nervous System

ANATOMY AND TERMINOLOGY

Controlling, regulating, and communicating system

Organization
- Central nervous system (CNS), brain and spinal cord
- Peripheral nervous system (PNS), cranial and spinal nerves
  - Autonomic nervous system—motor and sensory nerves of viscera (involuntary)
  - Somatic nervous system—motor and sensory nerves of skeletal muscles

Cells of the Nervous System (Fig. 12.1)

Neurons—Primary Cells of Nervous System

Classified according to function (afferent [sensory], efferent [motor], interneurons [associational])
- Dendrites (receive signals)
- Cell body (nucleus, within cell body)
- Axon (carries signals from cell body)
- Myelin sheath (insulation around axon)

Glia

Astrocytes
   Star shaped—transport water and salts between capillaries and neurons
Microglia
   Multiple branching processes—protect neurons from inflammation
Oligodendrocytes
   Form myelin sheath
Ependymal
   Lining membrane of brain and spinal cord where central spinal fluid circulates

Divisions of Central Nervous System (CNS) (Fig. 12.2)

Brain—Housed in Cranium (Box Comprising 8 Bones)—Functioning to Enclose and Protect

Listing from inferior to superior

Brainstem
Medulla oblongata—crossover area left to right and center of respiratory and cardiovascular systems
Pons—connection of nerves (face and eyes)
Midbrain

Diencephalon
Hypothalamus controls autonomic nervous system, body temperature, sleep, appetite, and control of pituitary
Thalamus relays impulses to cerebral cortex for sensory system (pain)

Cerebellum
Controls voluntary movement and balance

Cerebrum
Largest part of brain

Functions
Mental processes, personality, sensory interpretation, movements, and memory

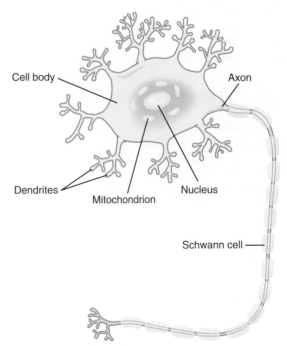

• Figure 12.1 Myelinated axon.

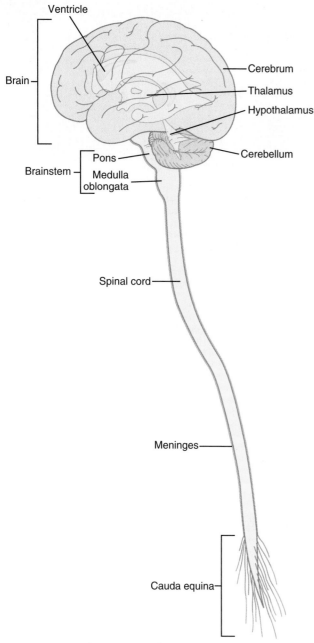

• **Figure 12.2** Brain and spinal cord.

Two Hemispheres
Right controls left side of body
Left controls right side of body

Divided Into Five Lobes
- Frontal
- Parietal
- Temporal
- Occipital
- Insula

Vertebral Column—33 Vertebrae

7 cervical
12 thoracic
5 lumbar
5 sacrum (fused)
4 coccygeal (fused)—tailbone

Spinal Cord—Housed Within Vertebrae From Medulla Oblongata to Second Lumbar

Spinal and brain meninges (coverings—dura mater [external], arachnoid, pia mater [internal])
  Spine and brain spaces bathed by cerebrospinal fluid (CSF) (subarachnoid space)
Cavities within brain contain cerebrospinal fluid (ventricles)

Peripheral Nervous System (PNS)

Cranial nerves, 12 pairs
Spinal nerves, 31 pairs

Autonomic Nervous System (ANS)— Housed Within Both PNS and CNS

Two divisions
- Sympathetic system—functions in fight and flight (stress)
- Parasympathetic system—functions to restore and conserve energy

TABLE 12-1	
Combining Forms	
Combining Form	**Meaning**
1. cephal/o	head
2. cerebell/o	cerebellum
3. cerebr/o	cerebrum
4. crani/o	cranium
5. dur/o	dura mater
6. encephal/o	brain
7. gangli/o	ganglion
8. ganglion/o	ganglion
9. gli/o	glial cells
10. lept/o	slender
11. mening/o	meninges
12. meningi/o	meninges
13. ment/o	mind
14. mon/o	one
15. myel/o	bone marrow, spinal cord
16. neur/o	nerve
17. phas/o	speech
18. phren/o	mind
19. poli/o	gray matter
20. pont/o	pons
21. psych/o	mind
22. quadr/i	four
23. radic/o	nerve root
24. radicul/o	nerve root
25. rhiz/o	nerve root
26. vag/o	vagus nerve

TABLE 12-2

Prefixes

Prefix	Meaning
1. hemi-	half
2. per-	through
3. quadri-	four
4. tetra-	four

TABLE 12-3

Suffixes

Suffix	Meaning
1. -algesia	pain sensation
2. -algia	pain
3. -cele	hernia
4. -esthesia	feeling
5. -iatry	medical treatment
6. -ictal	pertaining to
7. -kines/o	movement
8. -paresis	incomplete paralysis
9. -plegia	paralysis

TABLE 12-4

Medical Abbreviations

Abbreviation	Meaning
1. ANS	autonomic nervous system
2. CNS	central nervous system
3. CSF	cerebrospinal fluid
4. CVA	stroke/cerebrovascular accident
5. EEG	electroencephalogram
6. LP	lumbar puncture
7. PNS	peripheral nervous system
8. TENS	transcutaneous electrical nerve stimulation
9. TIA	transient ischemic attack

TABLE 12-5

Medical Terms

Term	Meaning	Term	Meaning
Burr	Drill used to create an entry into the cranium	Shunt	An artificial passage
Central nervous system	Brain and spinal cord	Skull	Entire skeletal framework of the head
Craniectomy	Permanent, partial removal of skull	Somatic nerve	Sensory or motor nerve
Craniotomy	Opening of the skull	Stereotaxis	Method of identifying a specific area or point in the brain
Cranium	That part of the skeleton that encloses the brain	Sympathetic nerve	Part of the peripheral nervous system that controls automatic body function and sympathetic nerves activated under stress
Discectomy	Removal of a vertebral disc		
Electroencephalography	Recording of the electric currents of the brain by means of electrodes attached to the scalp	Trephination	Surgical removal of a disk of bone
Laminectomy	Surgical excision of posterior arch of vertebra—includes spinal process	Vertebrectomy	Removal of vertebra
Peripheral nerves	12 pairs of cranial nerves, 31 pairs of spinal nerves, and autonomic nervous system; connects peripheral receptors to the brain and spinal cord		

Chapter 12: Anatomy and Terminology Quiz

(Quiz Answers Are Located in Appendix B)

1. Portion of nervous system that contains cranial and spinal nerves:
   a. central
   b. peripheral
   c. autonomic
   d. parasympathetic
2. Part of neuron that receives signals:
   a. dendrites
   b. cell body
   c. axon
   d. myelin sheath
3. NOT associated with glia:
   a. monocytes
   b. astrocytes
   c. microglia
   d. oligodendrocytes
4. Largest part of brain:
   a. cerebellum
   b. cerebrum
   c. cortex
   d. pons
5. Divided into two hemispheres:
   a. cerebellum
   b. cerebrum
   c. cortex
   d. pons
6. Number of pairs of cranial nerves:
   a. 10
   b. 11
   c. 12
   d. 13
7. Controls right side of body:
   a. left cerebrum
   b. right cerebrum
   c. right cortex
   d. left cortex
8. Combining form that means "brain":
   a. mening/o
   b. mon/o
   c. esthesi/o
   d. encephal/o
9. Prefix that means "four":
   a. per-
   b. tetra-
   c. para-
   d. bi-
10. Combining form that means "speech":
    a. phas/o
    b. rhiz/o
    c. poli/o
    d. myel/o

PATHOPHYSIOLOGY

Dementias—Classified by Causative Factor

Cognitive deficiencies

Causes

Alzheimer's disease
Vascular disease
Head trauma
Tumors
Infection
Toxins
Substance abuse
AIDS

Alzheimer's Disease

Most common type of dementia
Progressive intellectual impairment
- Results in damage to neurons (neurofibrillary tangles)
- Fatal within 3 to 20 years

Causes
Mostly unknown
Perhaps genetic defect, autoimmune reaction, or virus

Symptoms
Behavior change
Memory loss
Confusion
Disorientation
Restlessness
Speech disturbances
Personality change—anxiety, depression
Irritability
Inability to complete activities of daily living

Treatment
- No cure
- Aricept (drug has modest effect in early stages)
- Symptomatic treatment
- Support for family

Vascular Dementia

Result of brain infarctions (vascular occlusion resulting in loss of brain function)

Nutritional Degenerative Disease

Deficiency
- B vitamins
- Niacin
- Pantothenic acid

Associated with alcoholism

Amyotrophic Lateral Sclerosis (ALS)

Motor neuron disease (MND)
Also known as Lou Gehrig's disease
- Baseball player who died of ALS

Deterioration of neurons of spinal cord and brain
Results in atrophy of muscles and loss of fine motor skills
Difficulty walking, talking, and breathing
Mental functioning remains normal
Survival is 2 to 5 years after diagnosis
Genetic cause—familial chromosome 21 aberration
- Death usually results from respiratory failure

Treatment

Symptomatic only
Emotional support
No cure

Huntington's Disease—Chorea

Inherited progressive atrophy of cerebrum

Symptoms

Restlessness
Rapid, jerky movements in arms and face (uncontrollable jerking and facial grimacing)
Rigidity
Intellectual impairment, bradyphrenia, apathy

Treatment

Genetic defect of chromosome 4
No cure
Symptomatic

Parkinson's Disease (Parkinsonism)

Decreased secretion of dopamine
Typically occurs after age 40
Cause unknown

Symptoms

Muscle rigidity and weakness
Bradykinesia—slow voluntary movements
Postural instability, stooped
Shuffling gait
Tremors at rest
Masklike facial appearance
Depression

Treatment

Medications to reduce symptoms
Dopamine replacement

Multiple Sclerosis (MS)

Common neurologic condition
- Demyelination of central nervous system—replaced by sclerotic tissue

Diagnosed in young adults 20–40 years old

Results in myelin destruction and gliosis of white matter of central nervous system
Speculation that it is an autoimmune condition or result of a virus
Exacerbations and remission patterns

Symptoms

Precipitated by "an event," e.g., infection, pregnancy, stress
Loss of feeling (paresthesias)
Vision problems
Bladder disorder
Mood disorders
Weakness of limbs—unsteady gait and paralysis

Treatment

Symptomatic
Management of relapses
Reducing relapses and disease progression—disease-modifying drugs (DMDs)

Myasthenia Gravis (MG)

Means grave muscle weakness
Autoimmune neuromuscular condition—antibodies block neurotransmission to muscle cells
Most have pathologic changes of thymus

Symptoms

Insidious
Muscle weakness and fatigability
May be localized or generalized
Often affects
- Swallowing
- Breathing
- Compromised swallowing and breathing may lead to crisis

Treatment

Anticholinesterase drugs
- Restores normal muscle strength and recoverability after fatigue

Corticosteroids (prednisone) and immunosuppressive drugs
Thymectomy

Tourette Syndrome

Symptoms

Spasmodic, twitching movements, uncontrollable vocal sounds, inappropriate words
Begins with twitching eyelids and facial muscles (tics)
Verbal outbursts

Causes

Unknown
Excess dopamine or hypersensitivity to dopamine

Treatment

Antipsychotic drugs

Antidepressant drugs
Mood-elevating drugs

Poliomyelitis

Contagious viral disease
Affects motor neurons
Causes paralysis and respiratory failure
Prevent with vaccination

Postpolio Syndrome (PPS)

Also known as postpoliomyelitis neuromuscular atrophy
Progressive muscle weakness
- Past history of paralytic polio

Symptoms

Muscle weakness and fatigability
- May include atrophy and muscle twitching

Treatment

Symptomatic
Maintenance of respiratory function

Guillain-Barré Syndrome

Also known as
- Idiopathic polyneuritis
- Acute inflammatory polyneuropathy
- Landry's ascending paralysis
Demyelination of peripheral nerves—acquired disease

Symptoms

Primary ascending motor paralysis
Variable sensory disturbances

Treatment

Supportive

Congenital Neurologic Disorders

Hydrocephalus

Excessive amounts of circulating cerebrospinal fluid in ventricles of brain
Circulation is impaired in brain or spinal cord
Compresses brain

Treatment

Surgical placement of a shunt

Spina Bifida (Fig. 12.3)

Developmental birth defect that causes incomplete development of spinal cord and its coverings
Vertebrae overlying open portions of spinal cord do not fully form and remain unfused and open
- Spina bifida occulta—may not be noticed, no protrusion through defect
- Spina bifida manifesta, which includes:

- Myelomeningocele (spina bifida cystica)
  - Meninges and spinal cord protrude through defect
- Meningocele
  - Meninges herniated through defect
Results in neurologic deficiencies

Treatment

Surgical repair

Mental Disorders

Schizophrenia

Variety of syndromes
Results in changes in brain
Hereditary factors are considered a cause
- Also, fetal brain damage caused by viral infections, complications of pregnancy, nutritional deficiencies
Stress usually precipitates onset

Symptoms

Delusions of persecution and/or grandeur
Disorganized thought
Repetitive behaviors
Behavior issues
Decreased speech
Decreased ability to solve problems
Loss of emotions/flat affect
Hallucinations
Types are based on characteristics

Treatment

Antipsychotic drugs
  Drugs have very unpleasant side effects, such as tardive dyskinesia, with symptoms as follows:
  - Excessive movement
  - Grimacing
  - Jerking
  - Tremors
  - Shuffling gait
  - Dry mouth
  - Blurred vision

Depression

Mood (sustained emotional state) disorder
Exact cause is unknown

Symptoms

Sadness
Hopelessness
Lethargy
Insomnia
Anorexia

Treatment

Antidepressant drugs
Electroconvulsive therapy

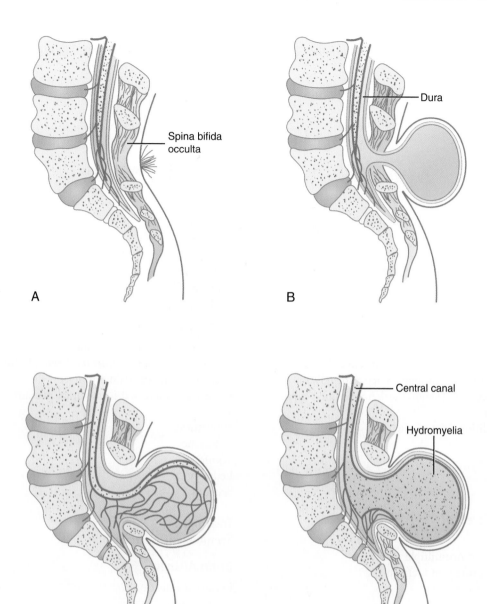

• **Figure 12.3 A.** Spina bifida occulta. **B.** Meningocele. **C.** Myelomeningocele. **D.** Myelocystocele or hydromyelia.

Central Nervous System (CNS) Disorders

Vascular Disorder

Transient Ischemic Attack (TIA)

Temporary reduction of blood flow to brain that produces strokelike symptoms but no lasting damage
  Often a warning sign before cerebrovascular accident

Symptoms

Depend on location of ischemia
• Usual recovery within 24 hours
No loss of consciousness
Slurred, indiscernible speech

May display muscle weakness in legs/arms
Paresthesia (numbness) of face
Mental confusion may be present
Repeated attacks common in the presence of atherosclerotic disease

Cerebrovascular Accident (CVA) or Stroke

Infarction of brain due to lack of blood/oxygen flow
  Necrosis of tissue with total occlusion of vessel

Causes

Atherosclerotic disease—thrombus formation
  Embolus
  Hemorrhage—arterial aneurysm

Symptoms

Depend on location of obstruction

- Thrombus
  - Gradual onset
  - Often occurs at rest
  - Intracranial pressure (ICP) minimal
  - Localized damage
- Embolus
  - Sudden onset
  - Occurs anytime
  - ICP minimal
  - Localized damage unless multiple emboli
- Hemorrhage
  - Sudden onset
  - Occurs most often with activity
  - ICP high
  - Widespread damage
  - May be fatal

Treatment

Anticoagulant drugs (clot dissolving) if caused by thrombus or embolus—tissue plasminogen activator (tPA)

Carotid endarterectomy (removes artherosclerotic plaque)

Oxygen treatment

Underlying condition treated, such as

- Hypertension
- Atherosclerosis
- Thrombus

Aneurysm—Cerebral

Dilation of artery

- May be localized or multiple

Rupture possible, often on exertion

- Fatal if rupture is massive

Symptoms

May display visual effects, such as

- Loss of visual fields
- Photophobia
- Diplopia
- Headache
- Confusion
- Slurred speech
- Weakness
- Stiff neck (nuchal rigidity)

Treatment

Dependent on diagnosis prior to rupture

Surgical intervention

Encephalitis

Infection of parenchymal tissue of brain or spinal cord

- Often viral

Accompanying inflammation

Usually results in some permanent damage

Symptoms

Stiff neck

Headaches

Vomiting

Fever

May have seizure

Lethargy

Some Types of Encephalitis

Herpes simplex

Lyme disease

West Nile fever

Western equine

Treatment

Symptomatic

Supportive

Reye's Syndrome

Associated with viral infection

- Especially when aspirin has been administered

Changes occur in brain and liver

- Leads to increased intracranial pressure

Symptoms

Headaches

Vomiting

Lethargy

Seizures

Treatment

Symptomatic treatment

Brain Abscess

Localized infection

Necrosis of tissue

Usually spread from infection elsewhere, such as ears or sinus

Symptoms

Neurologic deficiencies

Increased intracranial pressure

Treatment

Antibiotics for bacterial infections

Surgical drainage

Epilepsies

Chronic seizure disorder

Types

Partial Seizures (Focal)

State of altered focus but conscious—simple

Impaired consciousness—complex

Specialized epileptic seizures

Aura

- Auditory or visual sign that precedes a seizure

Generalized Seizures

Absence seizures—petit mal
- Brief loss of awareness
- Most common in children (febrile causation)

Tonic-clonic—grand mal or ictal event
- Loss of consciousness
- Alternate contraction and relaxation
- Incontinence
- No memory of seizure

Causes

Tumor
Hemorrhage
Trauma
Edema
Infection
Excessive cerebrospinal fluid
High fever

Treatment

Correct cause
Anticonvulsant drugs
Neurosurgery
Postictal event—after seizure—neurologic symptoms (weakness, etc.)

Trauma

Head Injury—Traumatic Brain Injury (TBI)

Concussion

Mild blow to head
Temporary axonal disturbances
    Grade 1: temporary confusion and amnesia (brief)
    Grade 2: memory loss for very recent events and confusion
    Grade 3: amnesia for recent events and disorientation (longer duration)
Results in reversible interference with brain function
- Recovery within 24 hours with no residual damage

Contusion

Bruising of brain
Force of blow determines outcome

Hematomas—Blood Accumulation (Clot)

Compresses surrounding structures

Classified based on location
- Epidural
  - Develops between dura and skull
- Subdural
  - Develops between dura and arachnoid
    - Development within 24 hours is acute
    - Development within a week is subacute
  - ICP increases with enlargement of hematoma
- Subarachnoid
  - Develops between pia and arachnoid
  - Blood mixes with cerebrospinal fluid
    - No localized hematoma forms

- Intracerebral
  - As a result of a contusion

Symptoms

Increased ICP
Others dependent on location and severity of injury

Treatment

Identification of the location of hematoma
Medications to decrease edema
Antibiotics
Surgical intervention—burr hole if necessary to decrease the ICP

Spinal Cord Injury

Result of trauma to vertebra, cord, ligaments, intervertebral disc

Vertebral Injuries Classified As
- Simple—affects spinous or transverse process
- Compression—anterior fracture of vertebrae
- Comminuted—vertebral body is shattered
- Dislocation—vertebrae are out of alignment
- Flexion injury in which hyperflexion compresses vertebra

Dislocation
Rotation

Symptoms

Depend on vertebral level and severity
Paralysis
Loss of sensation
Drop in blood pressure
Loss of bladder and rectal control
Decreased venous circulation

Treatment

Identification of area of injury
Immobilization
Corticosteroids to decrease edema
Bladder and bowel management
Rehabilitation

Tumors of Brain and Spinal Cord

Increases ICP
Life threatening
Rarely metastasize outside of central nervous system
Secondary brain tumors are common
Metastasis from lung or breast

Gliomas Common Type

Primary malignant tumor—encapsulated and invasive
Types based on cell from which tumor arises and location of tumor

Glioblastoma

Located in cerebral hemispheres (deep in white matter)
Highly aggressive

Oligodendrocytoma
Usually located in frontal lobes
Oligodendroblastoma, more aggressive form

Ependymoma
Located in ventricles
Most often occurs in children
Ependymoblastoma, more aggressive form

Astrocytoma
Located anywhere in brain and spinal cord
Invasive but slow growing

Pineal Region

Germ Cell Tumors
Usually in adolescents
Rare
Variable growth rate

Several Other Pineal Tumors
Pineocytoma
Teratoma
Germinoma

Blood Vessel

Angioma
Usually located in posterior cerebral hemispheres
Slow growing

Hemangioblastoma
Located in cerebellum
Slow growing

Medulloblastoma
Aggressive tumor
Located in posterior cerebellar vermis (fourth ventricle)

Meningioma
Originates in arachnoid
Slow growing

Pituitary Tumor
Related to aging
Slow growing
• Such as macroadenomas

Cranial Nerve Tumors
Neurilemmomas most common location: cranial nerve VIII
Slow growing
Metastatic

Spinal Cord Tumors
Symptoms are based on location of spinal compression
Intramedullary
• Originates in neural tissue
Extramedullary
• Originates outside the spinal cord
Metastatic tumors of spinal cord are more common
• Myeloma—marrow
• Lymphoma—lymph
• Carcinomas—lung, breast, prostate
Most common type of primary extramedullary tumor
• Meningiomas—anyplace in spine
• Neurofibromas—common in thoracic and lumbar regions

Chapter 12: Pathophysiology Quiz

(Quiz Answers Are Located in Appendix B)

1. Most common dementia is:
   a. Alzheimer's disease
   b. secondary
   c. nutritional degenerative disease
   d. Lou Gehrig's disease
2. MND stands for:
   a. maximal neuron disorder
   b. migrating niacin disorder
   c. motor neuron disease
   d. motor neuropathic disorder
3. Dopamine replacement is useful in treating:
   a. multiple sclerosis
   b. Parkinson's disease
   c. Huntington's disease
   d. CVA
4. Condition in which primary symptoms are muscle weakness and fatigability:
   a. amyotrophic lateral sclerosis
   b. multiple sclerosis
   c. dyskinesis
   d. myasthenia gravis
5. Another name for idiopathic polyneuritis is:
   a. Guillain-Barré syndrome
   b. multiple sclerosis
   c. amyotrophic lateral sclerosis
   d. postpolio syndrome
6. This condition is thought to be caused by genetic factors and, possibly, fetal brain damage:
   a. Parkinson's
   b. schizophrenia
   c. spina bifida
   d. Guillain-Barré syndrome

7. This condition is associated with viral infection, especially when aspirin has been administered:
   a. Reye's syndrome
   b. Guillain-Barré syndrome
   c. Lou Gehrig's disease
   d. Conn's syndrome
8. Concussion is a mild blow to the head in which recovery is expected within _____.
   a. 12 hours
   b. 24 hours
   c. 48 hours
   d. 1 week

9. ICP means:
   a. intercranial pressure
   b. intracranial pressure
   c. interior cranial pressure
   d. intensive cranial pressure
10. In this type of hematoma, blood mixes with cerebrospinal fluid:
   a. epidural
   b. subdural
   c. subarachnoid
   d. intracerebral

13

Senses

ANATOMY AND TERMINOLOGY

Sight	Eyes
Hearing	Ears
Smell	Nose
Taste	Tongue
Touch	Skin

Sight: Three Layers of Eye (Fig. 13.1)

Cornea (Outer Layer)

Fibrous, transparent layer that extends over dome of eye
Refracts (bends) light to focus on receptor cells (posterior eye)
Avascular (nourished by aqueous humor and tears)

Sclera (Extension of Outer Layer)

White of eye

Extends from edge of cornea (anterior surface) to optic nerve (posterior surface)
• Lies over choroid

Choroid (Middle Layer)

Vascular layer between sclera and retina
• Supplies nutrients

Retina (Inner Layer)

Contains rods and cones
• Rods provide night and peripheral vision
• Cones provide day and color vision and are stimulated by primary colors of red, green, and blue

Conjunctiva

Covers anterior sclera and lines eyelid (contiguous layer)

Lens

Behind pupil
Lens is connected by zonules to ciliary body
Ciliary body muscles cause lens to change shape to refract light rays (accommodation)

Fluids

Aqueous humor (front of lens)—watery substance secreted by ciliary body

Maintains shape of front portion of eye
Refracts light
Nourishes cornea

Vitreous humor (behind lens)—gel-like substance (not readily re-formed) filling large space behind lens

Maintains shape of eyeball
Refracts light

Optic Nerve

Light rays from rods and cones travel from eye to brain via optic nerve

Optic nerve meets retina in optic disc (no light receptors)—blind spot
Pathway of light ray
• Cornea—refraction site
• Anterior chamber (aqueous humor)—refraction site
• Pupil
• Lens—refraction site
• Posterior chamber (vitreous humor)—refraction site
• Retina (rods and cones)
• Optic nerve fibers—nerve cells act as a cable connecting the eye with the brain
• Optic chiasm
• Thalamus
• Cerebral cortex (occipital lobe)—light is interpreted

Hearing, Three Divisions of Ear

External Ear

Auricle (pinna)—sound waves enter ear
External auditory canal—tunnel from auricle to middle ear

Middle Ear

Begins with tympanic membrane (eardrum)

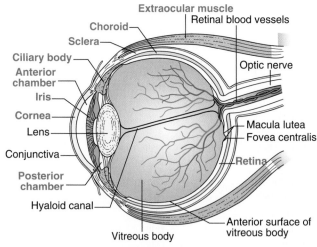

• **Figure 13.1** Eye and ocular adnexa.

Ossicles—small bones conducting sound waves from middle to inner ear
• Malleus
• Incus
• Stapes
Eustachian tube—leads to pharynx

Inner Ear (Labyrinth)

Vestibule

Semicircular canals/vestibular apparatus
Cochlea contains perilymph and endolymph (liquids through which sound waves are conducted)
• Organ of Corti—auditory receptor area
  Auditory nerve—electrical impulse is conducted to cerebral cortex for interpretation (hearing)

Pathway of sound vibration (exterior to brain)
• Pinna
• External auditory canal
• Tympanic membrane
• Malleus
• Incus
• Stapes

• Oval window
• Cochlea
• Auditory fluid/receptors in organ of Corti
• Auditory nerve
• Cerebral cortex

Smell

Olfactory Sense Receptors

Located in nasal cavity

Closely related to sense of taste
Cranial nerve I

Taste

Gustatory sense—sweet, salty, and sour differentiated
  Taste buds located on anterior portion of tongue
  Cranial nerves VII and IX

Touch

Mechanoreceptors

Widely distributed throughout body

React to touch and pressure
• Meissner corpuscles (touch)
• Pacinian corpuscles (pressure)

Proprioceptors

Position and orientation

Dysfunctions
• Vestibular nystagmus—involuntary movement of eyes
• Vertigo—sense of spinning/dizziness

Thermoreceptors

Under skin
  Sense temperature changes

Nociceptors

Pain sensors
  In skin and internal organs

TABLE 13-1

Combining Forms

Combining Form	Meaning	Combining Form	Meaning
1. ambly/o	dim, dullness	20. opt/o	eye, vision
2. aque/o	water	21. optic/o	eye
3. audi/o	hearing	22. ot/o	ear
4. blephar/o	eyelid	23. palpebr/o	eyelid
5. conjunctiv/o	conjunctiva	24. papill/o	optic nerve
6. cor/o, core/o	pupil	25. phac/o	eye lens
7. corne/o	cornea	26. phak/o	eye lens
8. cycl/o	ciliary body	27. phot/o	light
9. dacry/o	tear	28. presby/o	old age
10. essi/o, esthesi/o	sensation	29. pupill/o	pupil
11. glauc/o	gray	30. retin/o	retina
12. ir/o	iris	31. scler/o	sclera
13. irid/o	iris	32. scot/o	darkness
14. kerat/o	cornea	33. staped/o	stapes
15. lacrim/o	tear	34. tympan/o	eardrum
16. mi/o	smaller	35. uve/o	uvea
17. myring/o	eardrum	36. vitre/o	glassy
18. ocul/o	eye	37. xer/o	dry
19. ophthalm/o	eye		

TABLE 13-2

Prefixes

Prefix	Meaning
1. audi-	hearing
2. eso-	inward
3. exo-	outward

TABLE 13-3

Suffixes

Suffix	Meaning
1. -opia	vision
2. -omia	smell
3. -tropia	to turn

TABLE 13-4

Medical Abbreviations

Abbreviation	Meaning
1. AD	right ear
2. AS	left ear
3. AU	both ears
4. H or E	hemorrhage or exudate
5. IO	intraocular
6. IOL	intraocular lens
7. OD	right eye
8. OS	left eye
9. OU	each eye
10. PERL	pupils equal and reactive to light
11. PERRL	pupils equal, round, and reactive to light
12. PERRLA	pupils equal, round, and reactive to light and accommodation
13. REM	rapid eye movement
14. TM	tympanic membrane

TABLE 13-5

Medical Terms

Term	Meaning	Term	Meaning
Anterior segment	Those parts of eye in the front of and including lens (cornea, iris, ciliary body, aqueous humor)	Labyrinth	Inner connecting cavities, such as internal ear
		Labyrinthitis	Inner ear inflammation
Apicectomy	Excision of a portion of temporal bone	Lacrimal	Related to tears
Astigmatism	Condition in which refractive surfaces of eye are unequal	Mastoidectomy	Removal of mastoid bone
		Ménière's disease	Condition that causes dizziness, ringing in ears, and deafness
Aural atresia	Congenital absence of external auditory canal	Myopia	Nearsightedness, eyeball too long from front to back
Blepharitis	Inflammation of eyelid	Myringotomy	Incision into tympanic membrane
Cataract	Opaque covering on or in lens	Ocular adnexa	Orbit, extraocular muscles, and eyelid
Chalazion	Granuloma around sebaceous gland	Ophthalmoscopy	Examination of the interior of eye by means of a scope, also known as fundoscopy
Cholesteatoma	Tumor that forms in middle ear		
Conjunctiva	The lining of eyelids and covering of anterior sclera	Otitis media	Noninfectious inflammation of middle ear; serous otitis media produces liquid drainage (not purulent), and suppurative otitis media produces purulent (pus) matter
Dacryocystitis	Blocked, inflamed infection of nasolacrimal duct		
Dacryostenosis	Narrowing of lacrimal duct		
Ectropion	Eversion (outward sagging) of eyelid		
Entropion	Inversion of eyelid (lashes rubbing cornea)	Otoscope	Instrument used to examine ear
Enucleation	Removal of an organ or organs from a body cavity	Papilledema	Swelling of optic disc (papilla)
		Posterior segment	Those parts of eye behind lens
Episclera	Connective covering of sclera	Ptosis	Drooping of upper eyelid
Exenteration	Removal of an organ all in one piece, commonly used to describe radical excision	Sclera	Outer covering of eye
		Strabismus	Extraocular muscle deviation resulting in unequal visual axes
Exophthalmos	Protrusion of eyeball	Tarsorrhaphy	Suturing together of eyelids
Exostosis	Bony growth	Tinnitus	Ringing in the ears
Fenestration	Creation of a new opening in inner wall of middle ear	Transmastoid	Creates an opening in mastoid for drainage antrostomy
Glaucoma	Eye diseases that are characterized by an increase of intraocular pressure	Tympanolysis	Freeing of adhesions of the tympanic membrane
		Tympanometry	Test of the inner ear using air pressure
Hordeolum	Stye—infection of sebaceous gland (nodule on lid margin)	Tympanostomy	Insertion of ventilation tube into tympanum
Hyperopia	Farsightedness, eyeball is too short from front to back	Uveal	Vascular tissue of the choroid, ciliary body, and iris
Keratomalacia	Softening of cornea associated with a deficiency of vitamin A	Vertigo	Dizziness
Keratoplasty	Surgical repair of the cornea	Xanthelasma	Yellow plaque on eyelid (lipid disorder)

Chapter 13: Anatomy and Terminology Quiz

(Quiz Answers Are Located in Appendix B)

1. The middle layer of the eye:
   a. sclera
   b. retina
   c. episclera
   d. choroid
2. The covering of the anterior sclera and lining of eyelid:
   a. aqueous humor
   b. ossicles
   c. vitreous
   d. conjunctiva
3. Which of the following is NOT a bone of the middle ear?
   a. cochlea
   b. stapes
   c. malleus
   d. incus
4. This cranial nerve controls the sense of smell:
   a. I
   b. II
   c. III
   d. IV
5. Which of the following is NOT part of the inner ear?
   a. pinna
   b. vestibule
   c. semicircular canals
   d. cochlea
6. These receptors react to touch:
   a. nociceptors
   b. mechanoreceptors
   c. proprioceptors
   d. thermoreceptors
7. These receptors react to position and orientation:
   a. nociceptors
   b. mechanoreceptors
   c. proprioceptors
   d. thermoreceptors
8. Combining form meaning "eyelid":
   a. aque/o
   b. blephar/o
   c. optic/o
   d. uve/o
9. Combining form meaning "eye lens":
   a. cor/o
   b. irid/o
   c. ocul/o
   d. phak/o
10. Abbreviation meaning the pupils are equal, round, and reactive to light and accommodation:
    a. PERRLA
    b. PERRL
    c. PERL
    d. PURL

PATHOPHYSIOLOGY

Eye

Visual Disturbances

Astigmatism

Irregular curvature of refractive surfaces (cornea or lens) of eye

Can be congenital or acquired (as a result of disease or trauma)

Image is distorted

Treatment

Corrected with cylindrical lens

Diplopia

Double vision

Amblyopia

Dimness of vision—impairment of vision without detectable organic lesion of eye

Hyperopia

Farsightedness

Shortened eyeball
• Can see objects in distance, not close up

Treatment

Corrected with convex lens

Presbyopia

Age-related farsightedness

Treatment

Magnification (reading glasses or bifocals)

Myopia

Nearsightedness

Elongated eyeball
• Can see objects up close, not in distance

Treatment

Corrected with concave lens thicker at periphery

Nystagmus—Unilateral or Bilateral

Rapid, involuntary eye movements

Movements can be
- Vertical
- Horizontal
- Rotational
- Combination of above

Cause

Brain tumor or inner ear disease
Normal in newborns
Due to underlying condition or adverse effect of drug
Various types, such as
- Vestibular nystagmus
- Rhythmic eye movements

Strabismus

Cross-eyed

Due to muscle weakness or neurologic defect
Forms of strabismus
- Hypotropia (downward deviation of one eye)
- Hypertropia (upward deviation of one eye)
- Estropia (one eye turns inward)
- Exotropia (one eye turns outward)

Treatment
- Eye exercises/patching of normal eye
- Surgery to establish muscle balance

Infections

Conjunctivitis (Pink Eye)

Inflammation of conjunctival lining of eyelid or covering of sclera

Due to
- Infection
- Allergy
- Irritation

Treatment
- Varies with cause
- Antibiotic eye drops

Hordeolum (Stye)

Bacterial infection of eyelid hair follicle
- Usually Staphylococcus
- Results in mass on eyelid

Treatment
- Antibiotics
- Incision and drainage may be necessary

Keratitis

Corneal inflammation

May be caused by herpes simplex virus, contact lens issue, or exposure
Causes tearing and photophobia, pain

Macular Degeneration

Destruction of fovea centralis
- Fovea centralis is small pit in center of retina (fovea centralis retinae)

Usually age related—leading cause of blindness in elderly
Results from exposure to ultraviolet rays or drugs
Also may have a genetic component
Central vision is lost
Two types of macular degeneration
- Wet—development of new vascularization and leaking blood vessels near macula
- Dry (85% of cases)—atrophy and degeneration of retinal cells and deposits of drusen (clumps of extracellular waste)

Treatment

None for "dry" macular degeneration

Surgical intervention with laser for "net" macular degeneration to coagulate leaking vessels; success is limited
Medications

Detached Retina

Retinal tear—two layers of retina separate from each other
- Vitreous humor then leaks behind retina
- Retina then pulls away from choroid

Results in increasing blind spot in visual field
Condition is painless
Pressure continues to build if left unattended
Final result is blindness

Treatment

Surgical intervention with laser to repair tear (emergency/ urgency)—photocoagulation for small tears
Scleral buckle for large retinal detachments
Pneumatic retinopexy for medium to large retinal detachment. Gas bubble is injected into vitreous cavity; pressure to tear resulting in retinal reattachment.

Cataracts

Lens becomes opaque with protein aggregates

Classified by Morphology

Size
Shape
Location
Also may be classified by etiology (cause) or time cataract occurs

Examples of Classification

Congenital cataract
- Bilateral opacity present at birth
- Also known as developmental cataract

Heat cataract
- Also known as glassblowers' cataract
- Caused by exposure to radiation

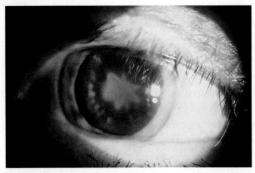

• **Figure 13.2** A concussive injury that resulted in a traumatic cataract.

Traumatic cataract (Fig. 13.2)
• Result of injury to eye
Senile cataract
• Age related
• Usually forms on anterior lens

Symptoms
Blurring of vision
Halos around lights

Treatment
Removal of cataract with intraocular lens implantation
If no intraocular lens implant, then glasses or contact lenses for refraction

Glaucoma
Excess accumulation of intraocular aqueous humor
• High pressure results in decreased blood flow and edema
• Damages retinal cells and optic nerve

Stages of Glaucoma
Mild, moderate, severe
• Based on visual field loss caused by disease

Narrow-Angle Glaucoma
Acute type of glaucoma

Rapid onset is painful

Chronic Glaucoma
Also known as
• Wide-angle glaucoma
• Open-angle glaucoma
Asymptomatic
Diagnosed in eye examination using tonometry to test anterior chamber pressure and visual field exams

Treatment
Medications that decrease output of aqueous humor and decrease intraocular pressure (IOP)
Laser treatment to provide drainage

Ear

Infections

Otitis Media
Infection or inflammation of middle ear cavity

Chronic infection produces adhesions
Results in loss of hearing
Often occurs in children in combination with URI (upper respiratory infection)
Causes severe ear pain (otalgia)

Treatment
Antibiotics
Surgical intervention with placement of tubes to allow for drainage
• Useful in patients with recurrent infection

Otitis Externa
Also known as swimmer's ear

Infection of external auditory canal and pinna (exterior ear)
Caused by bacteria or fungus
Results in pain and discharge

Treatment
Antibiotic
Encouraged to keep ear dry

Hearing Loss

Conductive Hearing Loss
Due to a defect of sound-conducting apparatus
• Accumulation of wax
• Scar tissue on tympanic membrane
Also known as:
• Transmission hearing loss
• Conduction deafness

Treatment
Hearing aids

Sensorineural
Due to a lesion of cochlea or central neural pathways

Also known as
• Perceptive deafness
May be divided into
• Cochlear hearing loss
  • Due to a defect in receptor or transducing mechanisms of cochlea
• Retrocochlear hearing loss
  • Due to defect located proximal to cochlea (vestibulocochlear nerve or auditory area of brain)
Presbycusis is age-related sensorineural hearing loss

Treatment
- Medication, implant, surgery

Ototoxic Hearing Loss

Caused by ingestion of toxic substance
Also known as toxic deafness

Ménière's Disease

Inner ear disturbance
Also known as idiopathic endolymphatic hydrops
Cause unknown
Common cause of vertigo (dizziness)
Other symptoms include hearing loss and tinnitus

Chapter 13: Pathophysiology Quiz

(Quiz Answers Are Located in Appendix B)

1. This condition can be acquired or congenital and results in an irregular curvature of the refractive surfaces of the eye:
   a. diplopia
   b. hyperopia
   c. nystagmus
   d. astigmatism
2. In this condition, the eyeball is shorter than normal and results in being able to see objects in the distance but not close up:
   a. diplopia
   b. hyperopia
   c. nystagmus
   d. astigmatism
3. Rapid, involuntary eye movement is the predominant symptom of this condition:
   a. diplopia
   b. hyperopia
   c. nystagmus
   d. astigmatism
4. Age-related farsightedness is:
   a. presbyopia
   b. hyperopia
   c. diplopia
   d. myopia
5. Another name for a stye is:
   a. keratitis
   b. hordeolum
   c. hyperopia
   d. strabismus
6. An inflammation of the cornea that is caused by herpes simplex virus is:
   a. keratitis
   b. hordeolum
   c. hyperopia
   d. strabismus
7. In this condition there is destruction of the fovea centralis:
   a. macular degeneration
   b. detached retina
   c. glaucoma
   d. cataract
8. This is an infection that occurs in the middle ear cavity:
   a. otitis media
   b. otitis externa
   c. ototoxic hearing loss
   d. retrocochlear hearing loss
9. The hearing loss that can be due to a lesion on the cochlea is:
   a. conductive
   b. sensorineural
   c. ototoxic
   d. transmission
10. This condition is also known as perceptive deafness:
    a. conductive
    b. sensorineural
    c. otitis media
    d. transmission

PART 2

Physician-based Reimbursement Issues

14

Physician-based Reimbursement Issues

Your Responsibility

Ensure accurate coding based upon services provided and documented

Obtain correct reimbursement for services rendered

Recognize upcoding (maximizing) or downcoding is never appropriate

Stay abreast of current and changing
- Reimbursement policies
- Coding guidelines

Health Insurance Portability and Accountability Act of 1996 (HIPAA)
- HIPAA changes are based on various resources such as
  - Centers for Medicare and Medicaid Policy Manuals
  - National Correct Coding Guidelines

Population Changing = Reimbursement Change

According to the U.S. Census Bureau (www.census.gov/prod/2014pubs/p25-1141.pdf, www.census.gov/content/dam/Census/library/publications/2014/demo/p25-1140.pdf):
- By 2030, more than 20% of U.S. residents projected to be aged 65+.
- Population aged 65+ is projected to be 83.7 million by 2050.
  - Almost double from 43.1 million in 2012.
  Medicare primarily for elderly

Medicare

Those Covered

Originally established for those 65 and older; implemented in 1966

Disabled and permanent renal disease (end-stage renal disease or transplant) patients added in 1972

Persons covered are called "beneficiaries"

Basic Structure

Medicare program established in 1965

Part A: Hospital and Institutional Care Coverage
- This is the part that most inpatient coders will work with

Part B: Supplemental—nonhospital

Example: Physician services and medical equipment
- This is the part that most outpatient coders will work with

Part C: Medicare Advantage Organizations (MAO) plans—combines parts A and B; added in 1997 through Balanced Budget Act

Plans include

Medicare Health Maintenance Organization (HMO)

Medicare Preferred Provider Organizations (PPO)

Medicare Private Fee-for-Service (PFFS)

Medicare Special Needs Plans (SNPs)

Medicare Medical Savings Account (MSA)

HMO Point of Service (HMOPOS)

Part D: Prescription Drug Plan (PDP)

Plans include
- Medicare Advantage Prescription Drug Plan (MA-PD)
- Private prescription drug plans (PDPs)
- Premium paid by beneficiary

Officiating Office

Department of Health and Human Services (DHHS) (www.hhs.gov)

Delegated to Centers for Medicare and Medicaid Services (CMS) (formerly HCFA)
- CMS runs Medicare and Medicaid
- CMS delegates daily operation to Medicare Administrative Contractors (MACs)
- MACs are usually insurance companies
- The Medicare Prescription Drug Improvement and Modernization Act of 2003 allowed CMS to reduce the 48 Fiscal Intermediaries to 15 Medicare Administrative Contractors (MACs)
  - CMS further reduced the total number of jurisdictions to 12 MACs and 4 DME MACs, with no plans for further reductions

Funding for Medicare

Social Security taxes
Equal match from government
CMS sends money to MACs
MACs handle paperwork and pay claims

Medicare Covers

Medical Necessity and Frequency Limitations

Defined in
- LCDs (Local Coverage Determinations)
- NCDs (National Coverage Determinations)

Beneficiary Pays

20% of Medicare-approved amount after deductible is met
    Part A and B annual deductible

Medicare Pays

Part A all covered costs except deductible
Part B 80% of Medicare-allowed amount of covered services
    after deductible is met
Preventive Services
- Initial Preventative Physical Examination (IPPE) (G0402)—no deductible (Welcome to Medicare)
- Annual Wellness Visit (AWV) co-pay and deductible waived in all POS (G0438—first visit; G0439—subsequent visit)
- Ultrasound Screening for Abdominal Aortic Aneurysm (AAA) (G0389)—no deductible
- Cardiovascular Disease Screenings (80061)—Lipid Panel; 82465—Cholesterol; 83718—Lipoprotein; 84478—Triglycerides—no copayment/coinsurance, no deductible
- Diabetes Screening Tests (82947)—Glucose, quantitative, blood (except reagent strip)
- 82950—Glucose, post-glucose dose (includes glucose); 82951—Glucose Tolerance Test (GTT), three specimens (includes glucose)—no copayment/coinsurance, no deductible
- Screening PAP—no deductible
- Screening pelvic exam—no deductible
- Screening mammogram—no deductible

Participating Providers

Signed Quality Improvement Organization (QIO) agreement with MACs to accept assignment on Medicare claims

Provider agrees to accept the Medicare Fee Schedule amount as payment in full
- Accepting assignment
Block 27 CMS-1500 (Fig. 14.1)

National Provider Identification (NPI)

10-digit number assigned to all covered health care providers
- Designed to provide one unique identifier for all providers as part of HIPAA

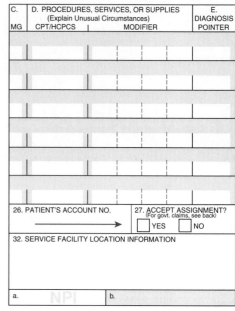

• **Figure 14.1** Block 27, Accept Assignment on the CMS-1500 (02/02), Health Insurance Claim Form.

- Eliminates the need for additional numbers by other carriers

Good Reasons to Participate

- Significant decrease in reimbursement amount for non-participating providers
- Participating providers receive approximately 5% more from Medicare than non-PAR providers
- Check sent directly from MACs to QIO providers
- Faster claims processing
- Provider names listed in QIO directory
- Sent to all beneficiaries

Part A, Hospital Inpatient

Hospitals submit charges electronically or, if an exempt facility, on CMS-1450 (UB-04) form
- MS-DRG basis for payment for Medicare patients
- Using principal diagnosis or principal procedure

Covered In-Hospital Expenses

Semiprivate room
Meals and special diets in hospital
All medically necessary services

Noncovered In-Hospital Expenses

Personal convenience items

Example: Slippers, TV
Any service or procedure determined to be "not medically necessary"

Types of Covered Expenses

Rehabilitation

Skilled nursing
Some personal convenience items for long-term illness or disabilities
Home health visits
Hospice care
Not automatically covered
- Must meet certain criteria

Part B, Supplemental

Part B pays services and supplies not covered under Part A

Not automatic
Beneficiaries purchase
- Pay monthly premiums

Types of Items Covered in Part B
Physician services
Outpatient hospital services
Ambulatory surgical services
Home health care
Medically necessary supplies and equipment

Coding for Medicare Part B Services
Three coding systems used to report Part B
- CPT (procedures and service)
- HCPCS (drugs, supplies, equipment, and special services)
- ICD-10-CM (diagnosis codes)

Electronic Transactions

HIPAA
- Created to govern health care portability
- Electronic data interchange (EDI)
  Transactions
- Activities involving transfer of health care information
  Transmission
- Movement of electronic data between two entities
  Today 99% Part A and 95% Part B claims filed electronically
- Using Electronic Remittance Advice (ERA)
  The software that supports electronic transmissions
- 5010 version

National Correct Coding Initiative (NCCI)

Developed by the Centers for Medicare and Medicaid Services to
- Promote national correct coding methods
- Control improper coding that results in inappropriate payment of Part B claims (physician) and hospital outpatient claims
- Complete list may be found at www.cms.gov/National CorrectCodInitEd/

Unbundling

CMS defines unbundling as

- Billing multiple procedure codes for a group of procedures that are covered by a single comprehensive code
  Example: Dividing one service into parts and coding for each part separately, such as:
  - Reporting bilateral procedures unilaterally
  Reporting 31231, bilateral or unilateral diagnostic nasal endoscopy, with modifier -50 (bilateral procedure), rather than correctly as 31231, no modifier
  - Downcoding to use an additional code
  Reporting one of two lacerations of the same complexity and site with a lesser code to enable reporting two separate repairs
  - Separating the surgical approach from the major surgical service
  Coding separately for a thoracic approach during an anterior spine procedure

Federal Register

Government publishes updates, revisions (changes), deletions in laws (Fig. 14.2) (www.federalregister.gov/ or https://www.govinfo.gov/)
  November and December issues contain major outpatient facility updates

Quality Improvement Organizations (QIO)

Part of U.S. Department of Health and Human Services (HHS) strategy for "providing better care and better health at a lower cost"
Core functions:
- To ensure quality of patient care
- Protect beneficiaries by addressing complaints and appeals
- Ensure Medicare pays only for reasonable and necessary services

Two Types of QIOs
Beneficiary and Family Centered Care (BFCC)
- Assists beneficiaries directly
- Quality of care reviews
- Filing complaints or appeals

Quality Innovation Network (QIN)
- Organizes beneficiaries, providers, and community members for improvement initiatives
- Data-driven approach
- Focus on safety, health quality, and care coordination

Resource-Based Relative Value Scale (RBRVS)

Physician payment reform implemented in 1992
Prior to reform, physicians were paid lowest of
- Physician's charge for service
- Physician's customary charge
- Prevailing charge in locality

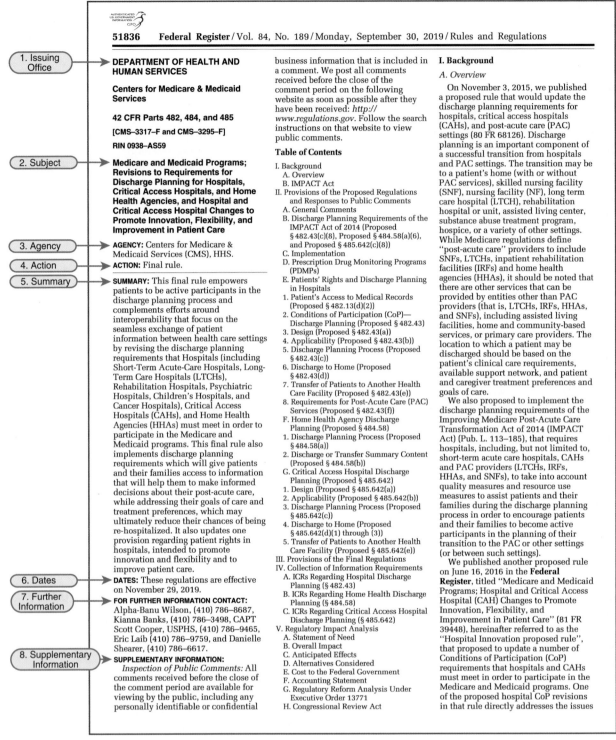

51836 Federal Register / Vol. 84, No. 189 / Monday, September 30, 2019 / Rules and Regulations

1. Issuing Office →

DEPARTMENT OF HEALTH AND HUMAN SERVICES

Centers for Medicare & Medicaid Services

42 CFR Parts 482, 484, and 485

[CMS–3317–F and CMS–3295–F]

RIN 0938–AS59

2. Subject →

Medicare and Medicaid Programs; Revisions to Requirements for Discharge Planning for Hospitals, Critical Access Hospitals, and Home Health Agencies, and Hospital and Critical Access Hospital Changes to Promote Innovation, Flexibility, and Improvement in Patient Care

3. Agency →

AGENCY: Centers for Medicare & Medicaid Services (CMS), HHS.

4. Action →

ACTION: Final rule.

5. Summary →

SUMMARY: This final rule empowers patients to be active participants in the discharge planning process and complements efforts around interoperability that focus on the seamless exchange of patient information between health care settings by revising the discharge planning requirements that Hospitals (including Short-Term Acute-Care Hospitals, Long-Term Care Hospitals (LTCHs), Rehabilitation Hospitals, Psychiatric Hospitals, Children's Hospitals, and Cancer Hospitals), Critical Access Hospitals (CAHs), and Home Health Agencies (HHAs) must meet in order to participate in the Medicare and Medicaid programs. This final rule also implements discharge planning requirements which will give patients and their families access to information that will help them to make informed decisions about their post-acute care, while addressing their goals of care and treatment preferences, which may ultimately reduce their chances of being re-hospitalized. It also updates one provision regarding patient rights in hospitals, intended to promote innovation and flexibility and to improve patient care.

6. Dates →

DATES: These regulations are effective on November 29, 2019.

7. Further Information →

FOR FURTHER INFORMATION CONTACT:
Alpha-Banu Wilson, (410) 786–8687, Kianna Banks, (410) 786–3498, CAPT Scott Cooper, USPHS, (410) 786–9465, Eric Laib (410) 786–9759, and Danielle Shearer, (410) 786–6617.

8. Supplementary Information →

SUPPLEMENTARY INFORMATION:
Inspection of Public Comments: All comments received before the close of the comment period are available for viewing by the public, including any personally identifiable or confidential business information that is included in a comment. We post all comments received before the close of the comment period on the following website as soon as possible after they have been received: *http://www.regulations.gov.* Follow the search instructions on that website to view public comments.

Table of Contents

I. Background
  A. Overview
  B. IMPACT Act
II. Provisions of the Proposed Regulations and Responses to Public Comments
  A. General Comments
  B. Discharge Planning Requirements of the IMPACT Act of 2014 (Proposed § 482.43(c)(8), Proposed § 484.58(a)(6), and Proposed § 485.642(c)(8))
  C. Implementation
  D. Prescription Drug Monitoring Programs (PDMPs)
  E. Patients' Rights and Discharge Planning in Hospitals
  1. Patient's Access to Medical Records (Proposed § 482.13(d)(2))
  2. Conditions of Participation (CoP)—Discharge Planning (Proposed § 482.43)
  3. Design (Proposed § 482.43(a))
  4. Applicability (Proposed § 482.43(b))
  5. Discharge Planning Process (Proposed § 482.43(c))
  6. Discharge to Home (Proposed § 482.43(d))
  7. Transfer of Patients to Another Health Care Facility (Proposed § 482.43(e))
  8. Requirements for Post-Acute Care (PAC) Services (Proposed § 482.43(f))
  F. Home Health Agency Discharge Planning (Proposed § 484.58)
  1. Discharge Planning Process (Proposed § 484.58(a))
  2. Discharge or Transfer Summary Content (Proposed § 484.58(b))
  G. Critical Access Hospital Discharge Planning (Proposed § 485.642)
  1. Design (Proposed § 485.642(a))
  2. Applicability (Proposed § 485.642(b))
  3. Discharge Planning Process (Proposed § 485.642(c))
  4. Discharge to Home (Proposed § 485.642(d)(1) through (3))
  5. Transfer of Patients to Another Health Care Facility (Proposed § 485.642(e))
III. Provisions of the Final Regulations
IV. Collection of Information Requirements
  A. ICRs Regarding Hospital Discharge Planning (§ 482.43)
  B. ICRs Regarding Home Health Discharge Planning (§ 484.58)
  C. ICRs Regarding Critical Access Hospital Discharge Planning (§ 485.642)
V. Regulatory Impact Analysis
  A. Statement of Need
  B. Overall Impact
  C. Anticipated Effects
  D. Alternatives Considered
  E. Cost to the Federal Government
  F. Accounting Statement
  G. Regulatory Reform Analysis Under Executive Order 13771
  H. Congressional Review Act

I. Background

A. Overview

On November 3, 2015, we published a proposed rule that would update the discharge planning requirements for hospitals, critical access hospitals (CAHs), and post-acute care (PAC) settings (80 FR 68126). Discharge planning is an important component of a successful transition from hospitals and PAC settings. The transition may be to a patient's home (with or without PAC services), skilled nursing facility (SNF), nursing facility (NF), long term care hospital (LTCH), rehabilitation hospital or unit, assisted living center, substance abuse treatment program, hospice, or a variety of other settings. While Medicare regulations define "post-acute care" providers to include SNFs, LTCHs, inpatient rehabilitation facilities (IRFs) and home health agencies (HHAs), it should be noted that there are other services that can be provided by entities other than PAC providers (that is, LTCHs, IRFs, HHAs, and SNFs), including assisted living facilities, home and community-based services, or primary care providers. The location to which a patient may be discharged should be based on the patient's clinical care requirements, available support network, and patient and caregiver treatment preferences and goals of care.

We also proposed to implement the discharge planning requirements of the Improving Medicare Post-Acute Care Transformation Act of 2014 (IMPACT Act) (Pub. L. 113–185), that requires hospitals, including, but not limited to, short-term acute care hospitals, CAHs and PAC providers (LTCHs, IRFs, HHAs, and SNFs), to take into account quality measures and resource use measures to assist patients and their families during the discharge planning process in order to encourage patients and their families to become active participants in the planning of their transition to the PAC or other settings (or between such settings).

We published another proposed rule on June 16, 2016 in the **Federal Register**, titled "Medicare and Medicaid Programs; Hospital and Critical Access Hospital (CAH) Changes to Promote Innovation, Flexibility, and Improvement in Patient Care" (81 FR 39448), hereinafter referred to as the "Hospital Innovation proposed rule", that proposed to update a number of Conditions of Participation (CoP) requirements that hospitals and CAHs must meet in order to participate in the Medicare and Medicaid programs. One of the proposed hospital CoP revisions in that rule directly addresses the issues

• **Figure 14.2** Example of page from the *Federal Register*.

National Fee Schedule (NFS)

RBRVS payment method
Termed Medicare Fee Schedule (MFS)
Payment 80% of MFS, after patient deductible
Used for physicians and suppliers

Relative Value Units (RVUs)

Assigns national unit values to each CPT code
  Local adjustments made
• Work and skill required
• Overhead costs

- Malpractice costs
  Often referred to as fee schedule
  Annually, CMS updates RVU based on national and local factors

Medicare Fraud and Abuse

Program established by Medicare
- To decrease and eliminate fraud and abuse
  Beneficiary signatures on file
- Service, charges submitted without need for patient signature
Presents opportunity for fraud

Fraud

Intentional deception to benefit

Example: Submitting for services not provided
Anyone who submits for Medicare services can be violator
- Physicians
- Hospitals
- Laboratories
- Billing services
- YOU

Fraud Can Be

Billing for services not provided
Misrepresenting diagnosis or CPT/HCPCS codes
Kickbacks
Unbundling services
Falsifying medical necessity
Systematic waiver of copayment or deductible

Office of the Inspector General (OIG)

Develops and publishes Work Plan monthly
(https://oig.hhs.gov/reports-and-publications/workplan/index.asp)
Outlines Medicare monitoring program
MACs monitor those areas identified in plan

Complaints of Fraud or Abuse

Submitted orally or in writing to MACs or OIG

Allegations made by anyone against anyone
Allegations followed up by MACs or OIG

Abuse

Generally involves
- Impropriety
- Lack of medical necessity for services reported
Review takes place after claim submitted
- MACs do historical review of claims

Kickbacks

Bribe or rebate for referring patient for any service covered by Medicare

Any personal-gain kickback
A felony
- $25,000 fine or
- 5 years in jail or
- Both

Protect Yourself

Use your common sense

Submit only truthful and accurate claims
- Stay current with all coding changes
If you are unsure about charges, services, or procedures
- Check with physician or supervisor

Managed Health Care

Network health care providers that offer health care services under one organization

Group hospitals, physicians, or other providers
Majority of people with health care coverage are covered by a Managed Health Care Organization (e.g., HMO, PPO, POS)

Managed Care Organizations

Responsible for health care services to an enrolled group or person
Coordinate various health care services
Negotiate with providers and groups

Preferred Provider Organization (PPO)

Providers form network to offer health care services as group
Enrollees who seek health care outside PPO pay more

Point of Service (POS)
In-network or out-of-network providers may be used
Benefits are paid at a higher rate to in-network providers
Subscribers are not limited to providers, but to amount covered by plan

Health Maintenance Organization (HMO)
Total package health care
Out-of-pocket expenses minimal
Assigned physician acts as gatekeeper to refer patient to outside organization

TABLE 14-1

Reimbursement Terminology

Term	Meaning	Term	Meaning
Advance Beneficiary Notice	ABN, notification in advance of services that Medicare probably will not pay for and the estimated cost to patient (Fig. 14.3) (formerly WOL, waiver of liability)	Coordination of Benefits	COB, management of multiple third-party payments to ensure overpayment does not occur
Ancillary Service	A service that is supportive of care of a patient, such as laboratory services	Co-payment	Cost-sharing between beneficiary and payer
Assignment	A legal agreement that allows the provider to receive direct payment from a payer and the provider to accept payment as payment in full for covered services	Deductible	That portion of covered services paid by the beneficiary before third-party payment begins
Attending Physician	The physician legally responsible for oversight of an inpatient's care (in residency programs, the teaching physician that monitors the resident's work)	Denial	Statement from a payer that coverage is denied
		Documentation	Detailed chronology of facts and observations, procedures, services, and diagnoses relative to the patient's health
Beneficiary	The person who benefits from insurance coverage; also known as subscriber, dependent, enrollee, member, or participant	Durable Medical Equipment	DME, medically related equipment that is not disposable, such as wheelchairs, crutches, and vaporizers
Birthday Rule	When both parents have insurance coverage, the parent with the birthday earlier in the year carries the primary coverage for a dependent	Electronic Data Interchange	EDI, computerized submission of health care insurance information exchange
Certified Registered Nurse Anesthetist	CRNA, an individual with specialized training and certification in nursing and anesthesia administration	Employer Identification Number	EIN, Internal Revenue Service (IRS)–issued identification number used on tax documents
"Clean Claim"	A properly completed claim submitted to a payer with all data fields containing current and accurate information and submitted within the timely filing period required by the insurer	Encounter Form Superbill	Medical document that contains information regarding a patient visit for health care services, can serve as a billing and/or coding document
Coinsurance	Cost-sharing of covered services	Explanation of Benefits	EOB or EOMB, written, detailed listing of medical service payments by third-party payer to inform beneficiary and provider of payment
Compliance Plan	Written strategy developed by medical facilities to ensure appropriate, consistent documentation within the medical record and ensure compliance with third-party payer guidelines and the Office of the Inspector General (OIG) Workplan guidelines	Fee Schedule	List of established payment for medical services arranged by CPT and HCPCS codes
		Follow-up Days	FUD, established by third-party payers and listing the number of days after a procedure for which a provider must provide services to a patient for no fee. Also known as *global days*, *global package*, and *global period*
Concurrent Care	More than one physician providing care to a patient at the same time	Group Provider Number	GPN, a numeric designation for a group of providers that is used instead of the individual provider number

TABLE 14-1

Reimbursement Terminology—cont'd

Term	Meaning	Term	Meaning
HMO	Health Maintenance Organization	Provider Identification Number	PIN, a number assigned by a third-party payer to providers to be used for identification purposes when submitting claims
Invalid Claim	Claim that is missing necessary information and cannot be processed or paid		
Medical Record	Documentation about the health care of a patient to include diagnoses, services, and procedures rendered	Reimbursement	Payment from a third-party payer for services rendered to a patient covered by the payer's health care plan
National Provider Identifier	NPI, 10-digit number assigned to provider by CMS and National Plan and Provider Enumeration System (NPPES) and used for identification purposes when submitting services to third-party payers	Rejection/Denial	A claim that did not pass the edits and is returned to the provider as rejected
		Resource-Based Relative Value Scale	RBRVS, a list of physician services with assigned units of monetary value
Noncovered Services	Any service not included by a third-party payer in the list of services for which payment is made	State License Number	Identification number issued by a state to a physician who has been granted the right to practice in that state
Point of Service	POS, a plan in which either an in-network or out-of-network provider may be used with a higher rate paid to in-network providers	UPIN	Unique provider identification number was replaced by the NPI
Preferred Provider Organization	PPO, providers form a network to offer health care services to a group	Usual, Customary, and Reasonable	UCR, used by some third-party payers to establish a payment rate for a service in an area with the usual (standard fee in area), customary (standard fee by the physician), and reasonable (as determined by payer) fee amounts
Prior Authorization	Also known as preauthorization, which is a requirement by the payer to receive written permission prior to patient services in order to be considered for payment by the payer		

A. Notifier:

B. Patient Name: C. Identification Number:

Advance Beneficiary Notice of Noncoverage (ABN)

<u>NOTE:</u> If Medicare doesn't pay for **D.** _____ below, you may have to pay.
Medicare does not pay for everything, even some care that you or your health care provider have good reason to think you need. We expect Medicare may not pay for the **D.** _____ below.

D.	E. Reason Medicare May Not Pay:	F. Estimated Cost

WHAT YOU NEED TO DO NOW:
- Read this notice, so you can make an informed decision about your care.
- Ask us any questions that you may have after you finish reading.
- Choose an option below about whether to receive the **D.** _____ listed above.
  Note: If you choose Option 1 or 2, we may help you to use any other insurance that you might have, but Medicare cannot require us to do this.

G. OPTIONS: Check only one box. We cannot choose a box for you.

☐ **OPTION 1.** I want the **D.** _____ listed above. You may ask to be paid now, but I also want Medicare billed for an official decision on payment, which is sent to me on a Medicare Summary Notice (MSN). I understand that if Medicare doesn't pay, I am responsible for payment, but **I can appeal to Medicare** by following the directions on the MSN. If Medicare does pay, you will refund any payments I made to you, less co-pays or deductibles.

☐ **OPTION 2.** I want the **D.** _____ listed above, but do not bill Medicare. You may ask to be paid now as I am responsible for payment. **I cannot appeal if Medicare is not billed**.

☐ **OPTION 3.** I don't want the **D.** _____ listed above. I understand with this choice I am **not** responsible for payment, and **I cannot appeal to see if Medicare would pay.**

H. Additional Information:

This notice gives our opinion, not an official Medicare decision. If you have other questions on this notice or Medicare billing, call **1-800-MEDICARE** (1-800-633-4227/**TTY:** 1-877-486-2048).
Signing below means that you have received and understand this notice. You also receive a copy.

I. Signature:	J. Date:

CMS does not discriminate in its programs and activities. To request this publication in an alternative format, please call: 1-800-MEDICARE or email: AltFormatRequest@cms.hhs.gov.

According to the Paperwork Reduction Act of 1995, no persons are required to respond to a collection of information unless it displays a valid OMB control number. The valid OMB control number for this information collection is 0938-0566. The time required to complete this information collection is estimated to average 7 minutes per response, including the time to review instructions, search existing data resources, gather the data needed, and complete and review the information collection. If you have comments concerning the accuracy of the time estimate or suggestions for improving this form, please write to: CMS, 7500 Security Boulevard, Attn: PRA Reports Clearance Officer, Baltimore, Maryland 21244-1850.

Form CMS-R-131 (Exp. 03/2020)   Form Approved OMB No. 0938-0566

• **Figure 14.3** Centers for Medicare and Medicaid Services Advance Beneficiary Notice (ABN).

Chapter 14: Reimbursement Quiz

(Quiz Answers Are Located in Appendix B)

1. Any person who is identified as receiving life or medical benefits:
   a. primary
   b. beneficiary
   c. participant
   d. recipient

2. According to the Birthday Rule, if both parents are covered by an employer-provided health policy, the insurance policy that would be primary for reporting their child's health services is:
   a. parent with the birthday earlier in the year
   b. parent with the birthday later in the year
   c. either parent
   d. parent whose birthday is closer to the child's

3. Abbreviation for durable medical equipment is:
   a. DRG
   b. CRN
   c. DME
   d. DIM
4. Management of multiple third-party payments to ensure that overpayment does not occur:
   a. PRO
   b. COB
   c. DME
   d. FUD
5. CMS delegates the daily operation of the Medicare program to:
   a. DHHS
   b. QIO
   c. RVU
   d. MACs
6. A QIO provider is one who:
   a. ensures quality of patient care
   b. submits charges directly to CMS
   c. receives 5% less than some other physicians
   d. can bill the patient the total remaining balance after payment from Medicare

7. This part of Medicare covers the inpatient portion of covered costs after the deductible has been paid:
   a. Part A
   b. Part B
   c. Part C
   d. Part D
8. This issue of the *Federal Register* contains outpatient major facility changes for CMS programs for the coming year:
   a. October/November
   b. November/December
   c. December/October
   d. November/August
9. This is the RBRVS payment method:
   a. RAI
   b. OPPS
   c. APC
   d. NFS
10. Entity responsible for development of the plan that outlines monitoring of the Medicare program:
    a. MACs
    b. OIG
    c. DHSS
    d. HEW

PART 3

Facility-based Reimbursement Issues

15

Facility-based Reimbursement Issues

Your Responsibility

Accurately code services that are provided and supported by documentation

Submit complete, accurate, and compliantly coded claims to obtain correct reimbursement for services rendered

Recognize upcoding (maximizing) or downcoding is never appropriate

Stay abreast of continuing changes

- Reimbursement and coverage policies, i.e., Local Coverage Determinations (LCD), or National Coverage Determinations (NCD)
- Coding guidelines from authoritative sources, i.e., AHA's *Coding Clinic for ICD-10-CM;* AHA's *Coding Clinic for HCPCS; UHDDS (Uniform Hospital Discharge Data) Guidelines;* and AMA's *CPT Assistant*
- Stay current with regulatory and Medicare Requirements. The CMS website (www.cms.gov/) offers links to many regulations for specific settings, including hospitals and physician practices. Some examples are:

Regulations such as the Health Insurance Portability and Accountability Act (HIPAA)

  - Centers for Medicare and Medicaid Policy Manuals
  - National Correct Coding Guidelines
  - MedLearn Matters Alerts and Educational Material https://www.cms.gov/files/document/november-15-2019-2020-mln-mattersr-articles-index.pdf
- Health Information Management Professionals are bound by the AHIMA Code of Ethics and the Standards of Ethical Coding (www.ahima.org/about/aboutahim a?tabid=ethics)

> **NOTE**
>
> For the certification examination:
>   You need a working knowledge of national reimbursement and regulatory guidelines.

Population Change = Reimbursement Change

According to the U.S. Census Bureau (www.census.gov/prod/2014pubs/p25-1141.pdf, www.census.gov/content/dam/Census/library/publications/2014/demo/p25-1140.pdf),)

- By 2030, more than 20% of U.S. residents projected to be aged 65+.

- Population aged 65+ is projected to be 83.7 million by 2050.
- Almost double from 43.1 million in 2012.

Elderly compose the fastest growing segment of our population and this growth will place additional demands on health care providers and facilities.

Medicare is the primary insurance for the elderly.

Medicare

Getting Bigger All the Time!

According to the CMS NHE Fact Sheet Projected NHE for 2018-2027 (www.cms.gov/Research-Statistics-Data-and-Systems/Statistics-Trends-and-Reports/NationalHealth ExpendData/NHE-Fact-Sheet.html)

- By 2027, spending is projected to grow at an average rate of 5.5% per year for 2018-27 and to reach nearly $6.0 trillion
- Comparatively higher projected enrollment growth, average annual spending growth in Medicare (7.4%) is expected to exceed that of Medicaid (5.5%) and private health insurance (4.8%)
- Medicare enrollment impacts are the key reason the share of health care spending sponsored by federal, state, and local governments, expected to increase by 2% points over the projection period, reaching 47% by 2027
- Job security for coders!

Those Covered—Beneficiaries

Originally established in 1965 for those 65 and older, and implemented in 1966

Added coverage for disabled and permanent renal disease (end-stage renal disease or transplant) in 1972

Persons covered are called "beneficiaries"

Basic Structure

Part A: Hospital and Institutional Care Coverage

Determine Service Provided

Institutional (facility) services, professional (physician or other individual) services, or supplies

- Professionals must report where services are performed with place of service code (www.cms.gov/Medicare/Coding/place-of-service-codes/Place_of_Service_Code_Set.html)

Institutional service may be inpatient (hospital bed for >24 hours) or outpatient (ambulatory surgical center, emergency room, etc.)

> **NOTE**
>
> For the certification examination:
> You need to know what is covered and not covered under Part A and what can be reported outside the MS-DRG payment.

Covered Inpatient Expenses Include

Room

Semiprivate room rate

- Pays the same amount whether the patient has a private room that is or is not medically necessary
- Semiprivate room
- Ward accommodations
- Accommodations must meet program standards

Patient Pays the Difference between Private and Semiprivate Room When

- Private room is not medically necessary
- Patient has requested the private room
  - Provider must inform patient of the additional charge for private room

Patient Does Not Pay the Difference between Private and Semiprivate Room When Isolation is Required to Avoid Jeopardizing the Health or Recovery of the Patient or Others

Example:
- Communicable diseases
- Heart attacks
- Cerebrovascular accidents
- Psychotic episodes
- Hospital has no semiprivate or ward accommodations available at the time of admission

Patients May be Assigned to Ward Accommodations if

- All semiprivate accommodations are occupied
- Facility has no semiprivate accommodations
- Patient requires immediate hospitalization
- Patient must be moved to semiprivate room when one is available
  - Accommodations must meet program standards

Nursing Services and Other Related Services

Defined as use of hospital facilities and medical social services ordinarily furnished by the hospital for the care/treatment of inpatients

- Meals and special diets during hospitalization
  Blood transfusion
- Patient pays all costs for the first three pints of blood or equivalent units of packed red cells
  - Patient pays 20% for each additional pint
- Coverage starts with 4th pint of blood in hospital or skilled nursing facility

Drugs, Biologicals, Supplies, Appliances, and Equipment

FDA-approved drugs and biologicals for use in the hospital

- Must usually be furnished by the hospital for the care/treatment of inpatients
  Supplies, appliances, and equipment
- Must be used for care/treatment solely during the inpatient hospital stay
  OR
  When unreasonable or impossible to limit the use to the inpatient period
  Example:
  - Items permanently installed in/attached to the patient's body while an inpatient, such as cardiac valves, cardiac pacemakers, and artificial limbs
  - Items that are temporarily installed in/attached to the patient's body while an inpatient and are necessary to permit the patient's release from the hospital, such as tracheotomy or drainage tubes

Hospital must have purchased the item

- A cost was incurred by the hospital for the item
  - Excluded are items given to the hospital
  Example:
- Free pharmaceutical samples

Certain Other Covered Diagnostic or Therapeutic Services

Diagnostic or therapeutic items/services ordinarily furnished to inpatients by hospital

- This includes the supply by others under arrangements made by the hospital
  Example:
  - Diagnostic or therapeutic services of an audiologist provided off the hospital premises but billed for by the hospital
  - Surgical dressings and splints, casts, and other devices used for the reduction of fractures and dislocations

Prosthetic devices are covered that replace all/part of an organ

- The function of a permanently inoperative or malfunctioning internal body organ
  Example:
  - Braces, trusses, artificial replacements (legs, arms, and eyes)

Diagnostic/therapeutic inpatient services of a psychologist/physical therapist

- Must be a salaried member of the staff of a hospital
  Inpatient diagnostic services furnished by an independent, certified clinical lab under arrangements with the hospital
- Lab certified under CLIA
  - CLIA = Clinical Laboratories Improvement Act
  Reasonable cost of medical/surgical services of medical/osteopathic interns or residents under an approved teaching program
- Transportation services
  Includes transport by ambulance to another facility for testing and/or treatment

Additionally Covered Expenses When They Meet Certain Criteria

Inpatient rehabilitation

Skilled nursing

Some personal convenience items for long-term illness/disability

Home health visit

Hospice care

Noncovered Inpatient-Hospital Expenses

Non–medically necessary services or supplies

Private-duty nurse or other private-duty attendant

Deluxe or non-medically necessary private room

Personal convenience items

• Those not routinely furnished to patients

Non-physician inpatient services that have not been provided directly or arranged for by hospital staff

Coverage Under Part A is Compulsory

Paid for by Social Security tax

Eligibility is determined by the Social Security Administration (SSA)

Reimbursement is for all covered and medically necessary services

• After annual deductible is met

ICD-10-CM diagnosis and procedure codes are basis for Part A payment

Charges are submitted electronically

Administrative Simplification Compliance Act (ASCA) prohibits payment of initial health care claims not sent electronically, except in limited situations

• Such as providers who have 25 or fewer full-time employees, or

• Claims from providers that submit fewer than 10 claims per month on average during a calendar year

Claim electronically transmitted in data "packets" over telephone line

• Medicare contractors perform series of edits

• Initial edits determine if batch of claims meets HIPAA standards

• Errors detected, entire batch of claims rejected and returned to provider to correct and resubmit

• Claims that pass initial edits are then edited against implementation guide requirements in HIPAA standards

• Errors detected, individual claims with errors rejected and returned to provider to correct and resubmit

• If first two levels of edits are passed, each claim is edited for compliance with Medicare coverage and payment policy requirements

• After successful transmission, an acknowledgment report is generated back to provider

Exempt providers may submit paper billing

Part B: Supplemental

Provides Coverage for Non-Hospital Charges

Physician services

Outpatient hospital services

Home health care

Medically necessary supplies and equipment

Those services and supplies not covered under Part A that are medically necessary

Payment for the hospital stay if the patient has exhausted all Part A benefits prior to admission

Beneficiaries Purchase Coverage with Monthly Premiums
Three Coding Systems Used to Report Part B Services and Supplies That are Medical Necessity for Services

HCPCS Level I = CPT—services

HCPCS Level II (also known as National Codes)—supplies, services, and drugs not included or covered by CPT coding system

On the certification examination, HCPCS Level II are only on the theory portion of the examination, not on the practical portion of the examination.

ICD-10-CM—diagnoses

Part C: Medicare Advantage Plans

Variety of health care options are available

• Health Maintenance Organization (HMO)

• Preferred Provider Organization (PPO)

• Private Fee-for-Service (PFFS)

• Special Needs Plans (SNPs)

• HMO Point of Service (HMOPOS)

Added after Part A and B

Part D: Prescription Drug, Improvement, and Modernization Act of 2003

Prescription drug plan

Premium paid by beneficiary

—Reimbursements based on the diagnoses of patients within the plan

Officiating Office

Department of Health and Human Services (DHHS)

Delegated to Centers for Medicare and Medicaid Services (CMS)

CMS runs Medicare and Medicaid

CMS delegates daily operation for Part A and Part B to Medicare Administrative Contractors (MACs)

• The Medicare Prescription Drug Improvement and Modernization Act of 2003 allowed CMS to reduce 48 fiscal intermediaries (FIs) to 15 Medicare Administrative Contractors (MACs).

• CMS further reduced the total number of jurisdictions to 12 MACs and 4 DME MACs, with no plans for further reductions.

Funding for Medicare

Social security taxes

Equal match from government

CMS sends money to MACs

MACs handle paperwork and pay claims

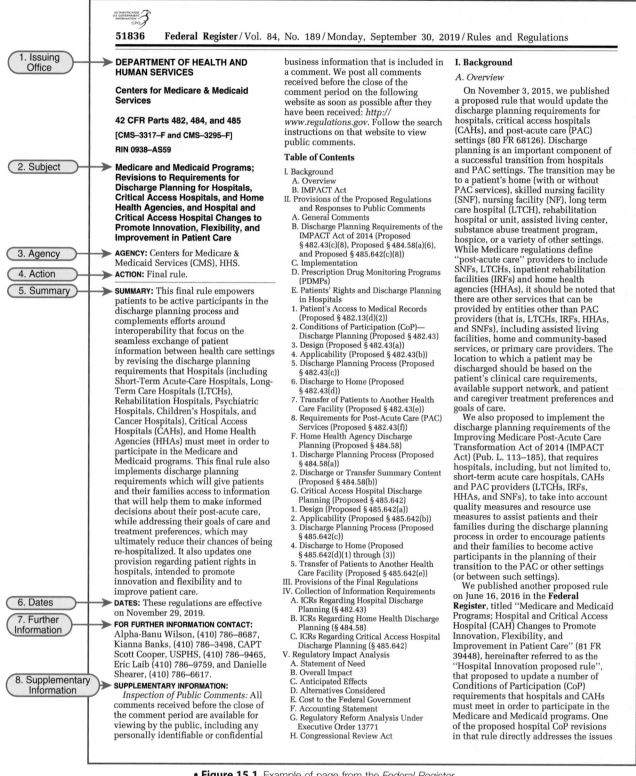

Federal Register / Vol. 84, No. 189 / Monday, September 30, 2019 / Rules and Regulations

51836

1. Issuing Office

DEPARTMENT OF HEALTH AND HUMAN SERVICES

Centers for Medicare & Medicaid Services

42 CFR Parts 482, 484, and 485

[CMS–3317–F and CMS–3295–F]

RIN 0938–AS59

2. Subject

Medicare and Medicaid Programs; Revisions to Requirements for Discharge Planning for Hospitals, Critical Access Hospitals, and Home Health Agencies, and Hospital and Critical Access Hospital Changes to Promote Innovation, Flexibility, and Improvement in Patient Care

3. Agency

AGENCY: Centers for Medicare & Medicaid Services (CMS), HHS.

4. Action

ACTION: Final rule.

5. Summary

SUMMARY: This final rule empowers patients to be active participants in the discharge planning process and complements efforts around interoperability that focus on the seamless exchange of patient information between health care settings by revising the discharge planning requirements that Hospitals (including Short-Term Acute-Care Hospitals, Long-Term Care Hospitals (LTCHs), Rehabilitation Hospitals, Psychiatric Hospitals, Children's Hospitals, and Cancer Hospitals), Critical Access Hospitals (CAHs), and Home Health Agencies (HHAs) must meet in order to participate in the Medicare and Medicaid programs. This final rule also implements discharge planning requirements which will give patients and their families access to information that will help them to make informed decisions about their post-acute care, while addressing their goals of care and treatment preferences, which may ultimately reduce their chances of being re-hospitalized. It also updates one provision regarding patient rights in hospitals, intended to promote innovation and flexibility and to improve patient care.

6. Dates

DATES: These regulations are effective on November 29, 2019.

7. Further Information

FOR FURTHER INFORMATION CONTACT: Alpha-Banu Wilson, (410) 786–8687, Kianna Banks, (410) 786–3498, CAPT Scott Cooper, USPHS, (410) 786–9465, Eric Laib (410) 786–9759, and Danielle Shearer, (410) 786–6617.

8. Supplementary Information

SUPPLEMENTARY INFORMATION:
Inspection of Public Comments: All comments received before the close of the comment period are available for viewing by the public, including any personally identifiable or confidential

business information that is included in a comment. We post all comments received before the close of the comment period on the following website as soon as possible after they have been received: *http://www.regulations.gov.* Follow the search instructions on that website to view public comments.

Table of Contents

I. Background
  A. Overview
  B. IMPACT Act
II. Provisions of the Proposed Regulations and Responses to Public Comments
  A. General Comments
  B. Discharge Planning Requirements of the IMPACT Act of 2014 (Proposed § 482.43(c)(8), Proposed § 484.58(a)(6), and Proposed § 485.642(c)(8))
  C. Implementation
  D. Prescription Drug Monitoring Programs (PDMPs)
  E. Patients' Rights and Discharge Planning in Hospitals
    1. Patient's Access to Medical Records (Proposed § 482.13(d)(2))
    2. Conditions of Participation (CoP)—Discharge Planning (Proposed § 482.43)
    3. Design (Proposed § 482.43(a))
    4. Applicability (Proposed § 482.43(b))
    5. Discharge Planning Process (Proposed § 482.43(c))
    6. Discharge to Home (Proposed § 482.43(d))
    7. Transfer of Patients to Another Health Care Facility (Proposed § 482.43(e))
    8. Requirements for Post-Acute Care (PAC) Services (Proposed § 482.43(f))
  F. Home Health Agency Discharge Planning (Proposed § 484.58)
    1. Discharge Planning Process (Proposed § 484.58(a))
    2. Discharge or Transfer Summary Content (Proposed § 484.58(b))
  G. Critical Access Hospital Discharge Planning (Proposed § 485.642)
    1. Design (Proposed § 485.642(a))
    2. Applicability (Proposed § 485.642(b))
    3. Discharge Planning Process (Proposed § 485.642(c))
    4. Discharge to Home (Proposed § 485.642(d)(1) through (3))
    5. Transfer of Patients to Another Health Care Facility (Proposed § 485.642(e))
III. Provisions of the Final Regulations
IV. Collection of Information Requirements
  A. ICRs Regarding Hospital Discharge Planning (§ 482.43)
  B. ICRs Regarding Home Health Discharge Planning (§ 484.58)
  C. ICRs Regarding Critical Access Hospital Discharge Planning (§ 485.642)
V. Regulatory Impact Analysis
  A. Statement of Need
  B. Overall Impact
  C. Anticipated Effects
  D. Alternatives Considered
  E. Cost to the Federal Government
  F. Accounting Statement
  G. Regulatory Reform Analysis Under Executive Order 13771
  H. Congressional Review Act

I. Background

A. Overview

On November 3, 2015, we published a proposed rule that would update the discharge planning requirements for hospitals, critical access hospitals (CAHs), and post-acute care (PAC) settings (80 FR 68126). Discharge planning is an important component of a successful transition from hospitals and PAC settings. The transition may be to a patient's home (with or without PAC services), skilled nursing facility (SNF), nursing facility (NF), long term care hospital (LTCH), rehabilitation hospital or unit, assisted living center, substance abuse treatment program, hospice, or a variety of other settings. While Medicare regulations define "post-acute care" providers to include SNFs, LTCHs, inpatient rehabilitation facilities (IRFs) and home health agencies (HHAs), it should be noted that there are other services that can be provided by entities other than PAC providers (that is, LTCHs, IRFs, HHAs, and SNFs), including assisted living facilities, home and community-based services, or primary care providers. The location to which a patient may be discharged should be based on the patient's clinical care requirements, available support network, and patient and caregiver treatment preferences and goals of care.

We also proposed to implement the discharge planning requirements of the Improving Medicare Post-Acute Care Transformation Act of 2014 (IMPACT Act) (Pub. L. 113–185), that requires hospitals, including, but not limited to, short-term acute care hospitals, CAHs and PAC providers (LTCHs, IRFs, HHAs, and SNFs), to take into account quality measures and resource use measures to assist patients and their families during the discharge planning process in order to encourage patients and their families to become active participants in the planning of their transition to the PAC or other settings (or between such settings).

We published another proposed rule on June 16, 2016 in the **Federal Register**, titled "Medicare and Medicaid Programs; Hospital and Critical Access Hospital (CAH) Changes to Promote Innovation, Flexibility, and Improvement in Patient Care" (81 FR 39448), hereinafter referred to as the "Hospital Innovation proposed rule", that proposed to update a number of Conditions of Participation (CoP) requirements that hospitals and CAHs must meet in order to participate in the Medicare and Medicaid programs. One of the proposed hospital CoP revisions in that rule directly addresses the issues

• **Figure 15.1** Example of page from the *Federal Register*.

Federal Register

Government publishes updates, revisions, deletions (changes) in *Federal Register* (Fig. 15.1)
- CMS website (www.cms.gov) also contains published changes

Updates to payment systems occur throughout the year
Part A hospital inpatient payment changes are effective October 1
Hospital outpatient facility payment changes and physician payment system changes are effective January 1, published November/December

Quarterly revisions to HCPCS are published by CMS
- AMA publishes changes to CPT Category III codes effective January 1 and July 1

Electronic Transactions

HIPAA
- Created to govern health care portability
  -electronic data interchange (EDI)
  -requiring security of information and privacy of patient information
  -establishing code sets appropriate for electronic reporting

Transactions
- Activities involving transfer of health care information

Transmission
- Movement of electronic data between two entities

Today 99% of Part A and 95% Part B claims filed electronically
- Data entered electronically or onto paper CMS-1500 form
- Response is Electronic Remittance Advice (ERA) with the electronic fund transfer (EFT)

The format that supports electronic transmissions
- 5010 version

National Correct Coding Initiative (NCCI)

Developed by the Centers for Medicare and Medicaid Services to
- Promote national correct coding methods, to reduce/alleviate separate reporting of bundled services
- Control improper multiple procedure coding that leads to inappropriate payment of Part B physician claims and hospital outpatient claims
- Complete list may be found at www.cms.gov/NationalCorrectCodInitEd/

Unbundling

CMS defines unbundling as
- Billing separately each component of an all-inclusive procedure
  Example:
  Billing 15260, Full thickness graft, free, including direct closure of donor site; nose, ears, eyelids and/or lips PLUS 12016, Simple repair of superficial wounds of face, ears, eyelids, nose, lips … when code 15260 states "including direct closure of donor site"

Prospective Payment Systems (PPS)

For services provided to Medicare patients in inpatient or ambulatory surgical centers
Established by Tax Equity and Fiscal Responsibility Act (TEFRA) of 1982

Social Security amendments passed use of inpatient PPS in 1983
For services provided in
- Acute care hospitals
- Skilled nursing facilities
- Inpatient rehabilitation facilities
- Long-term care hospital settings
  - Psychiatric hospitals or exempt psychiatric units
  Hospital/facility paid fixed amount for patient discharged in a treatment category
  Excludes these hospitals:
- Children's
- Rehabilitation
- Cancer

Ambulatory Payment Classifications (APCs)

Omnibus Budget Reconciliation Act of 1986 (OBRA)

Prior to OBRA, Medicare hospital outpatient services paid on a cost-based system
- Also known as a retrospective system

Act Mandated

Replacement of cost-based system with a PPS (Prospective Payment System)
Medicare hospital-based outpatient facilities report services and some supplies/drugs on claims using CMS Healthcare Common Procedure Coding System (HCPCS), which includes CPT codes
- CMS uses claims data to determine future payment rates/coverage policies
- Data sources were used to develop Outpatient Prospective Payment System (OPPS)

Developed Ambulatory Patient Groups (APGs)

Grouped outpatient services
Differs from MS-DRGs because an outpatient can be assigned multiple APGs
Outpatient claims may have multiple APGs on any given day, but only one MS-DRG is paid for the entire inpatient encounter

Final Version of the Classification System Was Ambulatory Payment Classifications (APCs)

Implementation on August 1, 2000

APCs Mandatory for
- Most Medicare hospital outpatient services

  Some exceptions are lab and therapy services that are paid by a separate fee schedule
- Inpatient services covered under Part B
  - If beneficiary has exhausted Part A benefits
- Inpatient services not covered by Part A

- Partial hospitalization services
Furnished by community mental health centers and some hospitals

APCs are Used for Reimbursement for Hospital-Based Outpatient Services

Such as:
- Outpatient surgery
- Hospital-based outpatient clinics
- Emergency departments
- Outpatient ancillary services
  Example: Radiology (Laboratory is paid on a separate fee schedule)

APC Structure

Consists of over 760 groups of services
- Each HCPCS code is assigned to an APC and has a status indicator defining how and whether separate payment is made (Fig. 15.2)

Services in each APC are alike:
- Clinically
- In resources required to provide the services

APC Includes Some Items/Services That Contribute to Cost of the Service but Medicare Does Not Usually Reimburse Separately

- These incidentals are packaged into the APC payment
  Example:
  - Supplies
  - Observation services (limited exceptions)

- Specific drugs
- Blood
- Medical visits on the same day of service or procedure unless separately identifiable and modified
- Guidance services (e.g., stereoscopic x-rays)

Medicare does reimburse separately for some items and services that are not packaged, such as casting, splinting, and strapping services

Further APC information is available at www.cms.gov/HospitalOutpatientPPS/

Pass-Through Codes

Services, procedures, and/or supplies not included in APC package

Paid an additional pass-through APC payment

Payment Rate and Co-Insurance

Co-insurance amount is 20% of the median charge for all services in the APC
- This means the payment rate and co-insurance will not change until the co-insurance amount becomes 20% of the total APC payment

APC Payment Status Indicators (SI) (Fig. 15.3)

One letter or one letter followed by a number (i.e., Q1) designating a status indicator is assigned to each HCPCS/CPT code

Indicates if service, procedure, or supply is reimbursable under the Outpatient Prospective Payment System (OPPS) or other fee schedule

APC	HCPCS Code	HCPCS Description	SI	Rel. Wt.	Pay Rate	Min. Coin.
5051	10060	Drainage of skin abscess	T	2.1627	$174.73	$34.95
5051	11057	Trim skin lesions over 4	T	2.1627	$174.73	$34.95
5051	11102	Tangntl bx skin single les	T	2.1627	$174.73	$34.95
5051	17270	Destruction of skin lesions	T	2.1627	$174.73	$34.95
5051	17271	Destruction of skin lesions	T	2.1627	$174.73	$34.95
5051	26010	Drainage of finger abscess	T	2.1627	$174.73	$34.95
5051	46916	Cryosurgery anal lesion(s)	T	2.1627	$174.73	$34.95
5051	97597	Rmvl devital tis 20 cm/<	T	2.1627	$174.73	$34.95
5071	10080	Drainage of pilonidal cyst	T	7.5503	$610.01	$122.01
5071	11010	Debride skin at fx site	T	7.5503	$610.01	$122.01
5071	11011	Debride skin musc at fx site	T	7.5503	$610.01	$122.01
5071	20103	Explore wound extremity	T	7.5503	$610.01	$122.01
5071	23330	Remove shoulder foreign body	T	7.5503	$610.01	$122.01
5071	28190	Removal of foot foreign body	T	7.5503	$610.01	$122.01
5071	40800	Drainage of mouth lesion	T	7.5503	$610.01	$122.01
5071	42400	Biopsy of salivary gland	T	7.5503	$610.01	$122.01
5071	60100	Biopsy of thyroid	T	7.5503	$610.01	$122.01

• **Figure 15.2** Final 2020 APC grouping of HCPCS codes (February, 2020).

	ADDENDUM D1. – OPPS PAYMENT STATUS INDICATORS FOR CY 2020	
Indicator	**Item/Code/Service**	**OPPS Payment Status**
A	Service furnished to a hospital outpatient that are paid under a fee schedule or payment system other than OPPS, for example:	Not paid under OPPS. Paid by fiscal intermediaries/MACS under a fee schedule or payment system other than OPPS.
	• Ambulance Services	
	• Clinical Diagnostic Laboratory Services	Not subject to deductible or coinsurance.
	• Non-Implantable Prosthetic and Orthotic Devices	
	• EPO for ESRD Patients	
	• Physical, Occupational, and Speech Therapy	
	• Routine Dialysis Services for ESRD Patients Provided in a Certified Dialysis Unit of a Hospital	
	• Diagnostic Mammography	Not subject to deductible or coinsurance.
	• Screening Mammography	
B	Codes that are not recognized by OPPS when submitted on an outpatient hospital Part B bill type (12x and 13x).	Not paid under OPPS.
		• May be paid by fiscal intermediaries/MACs when submitted on a different bill type, for example, 75x (CORF), but not paid under OPPS.
		• An alternate code that is recognized by OPPS when submitted on an outpatient hospital Part B bill type (12x and 13x) may be available.
C	Inpatient Procedures	Not paid under OPPS Admit patient. Bill as inpatient.
D	Discontinued Codes	Not paid under OPPS or any other Medicare payment system.
E	Items, Codes, and Services:	Not paid by Medicare when submitted on outpatient claims (any outpatient bill type).
	• That are not covered by any Medicare outpatient benefit based on statutory exclusion.	
	• That are not covered by any Medicare outpatient benefit for reasons other than statutory exclusion.	
	• That are not recognized by Medicare for outpatient claims but for which an alternate code for the same item or service may be available.	
	For which separate payment is not provided on outpatient claims.	
F	Corneal Tissue Acquisition; Certain CRNA Services and Hepatitis B Vaccines	Not paid under OPPS. Paid at reasonable cost.
G	Pass-Through Drugs and Biologicals	Paid under OPPS; separate APC payment.
H	Pass-Through Device Categories	Separate cost-based pass-through payment; not subject to copayment.
K	Nonpass-Through Drugs and Nonimplantable Biologicals, Including Therapeutic Radiopharmaceuticals	Paid under OPPS; separate APC payment.
L	Influenza Vaccine; Pneumococcal Pneumonia Vaccine	Not paid under OPPS. Paid at reasonable cost; not subject to deductible or coinsurance.
M	Items and Services Not Billable to the Fiscal Intermediary/MAC	Not paid under OPPS.
N	Items and Services Packaged into APC Rates	Paid under OPPS; payment is packaged into payment for other services. Therefore, there is no separate APC payment.
P	Partial Hospitalization	Paid under OPPS; per diem APC payment.
Q1	STVX-Packaged Codes	Paid under OPPS; Addendum B displays APC assignments when services are separately payable.
		(1) Packaged APC payment if billed on the same date of service as a HCPCS code assigned status indicator "S," "T," "V," or "X."
		(2) In all other circumstances, payment is made through a separate APC payment.
Q2	T-Packaged Codes	Paid under OPPS; Addendum B displays APC assignments when services are separately payable.
		(1) Packaged APC payment if billed on the same date of service as a HCPCS code assigned status indicator "T."
		(2) In all other circumstances, payment is made through a separate APC payment.
Q3	Codes That May Be Paid Through a Composite APC	Paid under OPPS; Addendum B displays APC assignments when services are separately payable.
		Addendum M displays composite APC assignments when codes are paid through a composite APC.
		(1) Composite APC payment based on OPPS composite-specific payment criteria. Payment is packaged into a single payment for specific combinations of service.
		(2) In all other circumstances, payment is made through a separate APC payment or packaged into payment for other services.
R	Blood and Blood Products	Paid under OPPS; separate APC payment.
S	Significant Procedure, Not Discounted when Multiple	Paid under OPPS; separate APC payment.
T	Significant Procedure, Multiple Reduction Applies	Paid under OPPS; separate APC payment.
U	Brachytherapy Sources	Paid under OPPS; separate APC payment.
V	Clinic or Emergency Department Visit	Paid under OPPS; separate APC payment.
X	Ancillary Services	Paid under OPPS; separate APC payment.
Y	Non-Implantable Durable Medical Equipment	Not paid under OPPS. All institutional providers other than home health agencies bill to DMERC.

• **Figure 15.3** Payment Status Indicators for the Hospital Outpatient Prospective Payment System Addendum.

Also identifies if reimbursement is bundled or separately payable and/or discounted

Example:
- HCPCS/CPT codes under SI "A" are not paid under OPPS but are paid under a fee schedule or another payment method
- Such as: 77057, mammogram screening (SI "A")
- Routine Dialysis Services
- Ambulance Services

Each APC is assigned a co-insurance amount and payment rate
- Adjusted by hospital's wage index (labor costs)

Fig. 15.4 illustrates the payment rate and co-insurance amounts

Example:
- Drainage of skin abscess (10060) is paid at $174.73, co-insurance amount of 20% ($34.95)
- Red blood cell deglycerolization (P9039) is paid at $320.46, co-insurance amount of 20% ($64.10)

Can receive payment for multiple services provided on the same day

Multiple procedures that have status indicator "S" are reimbursed at 100%

Multiple significant surgical procedures performed on the same day that have a status indicator of "T" are discounted
- Full payment made for the highest reimbursed procedure APC
- Multiple procedure payment reduction applies when two or more services with status indicator "T" are billed on the same date of service

-CA Modifier

Used with status indicator "C" services, these are inpatient procedures provided on an emergency basis in the outpatient setting
- Patient expires before admission to the hospital

-CA is assigned to inpatient-only procedure

Payment is allowed for only one procedure

Transitional Pass-Through Payments for Certain Devices and Items

Payments made for certain innovative devices, drugs, and biologicals

Paid as an additional APC payment

Example:
- Chemotherapeutic agents
  - Including supportive and adjunctive drugs
- Implantable devices
- Immunosuppressive drugs
- Orphan drugs
- Some new drugs
- Certain drugs given in the emergency room for heart attacks

Have co-insurance amounts that can be less than 20% of the Average Wholesale Price (AWP)

Payments for pass-throughs made for at least 2 years but not more than 3 years

Report devices and drugs with HCPCS C or J codes and SI "G," "H," or "K"

When a pass-through transitional payment has expired:
- C code removed from HCPCS and is usually given an applicable "J" code
- Separate payment is no longer made for item

Current HCPCS codes, including C codes, can be viewed and/or downloaded from the CMS website at www.cms.gov/Medicare/Coding/HCPCSReleaseCodeSets/Alpha-Numeric-HCPCS.html

Pass-through items for which separate payment expires should be reported on claim to identify cost to CMS

HCPCS codes for drugs, biologicals, devices, and radiopharmaceuticals that have a separate APC payment are listed in Final Annual Rule

Currently, very few devices are paid separately

Drugs and biologicals with final pass-through status for 2020 are displayed in Fig. 15.5

Most devices have no separate APC payment because the item is packaged into APC payment for procedure. Although hospitals do not receive additional payment for these devices, they are encouraged to report HCPCS codes on claim

In some cases, hospitals are required to report device HCPCS code. (See the following section "Device-Dependent Procedures")

Most recent information concerning applications and requirements for APC payments for new technologies, additional device categories, and pass-through payments for

HCPCS Code	Short Description	SI	APC	Relative Weight	Payment Rate	Minimum Unadjusted Copayment
10060	Drainage of skin abscess	T	5051	2.1627	$174.73	$34.95
10061	Drainage of skin abscess	T	5052	3.9547	$319.15	$63.91
10080	Rbc leukoreduced irradiated	T	5071	7.5503	$610.01	$122.01
10081	Drainage of pilonidal cyst	T	5071	7.5503	$610.01	$122.01
P9038	Rbc irradiated	R	9505	2.3618	$190.82	$38.17
P9039	Rbc deglycerolized	R	9504	3.9664	$320.46	$64.10
P9040	Rbc leukoreduced irradiated	R	9522	3.2523	$262.76	$52.56

• **Figure 15.4** Final APC payment rate and co-insurance amount (February, 2020).

CY 2019 HCPCS Code	CY 2020 HCPCS Code	CY 2020 Long Descriptor	Final CY 2020 SI	Final CY 2020 APC
A9584	A9584	Iodine I-123 ioflupane, diagnostic, per study dose, up to 5 millicuries	N	N/A
C9285	C9285	Lidocaine 70 mg/tetracaine 70 mg, per patch	N	N/A
J0485	J0485	Injection, belatacept, 1 mg	K	9286
J9042	J9042	Injection, brentuximab vedotin, 1 mg	K	9287
J0716	J0716	Injection, centruroides immune f(ab)2, up to 120 milligrams	K	1431
J9019	J9019	Injection, asparaginase (erwinaze), 1,000 iu	K	9289
C9290	C9290	Injection, bupivicaine liposome, 1 mg	N	N/A
C9293	C9293	Injection, glucarpidase, 10 units	N	9293
Q4132	Q4132	Grafix core, per square centimeter	N	N/A
Q4133	Q4133	Grafix prime, per square centimeter	N	N/A
J0131	J0131	Injection, acetaminophen, 10 mg	N	N/A
J0490	J0490	Injection, belimumab, 10 mg	K	1353
J0638	J0638	Injection, canakinumab, 1 mg	K	1311
J0712	J0712	Injection, ceftaroline fosamil, 10 mg	K	1824

• **Figure 15.5** Final 2020 Drugs and Biologicals with Pass-Through Status.

drugs and biologicals is located on the CMS website at www.cms.gov/HospitalOutpatientPPS

Device-Dependent Procedures

When hospitals report certain procedure codes that require the use of devices

- Must also report the applicable HCPCS codes and charges for all devices used to perform the procedures
- This information is used in calculating future OPPS payment amounts

If such a procedure is reported without at least one device HCPCS code, claim will be returned to provider

Procedures that require device HCPCS codes are listed in Device to Procedure Edits document

Download from CMS the device edits: www.cms.gov/HospitalOutpatientPPS/01_overview.asp

(On left side of screen click link: "Device, Radiolabeled Product, and Procedure Edits" and on Downloads page click "Device to Procedure Edits")

Discounting

Multiple surgical procedures during the same operative procedure

- Status indicator "T" indicates multiple procedure payment reduction applied

Highest weighted procedure APC paid at 100% (after applicable co-pay and deductible)

- Multiple procedure payment reduction applies when two or more services with status indicator "T" are billed on the same date of service

Terminated surgical procedures before the induction of anesthesia paid at 50%

- Indicated by use of modifier -73 added to surgical procedure code

Outlier Adjustments

Some costs that exceed 1.75 times the payment rate and exceed the APC payment rate plus a $2,025 fixed threshold receives an adjusted higher reimbursement

Inpatient-Only Procedures with Status Indicator "C"

CMS publishes a list of procedures that are "inpatient-only" procedures

- Procedures that are life-threatening and require substantial mortality risks as an outpatient

Visit www.cms.gov/HospitalOutpatientPPS and click link "Hospital Outpatient Regulations and Notices" for most current notices. (Select "Hospital Outpatient Prospective Payment- Final Rule with Comment" and then select "CY2020 OPPS Addenda"; when file opens, locate Addendum E)

Example:

Status Indicator "C" procedures are those that are not paid under OPPS

- 28080   Excision, interdigital (Morton) neuroma, single, each
- 32900   Resection of ribs, extrapleural, all stages
- 33535   Coronary artery bypass, using arterial graft(s); 3 coronary arterial grafts

Ambulatory Surgical Procedures

CMS publishes a list of procedures approved for ambulatory surgery center (ASC) procedures www.cms.gov/ASCPayment/

Example:
Approved ASC procedures are those that are paid under OPPS

- 10121 Incision and removal of foreign body, subcutaneous tissues; complicated
- 19340 Insertion of breast implant on the same day of mastectomy (i.e., immediate)
- 23155 Excision or curettage of bone cyst or benign tumor of proximal humerus; with autograft (includes obtaining graft)

Observation Status

Complete OPPS program information for 2020 was in the *Federal Register*, January 3, 2020, Vol. 85, No. 2
Historically, observation services were paid only for chest pain, congestive heart failure, and asthma
Beginning in 2008, observation services were paid for any diagnosis when other observation criteria were met
Time begins when the patient is admitted to the observation unit and ends when the patient is discharged or admitted as an inpatient

Outpatient Code Editor (OCE)

General functions of the OCE system
- Reviews claim data to identify errors and returns an edit flag(s)
- Edits are based upon HCPCS and ICD-10-CM codes
Assigns an APC number to each service covered under OPPS

Medicare Severity Diagnosis-Related Groups (MS-DRGs)

System of Classifying Patients into Groups by Related Diagnoses

For payment of operating costs based on prospectively set rates
For acute care hospital inpatient stays under Medicare Part A
Each diagnosis and procedure codes are categorized into an MS-DRG
MS-DRGs have relative weights assigned based on the average resources used to treat patients in that MS-DRG
- Similar types of patients
- Similar types of illnesses or injuries
- Severity of illness
- Treatments provided
  - Similar use of resources
Each facility has its own payment rate assigned by Centers for Medicare and Medicaid Services (CMS)

Although hospitals assign MS-DRGs for internal resource and financial management, the official MS-DRG for payment is calculated by Medicare from ICD-10-CM/CD-10-PCS codes that are assigned at the hospital.

System Based on

Principal diagnosis
Principal procedure
Any qualifying complication(s) or comorbidity(ies)

Structure of MS-DRGs

Divides All Principal Diagnoses into 25 Major Diagnostic Categories (MDCs) (Fig. 15.6)

Most MDCs correspond to major organ systems
   Example:
   - Respiratory System
   - Digestive System
   - Nervous System
Some MDCs correspond to an etiology (cause)
   Example:
   - Neoplasms
   - Human Immunodeficiency Virus Infections

MS-DRGs are Then Further Defined by a Particular Set of Patient Attributes Defined in the Uniform Hospital Discharge Data Set (UHDDS)

By Diagnosis

Principal diagnosis	Defined as "that condition established after study to be chiefly responsible for occasioning the admission of the patient to the hospital for care"
Secondary diagnosis	Conditions that co-exist at the time of admission, that develop subsequently to the admission, or that affect the treatment received and/or length of stay

By Procedure

Principal procedure	A procedure that is performed for definitive treatment rather than for diagnostic or exploratory purposes or that is necessary in order to take care of a complication
Significant procedure	Medicare defines a significant procedure as one that is • Surgical in nature • Carries an anesthetic/procedural risk, and • Requires specialized training
Discharge status	Condition and/or place to which the patient is being discharged, such as to home, skilled nursing facility, rehabilitation, home health care, long-term care

Birth weight: MS-DRGs for newborns may be affected by infant's birth weight

Example: MDC 15, Newborns & Other Neonates with Conditions Originating in the Perinatal Period Prematurity,

Major Diagnostic Categories

MDC 01 Diseases & Disorders of the Nervous System
MDC 02 Diseases & Disorders of the Eye
MDC 03 Diseases & Disorders of the Ear, Nose, Mouth & Throat
MDC 04 Diseases & Disorders of the Respiratory System
MDC 05 Diseases & Disorders of the Circulatory System
MDC 06 Diseases & Disorders of the Digestive System
MDC 07 Diseases & Disorders of the Hepatobiliary System & Pancreas
MDC 08 Diseases & Disorders of the Musculoskeletal System & Connective Tissue
MDC 09 Diseases & Disorders of the Skin, Subcutaneous Tissue & Breast
MDC 10 Endocrine, Nutritional & Metabolic Diseases & Disorders
MDC 11 Diseases & Disorders of the Kidney & Urinary Tract
MDC 12 Diseases & Disorders of the Male Reproductive System
MDC 13 Diseases & Disorders of the Female Reproductive System
MDC 14 Pregnancy, Childbirth & the Puerperium
MDC 15 Newborns & Other Neonates with Conditions Originating in Perinatal Period
MDC 16 Diseases & Disorders of Blood, Blood Forming Organs, Immunologic Disorders
MDC 17 Myeloproliferative Diseases & Disorders, Poorly Differentiated Neoplasms
MDC 18 Infectious & Parasitic Diseases, Systemic or Unspecified Sites
MDC 19 Mental Diseases & Disorders
MDC 20 Alcohol/Drug Use & Alcohol/Drug Induced Organic Mental Disorders
MDC 21 Injuries, Poisonings & Toxic Effects of Drugs
MDC 22 Burns
MDC 23 Factors Influencing Health Status & Other Contacts with Health Services
MDC 24 Multiple Significant Trauma
MDC 25 Human Immunodeficiency Virus Infections

• **Figure 15.6** MDCs of the ICD-10-CM/PCS MS-DRGs.

Fig. 15.7, illustrates DRGs 791 and 792 are affected by low birth weight and/or preterm
MS-DRGs are not affected by age
  Exception: MS-DRGs for newborns

Surgical Classes in Each MDC Are Defined in a Hierarchical (Least-to-Most Resource Intense) Order

Multiple procedures related to principal diagnosis during hospital stay are assigned to only the highest surgical class in the hierarchy

- MS-DRG Grouper performs assignment
  - Grouper = Computer software

CASE STUDY

The principal diagnosis is congestive heart failure (I50.9). Additional diagnoses are morbid obesity due to excess calories (E66.01), Type 2 diabetes without complications (E11.9), atherosclerotic heart disease (I25.10), psoriasis (L40.9), depressive disorder (F32.9), unspecified personality disorder (F60.9), pure hypercholesterolemia (E78.0), cardiomegaly (I51.7), and initial episode of acute subendocardial myocardial infarction (I21.4). If I21.4 had been listed within the top nine diagnoses, the reimbursement would have been based on MS-DRG 293 compared to 282 (for which the reimbursement is significantly greater) if the complication of subendocardial infarction had been correctly listed. Review the principal reason for admission and the principal diagnosis assignment after study for correct MS-DRG assignment.

MS-DRGs MCC and CC

- All diagnoses were reviewed to determine if they qualify as a CC or non-CC
- Key criterion being the increase in hospital resources
- All diagnoses were divided into three severity levels:
  - Major complications or comorbidities (MCC)
  - Complications or comorbidities (CC)
  - Non-CCs—do not affect MS-DRG assignment

The MS-DRG system is 001-998 with allowances for future changes

Chronic conditions may have to be decompensated or in exacerbation to qualify as a CC for MS-DRGs

The following codes are MCCs only if patient is discharged alive:

I46.2	Cardiac arrest due to underlying cardiac condition
I46.8	Cardiac arrest due to other underlying condition
I46.9	Cardiac arrest, cause unspecified
I49.01	Ventricular fibrillation
R09.2	Respiratory arrest
R57.0	Cardiogenic shock
R57.1	Hypovolemic shock
R57.8	Other shock

A hospital's reimbursement depends even more on complete documentation and accurate coding with MS-DRGs
MS-DRGs are affected by the CC exclusions list

- Lists certain diagnoses that would not be considered CCs when coded as a secondary diagnosis with a certain principal diagnosis

MDC 15 Newborns & Other Neonates with Conditions Originating in Perinatal Period
Prematurity

Major Problems	DRG
Yes	791
No	792

DRG 791 PREMATURITY W MAJOR PROBLEMS
DRG 792 PREMATURITY W/O MAJOR PROBLEMS

PREMATURITY
PRINCIPAL OR SECONDARY DIAGNOSIS

P0700	Extremely low birth weight newborn, unspecified weight
P0710	Other low birth weight newborn, unspecified weight
P0714	Other low birth weight newborn, 1000-1249 grams
P0715	Other low birth weight newborn, 1250-1499 grams
P0716	Other low birth weight newborn, 1500-1749 grams
P0717	Other low birth weight newborn, 1750-1999 grams
P0718	Other low birth weight newborn, 2000-2499 grams
P0726	Extreme immaturity of newborn, gestational age 27 completed weeks
P0730	Preterm newborn, unspecified weeks of gestation
P0731	Preterm newborn, gestational age 28 completed weeks
P0732	Preterm newborn, gestational age 29 completed weeks
P0733	Preterm newborn, gestational age 30 completed weeks
P0734	Preterm newborn, gestational age 31 completed weeks
P0735	Preterm newborn, gestational age 32 completed weeks
P0736	Preterm newborn, gestational age 33 completed weeks
P0737	Preterm newborn, gestational age 34 completed weeks
P0738	Preterm newborn, gestational age 35 completed weeks
P0739	Preterm newborn, gestational age 36 completed weeks

MAJOR PROBLEMS
See Major Problem Diagnoses Listed under DRG 793

• **Figure 15.7** MDC 15, Newborns & Other Neonates with Conditions Originating in the Perinatal Period, Prematurity.

- Example: J82 (Eosinophilic pneumonia) is excluded as a CC when most of the pneumonia codes are assigned as principal diagnosis
- Good documentation and accurate coding will be even more important to obtain the optimum reimbursement for the hospital

Challenges for coding staff include:

- It may take more time to review and code a record resulting in decreased productivity
- Greater specificity in code assignment is necessary with ICD-10-CM/PCS and MS-DRGs
- There will be an increase in physician queries and communications
- Assigning POA (present on admission) indicators requires extra attention and may decrease productivity
- The coder must have a strong knowledge base about clinical conditions and disease to effectively use the MS-DRG system

MS-DRG Classification

Begins with diagnosis and pre-MDC (Fig. 15.8)

Pre-Major Diagnostic Categories (Pre-MDCs)

Pre-MDC MS-DRGs are very resource intensive
Services for these MS-DRGs may be performed for diagnoses in many different MDCs
Assigned independently of the MDC to indicate the procedure performed
Cases are assigned to these MS-DRGs before they are assigned a MDC

DRG	DRG Description
001	Heart transplant or implant of heart assist system w MCC
002	Heart transplant or implant of heart assist system w/o MCC

See Fig. 15.9 for the Pre-MDC table for DRG 001 and DRG 002.
There are 2 MDCs based on **both** principal diagnosis and secondary diagnosis

- MDC 24   Multiple Significant Trauma
- MDC 25   Human Immunodeficiency Virus Infections

Pre-MDC

ALL PATIENTS

Heart Transplant or Implant of Heart Assist System

MCC	DRG
Yes	001
No	002

ECMO or Tracheostomy with MV >96 Hours or PDX Except Face, Mouth and Neck

ECMO	Tracheostomy	MV>96	PDX Exc Face, Mouth, Neck	Major O.R. Procedure	DRG
Yes	n/a	n/a	n/a	n/a	003
No	Yes	Yes		Yes	003
No	Yes		Yes	Yes	003
No	Yes	Yes		No	004
No	Yes		Yes	No	004

Liver or Intestinal Transplant

Liver Transplant	Intestinal Transplant	MCC	DRG
Yes	Yes	n/a	005
No	Yes	n/a	005
Yes	No	Yes	005
Yes	No	No	006

Allogeneic Bone Marrow Transplant

DRG
014

Lung Transplant

DRG
007

Simultaneous Pancreas/Kidney Transplant

DRG
008

Autologous Bone Marrow Transplant or T-cell Immunotherapy

T-cell Immunotherapy	Bone Marrow Transplant	CC or MCC	DRG
Yes	n/a	n/a	016
No	Yes	Yes	016
No	Yes	No	017

Pancreas Transplant

DRG
010

Tracheostomy for Face, Mouth and Neck Diagnoses or Laryngectomy

MCC	CC	DRG
Yes	n/a	011
No	Yes	012
No	No	013

• **Figure 15.8** Pre-MDC in ICD-10-CM/PCS MS-DRG.

Pre-MDC
Heart Transplant or Implant of Heart Assist System

MCC	DRG
Yes	001
No	002

DRG 001 HEART TRANSPLANT OR IMPLANT OF HEART ASSIST SYSTEM W MCC
DRG 002 HEART TRANSPLANT OR IMPLANT OF HEART ASSIST SYSTEM W/O MCC

HEART TRANSPLANT
OPERATING ROOM PROCEDURES

02YA0Z0	Transplantation of Heart, Allogeneic, Open Approach
02YA0Z1	Transplantation of Heart, Syngeneic, Open Approach
02YA0Z2	Transplantation of Heart, Zooplastic, Open Approach
02RK0JZ	Replacement of Right Ventricle with Synthetic Substitute, Open Approach
with 02RL0JZ	Replacement of Left Ventricle with Synthetic Substitute, Open Approach

IMPLANT OF HEART ASSIST SYSTEM

02HA0QZ	Insertion of Implantable Heart Assist System into Heart, Open Approach
02HA3QZ	Insertion of Implantable Heart Assist System into Heart, Percutaneous Approach
02HA4QZ	Insertion of Implantable Heart Assist System into Heart, Percutaneous Endoscopic Approach
02HA0RS	Insertion of Biventricular Short-term External Heart Assist System into Heart, Open Approach
with 02PA0RZ	Removal of Short-term External Heart Assist System from Heart, Open Approach
02HA0RS	Insertion of Biventricular Short-term External Heart Assist System into Heart, Open Approach
with 02PA3RZ	Removal of Short-term External Heart Assist System from Heart, Percutaneous Approach
02HA0RS	Insertion of Biventricular Short-term External Heart Assist System into Heart, Open Approach
with 02PA4RZ	Removal of Short-term External Heart Assist System from Heart, Percutaneous Endoscopic Approach
02HA0RZ	Insertion of Short-term External Heart Assist System into Heart, Open Approach
with 02PA0RZ	Removal of Short-term External Heart Assist System from Heart, Open Approach

• **Figure 15.9** Example of Pre-MDCs in ICD-10-CM/PCS MS-DRG, DRG 001 and 002.

Example: Patient with HIV (B20), admitted for treatment of pneumonia due to pseudomonas (J15.1). The principal diagnosis is HIV with secondary diagnosis of pneumonia. The assignment of MS-DRG 976 HIV with Major Related Condition without CC/MCC is affected by the secondary diagnosis of J15.1.

Use surgical procedure MS-DRG if surgery was performed
• Surgical procedures pay more than nonsurgical MDCs

Fig. 15.10 illustrates MDC 1, Diseases and Disorders of the Nervous System
• Contains DRGs 020-036 with selection based on with or without a major complication or comorbidity (MCC)
    with or without complication or comorbidity (CC)
Fig. 15.11 illustrates MDC 1, DRGs 020-022.
• Surgical procedures with or without MCC or CC

Use principal diagnosis to select MS-DRG if no surgery was performed

MS-DRG Selection if No Surgical Procedure is Performed is Based on:

• Qualifying MCC/CC
    • An MCC/CC is likely to result in increased use of hospital resources
    • Pneumonia is an MCC; benign hypertension is not an MCC or a CC
    • Discharge disposition may make a difference in the MS-DRG assigned
• **May be excluded as MCC/CC**
    • Chronic and acute manifestations of the same disease (not CCs for one another)
    • Is closely related to the principal diagnosis

MDC 1 Diseases & Disorders of the Nervous System
Intracranial Vascular Procedures with PDX Hemorrhage

MCC	CC	DRG
Yes	n/a	020
No	Yes	021
No	No	022

DRG 020 INTRACRANIAL VASCULAR PROCEDURES W PDX HEMORRHAGE W MCC
DRG 021 INTRACRANIAL VASCULAR PROCEDURES W PDX HEMORRHAGE W CC
DRG 022 INTRACRANIAL VASCULAR PROCEDURES W PDX HEMORRHAGE W/O CC/MCC

INTRACRANIAL VASCULAR PROCEDURES
OPERATING ROOM PROCEDURES

031H09G	Bypass Right Common Carotid Artery to Intracranial Artery with Autologous Venous Tissue, Open Approach
031H0AG	Bypass Right Common Carotid Artery to Intracranial Artery with Autologous Arterial Tissue, Open Approach
031H0JG	Bypass Right Common Carotid Artery to Intracranial Artery with Synthetic Substitute, Open Approach
031H0KG	Bypass Right Common Carotid Artery to Intracranial Artery with Nonautologous Tissue Substitute, Open Approach
031H0ZG	Bypass Right Common Carotid Artery to Intracranial Artery, Open Approach
031J09G	Bypass Left Common Carotid Artery to Intracranial Artery with Autologous Venous Tissue, Open Approach
031J0AG	Bypass Left Common Carotid Artery to Intracranial Artery with Autologous Arterial Tissue, Open Approach
031J0JG	Bypass Left Common Carotid Artery to Intracranial Artery with Synthetic Substitute, Open Approach
031J0KG	Bypass Left Common Carotid Artery to Intracranial Artery with Nonautologous Tissue Substitute, Open Approach
031J0ZG	Bypass Left Common Carotid Artery to Intracranial Artery, Open Approach

• **Figure 15.10** Example of MDC 1 Diseases & Disorders of the Nervous System. Surgical DRGs.

Example:
- Cardiomyopathy is not considered a CC with congestive heart failure
- Urinary tract infection is considered a CC with congestive heart failure

Certain ICD-10-CM diagnosis codes include both an acute manifestation or complication with the underlying condition in one code.

Example:
- Exacerbation of Crohn's disease of small intestine with abscess: K50.014 (MS-DRG 386 Inflammatory Bowel Disease w CC)

MCC/CCs for MS-DRGs

CMS publishes a list of ICD-10-CM codes that are MCCs and CCs

Post Acute Transfer

CMS thought it was overpaying the acute care hospital for these patients at the full MS-DRG rates, so a reduction in payment formula was implemented
- Medicare developed special rules that apply to particular MS-DRGs in which patients are frequently discharged immediately to a rehab hospital, skilled nursing facility, a long-term care hospitals or home health care
- Termed transfer MS-DRGs
- Part of the Balanced Budget Act of 1997

Payment is adjusted when the covered days preceding the "transfer" are less than the Geometric Mean Length of Stay (GMLOS) of the assigned MS-DRG
- The facility is reimbursed on a per diem rate that is calculated by taking the hospital's normal reimbursement for the MS-DRG divided by the GMLOS

There are three types of transfers that are affected:
- Transfers to another acute care hospital
  - The transferring hospital receives double the per diem rate for the first day plus the per diem rate for each subsequent day prior to the transfer
  - Not to exceed the total MS-DRG payment
- Designated MS-DRGs transferred to a post acute care setting
  - The same formula as a transfer to another acute care hospital
- Designated special pay MS-DRGs transferred to a post acute care setting
  - The transferring hospital receives the per diem rate for the first day plus one-half the per diem rate for each subsequent day prior to the transfer

MDC 1 Diseases & Disorders of the Nervous System

MDC 1 Assignment of Diagnosis Codes

Surgical DRGs. O.R. Procedure of ...

Intracranial Vascular Procedures with PDX Hemorrhage

MCC	CC	DRG
Yes	n/a	020
No	Yes	021
No	No	022

Craniotomy with Major Device Implant or Acute Complex CNS PDX

Major Device Implant or Acute Complex CNS PDX	Chemotherapy Implant	PDX Epilepsy w/ Neurostim	MCC	DRG
	Yes	No	n/a	023
Yes	No	No	Yes	023
	No	Yes	n/a	023
Yes	No	No	No	024

Spinal Procedures

MCC	CC	Spinal Neurostimulator Combinations	DRG
Yes	n/a	n/a	028
No	Yes	n/a	029
No	No	Yes	029
No	No	No	030

Ventricular Shunt Procedures

MCC	CC	DRG
Yes	n/a	031
No	Yes	032
No	No	033

Carotid Artery Stent Procedures

MCC	CC	DRG
Yes	n/a	034
No	Yes	035
No	No	036

• **Figure 15.11** MDC 1 Diseases & Disorders of the Nervous System. DRG 020, 021, and 022.

Present on Admission Indicator (POA)

Hospitals submit Medicare inpatient claims with a Present On Admission (POA) indicator for nearly every diagnosis Exempt are:
- Critical access hospitals
- Maryland waiver hospitals*
- Long-term care hospitals

- Cancer and inpatient psychiatric hospitals
- Inpatient rehabilitation facilities
- Children's inpatient facilities
- Rural health clinics
- Federally qualified health centers
- Religious non-medical health care institutions
- Veterans Administration/Department of Defense hospitals Medicare returns claims without POA codes
- Hospitals must correct and resubmit a claim POA guidelines are provided in Appendix I of the *ICD-10-CM Official Guidelines for Coding and Reporting*

*No longer exempt from reporting requirements, but report does not calculate into payment.

POA defined as present at the time the order for inpatient admission occurs

- Conditions that develop during an outpatient encounter are considered as Present On Admission
  - Example: Emergency room, observation, outpatient surgery

The reporting options are:

Y Yes (this diagnosis was present at the time of admission)

N No (this diagnosis was not present at the time of admission)

U Unknown (documentation is insufficient to determine if condition was present at time of inpatient admission)

  - N and U indicators report as Not Present on Admission (NPOA) and do not cause an increased payment at the CC/MCC level

W Clinically undetermined (provider is unable to clinically determine whether the condition was present at the time of admission or not)

Unreported/Not used – (Exempt from POA reporting)

Hospitals report ICD-10-CM/CD-10-PCS codes for procedures and diagnoses, and CMS determines the MS-DRG and payment

Hospitals also calculate MS-DRGs to estimate accounts receivable, occupancy rates, and case mix

Hospital-Acquired Conditions (HAC)

Medicare will not reimburse a higher-payment MS-DRG if one of the following hospital-acquired or preventable conditions occurs after the patient's admission to the hospital:

*No longer exempt from reporting requirements, but report does not calculate into payment

- Foreign object retained after surgery
- Air embolism
- Blood incompatibility
- Pressure ulcer stages 3 and 4
- Falls and trauma
- Catheter-associated urinary tract infection
- Vascular catheter-associated infection
- Manifestations of poor glycemic control
- Surgical site infection following surgery
  - Coronary artery bypass graft (CABG)
  - Orthopedic procedures
  - Bariatric surgery
  - Cardiac electronic device implant
- Deep vein thrombosis and pulmonary embolism following certain orthopedic procedures
- Iatrogenic pneumothorax with venous catheterization

These diagnoses will not qualify as MCC/CC if not present at the time of admission, thus reducing facility reimbursement

- Proposal for HAC Reduction Program that will adjust payment when HAC occurs

72-Hour Rule

Also known as the "3-day window"

Part of Medicare's Prospective Payment System (PPS)

- IRF (Inpatient Rehabilitation Facilities) and PPS providers not subject to 72-hour rule

States that reimbursement for any hospital outpatient diagnostic or other services provided for the same diagnosis occasioning the admission 3 days prior to admission is included in the MS-DRG payment for that hospital stay.

- Hospitals must demonstrate with supporting documentation that the services (outpatient) were unrelated to the diagnoses/reason for admission to report these services as an outpatient account.

Monitoring MS-DRG Reimbursement

Accounts Receivable (AR)

List of high-dollar cases

List of unbilled accounts/claims

Remittance Advice

Sent by MACs listing amounts paid to hospital

Always verify correct MS-DRG was paid based on MS-DRG initially submitted

Audit for underpayments of transfer MS-DRGs

Resource Utilization Groups (RUGs)

Reimbursement system used in long-term skilled health care settings

- Long-term care hospitals (LTCH) are defined as those with average stays greater than 25 days

Based on resources

Utilizes information from the minimum data set (MDS)

- Rehabilitation services
- Special care needs
- Clinical requirements
- Activity of daily living
- Cognitive function
- Behavioral symptoms and resident's distressed mood

Assessment of patient must be on days 5, 14, 30, 60, and 90

- Defined by federal law

Home Health Prospective Payment System (HHPPS)

Reimbursement system used in home care agencies

Based on information in Outcome and Assessment Information Set (OASIS)

Payment based on visit

Home Assessment Validation and Entry (HAVEN) is the CMS free-data entry software utilized by most Home Health Agencies (HHA)

Inpatient Rehabilitation Facility (IRF) Prospective Payment System

Paid on a per-discharge basis

Utilizes information from an Inpatient Rehabilitation Facility Patient Assessment Instrument (IRF PAI)

- Classifies patients into distinct groups based on clinical characteristics and expected resource needs

Inpatient Psychiatric Facility (IPF) Prospective Payment System

- Originally excluded from PPS
- Also excluded were rehabilitation, children's, cancer, and long-term care hospitals, rehabilitation and hospitals located outside the 50 states and Puerto Rico
- Referred to as TEFRA (Tax Equity and Fiscal Responsibility Act) facilities. Paid on a per diem amount
- Adjusted based on:
  1. Diagnosis-Related Group classification
  2. Patient age
  3. Length of stay
  4. Any comorbidities

Revenue Codes

Four digit classification system that
- Identifies services/procedures
- Identifies location where services were rendered
- Begins with 0 (zero)

Three Main Categories

1. Billing revenue codes
   Example:
   - 0137, replacement of a prior claim for a hospital outpatient charge

2. Accommodation revenue codes
   Example:
   - 0120, semiprivate room and board for obstetrical patient
3. Ancillary revenue codes
   Example:
   - 0314, laboratory pathological services for a biopsy

The Digits and Their Placement Further Define Elements of the Revenue Code

Example:

Revenue code for laboratory pathological service is 031X The fourth digit (X) is assigned from one of five subcategory digits
- Subcategory identifies type of service/procedure within category

Example:
- Fourth digit (4) identifies biopsy services (0314)

Medicare Determines Included and Excluded Services Based on Revenue Codes

Under the OPPS, Medicare requires use of HCPCS codes by hospital outpatient departments when a code for that service is available (see Fig. 15.12)

Data Quality

Charge Description Master

Database used by hospitals

Includes all services, procedures, supplies, and drugs with a
- Corresponding internal numbered description of everything utilized by the patient
- Revenue code
- CPT/HCPCS codes
- Charge (Fig. 15.13)

Revenue Code	Description	HCPCS Codes
0274	Prosthetic and orthotic devices	L9900, Orthotic
0331	Injected chemotherapy	96401, Chemotherapy administration
0481	Cardiac catheterization laboratory	93460, Combined heart cath
0623	Surgical dressing	G0168, Wound closure
0636	Pharmacy	J1645, Dalteparin sodium
0901	Electroshock treatment	90870, Electroconvulsive therapy

• **Figure 15.12** Example of some services that require HCPCS codes.

HCPCS	Description	Active Date	Revenue Code	Charge
Q2017	Teniposide, 50mg	01/01/2014	0636	$825.50
96413	Chemotherapy admin Infusion, up to one hour	01/01/2007	0261	$285.11
P9016	Red blood cells, leukocytes reduced, each unit	01/01/1994	0380	$189.45
96360	Infusion therapy, not chemotherapy drugs, 1 hr	01/01/2009	0450	$108.24
J0207	Amifostine, 500mg	01/01/1994	7000	$475.05

• **Figure 15.13** Example of basic charge description master.

Elements of a Charge Description Master

- Unique department code number
- Description number (charge code) that is internally assigned to identify each procedure, supply, drug, and service
- The charge code is a unique alpha or alphanumeric code that remains constant year after year
- Procedure/service description
- CPT/HCPCS codes—HCPCS code may change based on code changes and changes in payer requirements
- Revenue code—may change based on payer requirements
- Cost/Charge—generally evaluated and changed annually
- Hard-coded modifiers when applicable
- Charge master automatically enters appropriate modifier

Should be Reviewed Regularly and Updated as Needed to Assist in

- Reduction of claim denials
- Accurate reimbursement
- Compliance
- Better data management and quality
- Tracking of services and supplies

Review for

Invalid/inaccurate codes
- Unclear/incorrect descriptions
- Omitted procedures or supplies
- Correct service/supply and revenue code linkage
- Appropriate fees

Beneficiary signatures on file
- Service, charges submitted without need for patient signature

Things that may be perceived as fraudulent

Fraud

Intentional deception to benefit

Example: Submitting for services not provided

Anyone who submits for Medicare services can be violator, such as

- Physicians
- Hospitals
- Laboratories
- Billing services
- YOU

Fraud Can be

Billing for services not provided
Misrepresenting diagnosis, CPT, or HCPCS code(s)
Kickbacks
Unbundling services
Falsifying medical necessity
Systematic waiver of co-payment

Fraud Examples

Patient presents with chest pain and is treated.
    Progress note indicates myocardial infarction (MI) is to be ruled out.

Laboratory tests do not suggest or indicate MI.
    Coder assigns MI as PDx as the reason for encounter/admission.
Chest pain pays less than MI.
This is fraud!

Other Examples of Fraud

Upcoding is using a higher-level code for a lower-level service
Misrepresenting the diagnosis for a patient to justify the service or equipment furnished
Unbundling or exploding charge
    Example: Reporting multichannel lab tests (many tests in one process) to appear as if the individual tests were performed
Billing noncovered services
    Example: Routine foot care reported as more involved form of foot care that is paid under the Medicare program
Applying for duplicate payment
    Example: Patient has Medicare and another insurance and both are billed without indicating that there is another third-party payer

Office of the Inspector General (OIG)

Develops and publishes Work Plan annually
    Outlines Medicare monitoring program
    MACs monitor those areas identified in plan

Complaints of Fraud or Abuse

Submitted orally or in writing to MACs or OIG
Allegations made by anyone against anyone
Allegations followed up by MACs and/or OIG
www.oig.hhs.gov/reports-and-publications/workplan/index.asp

Abuse

Generally involves
- Impropriety
- Lack of medical necessity for services reported
Review takes place after claim is submitted
- MACs go back and do historical review of claims

Kickbacks

Bribe or rebate for referring patient for any service covered by Medicare
Any personal gain kickback
A felony
- $25,000 fine or
- 5 years in jail or
- Both

Protect Yourself

Use your common sense
Submit only truthful and accurate claims

If you are unsure about charges, services, or procedures check with physician or supervisor

Managed Health Care

Network health care providers and facilities that offer health care services under one organization

Group hospitals, physicians, or other providers

Majority of people with health care coverage are covered by a managed care organization (e.g., HMO, PPO, POS)

Managed Care Organizations

Responsible for health care services to an enrolled group or person

Coordinate various health care services

Negotiate with facilities and providers

Capitation method common in managed care

- Prepaid, fixed amount for each person in the plan
  - Regardless of resource use

Preferred Provider Organization (PPO)

Providers and facilities form network to offer health care services as group

Enrollees who seek health care outside PPO pay more

Point of Service (POS)

In-network or out-of-network providers may be used

Benefits are paid at a higher rate to in-network providers

Subscribers are not limited to providers, but to amount covered by plan

Health Maintenance Organization (HMO)

Total package health care

Out-of-pocket expenses minimal

Assigned physician acts as gatekeeper to refer patient outside organization

TABLE 15-1	
Abbreviations	

AMLOS	Arithmetic Mean Length of Stay	IRF	Inpatient Rehabilitation Facility
APCs	Ambulatory Patient Classifications	IRF PAI	Inpatient Rehabilitation Facility Patient Assessment Instrument
APGs	Ambulatory Patient Groups	LCD	Local Coverage Determination
AWP	Average Wholesale Price	LMRP	Local Medical Review Policies, replaced by LCD, Local Coverage Determination
CC	Complications and Co-morbidities		
CCI	Correct Coding Initiative (AKA, NCCI)	MCC	Major Complication/Comorbidity
CLIA	Clinical Laboratories Improvement Act	MDCs	Major Diagnostic Categories
DCN	Document Control Number	NCCI	National Correct Coding Initiative
DME	Durable Medical Equipment	NCD	National Coverage Decisions
DRG	Diagnosis-Related Groups	NCHS	National Centers for Health Statistics
EDI	Electronic Data Interchange	NPI	National Provider Identifier
EIN	Employer Identification Number	OASIS	Outcome and Assessment Information Set
EOB	Explanation of Benefits	OBRA	Omnibus Budget Reconciliation Act of 1986
ESRD	End Stage Renal Disease	OCE	Outpatient Code Editor
FL	Field Locators	OIG	Office of the Inspector General
FUD	Follow-up Days	OR	Operating Room
GMLOS	Geometric Mean Length of Stay	PDx	Principal Diagnosis
GPN	Group Provider Number	PIN	Provider Identification Number
HAC	Hospital-Acquired Condition	POA	Present on Admission
HAVEN	Home Assessment Validation and Entry	PPO	Preferred Provider Organization
HCPCS	Healthcare Common Procedural Coding System	PPS	Prospective Payment System
HHA	Home Health Agencies	PRO	Peer Review Organization, now QIO
HHPPS	Home Health Prospective Payment System	QIO	Quality Improvement Organization
HICN	Health Insurance Claim/Identification Number	RBRVS	Resource-Based Relative Value Scale
HIPAA	Health Insurance Portability and Accountability Act	RUGs	Resource Utilization Groups
		SI	Status Indicators
HMO	Health Maintenance Organization	UCR	Usual, Customary, and Reasonable
HOPPS	Hospital Outpatient Prospective Payment System	UHDDS	Uniform Hospital Discharge Data Set
HPMP	Hospital Payment Monitoring Program	WHO	World Health Organization
ICN	Internal Control Number		
IPF	Inpatient Psychiatric Facility		

TABLE 15-2

Reimbursement Terminology

Advance Beneficiary Notice	ABN, notification in advance of services that Medicare may not pay for them, including the estimated cost to the patient
Ancillary Service	A service that is supportive of care of a patient, such as laboratory services
APC	A classification system used to group like services based upon clinical similarities and resources utilized
Assignment	A legal agreement that allows the provider to receive direct payment from a payer and the provider to accept payment as payment in full for covered services
Attending Physician	The physician legally responsible for oversight of an inpatient's care
Beneficiary	The person who benefits from insurance coverage; also known as subscriber, dependent, enrollee, member, or participant
Birthday Rule	When both parents have insurance coverage, the parent with the birthday earliest in the year is the primary coverage for a dependent
Certified Registered Nurse Anesthetist	CRNA, an individual with specialized training and certification in nursing and anesthesia
Charge Description Master	Record of services, procedures, supplies, and drugs with corresponding codes, descriptions, and charges billed
Co-insurance	Cost-sharing of covered services
Compliance Plan	Written strategy developed by medical facilities to ensure appropriate, consistent documentation within the medical record and ensure compliance with third-party payer guidelines
Concurrent Care	More than one physician providing care to a patient at the same time
Coordination of Benefits	COB, management of multiple third-party payments to ensure overpayment does not occur
Co-payment	Cost-sharing between beneficiary and payer
Correct Coding Initiative	CCI, developed by CMS to control improper unbundling of CPT codes leading to inappropriate payment; also known as NCCI (National Correct Coding Initiative)
Deductible	That portion of covered services paid by the beneficiary before third-party payment begins
Denial	Statement from the payer that reimbursement is denied
Documentation	Detailed chronology of facts and observations regarding a patient's health
Diagnosis-Related Groups	DRGs, a case mix classification system established by CMS consisting of classes of patients who are similar clinically and in consumption of hospital resources; replaced with MS-DRGs
Durable Medical Equipment	DME, medically related equipment that is not disposable, such as wheelchairs, crutches, and vaporizers
Electronic Data Interchange	EDI, computerized submission of health care insurance information exchange
Employer Identification Number	EIN, an Internal Revenue Service (IRS)–issued identification number used on tax documents
Encounter Form	Medical document that contains information regarding a patient visit for health care services
Explanation of Benefits	EOB, written, detailed listing of medical service payments by third-party payer to inform beneficiary and provider of payment
Fee Schedule	Established list of payments for medical services, i.e., lab, physician services
Follow-up Days	FUD, established by third-party payers and listing the number of days after a procedure for which a provider must provide normal uncomplicated related services to a patient for no fee (also known as global days, global package, or global period)
Group Provider Number	GPN, numeric designation for a group of providers that is used instead of the individual provider number
Hospital Payment Monitoring System	HPMS, an inpatient PPS audit system used by CMS to reduce improper payments
Invalid Claim	Claim that is missing necessary information and cannot be processed or paid
Inpatient	CMS defines an inpatient as a person who has been formally admitted to a hospital with the expectation that he or she will remain at least overnight and occupy a bed even if it later develops that the patient can be discharged or transferred to another hospital and not actually use a hospital bed overnight
Medical Record	Documentation about the health care of a patient

Continued

TABLE 15-2

Reimbursement Terminology—cont'd

Medicare Administrative Contractors	MACs replaced Fiscal Intermediaries (FIs)
Medicare Severity Diagnosis-Related Groups	MS-DRG, classification system implemented October 2007 that is based on the principal diagnosis and the medical or surgical service provided to the Medicare inpatient in which the hospital/facility is paid a fixed amount for each patient discharged in a treatment category
National Correct Coding Initiative	Developed by CMS to control improper unbundling of CPT codes leading to inappropriate payment; also known as CCI (Correct Coding Initiative)
Noncovered Services	Any service not included by a third-party payer in the list of services for which payment is made
National Provider Identifier	NPI, 10-digit number assigned to provider and used for identification purposes when submitting services to third-party payers
Hospital Outpatient	An individual who is not an inpatient of a hospital but who is registered as an outpatient at the hospital
Prior Authorization	Also known as preauthorization, which is a requirement by the payer to receive written permission prior to patient services if the service is to be considered for payment by the payer
Provider Identification Number	PIN, or UPIN, assigned by the third-party payer to providers to be used for identification purposes when submitting services to third-party payers
Rejection	A claim that does not pass edits and is returned to the provider as rejected
Reimbursement	Payment from a third-party payer for services rendered to a patient covered by the payer's health care plan
State License Number	Identification number issued by a state to a physician who has been granted the right to practice in that state
Usual, Customary, and Reasonable	UCR, used by third-party payers to establish a payment rate for a service in an area with the usual (standard fee in area), customary (standard fee by the physician), and reasonable (as determined by payer) rate

Chapter 15: Reimbursement Quiz

(Quiz Answers are located in Appendix B)

1. Any person who is identified as receiving life insurance or medical benefits:
   a. primary
   b. beneficiary
   c. participant
   d. recipient
2. TEFRA of 1982 established the _____, which pays a fixed amount intended to cover the cost of treating a typical patient for a particular DRG.
   a. OPPS
   b. NPI
   c. DRG
   d. PPS
3. The set of patient attributes that is used to define each MS-DRG consists of:
   a. principal diagnosis, secondary diagnosis, insurance policy rules, principal procedure, and patient age
   b. principal procedure, discharge status, patient age and sex, and principal diagnosis
   c. principal and secondary diagnosis, principal procedure, patient age and sex, and discharge status
   d. principal diagnosis, secondary diagnosis, medical or surgical service (principal or significant), and any qualifying complication(s)/comorbidity(ies), discharge status
4. A four-digit classification system that identifies and explains services or procedures and the location in which they were rendered is called a(n):
   a. ancillary code
   b. revenue code
   c. billing code
   d. accommodation code
5. CMS delegates the daily operation of the Medicare program to:
   a. DHHS
   b. QIO
   c. RVU
   d. MACs

6. The Omnibus Budget Reconciliation Act of 1986 required a PPS-based payment system to replace the one based on existing outpatient hospital cost. This system is what classification system?
   a. MS-DRGs
   b. APCs
   c. CPT
   d. ICD-10-CM

7. This part of Medicare covers the inpatient hospital portion:
   a. Part A
   b. Part B
   c. Part C
   d. Part D

8. This issue of the *Federal Register* contains major outpatient facility changes for CMS programs for the coming year:
   a. October/November
   b. November/December
   c. December/October
   d. November/August

9. This is the number of MS-DRGs:
   a. 001-502
   b. 001-999
   c. 001-998
   d. 001-604

10. Entity responsible for development of the plan that outlines monitoring of the Medicare program:
   a. MACs
   b. OIG
   c. DHSS
   d. HEW

PART **4**

CPT and HCPCS Coding

16

Introduction to CPT

Introduction to Medical Coding

Translates services/procedures/supplies/drugs into CPT/HCPCS codes

Translates diagnosis(es) into ICD-10-CM codes

Two Levels of Service Codes

1. Level I CPT
2. Level II HCPCS, National Codes

Diagnosis Codes, ICD-10-CM

ICD-10-CM, International Classification of Diseases, 10th Revision, Clinical Modification

- Classification system
- Translates diagnosis(es) (dx) into standardized codes that explain why service was provided
- Very specific in nature
- May be up to seven characters
- Example: Diabetes becomes E11.9

CPT

Developed by the AMA in 1966

Five-digit codes to report services provided to patients

Updated each November for use January 1

- Historically in numerical order
- Not the case for more than 100 codes
- Pound symbol (#) appears before the resequenced codes
  Example: In the 51725-51798 range, code 51797 follows 51729 (in numeric order). Code 51797 also appears in correct numeric order in the CPT, but next to the code a note states "Code is out of numerical sequence. See 51725-51798."

See Appendix N of the CPT for a complete list of the resequenced codes.

Types of CPT Codes

- Medical
- Surgical
- Diagnostic services

- Anesthesia
- Evaluation and Management

CPT Codes

Allow communication that is both effective and efficient
Inform third-party payers of services/procedures provided
Used as a basis of payment

Incorrect Coding

Results in providers being paid inappropriately (either overpayment or underpayment)

Outpatient Physician (Non-Hospital) Services

Reported on standardized insurance form
CMS-1500 example (Fig. 16.1)

CPT Format

Symbols

Used to convey information
- ● Bullet = New code symbol
- ▲ Triangle = Revised code
- ►◄ Right and left triangles = Beginning and ending of text change
- + Plus = Add-on code
  - Full list in Appendix D of CPT
- ⊘ Circle with line = Modifier -51 exempt code
  - Modifier -51 cannot be used with these codes
  - Full list in Appendix E of CPT
- ★ Star = Telemedicine Services
  - Such as 97802, medical nutrition therapy
  - Full list in Appendix P of CPT
- ⚡ Lightning bolt symbol = Codes for which the FDA status is pending
  - Full list in Appendix K of CPT
- # Number sign = Resequenced CPT codes
  - Such as 21552, excision of tumor, 3 cm or greater, resequenced code in 2010
  - Full list in Appendix N
- ○ Circle = Recycled/reinstated code

HEALTH INSURANCE CLAIM FORM

APPROVED BY NATIONAL UNIFORM CLAIM COMMITTEE (NUCC) 02/12

| | PICA | | | | | | | | PICA | |

1. MEDICARE □ (Medicare#)   MEDICAID □ (Medicaid#)   TRICARE □ (ID#DoD#)   CHAMPVA □ (Member ID#)   GROUP HEALTH PLAN □ (ID#)   FECA BLK LUNG □ (ID#)   OTHER □ (ID#)   **1a.** INSURED'S I.D. NUMBER _____ (For Program in Item 1)

2. PATIENT'S NAME (Last Name, First Name, Middle Initial)

3. PATIENT'S BIRTH DATE   MM | DD | YY   SEX   M □   F □

4. INSURED'S NAME (Last Name, First Name, Middle Initial)

5. PATIENT'S ADDRESS (No., Street)

6. PATIENT RELATIONSHIP TO INSURED   Self □   Spouse □   Child □   Other □

7. INSURED'S ADDRESS (No., Street)

CITY _____ STATE   **8.** RESERVED FOR NUCC USE   CITY _____ STATE

ZIP CODE   TELEPHONE (Include Area Code) ( )

ZIP CODE   TELEPHONE (Include Area Code) ( )

9. OTHER INSURED'S NAME (Last Name, First Name, Middle Initial)

10. IS PATIENT'S CONDITION RELATED TO:

11. INSURED'S POLICY GROUP OR FECA NUMBER

a. OTHER INSURED'S POLICY OR GROUP NUMBER

a. EMPLOYMENT? (Current or Previous)   YES □   NO □

a. INSURED'S DATE OF BIRTH   MM | DD | YY   SEX   M □   F □

b. RESERVED FOR NUCC USE

b. AUTO ACCIDENT?   YES □   NO □   PLACE (State) ___

b. OTHER CLAIM ID (Designated by NUCC)

c. RESERVED FOR NUCC USE

c. OTHER ACCIDENT?   YES □   NO □

c. INSURANCE PLAN NAME OR PROGRAM NAME

d. INSURANCE PLAN NAME OR PROGRAM NAME

10d. CLAIM CODES (Designated by NUCC)

d. IS THERE ANOTHER HEALTH BENEFIT PLAN?   YES □   NO □   *If yes,* complete items 9, 9a, and 9d.

READ BACK OF FORM BEFORE COMPLETING & SIGNING THIS FORM.

12. PATIENT'S OR AUTHORIZED PERSON'S SIGNATURE I authorize the release of any medical or other information necessary to process this claim. I also request payment of government benefits either to myself or to the party who accepts assignment below.

SIGNED _____ DATE _____

13. INSURED'S OR AUTHORIZED PERSON'S SIGNATURE I authorize payment of medical benefits to the undersigned physician or supplier for services described below.

SIGNED _____

14. DATE OF CURRENT ILLNESS, INJURY, or PREGNANCY(LMP)   MM | DD | YY   QUAL. |

15. OTHER DATE   QUAL. | MM | DD | YY

16. DATES PATIENT UNABLE TO WORK IN CURRENT OCCUPATION   FROM MM | DD | YY   TO MM | DD | YY

17. NAME OF REFERRING PROVIDER OR OTHER SOURCE   17a. | 17b. NPI |

18. HOSPITALIZATION DATES RELATED TO CURRENT SERVICES   FROM MM | DD | YY   TO MM | DD | YY

19. ADDITIONAL CLAIM INFORMATION (Designated by NUCC)

20. OUTSIDE LAB?   YES □   NO □ $ CHARGES

21. DIAGNOSIS OR NATURE OF ILLNESS OR INJURY Relate A-L to service line below (24E)   ICD Ind. |

A. |____   B. |____   C. |____   D. |____
E. |____   F. |____   G. |____   H. |____
I. |____   J. |____   K. |____   L. |____

22. RESUBMISSION CODE _____ ORIGINAL REF. NO. _____

23. PRIOR AUTHORIZATION NUMBER

24. A. DATE(S) OF SERVICE From MM DD YY To MM DD YY	B. PLACE OF SERVICE	C. EMG	D. PROCEDURES, SERVICES, OR SUPPLIES (Explain Unusual Circumstances) CPT/HCPCS	MODIFIER	E. DIAGNOSIS POINTER	F. $ CHARGES	G. DAYS OR UNITS	H. EPSDT Family Plan	I. ID. QUAL.	J. RENDERING PROVIDER ID. #
1										NPI
2										NPI
3										NPI
4										NPI
5										NPI
6										NPI

25. FEDERAL TAX I.D. NUMBER   SSN □ EIN □

26. PATIENT'S ACCOUNT NO.

27. ACCEPT ASSIGNMENT? (For govt. claims, see back)   YES □   NO □

28. TOTAL CHARGE $

29. AMOUNT PAID $

30. Rsvd for NUCC Use

31. SIGNATURE OF PHYSICIAN OR SUPPLIER INCLUDING DEGREES OR CREDENTIALS (I certify that the statements on the reverse apply to this bill and are made a part thereof.)

SIGNED _____ DATE _____

32. SERVICE FACILITY LOCATION INFORMATION   a. NPI   b.

33. BILLING PROVIDER INFO & PH # ( )   a. NPI   b.

NUCC Instruction Manual available at: www.nucc.org   *PLEASE PRINT OR TYPE*   APPROVED OMB-0938-1197 FORM 1500 (02-12)

• Figure 16.1 The CMS-1500 Health Insurance Claim Form.

CPT Sections

1. Evaluation & Management (E/M)
2. Anesthesia
3. Surgery
4. Radiology
5. Pathology and Laboratory
6. Medicine

> **NOTE**
>
> During your examination, the front section of the CPT (Introduction and Illustrations) is an excellent resource on the format, definitions of terms, medical terms, and instructions in the CPT. Review these well before the examination to familiarize yourself with where to find the information that is contained in the front section.
>
> Also, flag the different sections of the CPT for easy access during the examination—for example, the list of illustrations section, E/M Guidelines, Appendices, and other major sections of the manual.

Categorized by

Sections
  Subsections
  Subheadings
  Categories
    Anatomy
      Knee or Shoulder
    Procedure
      Incision or Excision
    Condition
      Fracture or Dislocation
    Description
      Cast or Strap
    Surgical approach
      Anterior Cranial Fossa or Middle Cranial Fossa

Guidelines

Section-specific information begins each section
Provides instruction pertinent to entire section

Notes

Located throughout CPT
Provides instruction pertinent to specific subsection

Two Types of Code Descriptions

1. **Stand-alone:** Full description
   Example: 10080 Incision and drainage of pilonidal cyst; simple
2. **Indented:** Dependent on preceding stand-alone for meaning
   Example: 10080 Incision and drainage of pilonidal cyst; simple
          10081   complicated

Semicolon

- Description preceding semicolon is the common part of the description and applies to any indented codes under it
- You must return to stand-alone for full description
  Example: 10081 Incision and drainage of pilonidal cyst; complicated

Modifiers Add Information

CPT Modifier

Appended to the end of the CPT/HCPCS code
  Some modifiers are informational; others affect reimbursement
  Example: 43820 gastrojejunostomy
  - -62 two primary surgeons
  - 43820-62 two surgeons performed a gastrojejunostomy
  - Only used if both surgeons submit same CPT code and both surgeons dictate a separate operative report

Level II HCPCS Modifiers

"-AS" physician's assistant
  "-F1" Left hand, second digit
  All modifiers used on CPT or HCPCS codes
  All HCPCS modifiers begin with a letter
  Modifiers are placed in Block D, Modifier (see Fig. 16.1)

Unlisted Services

Codes usually end in "99" = "no specific code" in Category I or Category III
Used when a more specific code cannot be assigned
Written report must accompany claim form indicating
- Nature
- Extent
- Need
- Time
- Effort
- Equipment used

Category II Codes—Supplemental Tracking Codes

Used for performance measurements
- Optional unless practice participating in Quality Payment Program (QPP)
  These codes collect data concerning the quality of care and test results
  Alphanumeric and end in the letter "F" (0005F)
  Located after the Medicine section in CPT
- On CPC exam

Category III Codes—New Technology

Temporary codes—may be included in this section up to 5 years

Identify emerging technology, services, and procedures

Located after Category II codes

Alphanumeric and end in the letter "T" (0055T)

- May or may not receive future Category I code status
- Category I codes (00100-99607)
- Approved by AMA and the Food and Drug Administration (FDA)
- Proven clinical effectiveness (efficacy)
- Category III has not been approved and has no proven clinical effectiveness (efficacy)
- Use Category III code instead of unlisted code if no Category I code appropriate
- Use unlisted code if no Category III code exists
- On CPC exam

The Index

Used to locate service/procedure terms and codes

Speeds up code location

Uses dictionary format

- First entries and last entries on top of page
- Code display in index
  - Single code: 38115
  - Multiple codes: 26645, 26650
  - Range of codes: 22310-22325

Location Methods

Service/procedure: Repair, excision
Anatomic site: Meniscus, knee
Condition or disease: Cleft lip, clot
Synonym: Toe and interphalangeal joint

Eponym: Jones procedure, Heller operation
Abbreviation: ECG, PEEP (positive end-expiratory pressure)
"See" in Index
Cross-reference terms: "Look here for code"
Index: Stem, Brain: *See* Brainstem

Appendices of CPT

Appendix A: Modifiers

Appendix B: Summary of Additions, Deletions, and Revisions

Appendix C: Clinical Examples (E/M Codes)

Appendix D: Summary of CPT Add-on Codes

Appendix E: Summary of CPT Codes Exempt from Modifier -51

Appendix F: Summary of CPT Codes Exempt from Modifier -63

Appendix G: Summary of CPT Codes That Include Moderate (Conscious) Sedation (Deleted for 2017)

Appendix H: Alphabetical Clinical Topics Listing (AKA-Alphabetical Listing) (Moved to AMA CPT website at www.ama-assn.org/go/CPT)

Appendix I: Genetic Testing Code Modifiers (Deleted for 2013)

Appendix J: Electrodiagnostic Medicine Listing of Sensory, Motor, and Mixed Nerves

Appendix K: Product Pending FDA Approval

Appendix L: Vascular Families

Appendix M: Renumbered CPT Codes—Citations Crosswalk

Appendix N: Summary of Resequenced CPT Codes

Appendix O: Multianalyte Assays with Algorithmic Analyses

Appendix P: CPT Codes That May Be Used For Synchronous Telemedicine Services

Review information in the CPT appendices prior to examination

17

Evaluation and Management (E/M) Section (99202-99499)

Subsections by type of service
Types of service
- Consultation
- Office Services
- Hospital Services, etc.

Integral Factors When Selecting E/M Codes

1. Place of Service

Explains setting of service
- Office
- Emergency Department
- Nursing Home

2. Type of Service

Physicians provide many types of service
- Consultations (not reported for Medicare)
- Admissions
- Office visits

3. Patient Status

The four status types are
1. New patient
2. Established patient
3. Outpatient
4. Inpatient

New Patient

Has not received any professional service in last 3 years from the same physician or another physician of the same specialty and in the same group

New patients are more labor-intensive for physician, medical staff, and clerical staff

Established Patient

Has received professional services in last 3 years from the same physician or another physician of the same specialty in the same group

Medical record available with current, relevant information

Outpatient

One who has not been admitted to a health care facility
Example: Patient receives services at clinic, ED, or same-day surgery center

Inpatient

One who has been formally admitted to a health care facility

Example: Patient admitted to hospital or nursing home
Physician dictates
- Admission orders
- H&P (history and physical)
- Requests for consultations

Levels of E/M Service Based On

- Skill required to provide service
- Time spent
- Level of knowledge necessary to treat the patient
- Effort required
- Responsibility required/assumed

Levels of 99202-99215 Based Only On

- Medical decision making (MDM)
- Time spent

E/M Levels Divided Based On

Key Components (KC)

- History (Hx)
- Physical examination (PE)
- MDM

Contributory Factors (CF)

- Counseling
- Coordination of care
- Nature of presenting problem

Every Encounter Contains Varying Amount of KC and CF

More extensive component/factor
- Higher level of service
  - Less extensive component/factor
- Lower level of service

Key Components

Four Elements of a History

1. Chief Complaint (CC)
2. History of Present Illness (HPI)
3. Review of Systems (ROS)
4. Past, Family, and/or Social History (PFSH)

Chief Complaint (CC)—Subjective

Reason for encounter or presenting problem: Patient's current complaint in patient's own words
  Documented in medical record for each encounter

History of Present Illness (HPI)—Subjective

Description of development of current illness, e.g., date of onset
  Patient describes HPI
  Provider must personally document

Physician and Patient Dialogue

Development of a CC of Abdominal Pain (HPI):
"Started Thursday night and was mild. During the night, it got worse. Friday morning I went to work but had to leave because the pain got so bad."
  Location. Specific source of pain
    "Pain was in lower left-hand side, a little toward back."
  Quality. Is pain sharp, intermittent, burning?
    "Pain is really sharp and constant."
  Severity. Is pain intense, moderate, mild?
    "Pain is terrible, worst pain I have ever had." (intensity of pain/scale)
  *__Duration.__ How long has pain been present?
    "Pain has been going on now for 3 days."
  Timing. Is pain constant or does it come and go?
    "Pain just continues. It just doesn't go away."
  Context. When does it hurt most?
    "Pain is just there, it doesn't matter what I am doing."
  Modifying factors. Does anything make it better or worse?
    "Nothing I do makes it any better or any worse."

*Duration is not listed in CPT as HPI element.

Associated signs and symptoms. Does anything else feel different when pain is present?
  "Yes, I have nausea when pain is worst."

Review of Systems (ROS)—Subjective

Questions posed to the patient to identify signs and symptoms that have been or are being experienced relating to the HPI
  Organ systems (OS), e.g., respiratory system, cardiovascular system
  Extent of ROS depends on CC and patient status (new, established, inpatient, outpatient)

ROS Elements

Constitutional—General, fever, weight loss or gain
  Eyes—Organ System (OS)
  Ears, Nose, Mouth, Throat (OS)
  Cardiovascular (OS)
  Respiratory (OS)
  Gastrointestinal (OS)
  Genitourinary (OS)
  Musculoskeletal (OS)
  Integumentary (OS)
  Neurological (OS)
  Psychiatric (OS)
  Endocrine (OS)
  Hematologic/Lymphatic (OS)
  Allergic/Immunologic (OS)

Past, Family, and/or Social History (PFSH)
Past

Contains relevant information about past illness, injury, or treatment, including
- Major illnesses/injuries
- Operations
- Hospitalizations
- Allergies
- Immunizations
- Dietary status
- Current medications

Family History

Health status or cause of death of family members
- Parents
- Siblings
- Children
Family history items related to CC
- Hereditary diseases

Social History

Review of past and current activities
- Marital status
- Employment
- Occupational history
- Military history
- Use of drugs/alcohol/tobacco

- Educational activities
- Sexual history
- Other relevant or contributory factors

Four History Levels

1. Problem Focused (PF)
2. Expanded Problem Focused (EPF)
3. Detailed (D)
4. Comprehensive (C)

Problem-Focused History

CC
    Brief HPI
    No ROS
    No PFSH

Expanded Problem-Focused History

CC
    Brief HPI
    Problem Focused ROS
    No PFSH

Detailed History

CC
    Extended HPI
    Problem pertinent ROS, extended to include a limited number of additional systems
    Pertinent PFSH directly related to problem

Comprehensive History

CC
    Extended HPI
    Complete ROS directly related to CC, plus review of 10+ systems
    Complete PFSH
    Summary of elements required for each level of history (Fig. 17.1)

History Elements

Chief Complaint (CC)
Reason for the encounter in the patient's words

History of Present Illness (HPI)
Location
Quality
Severity
Duration*
Timing
Context
Modifying factors
Associated signs and symptoms

Review of Systems (ROS)
Constitutional symptoms (fever, weight loss, etc.)
Ophthalmologic (eyes)
Otolaryngologic (ears, nose, mouth, throat)
Cardiovascular
Respiratory
Gastrointestinal
Genitourinary
Musculoskeletal
Integumentary (skin and/or breast)
Neurologic
Psychiatric
Endocrine
Hematologic/Lymphatic
Allergic/Immunologic

Past, Family, and/or Social History (PFSH)
Past major illnesses, operations, injuries, and treatments
Family medical history for heredity and risk
Social activities, both past and current

Elements Required for Each Level of History

		Problem Focused	Expanded Problem Focused	Detailed	Comprehensive
History	HPI	Brief 1-3	Brief 1-3	Extended 4+	Extended 4+
	ROS	None	Problem-pertinent 1	Extended 2-9	Complete 10+
	PFSH	None	None	Pertinent 1	Complete 2-3

*Duration is not listed in the CPT E/M Guidelines, but is listed in the DGs.

• **Figure 17.1** History elements required for each level of history.

Four Examination Levels (Objective)

Problem-Focused Examination (1995 Documentation Guidelines [DG])

Limited examination of affected body area or organ system

Expanded Problem-Focused Examination (1995 DG)

Limited examination of affected body area or organ system
Other related body area(s) or organ system(s)

Detailed Examination (1995 DG)

Extended examination of affected body area(s) and other symptomatic or related organ system(s)

Comprehensive Examination (1995 DG)

Eight or more organ systems
Summary of elements required for each level of examination (Fig. 17.2)

Medical Decision Making Complexity (MDM)

Management Options

Based on number of possible diagnoses
Levels: Minimal, limited, multiple, or extensive

Data Reviewed

Laboratory, radiology; any test/procedure results are documented along with the data reviewed and the identity of the reviewer in medical record
- "Hemoglobin within normal limits."
- "Chest x-ray, negative."
  Old medical records (data) from others may be requested and reviewed
  Levels: Minimal, limited, moderate, or extensive

Risks

Risks of morbidity (poor outcome), complications, or mortality (death) associated with problem, diagnostic procedure

Other diseases or factors (co-morbidities)
- Diabetes
- Extreme age
Urgency relates to risks
- Myocardial infarction
- Ruptured appendix
Levels: Minimal, low, moderate, or high
See Fig. 17.3, CMS Table of Risk

Examination Elements

General (OS)
Constitutional

Body Areas (BA)
Head (including the face)
Neck
Chest (including breasts and axillae)
Abdomen
Genitalia, groin, buttocks
Back
Each extremity

Organ System (OS)
Ophthalmologic (eyes)
Otolaryngologic (ears, nose, mouth, throat)
Cardiovascular
Respiratory
Gastrointestinal
Genitourinary
Musculoskeletal
Integumentary
Neurologic
Psychiatric
Hematologic/Lymphatic/Immunologic

Elements Required for Each Level of Examination

	Problem Focused	Expanded Problem Focused	Detailed	Comprehensive
Examination	Limited to affected BA or OS	Limited to affected BA or OS and other related OS(s)	Extended of affected BA(s) and other related OS(s)	General multi-system (OSs only)

• **Figure 17.2** Examination elements required for each level of examination.

TABLE OF RISK
(Total = highest risk in any one category)

Level of risk	Presenting problem(s)	Diagnostic procedure(s) ordered	Management options selected
Minimal	• One self-limited or minor problem, e.g., cold, insect bite, tinea corpus	• Laboratory tests requiring venipuncture • Chest x-rays • EKG/EEG • Urinalysis • Ultrasound, e.g., echocardiography • KOH prep	• Rest • Gargles • Elastic bandages • Superficial dressings
Low	• Two or more self-limited or minor problems • One stable chronic illness, e.g., well controlled hypertension or non-insulin dependent diabetes, cataract, BPH • Acute uncomplicated illness or injury, e.g., cystitis, allergic rhinitis, simple sprain	• Physiologic tests not under stress, e.g., pulmonary function tests • Non-cardiovascular imaging studies with contrast, e.g., barium enema • Superficial needle biopsies • Clinical laboratory tests requiring arterial puncture • Skin biopsies	• Over-the-counter drugs • Minor surgery with no identified risk factors • Physical therapy • IV fluids without additives
Moderate	• One or more chronic illnesses with mild exacerbation, progression, or side effects of treatment • Two or more stable chronic illnesses • Undiagnosed new problem with uncertain prognosis, e.g., lump in breast • Acute illness with systemic symptoms, e.g., pyelonephritis, pneumonitis, colitis • Acute complicated injury, e.g., head injury with brief loss of consciousness	• Physiologic tests under stress, e.g., cardiac stress test, fetal contraction stress test • Diagnostic endoscopies with no identified risk factors • Deep needle or incisional biopsy • Cardiovascular imaging studies with contrast and no identified risk factors, e.g., arteriogram, cardiac catheterization • Obtain fluid from body cavity, e.g., lumbar puncture, thoracentesis, culdocentesis	• Minor surgery with identified risk factors • Elective major surgery (open, percutaneous, or endoscopic) with no identified risk factors • Prescription drug management • Therapeutic nuclear medicine • IV fluids with additives • Closed treatment of fracture or dislocation without manipulation
High	• One or more chronic illnesses with severe exacerbation, progression, or side effects of treatment • Acute or chronic illnesses or injuries that pose a threat to life or bodily function, e.g., multiple trauma, acute MI, pulmonary embolus, severe respiratory distress, progressive severe rheumatoid arthritis • Psychiatric illness with potential threat to self or others • Peritonitis • Acute renal failure • An abrupt change in neurologic status, e.g., seizure, TIA, weakness, or sensory loss	• Cardiovascular imaging studies with contrast with identified risk factors • Cardiac electrophysiological tests • Diagnostic endoscopies with identified risk factors • Discography	• Elective major surgery (open, percutaneous, or endoscopic) with identified risk factors • Emergency major surgery (open, percutaneous or endoscopic) • Parenteral controlled substances • Drug therapy requiring intensive monitoring for toxicity • Decision not to resuscitate or to de-escalate care because of poor prognosis

• **Figure 17.3** Centers for Medicare and Medicaid Services (CMS) Table of Risk.

Four Levels of MDM Complexity

1. Straightforward MDM

Number of diagnoses or management options: Minimal
Amount or complexity of data: Minimal/None
Risk of complications or death: Minimal

2. Low-Complexity MDM

Number of diagnoses or management options: Limited
Amount or complexity of data: Limited
Risk of complications or death: Low

3. Moderate-Complexity MDM

Number of diagnoses or management options: Multiple
Amount or complexity of data: Moderate
Risk of complications or death: Moderate

4. High-Complexity MDM

Number of diagnoses or management options: Extensive
Amount or complexity of data: Extensive
Risk of complications or death: High
Summary of elements required for each level of MDM
  (Fig. 17.4)
The diagnosis or management options, amount or complexity of data, and risk are totaled to arrive at the level of MDM

- Only two of three categories must meet or exceed each other in any level to assign the MDM
  Example: Moderate complexity for diagnosis or management options and moderate complexity of amount or complexity of data, but only a low risk would be assigned a moderate level MDM
  Example: Low risk of death, moderate diagnosis or management options, and high amount or complexity of data: Assign the moderate level of MDM

Contributory Factors

Counseling

Provided to patient or family members (synopsis must be stated in medical record)
  Discussion of diagnosis, test results, impressions, recommendations, prognosis, risks/benefits of treatment options or lack thereof, and risk factor reduction

Coordination of Care

Work done on behalf of patient by physician to provide care

Nature of Presenting Problem

Type of problem patient presents to physician with or reason for encounter

---

Medical Decision Making Elements

Number of Diagnoses or Management Options
Minimal
Limited
Multiple
Extensive

Amount or Complexity of Data to Review
Minimal/None
Limited
Moderate
Extensive

Risk of Complications or Death If Condition Goes Untreated
Minimal
Low
Moderate
High

Elements Required for Each Level of Medical Decision Making

	Straightforward	Low	Moderate	High
Number of diagnoses or management options	Minimal	Limited	Multiple	Extensive
Amount or complexity of data to review	Minimal/None	Limited	Moderate	Extensive
Risk	Minimal	Low	Moderate	High

- **Figure 17.4** Elements required for each level of medical decision making.

Levels of Presenting Problem

Minimal Presenting Problem

May not require a physician
   Example: A dressing change or removal of an uncomplicated suture

Self-Limiting or Minor Presenting Problem

Self-limiting problems are minor and with a good outcome and no complications predicted
   Example: Sore throat or a slightly irritated skin tag

Low-Severity Presenting Problem

Without treatment, low risk
   Example: A middle-aged, healthy male with an upper respiratory infection

Moderate-Severity Presenting Problem

Without treatment, moderate risk
   Example: An elderly male with bacterial pneumonia

High-Severity Presenting Problem

Without treatment, high risk
   Example: An elderly male in very poor health with diabetic ketoacidosis

Time

Direct face-to-face: Physician or Other Qualified Health Care Professional and patient together

Example: Clinic visit or at bedside in hospital
   Calculated for code assignment beginning and ending times documented in medical record
   Unit/Floor: Time spent by physician on patient's floor or unit, also at patient's bedside
Example: Reviewing patient records or at chart desk and then with patient

> **NOTE**
>
> Over 50% of the total time should include counseling and/or coordination of care, and the documentation must reflect the total time of the visit and the time spent counseling and/or in coordination of care to qualify to assign the code based on time.

Use of E/M Code

Codes are grouped by type of service and place of service
* Consultation
* Office visit
* Hospital admission
   Different codes are required for various levels of service assignment
   New patient (99202-99205) services to new patient in office or other outpatient setting

Selection of Level of E/M Services

For the following categories/subcategories, all three of the key components must meet or exceed the level stated in the code description:
* Office or Other Outpatient Services, New Patient
* Hospital Observation Services
* Initial Hospital Care
* Observation of Inpatient Care Services
* Office or Other Outpatient Consultations
* Inpatient Consultations
* Emergency Department Services
* Initial Nursing Facility Care
* Other Nursing Facility Services
* Domiciliary, Rest Home (e.g., Boarding Home), or Custodial Care Services, New Patient
* Home Services, New Patient
   For the following categories/subcategories, two of the three key components must meet or exceed the level stated in the code description:
* Office or Other Outpatient Services, Established Patient
* Subsequent Observation Care
* Subsequent Hospital Care
* Subsequent Nursing Facility Care
* Domiciliary, Rest Home (e.g., Boarding Home), Established Patient
* Home Services, Established Patient

New Patient (99202-99205)

All new patients must be seen by physician
Code selection based on MDM or time spent

Established Patient (99211-99215)

99211 may not require a physician's presence
   No such code in New Patient category; all new patients are seen by physician
   Code selection based on MDM or time spent

Hospital Observation Status (99217-99220, 99224-99226, 99234-99236)

Not officially admitted to "inpatient status"

Patient not ill enough to admit but is too ill not to be monitored or discharged
Read notes at beginning of subsection
Observation services are not codes for "inpatient" services
Observation admission can be reported only for first day of service
When patient admitted on observation status and discharged on same day:
* Assign code from 99234-99236 (Observation or Inpatient Care Services category including admission and discharge)
   Patient in hospital overnight for observation but less than 48 hours:
   * **First day:** 99218-99220 (Initial Observation Care)

- **Second day:** 99217 (Observation Care Discharge Services)

If observation stay longer than 48 hours:
- **First day:** 99218-99220 (Initial Observation Care)
- **Second day:** 99224-99226 (Subsequent Observation Care)
- **Third day:** 99217 (Observation Care Discharge Services)

Initial Observation Care

- Beginning of observation care service
- Does not require a specific hospital unit; can be a regular bed on a floor or in emergency department (ED)
- Status specified as "observation"
  E/M services immediately prior to admission bundled into observation service
  Example: Office visit prior to observation, bundled into observation service

Hospital Inpatient Services (99221-99239)

Officially admitted to a hospital setting
  Total (all day and night)
  Partial (all day and no night, all night and no day, or a variation)
  - Time in and out must be specified in medical record

Types of Physician Status

Attending: Primary or admitting physician
Consultant: Physician whose opinion and advice requested by attending physician
Referring: Physician requesting a consultation from another physician regarding a patient's health status

Types of Care

Concurrent care given to patient by more than one physician each of different specialties
  Example: Pulmonologist and cardiologist both treating patient for different conditions at same time

Three Types of Hospital Inpatient Services

Initial Hospital Care (99221-99223)

First service includes admission
  Initial paperwork
  Initial treatment plans and orders
  Used only once for each admission
  - Only one admission by the attending or admitting physician billable per hospitalization

Subsequent Hospital Care (99231-99233)

After initial service
  Physician reviews patient's progress using documentation, information received from nursing staff, examination of patient
  - May be reported by multiple physicians of different specialties managing different conditions

(concurrent care); only one per day per physician per specialty

Hospital Discharge Services (99238, 99239)

Final day of hospital stay when patient in hospital more than 1 day
Documentation indicates final patient status
Time based
- Total time
- Does not need to be continuous time
Beginning and ending time or total time spent must be documented to assign the extended discharge code or use lowest-level code

Final Status of Patient

Summary of Stay (Discharge)

Condition (final examination)
Medications
Plan for return (follow-up care) to physician
How hospital stay progressed
Discharged destination (to home, nursing facility, etc.)
Only attending physician can use discharge code (only one discharge per admission)
Code based on time spent in service
Beginning and ending time or total time spent must be documented to assign the extended discharge code or must use lowest-level code

Consultation Services (99241-99255)

One physician or appropriate source requests another physician's opinion or advice
Either inpatient or outpatient; outpatient consultations include those provided in ED
  Outpatient consultations (99241-99245)
  Inpatient consultations (99251-99255)
Effective January 1, 2010, CMS no longer recognized CPT consultation codes (ranges 99241-99245 and 99251-99255) for inpatient facility and office/outpatient settings.
Consultation services reported with:
New patient office/outpatient (99202-99205)
Established patient office/outpatient (99211-99215)
Initial hospital codes (99221-99223)

Third-Party-Payer Consultations

Request consult for
- Past medical treatment
- Current condition
- Payers may request prior to approving procedure
- Report services with -32, mandated services

Emergency Department Services (99281-99288)

No distinction between new and established patients
  Must be open 24 hours a day to qualify as ED (ER)
  ED services often require additional codes from Critical Care Services
  - Typically billed by ED physicians

Other Emergency Services (99288), reports two-way communication for emergency care

Critical Care Services (99291, 99292)

Example: Vital organ failure
Critical care services are provided to patients over 71 months of age in life-threatening (critically ill/injured) situations
Time-based codes
- Total time under 30 minutes reported with appropriate E/M code (e.g., ED)

Critical Care Services (99291, 99292)

Time must be documented in medical record to select from this code range; does not need to be continuous
- Over 71 months of age
  99291 and 99292 reports total length of time a physician spends caring for critically ill patient
- 99291: 30-74 minutes
- 99292: Each additional 30 minutes

Nursing Facility Services (99304-99318)

Non-hospital settings with professional staff
- Provide continuous health care services to patients who are not acutely ill
Formerly known as Skilled Nursing Facility (SNF), Intermediate Care Facility (ICF), and Long-Term Care Facility (LTCF)
Various levels of nursing facility services

Initial Nursing Facility Assessment (99304-99306)

Provided at time of patient's initial admission/readmission

Subsequent Nursing Facility Care Codes (99307-99310)

99307 stable, recovering, or improving
99308 not responding or minor complication
99309 significant complication or new problem
99310 significant new problem requiring immediate physician attention

Nursing Facility Discharge Services (99315, 99316)

For final discharge service
Time-based
- Total time, does not need to be continuous
  Other Nursing Facility Services (99318)
- Annual Nursing Facility Assessment

Domiciliary, Rest Home, or Custodial Care Services (99324-99337)

Health care services are not available on site
Types of services provided are lodging, meals, supervision, personal care, leisure activities
Residents cannot live independently
Codes for either new or established patients

Domiciliary, Rest Home, or Home Care Plan Oversight Services (99339, 99340)

Read notes at beginning of subsection

Reports individual physician supervision of patient in home or domiciliary rest home
Services not face-to-face
Time-based
- 99339 15-29 minutes
- 99340 30 minutes or more
Reported once per 30-day period

Home Services (99341-99350)

Care provided in patient's home
Travel time not separately billable
- Not included in determining CPT code
Services based on key components and contributory factors
Codes for new or established patients

Prolonged Services (99354-99360; 99415-99417)

Time codes for direct face-to-face and without direct face-to-face contact
Report time beyond the usual E/M service
- Time must be documented in medical record
Codes for first 30-74 minutes and each additional 30 minutes thereafter
If less than 30 minutes, do not report service as prolonged
Code 99417 reported with only 99205, 99215

Standby Services (99360)

Not caring for other patient(s) to use these codes
Standing by only for that patient, if needed
Standby requested by another physician
- Must be documented in medical record
Report in 30-minute increments
Less than 30 minutes—do not report
Can report for subsequent 30 minutes only if a full 30 minutes
Carriers have strict policies regarding reimbursement for this service

Case Management Services (99366-99368)

Medical Team Conferences (99366-99368)

Codes for with or without face-to-face patient/family contact
- Minimum of three health care professionals, different specialties/disciplines participate in team
- Each member must have performed face-to-face evaluation in past 60 days
- Documentation must reflect member's contribution of information and treatment recommendation
- Not reported for organization or facility contracted services
Time-based
Begins and ends at start and conclusion of review

Care Plan Oversight Services (99374-99380)

Used to report supervision of patient care in home health agency, hospice, domiciliary, or equivalent environment
Patient not present
Codes are time-based

- 15-29 minutes
- 30 minutes or more
- Time must be documented in medical record

Reported once for each 30-day period

Preventive Medicine Services (99381-99429)

Used to report services when patient is not currently ill
> *Example:* Annual checkup
> Codes divided by new or established and age
> If significant problem is encountered during preventive examination
>> - E/M code also reported, append modifier -25

Counseling Risk Factor Reduction and Behavior Change Intervention (99401-99429)

Patient is seen specifically to promote health and/or wellness
> *Example:* Diet, exercise program
> Patient without symptoms or an established diagnosis to use these codes
> Codes based on
>> - Time, individual or group, and physician review of assessment data

Non-Face-to-Face Services (99091, 99421-99423, 99441-99458, 99473-99474)

Physician E/M services provided remotely
- 99441-99443 telephone E/M services, 99421-99423 online digital E/M services
  Established patient, report based on documented time
  Billed for up to 7 days of cumulative time
- 99446-99449, 99451-99452 report interprofessional telephone/internet/electronic health record consultations
  - Usually provided on urgent/emergency basis
  - No face-to-face, based on total time

99091, 99453, 99454, 99473, 99474 report digitally stored data services and remote physiologic monitoring
- Examples include blood pressure, weight, pulse oximetry, respiratory flow rate
- 99453 reports initial setup and equipment education
- 99454 reports daily recording or transmissions, per 30-day timeframe
- Neither reported when monitoring is less than 16 days

99457-99458 reports treatment management related to remote physiologic services
- Health professional utilizes results of monitoring (99453, 99454)
- Manage patient's treatment plan

Special E/M Services (99450, 99455-99456)

- 99450 is reported for services provided for insurance or disability assessments
  Involves no treatment; any treatment provided would be coded separately

99455-99456 report work related or medical disability evaluation
Codes divided
- 99455: Assessment by treating physician
- 99456: Assessment by nontreating physician

Newborn Care (99460-99465)

Initial and subsequent care in/other than hospital or birthing center
For normal newborn infant
Per day, for E/M services
99463, initial hospital/birthing center when admission and discharge are same day

Delivery/Birthing Room Attendance and Resuscitation Services (99464-99465)

99464, attendance at delivery
> Documented request by attending in medical record
> Provides initial stabilization
99465, resuscitation and ventilation

Inpatient Neonatal Intensive Care Services and Pediatric and Neonatal Critical Care Services (99466-99486)

Pediatric Critical Care Patient Transport
99466-99467; 99485-99486
> Critically ill or injured patient
> 24 months or younger
> 99466, first 30-74 minutes
>> Each additional 30 minutes, 99467
> Reports face-to-face interfacility transport
> 99485, 99486, supervision by a control physician
>> First 30 minutes (99485) and each additional 30 minutes (99486)

Inpatient Neonatal and Pediatric Critical Care
99468-99476
> Divided by
>> Initial day
>> Subsequent day
> Divided by age
>> Neonatal (Age 28 days or younger)
>> Pediatric (29 days through 24 months)
>> Pediatric (2 through 5 years)

Initial and Continuing Intensive Care Services
99477-99480
> Hospital Care
> 99477 for neonate 28 days of age or younger
> 99478-99480 divided by birth weight
>> very low birth weight (VLBW) ≤1500 grams (≤3.3 pounds)
>> low birth weight (LBW) 1501-2500 grams (3.3-5.5 pounds)
>> normal birth weight 2501-5000 grams (5.51-11.01 pounds)

Subdivided on day
   Initial
   Subsequent

Care Management Services (99439, 99487-99491)

Chronic Care Management Services (99439, 99490-99491)

- Establishment, implementation, revision, or monitoring of a comprehensive care plan for a patient with 2+ chronic conditions
- Last at least one year or result in death

Complex Chronic Care Management Services (99487, 99489)

- Per month
- At least 60 minutes of physician directed clinical staff time
- Compliance with chronic care criteria
- Substantial revision of a comprehensive care plan

Psychiatric Collaborative Care Management Services (99492-99494)

- Treating physician reports, but services also include consultations with behavioral health care manager and psychiatric consultant.

- Several specific elements must be documented to report.
- Reported by month, time based
  - Initial month (99492)
    - 36 minutes-85 minutes
    - Less than 36 minutes not reported
  - Subsequent months (99493)
    - 31 minutes-75 minutes
    - Less than 31 minutes not reported
  - Additional 30 minutes, any month (99494)

Transitional Care Management Services (99495-99496)

- Patient transition clinical setting to community setting
- MDM is moderate or high with first face-to-face service

Advance Care Planning (99497-99498)

- Face-to-face physician services with a patient/surrogate to counseling and/or develop advance directives
- Time based, first 30 minutes/each additional 30 minutes

Other Evaluation and Management Services (99499)

- 99499 reports unlisted E/M services Accompanied by a special report

PRACTICE EXERCISE 17.1 PROGRESS NOTE, ACUTE AND CHRONIC RENAL FAILURE

Progress Note

LOCATION: Inpatient, Hospital
PATIENT: Mike Lumbardi
ATTENDING PHYSICIAN: George Orbitz, MD
NEPHROLOGY PROGRESS NOTE: Mike had no major events. He tolerated the angiogram very well. He had peripheral vascular disease, but nothing to bypass, unfortunately. The patient denies any chest pain, shortness of breath. He has no nausea or vomiting. He has no leg edema and no GI symptoms.

PHYSICAL EXAMINATION: His vital signs were stable this morning. Temperature 36.9°C. Blood pressure 165/85. Heart rate 52 per minute. Respirations 16 per minute. Sats were 96% on room air. The patient was not in any respiratory, cardiac, or neurologic distress. He had no increase in jugulovenous pressure; regular rate and rhythm. The lungs were clear bilaterally without any crackles. The abdomen was soft and nontender; no organomegaly. No edema, with decreased pulses bilaterally, with signs of chronic venous and arterial insufficiency.

Intake/output in the past 8 hours: 1286 in, 1050 out.

Labs are pending from this morning, but his creatinine yesterday was 1.3.

IMPRESSION
1. Acute on top of chronic renal failure related to intravascular volume depletion, with creatinine coming down from 1.6 to 1.3.
2. Peripheral vascular disease.
3. Hypertension.

RECOMMENDATIONS
1. Basic metabolic panel is pending today.
2. If his creatinine goes up over time, he might need to have a renal MRA to look for renal artery stenosis.
3. Since patient is making urine, I don't think that his creatinine will go up acutely after his angiogram yesterday.
   CPT Code(s): _____

   ICD-10-CM Code(s): _____

Abstracting Questions

1. Are all three key elements (history, examination, and MDM complexity) documented? _____
   _____

2. How many key elements are required for this type of service? _____

3. Should both acute and chronic renal failure be reported, and if so, which is reported first? _____
   _____

4. Is the volume depletion reported? _____
   _____

PRACTICE EXERCISE 17.2 CLINIC VISIT, DIARRHEA

Clinic Note

FOLLOW-UP CLINIC VISIT
SUBJECTIVE: This is a 3½-year-old girl who presents today. Mother states that patient has had diarrhea over the past 3-4 days. Yesterday she had about 4-5 stools. They have been mustard colored, real runny, sometimes in little slivers. No blood has been present. She threw up 3-4 days ago, but this has since ended. Her eating is down, although she is drinking a lot. She will complain of her stomach hurting. Her temperature was as high as 103° F, and that was about 3 days ago. She is taking Motrin.

OBJECTIVE: On general appearance: She is alert and does not appear to be in any acute distress. Temperature is 97.2°F. Weight is 42 pounds. **HEENT:** Eyes are clear. The right TM has some increased erythema present. Landmarks are still seen. The left TM is nice and clear with good landmarks. Oropharynx is unremarkable. Neck is supple. Heart reveals a regular rate and rhythm without murmur. GU: Normal female genitalia.

ASSESSMENT
1. Viral gastroenteritis.
2. Possibly early right otitis media.

PLAN: I did discuss with mother that we could put her daughter on an antibiotic now, but we also could wait to see if she starts complaining of right ear pain or if her fever comes back. If that is the case, I did give mother a prescription for Amoxicillin to have her daughter take 375 mg p.o. t.i.d. × 10 days, and I would want to recheck her ear in 3 weeks. If she does not have any complaints or fever, mother will hold off just so Amoxicillin does not worsen her diarrhea. Mother was in agreement with this plan.

CPT Code(s): _____

ICD-10-CM Code(s): _____

Abstracting Questions

1. What category of E/M codes is used to report this service? _____

2. What body system is reviewed in the statement "right TM"? _____

PRACTICE EXERCISE 17.3 VOMITING

Dr. Sutton is an employee of the hospital.

LOCATION: Outpatient, Hospital
PATIENT: Penny Karlin
PRIMARY CARE PHYSICIAN: Ronald Green, MD
ED PHYSICIAN: Paul Sutton, MD
SUBJECTIVE: This is a 50-year-old female who is presenting to the emergency department today with a complaint of vomiting.

HISTORY OF PRESENT ILLNESS: This patient has quite significant recent medical history; recently diagnosed with grade IV esophageal cancer. She has been to the Lato Clinic and evaluated there, as well as in Los Angeles with endoscopy, and eventually to the Lato Clinic for further workup. With her workup there they found that she had quite extensive cancer with metastatic disease to the bones as well as to the stomach and thought that palliative oncologic treatment was all that could be offered and she should return to the area for this. She is scheduled to have a central line placed tomorrow and also considerations to nutritional needs. She stated that over the past several days she has had some fundraisers and some events for her and she really wanted to attend even though she was not able to keep foods and fluids down. She has been taking only small sips at a time. It seems like her ability to swallow is getting quite impaired, and as a result she cannot swallow her pain pill, so she is having severe pain in her back, hip, and abdomen. She has had increasing fatigue, has vomited several times, and just is not doing well and comes in for this at this time.

PAST MEDICAL HISTORY: Remarkable for esophageal cancer grade IV adenocarcinoma, noted with pelvic mets.

MEDICATIONS: Oxycodone and promethazine.

ALLERGIES: NKA, other than latex.

SOCIAL HISTORY: No smoking or alcohol.

REVIEW OF SYSTEMS: Negative for fever or chills. No shortness of breath. No headache. Patient's got nausea and abdominal and lower chest pain as positives on her review of systems.

On admission to the emergency department today, the patient's vital signs show a temperature of 36.8, pulse of 99, respiratory rate at 18, and blood pressure 132/84. General: This is a 50-year-old female who is awake, alert, and cooperative. **HEENT:** Head is normocephalic and atraumatic. Pupils are reactive to light. Conjunctivae clear. Nares patent. TMs are clear. Mouth reveals a somewhat dry oropharynx with some chapping of the lips, which appear parched. Neck is supple. Trachea is midline. Examination of lungs reveals clear breath sounds. Cardiovascular: S1 and S2 without murmur, click, or rub. Abdomen is soft. There is mild tenderness to palpation in the epigastric region. No mass, guarding, or rigidity. Extremities are without deformity or edema. Skin exam shows no rash. Cranial nerves 2 through 12 grossly intact. No gross motor or sensory deficits noted at this time.

SUMMARY OF EMERGENCY DEPARTMENT COURSE: The patient is seen and evaluated for the above-mentioned complaint. Orthostatic blood pressures were obtained: lying 112/87 with a pulse of 78, sitting 108/74 with a pulse of 98, and standing 102/80 with a pulse of 117. So she had quite an increase in her heart rate with standing, which I believe is significant. I did start an IV here in the department with normal saline; I gave her a liter of normal saline and 4 mg of morphine for her pain, which did help her pain significantly. It came down from an 8 to a 3. Checked some blood counts and metabolic panel as well as giving her some Phenergan for nausea, and this did help take away the nausea. Her CBC shows a hemoglobin level of 9.1, white count is okay, and her electrolytes are normal. So I think she is on the cusp of dehydration; certainly some anemia present here. I spoke with Dr. Green, who is covering for Dr. White, the patient's oncologist here, and he agreed to come in and evaluate the patient and did admit the patient to his service for further evaluation and treatment.

ASSESSMENT
1. Acute nausea and vomiting and dehydration.
2. Adenocarcinoma of the esophagus with metastatic disease.

PLAN: As above, the patient will be admitted for further evaluation and treatment per Dr. Green, certainly to control her pain, and it looks to me that the patient is going to have to change her pain regimen from oral to either parenteral or transdermal delivery system. She is going to have a line placed tomorrow, and further evaluation and treatment will be based on Dr. Green's plan for the patient. These plans as mentioned above were reviewed with the patient, who was in agreement. She will be admitted in fair condition with poor prognosis.

CPT Code(s): _____

_____

ICD-10-CM Code(s): _____

_____

Abstracting Questions

1. What level of history was documented? _____

_____

2. What level of examination was documented? _____

_____

3. What level of medical decision making was documented?

_____

4. This case began in the emergency department, but what was the ultimate disposition of this patient? _____

_____

5. Why is a neoplasm code not the first-listed diagnosis?

_____

PRACTICE EXERCISE 17.4 WELL-CHILD CHECK

Clinic Note

LOCATION: Outpatient, Hospital
PATIENT: Bradley Wellingstone
PHYSICIAN: Rolando Ortez, MD

SUBJECTIVE: This is a 3-week-old former 32-week gestational male infant who was in RNICU from birth. He did have some mild respiratory difficulties, oxygen requirements that resolved without further sequelae. He was also there for sepsis and feeding difficulties as well as apnea. He was discharged home on caffeine citrate, home apnea monitoring. He did return 2 days ago to get his first dose of Synagis. He is here for general checkup otherwise.

OBJECTIVE: He is on 24-calorie Enfamil and is taking that well without difficulty, taking almost 2 ounces at feeding; urinating and stool schedule is normal. No other complaints from his mother.

ASSESSMENT: On exam, alert, in no distress, and afebrile. His weight is up to 2341 grams, which is up 150 grams. Fontanelle, eyes, ears, nose, and pharynx are clear. Neck is supple. Lungs are clear to auscultation. Heart is regular rate and rhythm without murmur. Abdomen benign. Extremities: Full range of motion. No hip abnormalities. Skin is without rash. Neurologic exam without defect.

IMPRESSION: Thriving former 32-weeker. Now 3 weeks old.

PLAN: Anticipatory guidance discussed. We talked about feeding issues, accident prevention, car seat use, sleeping position on the side or the back. We will see them back in 1 month for his next Synagis dose as well as a recheck. We will have him on caffeine citrate 10 mg/day along with home apnea monitoring with plans to stop the caffeine in 1 month. With any problems, they need to give us a call or come back in sooner for re-evaluation.

CPT Code(s): _____

_____

ICD-10-CM Code(s): _____

_____

Abstracting Questions

1. From what CPT section would a code be located to report this? _____

2. From what CPT subcategory would this service be reported? _____

3. Was the patient a new or established patient with the provider? _____

4. Does the age of the patient affect code assignment? _____
_____

5. What type of diagnosis code was reported? _____
_____

PRACTICE EXERCISE 17.5 NICU PROGRESS NOTE, VENTILATOR ASSIST

Dr. Ortez has been following this infant since birth.

LOCATION: Inpatient, Hospital

PATIENT: Loren Black

ATTENDING PHYSICIAN: Rolando Ortez, MD

SUBJECTIVE: Baby is currently 2 days old, slightly under 48 hours.

OBJECTIVE: Weight today is 1716 kg (decreased by 135 grams). He is down 5.1% of his weight since birth. OFC is 30 cm (decreased 0.5 cm). Intake yesterday was 152 cc, 82 cc/kg/day. Output was 170 cc, 3.8 cc/kg/hour. He has had no stools since birth. Vital signs reveal his temperature to be acceptable while on an open, radiant warmer. Heart rate is generally in the 110s-120s. Respiratory rate has generally been equal to the IMV (60). Mean blood pressures have generally been in the 40s-50s. Oxygen saturations have remained in the high 90s.

PHYSICAL EXAMINATION: In general, he is pink, on current ventilator settings. He does have slightly dysmorphic features with wide-set eyes and slightly down-slanting palpebral fissures. Ears are low set and posteriorly rotated. Endotracheal tube was in place. Neck was without masses. Chest reveals symmetric expansion and lungs are clear to auscultation on current ventilator settings. Cardiac Exam: Regular rate without murmur or click. Peripheral pulses are 2+ and symmetric. Abdominal Exam: UAC in place. Liver is palpable 1 cm below the right costal margin. No splenomegaly or masses were noted. Genital Exam: Normal male. Testes are not palpable. Extremity Exam: No fixed decreased range of motion, deformity, or joint abnormality. Neurologic Exam: Mild, diffuse hypotonia. No focal deficits are appreciated.

CURRENT MEDICATIONS

1. Ampicillin 90.4 mg IV q12h.
2. Gentamicin 5.4 mg IV q18h.
3. Morphine sulfate 0.18 mg IV q6h and q1h p.r.n.
4. Dopamine 5 mcg/kg/min.
5. Vecuronium 0.18 mg IV q1-2h p.r.n.

LABORATORY STUDIES: Last arterial blood gas was obtained on ventilator setting of IMV 60, pressures of 24/4, and FIO_2 of 0.5 revealed pH 7.27, PCO_2 51.1, PO_2 66.5, and bicarbonate 22.5. Chemistry panel this morning reveals sodium of 134, potassium of 4.9, chloride of 102, glucose of 111, BUN of 18, creatinine of 1.0, calcium of 7.5, magnesium of 3.8, phosphorus of 7.7, bilirubin of 7.8. CBC reveals a white count of 6190. Platelet count was 98,000. Chest x-ray continues to show significant evidence of hyaline membrane disease. Endotracheal tube is near the carina and has been withdrawn somewhat.

IMPRESSION/RECOMMENDATIONS

1. Two-day-old infant who was born at 30 weeks' gestation. He does have clinical features suggestive of Noonan syndrome.
2. Respiratory: Continues to show evidence of hyaline membrane disease with respiratory failure. He has received three doses of surfactant therapy. He does have echocardiographic evidence of PDA, and we will be treating this at this time. We will attempt to decrease his ventilator settings based on serial clinical examination, pulse oximetry, arterial blood gas determinations, and chest x-ray.
3. Cardiovascular: Status is acceptable at this time while on dopamine at 5 mcg/kg/min. Echocardiogram shows a patent ductus arteriosis. There also appears to be a slight abnormality to the pulmonary valve, which could be associated with his possible Noonan syndrome. He is going to receive indomethacin therapy.
4. Gastrointestinal: Abdominal exam remains benign. He is NPO. He does have mild hyperbilirubinemia. Direct antibody test was negative. We will begin phototherapy at this time.
5. Hematologic: Serial CBCs have been acceptable except for mild thrombocytopenia. We will continue to monitor, especially in light of the indomethacin therapy. He has not required any blood product transfusions since birth.
6. Infectious Disease: Blood culture remains negative at this time. We have discontinued his gentamicin, and he is being placed on cefotaxime because of the indomethacin.
7. Neurologic: Exam remains acceptable given his extreme prematurity. He will require screening intracranial ultrasound and long-term neurodevelopmental follow-up.
8. Renal/Metabolic: Urine output remains adequate and renal function studies are acceptable. Previous metabolic parameters are acceptable. We will repeat in the morning.
9. Fluids/Electrolytes/Nutrition: Weight loss is acceptable and electrolytes are in the more normal range today. We will adjust his TPN accordingly.
10. Apnea/Bradycardia: None since birth.
11. Health Care Maintenance: None yet.

SOCIAL HISTORY: Mom and dad are being kept up to date with regard to the patient's condition. Their questions have been answered, and they are in agreement with the outlined management plan.

CPT Code(s): _____

ICD-10-CM Code(s): _____

_____

Abstracting Questions

1. The surfactant therapy was given for which diagnosis?

   _____

2. What does PDA mean? _____

   _____

18

Anesthesia Section (00100-01999)

Anesthesiologist

Doctor of medicine specializing in anesthesia

Usually outside practices, e.g., Anesthesia Associates, Inc., or Pain Clinic, Ltd.
Professional services reported separately

CRNA

Certified Registered Nurse Anesthetist

Uses of Anesthesia

Manage unconscious patients, life functions, and resuscitation

Analgesia

Relieve pain

Some Methods of Anesthesia

Endotracheal: Through mouth (general anesthesia)
Local: Application to area (injection or topical)
Epidural: Between vertebral spaces—injection into epidural space
Regional: Field or nerve block
MAC: Monitored anesthesia care (service provided by an anesthesiologist or CRNA)
Patient is monitored, and if necessary, sedation (including general anesthesia) may be provided
Spinal: Anesthesia applied to the spinal cord area, outside the dura mater
General: State of unconsciousness accomplished through drug administration or by inhalation

Patient-Controlled Analgesia (PCA)

Patient self-administers drug
Used to relieve chronic pain or temporarily for severe pain following surgery

Moderate (Conscious) Sedation

Codes in Medicine Section of CPT

99151-99153 assigned when sedation is provided by same physician performing procedure
99155-99157 assigned when another physician administers sedation
- Trained observer must be present
  Decreased level of consciousness
  Codes divided by age (under 5, 5 and over) and time (15 minutes and each additional 15 minutes)

Anesthesia Formula

$(B + T + M) \times$ conversion factor = Anesthesia payment

B Is for Base Units

Published in *Relative Value Guide (RVG)* by American Society of Anesthesiologists
National unit values for anesthesia services based on complexity of service

T Is for Time

Patient record indicates time, e.g., 60 minutes

Usually, 15 minutes = 1 unit
Example: 60 minutes = 4 units
Some payers may indicate 1 unit = 1 minute
Begins: Anesthesiologist begins to prepare patient for induction—preoperative
Continues throughout procedure—intraoperative
Ends: Patient no longer under care of anesthesiologist—postoperative

M Is for Modifying Unit

Additional units based on physical status of patient (see modifiers that follow)

Physical Status Modifiers, P1-P6

Located in Anesthesia Guidelines

Not reported to Medicare
Help to show complexity of service
- P1 Normal healthy
- P2 Mild systemic disease
- P3 Severe systemic disease
- P4 Severe systemic disease is constant threat to life
- P5 Not expected to survive without the operation
- P6 Clinically brain dead

Qualifying Circumstances Codes (99100-99140)

Anesthesia services provided under difficult circumstances

Located in both Anesthesia Guidelines and Medicine section
Listed in addition to primary anesthesia code
More than one may be reported

Summing Up Formula

Base units (from *RVG*) based on CPT codes

Time units (usually 15 min is a unit)
- Total time ÷ 15 = time units
Modifiers [Qualifying Circumstances (99100-99140) and/or Physical Status (P1-P6)]

Conversion Factors

CMS anesthesia conversion factors

Sum of money allocated by payer, per unit for payment of anesthesia services

Anesthesia for Multiple Surgical Procedures

Once anesthetized, length of time, not number of procedures performed during session

Report highest *Relative Value Guide (RVG)* valued CPT code
Example: Two procedures during same session
- One, 10 base units; the other, 5 base units
- Report only 10 base units and combined time for all procedures

Anesthesia Modifiers

Anesthesia code reported twice
- Once for anesthesiologist
- Once for CRNA
Each reports service on separate claim form
- One claim for anesthesiologist's service
- One claim for CRNA's service
Anesthesia modifiers report supervision/direction circumstances
- AA, anesthesia services performed personally by anesthesiologist
- AD, medical supervision >4 concurrent procedures
- QK, medical direction of 2-4 concurrent procedures
- QX, CRNA service with medical direction
- QY, medical direction of 1 CRNA
- QZ, CRNA service without medical direction
Anesthesia modifier always precedes the physical status modifier

PRACTICE EXERCISE 18.1 PERFORATED APPENDICITIS

Assign anesthesia code(s) and any necessary modifiers. Do not assign surgery codes. Do not assign diagnosis codes. During this procedure the anesthesiologist was medically directing two CRNAs providing anesthesia for concurrent procedures. The patient's physical status is P2.
OPERATIVE REPORT
LOCATION: Inpatient, Hospital
PATIENT: Laurence Hooper
ATTENDING PHYSICIAN: Gary Sanchez, MD
SURGEON: Gary Sanchez, MD
PREOPERATIVE DIAGNOSIS: Perforated appendicitis.
POSTOPERATIVE DIAGNOSIS: Same.
ANESTHESIA: General.
ANESTHESIOLOGIST: Janice E. Larson, MD
  PROCEDURE: The patient was brought to the operating room, placed under general anesthesia, and prepped and draped sterilely. The patient's advanced age is a concern, since he is 92. A right lower quadrant skin incision was made with a #10 blade, and dissection was carried down through the subcutaneous tissue using electrocautery. The anterior sheath of the rectus fascia was opened. The rectus was retracted medially. The posterior sheath and peritoneum were grasped with curved clamps and sharply incised, allowing entry into the peritoneal cavity. There were a few adhesions, which we took down sharply. We then delivered the appendix up and into the wound. We took down the mesoappendix between Kelly clamps and tied the vascular pedicles with 2-0

silk free ties. The base of the appendix was then crushed. It was tied with 0 Vicryl. It was inverted into the base of the cecum with a 3–0 silk pursestring suture. The abdomen was then irrigated with saline until returns were clear. We closed the posterior sheath and peritoneum with running 0 Vicryl, closed the anterior sheath with interrupted 0 Vicryl, and closed the skin with subcuticular 4–0 undyed Vicryl. Steri-Strips and sterile Band-Aids were applied. All sponge and needle counts were correct. Before the patient left the operating room, the wound was anesthetized with a total of 30 cc of 0.50% Sensorcaine with epinephrine solution.

CPT Code(s): _____ _____

_____

Abstracting Questions

1. What is the main term referenced in the index of the CPT to locate the code? _____

_____

2. What was the subterm used in the CPT index to locate the anesthesia code? _____

_____

3. Does the quadrant entered to perform the surgical procedure affect CPT anesthesia code assignment? _____

_____

Continued

PRACTICE EXERCISE 18.1 PERFORATED APPENDICITIS—cont'd

4. Was the procedure at the abdominal wall or intraperitoneal?

_____

5. Were there any Qualifying Circumstances to report?

_____

6. Who decides what Physical Status Modifier should be reported? _____

_____

7. Was the anesthesiologist providing service or medically directing cases? _____

_____

PRACTICE EXERCISE 18.2 LEFT BREAST BIOPSY

Assign anesthesia code(s) only. Do not assign surgery codes. Do not assign diagnosis codes. The patient's physical status is P1.
OPERATIVE REPORT
LOCATION: Outpatient, Hospital
PATIENT: Adrienne Gardener
ATTENDING PHYSICIAN: Gary Sanchez, MD
SURGEON: Gary Sanchez, MD
PREOPERATIVE DIAGNOSIS: Left breast mass.
POSTOPERATIVE DIAGNOSIS: Same.
PROCEDURE PERFORMED: Left breast biopsy.
ANESTHESIA: Local with IV sedation and monitored anesthesia care.
ANESTHESIOLOGIST: Janice E. Larson, MD
PROCEDURE: The patient was brought to the operating room, given IV sedation, and then anesthetized with a total of 30 cc of 1% Sensorcaine with epinephrine solution. Incision was made over the top of the mass with a #15 blade, and dissection was carried down through subcutaneous tissues

sharply. We encountered the mass, which appeared to be a fibroadenoma. We excised this sharply. We got the entire lesion. We controlled bleeding with electrocautery. We then closed the skin with subcuticular 4–0 undyed Vicryl. Steri-Strips and sterile Band-Aids were applied. She tolerated this well and was taken to recovery room in stable condition.
  Pathology Report Later Indicated: Fibroadenoma.

CPT Code(s): _____

Abstracting Questions

1. Do you report the sedation with CPT anesthesia codes or medicine codes? _____

_____

2. Was the procedure superficial (subcutaneous) or deep (internal structures)? _____

_____

PRACTICE EXERCISE 18.3 TAKEDOWN COLOSTOMY AND CHOLECYSTECTOMY

Assign anesthesia code(s) only. Do not assign surgery codes. Do not assign diagnosis codes. The anesthesiologist was supervising two concurrent procedures. The patient's physical status is P2.
OPERATIVE REPORT
LOCATION: Inpatient, Hospital
PATIENT: Simon Sulten
ATTENDING PHYSICIAN: Gary Sanchez, MD
SURGEON: Gary Sanchez, MD
PREOPERATIVE DIAGNOSES
  1. Colostomy for obstructing colon cancer.
  2. Symptomatic cholelithiasis.
POSTOPERATIVE DIAGNOSES: Same.
PROCEDURE PERFORMED
  1. Takedown colostomy with end-to-end colorectostomy.
  2. Open cholecystectomy.
ANESTHESIA: General.
ANESTHESIOLOGIST: Janice E. Larson, MD
PROCEDURE: The patient was brought to the operating room, placed under general anesthesia, and prepped and draped sterilely. The previous midline was reopened with the #10 blade, and we excised the old scar. We carried out dissection through subcutaneous tissues using electrocautery. Midline fascia was divided sharply. We entered the peritoneal cavity and entered the midline fascia along the length of the incision. We took down numerous filmy adhesions and ran the small bowel from the terminal ileum to the ligament of Treitz, which appeared normal. First, we placed an Omni retractor and exposed the right upper quadrant. We identified the cystic

duct and cystic artery and tied them off with 0 silk ties proximally and distally before transecting them. We then shelled the gallbladder from its fossa using electrocautery. We placed a pack up by the liver bed. We then identified the rectal stump and dissected this free. We then made an elliptical incision around the colostomy opening and carried our dissection down to fascia, freed up the stoma, and fired our TLC 75 stapler across the descending colon. We sent the specimen to pathology for permanent. We mobilized the left colon along the avascular line of Toldt up and around the splenic flexure. Once we had adequate length, we placed a Glassman clamp proximally on the rectum and distally on the descending colon. We then performed a two-layer, hand-sewn, end-to-end anastomosis with an outer layer of 3–0 silk Lembert and inner layer of running 3–0 Vicryl. There was a patent anastomosis, and we could easily milk contents through with no evidence of spilling. We then closed the fascia from the colostomy site with interrupted 0 Vicryl and running 0 PDS. We closed the skin with skin clips. All sponge and needle counts were correct. Patient tolerated this well and was taken to recovery in stable condition.
  CPT Code(s): _____

Abstracting Question

1. Was a supervision modifier required? _____

_____

PRACTICE EXERCISE 18.4   INCISION AND DRAINAGE OF PERIRECTAL ABSCESS

Assign anesthesia code(s) only. Do not assign surgery codes. Do not assign diagnosis codes. The patient's physical status is P3.

OPERATIVE REPORT
LOCATION: Outpatient, Hospital
PATIENT: Suzy Tarsinski
ATTENDING PHYSICIAN: Gary Sanchez, MD
SURGEON: Gary Sanchez, MD
PREOPERATIVE DIAGNOSIS: Perirectal abscess.
POSTOPERATIVE DIAGNOSIS: Same.
PROCEDURE PERFORMED: Incision and drainage of perirectal abscess.
ANESTHESIA: Spinal.
ANESTHESIOLOGIST: Janice E. Larson, MD
   PROCEDURE: The patient was brought back to the operating room, and after a spinal anesthetic had been given, the area of the rectum was cleaned and draped in the usual fashion after the patient had been placed in a jackknife position. An incision was made over the top of this abscess with a #10-blade scalpel. We entered the abscessed cavity, which returned large amounts of purulent material. We broke up the loculations, debrided the necrotic tissue with a #10 blade, and irrigated with a liter of saline. We then were able to pack the cavity with sewed Kerlix. The patient tolerated the procedure well, and all sponges and needles were accounted for at the end of the procedure. Soon she could be transferred to the Post Anesthesia Care Unit in stable condition.

CPT Code(s): _____

_____

Abstracting Question

1. For the purpose of locating an anesthesia code in the CPT manual, what was the location of the I&D? _____

PRACTICE EXERCISE 18.5   INTRACEREBRAL HEMATOMA

Assign anesthesia code(s) only. Do not assign surgery codes. Do not assign diagnosis codes. The patient is not expected to survive without this procedure.

OPERATIVE REPORT
LOCATION: Inpatient, Hospital
PATIENT: Suzy Kunklemann
ATTENDING PHYSICIAN: Gary Sanchez, MD
SURGEON: Gary Sanchez, MD
PREOPERATIVE DIAGNOSIS: Intracerebral hematoma, right temporal lobe.
POSTOPERATIVE DIAGNOSIS: Intracerebral hematoma, right temporal lobe.
PROCEDURE PERFORMED: Osteoplastic craniotomy, right temporal area; evacuation of intracerebral hematoma.
ANESTHESIA: General.
   PROCEDURE: This patient is not expected to survive without this procedure, and at this point we have no other choice but to proceed. Under general anesthesia, the patient's head was placed in the Mayfield pins. The right frontal temporoparietal area was prepped and draped in the usual manner. A linear incision was made extending from the midline of the temporal fossa up to the midportion of the scalp. The skin was incised. The temporalis muscle was separated and divided off the bone. I did a craniotomy here the size of a half dollar coin and made a burr hole. I utilized the craniotome to elevate the bone flap, which was a free bone flap. This was then removed. We placed the Weitlaners into the wound and then incised the dura in a cruciate fashion over the temporal lobe. I then entered the middle temple gyrus, irrigated much of the clot from the temporal and posterior parietal areas, and evacuated the clot from the area. This took copious irrigation. We used cotton balls for hemostasis. I did this numerous times until all the bleeders were coagulated. I then lined the cystic cavity with Gelfoam and coagulated the edges of the raw brain. I closed the dura with 4–0 Vicryl. This was closed in a watertight fashion. I used 2–0 Vicryl to elevate the dura to the bone flap with Wurzburg plates, two of them, using plates and screws. I then closed the scalp in one layer using 0 Vicryl on the temporalis muscle and fascia, and the skin was approximated with 2–0 nylon interrupted mattress sutures. Dressing was applied, and the patient was on the ventilator and discharged to the surgical intensive care unit.

CPT Code(s): _____

_____

Abstracting Question

1. Would a physical status modifier be required? _____

19

CPT/HCPCS Level I Modifiers (-22 to -99)

Alter CPT or HCPCS code

Full list, CPT, Appendix A
- Two separate lists
  - One for physician use
  - One for hospital outpatient use

Modifier Functions

Altered (i.e., increased or reduced service)

Bilateral
Multiple
Only portions of service (i.e., professional service only)
More than one surgeon

-22 Increased Procedural Service

Indicates services significantly greater than usual

Accompanied by written report and supportive documentation

-23 Unusual Anesthesia

Use of general anesthesia where local or regional is norm

   Example: Highly agitated senile patient
Used only with anesthesia codes
Written report with submission of modifier

-24 Unrelated E/M Services by Same Physician or Other Qualified Health Care Professional During a Postoperative Period

Service not related to surgery
If E/M provided during postoperative global period, no payment considered without -24

-25 Significant, Separately Identifiable E/M Service, by Same Physician or Other Qualified Health Care Professional on the Same Day of the Procedure or Other Service

Documentation must support service
   Example: Patient seen for sinus congestion, provider performs H&P, prescribes decongestant, notes and removes lesion on back

Code: Procedure + E/M-25

-26 Professional Component

Professional component (physician, -26)
   Technical component (technician + equipment, -TC)

-32 Mandated Service

Mandated by payer, workers' comp, or official body or court of law
   Not request of patient, patient's family, or another physician
   Example: Workers' Compensation requests examination of person currently receiving disability benefits

-33 Preventive Services

Patient Protection and Affordable Care Act (PPACA) requires health insurance coverage of preventive services without cost
US Preventive Services Task Force (USPSTF) grades preventive services:
- Grade A: High certainty that the net benefit is substantial
- Grade B: High certainty that the net benefit is moderate or there is a moderate certainty that the next benefit is moderate to substantial

Task Force list located at: https://www.uspreventiveservices taskforce.org/Page/Name/uspstf-a-and-b-recommendations/ Example of services:

- Grade A
- Topic: Blood pressure screening
- Description: The USPSTF recommends screening for high blood pressure in adults aged 18 and older.

-47 Anesthesia by Surgeon

Surgeon administers regional or general anesthesia

Physician acts as both surgeon and anesthesiologist
Used only with Surgery codes

-50 Bilateral Procedure

Organs that are bilateral

Example: Procedure on kidneys
Caution: Some codes describe bilateral procedures
Typically not used on Integumentary System codes

-51 Multiple Procedure—Three Types

1. Same procedure, different sites
2. Multiple operation(s), same operative session
3. Procedure performed multiple times
   - List most resource-intense procedure first, then descending order of resource intensity
   - Next, other procedure(s) + -51 (unless code is -51 exempt or add-on code) Usual procedure payment: 1st 100%, 2nd 50%, 3rd 25%-50%, depending on payer

-52 Reduced Services

Service reduced or not performed to the extent described in code description

There is no other code that accurately reflects the service actually provided
Physician directed reduction
Documentation substantiates reduction
Not to be used for patient unable to pay
Submit regular charge amount, payer will adjust

-53 Discontinued Procedure

Surgical/diagnostic procedures

Procedure started, then stopped due to patient's condition
Does not apply to presurgical discontinuance
Submit regular charge, payer will adjust
DO NOT USE -53
- When patient cancels scheduled procedure
- With E/M codes
- With time-based code

-54 Surgical Care Only

Physician provides only procedure (intraoperative); other physician performs preoperative and postoperative service

Documented patient transfer must be in record
Some payers require copy of transfer order

-55 Postoperative Management Only

Physician provides only the care after hospital discharge; report surgical code + modifier -55

If transferred while patient hospitalized, report postoperative management with subsequent hospital codes 99231-99233
Documentation of transfer in medical record

-56 Preoperative Management Only

Physician provided only preoperative care; report surgical code + modifier -56

Not acceptable for Medicare
Usual reimbursement for portions, surgical package
- 10% preoperative
- 70% intraoperative
- 20% postoperative
Each payer determines reimbursement for portions

-57 Decision for Surgery

E/M, 99202-99499

Medicine, 92002, 92004, 92012, and 92014 ophthalmologic services
Medicare: Only for preoperative period of major surgery (day before or day of)

-58 Staged/Related Procedure or Service by Same Physician or Other Qualified Health Care Professional During Postoperative Period

Subsequent procedure planned at time of initial surgery
- During postoperative period of previous surgery in series
  Example: Multiple skin grafts completed in several sessions
- Do not use when code describes total sessions
  Example: 67208 destruction of lesion of retina, one or more sessions
- More extensive than original procedure or
- For therapy following diagnostic procedure (e.g., breast biopsy and subsequent mastectomy)

-59 Distinct Procedural Service

Used to report non-E/M services not normally reported together

- Different session or encounter
- Different procedure
- Different site

Separate incision, excision, lesion, injury

Example: Physician removes several lesions from patient's leg; also notes a suspicious lesion on torso and biopsies it

- Excision code for lesion removal + biopsy code for torso lesion with −59
- Indicates biopsy as distinct procedure, not part of lesion removal

CMS established four HCPCS subset modifiers:

- referred to as −X{EPSU} modifiers
- more descriptively define modifier -59
- payer specific

-62 Two Surgeons

Both function as cosurgeons (equals)

Usually of different specialties
Each reports same code + -62
Each dictates operative/procedure note for their portion
Total reimbursement = 125%; each physician = 62.5%

-63 Procedure Performed on Infants Less Than 4 kg

Kilogram = 2.2 pounds (4 kg = 8.8 lb)

Small size increases complexity
Use with all Surgery section codes except Integumentary System or directed otherwise (see parenthetical guideline following 63702)

-66 Surgical Team

Team: Several physicians with various specialties plus technicians and other support personnel

Very complex procedures
Payers may increase payment up to 50%

- Each physician's service must be documented in the medical record

-76 Repeat Procedure/Service by Same Physician or Other Qualified Health Care Professional

Assigned to indicate necessary service

Example: X-rays before and after fracture repair

-77 Repeat Procedure/Service by Another Physician or Other Qualified Health Care Professional

Performed by one physician, repeated by another physician

Submitted with written report to establish medical necessity and identity of performing physician

- Do not append to E/M codes

-78 Unplanned Return to Operating/Procedure Room by the Same Physician or Other Qualified Health Care Professional Following Initial Procedure for a Related Procedure During Postoperative Period

For complication of first procedure

Example: Patient had outpatient procedure in morning; was returned to operating room in afternoon with severe hemorrhage

Indicates not typographical error

- Medical record must specifically document need for service provided

-79 Unrelated Procedure or Service by Same Physician or Other Qualified Health Care Professional During Postoperative Period

Example: Several days after discharge for procedure, patient returns for unrelated problem

Diagnosis code would also be different

-80 Assistant Surgeon

Reimbursed at 15% to 30%

Payers identify procedures for which they reimburse assistant at surgery

-81 Minimum Assistant Surgeon

Services at a level less than that described in -80

Reimbursed at 10% if services reported with the modifier are recognized by payer

-82 Assistant Surgeon (When Qualified Resident Surgeon Not Available)

Teaching hospitals

- Have residents who assist as part of education
- Must demonstrate no qualified resident available to use -82
  - Unavailability must be documented in written report

-90 Reference (Outside) Laboratory

Physician has business relationship with outside lab

Physician pays lab
Physician bills payer for lab services

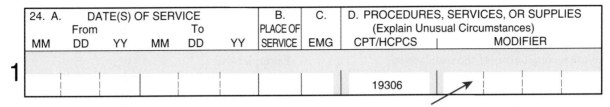

• **Figure 19.1** 3-6 CMS-1500 (02/12) allows for multiple placement of modifiers. (Courtesy U.S. Department of Health and Human Services, Centers for Medicare and Medicaid Services.)

-91 Repeat Clinical Diagnostic Laboratory Test

Repeat same laboratory tests on same day for multiple test results

- e.g., serial troponin levels for acute MI confirmation
  Not tests rerun to confirm or negate original test results
  Not assigned for malfunction of equipment, loss of specimen, or technician error

-92 Alternative Laboratory Platform Testing

Used to report a laboratory test using portable instrument or kit

Usually single use
  86701-86703 HIV testing

-95 Synchronous Telemedicine Services

Used when a provider and patient interact from separate locations

Star (★) symbol appears next to code.
  Reference full list of applicable codes in Appendix P.

-96 Habilitative Services

Used for services that help an individual with daily living skills and functions that are not yet developed, intent is to retain/improve over time.

-97 Rehabilitative Services

Used for services that help an individual regain daily living skills and functions that were lost/impaired because of injury/illness, intent is to retain/improve over time.

-99 Multiple Modifiers

Used when service needs more than one modifier but payer allows for only one modifier with each code

CMS-1500 (Fig. 19.1)

HCPCS Level II Modifiers

Examples of HCPCS Anatomical Modifiers

-LT Left side
-RT Right side

-E1 Upper left, eyelid
-E2 Lower left, eyelid
-E3 Upper right, eyelid
-E4 Lower right, eyelid
-FA Left hand, thumb
-F1 Left hand, second digit
-F2 Left hand, third digit
-F3 Left hand, fourth digit
-F4 Left hand, fifth digit
-F5 Right hand, thumb
-F6 Right hand, second digit
-F7 Right hand, third digit
-F8 Right hand, fourth digit
-F9 Right hand, fifth digit
-TA Left foot, great toe
-T1 Left foot, second digit
-T2 Left foot, third digit
-T3 Left foot, fourth digit
-T4 Left foot, fifth digit
-T5 Right foot, great toe
-T6 Right foot, second digit
-T7 Right foot, third digit
-T8 Right foot, fourth digit
-T9 Right foot, fifth digit
-LC Left circumflex coronary artery
-LD Left anterior descending coronary artery
-RC Right coronary artery
  Anatomical modifiers are not used with skin procedures
  Example: Removal of skin tags, any area
  Exception is with codes for procedures on sites including sweat glands, eyelids, and breasts

HCPCS Modifiers for Selective Identification of Subsets of Distinct Procedural Services (-59 Modifier)

-XE Separate Encounter

A service that is distinct because it occurred during a separate encounter

-XS Separate Structure

A service that is distinct because it was performed on a separate organ/structure

-XP Separate Practitioner

A service that is distinct because it was performed by a different practitioner

-XU Unusual Non-Overlapping Service

The use of a service that is distinct because it does not overlap usual components of the main service

Example: -XE

- Patient seen in the morning for a cardiovascular stress test and then later in the day patient returns for a rhythm ECG
- Patient is seen in the outpatient infusion center at 8:00 a.m. and seen again in the outpatient infusion center for another treatment at 6:00 p.m.

Example: -XS

- Patient seen for destruction and during procedure unrelated to the destruction the physician obtains tissue for pathologic examination

- Patient under goes a laparoscopy, surgical, ablation of one or more liver tumor(s) and during the surgery, patient has ultrasonic guidance for needle placement

Example: -XP

- Patient undergoes a hernia repair at 7:00 a.m. Later in the day the patient develops acute abdominal pain and returns for another physician to perform a surgical laparoscopic appendectomy

Example: -XU

- Patient seen for two separate lesions; a lipoma is excised on upper thigh region (3 cm), and a separate lipoma excised on the lower leg region (less than 3 cm)

PRACTICE EXERCISE 19.1 MASSIVE DEBRIDEMENT

OPERATIVE REPORT
LOCATION: Inpatient, Hospital
PATIENT: Pam Tieg
ATTENDING PHYSICIAN: Leslie Alanda, MD
SURGEON: Gary Sanchez, MD
PREOPERATIVE DIAGNOSES
1. Massive abdominal wound.
2. Status post multiple small-bowel fistula repair.
POSTOPERATIVE DIAGNOSES
1. Massive abdominal wound.
2. Status post multiple small-bowel fistula repair.
   SURGICAL FINDINGS: There was a 28 × 50-cm open wound in the abdomen extending predominantly to the right over past the midline on the left with a more inferior extension near the inguinal ligament. The primary areas of concern were pockets that were at least 8 to 10 cm in diameter in their total dimensions that had undermined in the retroperitoneal space behind the bowel. This contained malodorous fat necrosis and other necrotic tissue, and the odor smelled like Gram-negative organisms. We noted that the bowel was anterior in this space and probably came down on the psoas muscle posteriorly on the right side. Also, there were various areas of fat necrosis overlying the superficial aspect of the wound and fat necrosis along the edges of the wound that was quite malodorous. Multiple cultures and sensitivities were obtained, particularly of the area around the ileostomy site, the large area of fat necrosis in the left side of the abdomen, and the two undermined retroperitoneal areas. There was some extrusion of the mesh with the surrounding coagulative necrosis superiorly.
SURGICAL PROCEDURE: Massive debridement of open abdominal wound and status post multiple enterotomy repairs, small bowel.
ANESTHESIA: General, administered through tracheostomy tube.
ESTIMATED BLOOD LOSS: Approximately 50 cc.
ADDENDUM: Dr. White was called to observe the wound at his request and advised us regarding the dissection retroperitoneally in the proximity of the bowel in the area.
   PROCEDURE: The abdomen was prepped as well as possible considering the conditions with Betadine scrub and solution and draped in a routine sterile fashion. A major 3-cm area of fat necrosis was initially debrided, and I debrided multiple sites of fat necrosis over the exposed surface of the wound, and then along the marginal surface there were

multiple sites that were malodorous. Culture and sensitivity were obtained of the original fat necrosis area, the area around the ileostomy, and the more malodorous areas along the skin edges. We then, on the right side, lifted up the abdominal contents and dissected behind this, encountering foul-smelling, anaerobic-smelling collection of tissue, which probably consisted of old blood clot and fat necrosis. This was gently curetted out without entering the bowel. The bowel was in immediate proximity. We came down on what appeared to be the psoas area, which apparently connected with this pocket on the right side. We packed the right side with metronidazole-soaked Kerlix roll and vaginal packing, then also did the same on the left side. We covered the areas of the wound that were most accessible with fine mesh gauze soaked in metronidazole. ABD pads were then applied. The patient tolerated the procedure well and left the area in good condition.
CPT Code(s): _____

_____

ICD-10-CM Code(s): _____

_____

Abstracting Questions

1. Was debridement superficial, deep, or both? _____

   _____

2. Was the skin debridement code selection affected by the infection? _____

   _____

3. Does the skin debridement code include the retroperitoneal exploration? _____

   _____

4. Was there a CPT code for re-exploration of a recent abdominal surgery site? _____

   _____

5. Why would code 11008 not be reported? _____

   _____

6. Were there different diagnosis codes required to report the necrotic status of abdominal fat, skin, and retroperitoneum?

   _____

PRACTICE EXERCISE 19.2   NEVUS EXCISION

OPERATIVE REPORT

One week prior to this report, Dr. Erickson, plastic surgeon, removed a portion of a nevus from the right arm of Leonardo Zapata. Dr. Erickson believed that a further excision was necessary but wanted another opinion. Mr. Zapata was referred to Dr. Matalo to obtain his opinion on the further excision (staged procedure). Dr. Matalo recommended further excision, and today Dr. Erickson performed the other surgery. The follow-up for the first procedure was 10 days.

LOCATION: Outpatient, Hospital
PATIENT: Leonardo Zapata
PRIMARY CARE PHYSICIAN: Ronald Green, MD
SURGEON: Mark Erickson, MD

INDICATION: This patient had a 1-cm lesion excised from the right arm approximately 1 week ago. There was a question as to whether or not this was a Spitz nevus versus melanoma, and this was referred to Dr. Matalo at the New York Clinic for a second opinion. His opinion was that this was a Spitz nevus, and further conservative excision was recommended if that had not already been done. Since we only took a 5-mm margin, we are going to take about another 1 cm or so off around the previously excised area.

PREOPERATIVE DIAGNOSIS: Spitz nevus, right arm.
POSTOPERATIVE DIAGNOSIS: Spitz nevus, right arm.
SURGICAL FINDINGS: A healed incision of the right arm 2 cm in diameter.
ANESTHESIA: Six cc of 1% Xylocaine with 1:100,000 epinephrine.

PROCEDURE: The arm was prepped with Betadine solution and draped in the routine sterile fashion. The lesion was anesthetized and excised elliptically. Bleeders were electrocoagulated, and the wound was closed with interrupted subcuticular 3–0 Monocryl sutures and two twists of 4–0 Prolene. Half-inch Steri-Strips were applied. The patient tolerated the procedure well and left the area in good condition. He will use the sling that he used with his previous incision.

Pathology Report Later Indicated: Nevus, right arm, re-excision. Skin showing biopsy site with fibrosis, granulation tissue, and suture.

CPT Code(s): _____

ICD-10-CM Code(s): _____

_____

Abstracting Questions

1. Is a modifier required to indicate the patient is in the global period from a previous procedure? _____

_____

2. What modifier reports a more extensive procedure than the initial procedure performed during the global period of a previous procedure? _____

_____

3. What was the excised diameter of the initial excision?

_____

4. What is the excised diameter for the re-operation? _____

_____

PRACTICE EXERCISE 19.3   ECHOCARDIOGRAM

Remember to report only the profession portion of the service when the physician is not an employee of the facility in which the service is being provided.

ECHOCARDIOGRAM REPORT

LOCATION: Outpatient, Hospital
PATIENT: Loralee Branigan
ATTENDING/ADMIT PHYSICIAN: James Noonar, MD
RADIOLOGIST: Morton Monson, MD
PERSONAL PHYSICIAN: Ronald Green, MD

INDICATIONS: Valvular heart disease, atrial fibrillation, left ventricular dysfunction.

The M-Mode echo measurements are listed on the accompanying data sheet. They are essentially within normal limits.

The two-dimensional echocardiogram clearly demonstrates some thickening and calcification of the mitral valve leaflets as well as thickening of the aortic valve leaflets. The aortic valve opening is normal, and the mitral valve opening is probably normal as well. Left ventricular contractility is definitely diminished. The ejection fraction is in the range of about 20-25% only.

The Doppler and color Doppler studies do confirm the presence of mild tricuspid insufficiency. The RV systolic pressure is 32 mm Hg, which is consistent with mild pulmonary hypertension.

CONCLUSION: Depression of left ventricular function, as described above, with mild valvular pathology, as described above.

CPT Code(s): _____

_____

ICD-10-CM Code(s): _____

_____

Abstracting Questions

1. What approach was used for the cardiac echocardiogram?

_____

2. Is the Doppler study also reported? _____

_____

3. Is the Doppler color flow study reported? _____

_____

4. What modifier is required on the CPT code? _____

_____

PRACTICE EXERCISE 19.4 CERVICAL CERCLAGE PREOPERATIVE EXAMINATION

LOCATION: Outpatient, Clinic
PATIENT: Chandelle Jackson
ATTENDING PHYSICIAN: Andy Martinez, MD
SURGEON: Andy Martinez, MD
ADMITTING DIAGNOSIS: Decreased cervical length with suspected incompetent cervix.
PROCEDURE PLANNED: Cervical cerclage.

HISTORY OF PRESENT ILLNESS: The patient is a 26-year-old woman, gravida 5, para 2, whose last menstrual period was August 12 of this year, giving her an estimated date of confinement of May 17 of next year. This presently places her at 19 weeks and 3 days gestation. Her due date has been confirmed by pelvic ultrasound, the earliest of which was at 15 weeks gestation. We suspect possible incompetent cervix. The patient does have a history of two preterm deliveries, the first was 3 years ago in March when she delivered at 32 weeks after a 7-hour labor. Her previous obstetrician had therefore discussed with her that perhaps a cervical cerclage would be appropriate. Her history did not seem overly convincing for incompetent cervix. She had had LEEP procedure about 5 years ago. She then had a miscarriage the following year, for which she had a D&C, and then had a therapeutic abortion 2 years later. I have been following cervical length on this pregnancy. On initial scan at 15 weeks' gestation, cervical length was not performed but a week later was found to be 2.7 cm. Follow-up ultrasound done at 17 weeks' gestation showed cervical length to be 3.1 cm. The most recent ultrasound from 19 weeks' gestation showed cervical length decreased to 2.5 cm, and with the patient's questionable history the decision has been made to proceed with cervical cerclage.

OBSTETRIC AND GYNECOLOGIC HISTORY: As noted above.

PAST MEDICAL AND SURGICAL HISTORY: The patient had a tonsillectomy at age 14 and a hallux vagus correction at age 20.

MEDICATIONS: Prenatal vitamins.
PHYSICAL EXAMINATION: Blood pressure: 108/60. Height: 5'6". Weight: 132 lb. Lungs: Clear to auscultation bilaterally. Heart: Sounds normal. Abdomen: Gravid with uterus palpable at the level of the umbilicus. Fetal heart rate is in the 140s. Bimanual examination was carried out, and the cervix is long, soft, and closed.

ASSESSMENT AND PLAN: The patient has had two previous preterm deliveries with history questionable for incompetent cervix, and now has decreased cervical length of 2.5 cm on ultrasound at 19 weeks' gestation. After discussing risks and alternatives, the patient has consented to proceed with cervical cerclage. She is aware of the risks, such as general anesthetic, hemorrhage, infection, ruptured membranes, and ultimately loss of the pregnancy. She does, however, consent to proceed, and the surgery has been scheduled for tomorrow.

CPT Code(s): _____

_____

ICD-10-CM Code(s): _____

_____

Abstracting Questions

1. What section of the CPT would be referenced to locate a code to report the service provided in this report? _____

_____

2. Was the patient admitted to the hospital after the clinic examination? _____

_____

PRACTICE EXERCISE 19.5 ETHMOIDECTOMY, SPHENOIDOTOMY, AND SEPTOPLASTY

Ready for a challenge? This case will give your coding skills an excellent workout. There will be five service codes and five diagnosis codes. The most extensive procedure is the septoplasty, and that code will be sequenced first.
LOCATION: Outpatient, Hospital
PATIENT: Russell Price
ATTENDING PHYSICIAN: Jeff King, MD
SURGEON: Jeff King, MD
PREOPERATIVE DIAGNOSES
 1. Septal deviation.
 2. Bilateral sinonasal polyposis.
 3. Pansinusitis.
 4. Bilateral inferior turbinate hypertrophy.
 5. Nasal obstruction.
POSTOPERATIVE DIAGNOSIS: Same as Preoperative.
PROCEDURES PERFORMED
 1. Bilateral endoscopic total ethmoidectomy.
 2. Bilateral endoscopic maxillary antrostomy with removal of polyps from maxillary sinus.
 3. Bilateral endoscopic sphenoidotomy.
 4. Septoplasty.
 5. Bilateral inferior turbinate overfracture.
ANESTHESIA: Endotracheal.

INDICATIONS: A 43-year-old male with history of nasal trauma that resulted in a septal deviation. He also has a history of bilateral sinonasal polyposis and has undergone prior polypectomy and sinus surgery. The patient now has recurrent disease. This was confirmed on examination and the CT scan. He also has bilateral inferior turbinate hypertrophy. The patient also has a history of severe snoring. He is to undergo correction of his nasal obstruction and sinusitis to see if that will help. If not, further evaluation of his snoring will be done.

PROCEDURE: After consent was obtained, the patient was taken to the operating room and placed on the operating table in supine position. After an adequate level of general endotracheal anesthesia was obtained, the patient was positioned for nasal and sinus surgery. The patient's nose was packed with cotton pledgets soaked with 4% cocaine. After several minutes, 1% Xylocaine with 1:100,000 epinephrine was infiltrated into the nasal portion of the polyps as well as the septum bilaterally and the inferior turbinates. Nasal hairs were trimmed. Attention was first focused on the right side. Using the 5-degree sinuscope and the microdebrider, the nasal portions of the polyps were removed. Polyps were noted both medial and lateral to the middle turbinate. There was also some scarring from the middle turbinate to the lateral nasal

PRACTICE EXERCISE 19.5   ETHMOIDECTOMY, SPHENOIDOTOMY, AND SEPTOPLASTY—cont'd

wall. This scar tissue was also removed with a microdebrider. Subsequently, polyps in the middle meatus and anterior posterior ethmoid areas were removed with microdebrider.

The maxillary sinus ostia area was cleared of polyps, and then the ostium was widened in a posterior-to-inferior direction. Polyps within the sinus near the ostia were also removed. The area was then packed with cotton pledgets soaked with 1:50,000 units of epinephrine. Attention was then focused on the left side, where a similar procedure was performed. Again, polyps were noted to be both medial and lateral to the middle turbinate remnant. Polyps were obstructing the maxillary sinus drainage area and were also cleared. The left side was packed with a pledget soaked with epinephrine solution. Attention was refocused on the right side, where further polyps were removed from the sphenoid/ethmoid area. Remnant of the superior turbinate was also cleared of polyps. The sphenoid sinus ostium was cleared of polyps. The area was then packed with cotton pledget soaked with epinephrine solution. Similar procedure was then performed on the left side. Attention was then focused on the nasal septum. Utilizing a right hemitransfixion incision, mucoperichondrium and mucoperiosteal flaps were elevated. The cartilaginous septum was noted to be severely attenuated and deviated with several fractured areas. Deviated portions were removed. This does not leave much support for the nasal tip area. If this is a problem in the future, this will need to be reconstructed. The deviated portion of the bony septum and spurs off the maxillary crest were then removed.

Attention was then focused on the inferior turbinates, which were outfractured. The hemitransfixion incision was then closed with an interrupted 4–0 chromic suture. A quilting suture of 4–0 plain gut was then performed. The pledgets in the sinus area were then removed. There was some oozing from the ethmoid as well as the sphenoid sinus areas. As such, these areas were coated with FloSeal and then packed lightly with strips of Surgicel soaked with local solutions. Bacitracin ointment was then applied. Silastic splints were then placed on both sides of the nasal septum and secured with nylon suture. The nose was then packed bilaterally. Packs consisted of a Merocel sponge with a gloved finger coated with Bacitracin ointment. It was inflated with location solution. Nasal dressing was applied.

The patient tolerated the procedure well, and there was no break in technique. The patient was extubated and taken to the postanesthetic care unit in good condition. Fluids administered included 2000 cc RL. Blood loss was less than 150 cc. Preoperative medications included 12 mg Decadron and 1 gram Ancef IV.

CPT Code(s): _____

_____

ICD-10-CM Code(s): _____

_____

Abstracting Questions

1. Maxillary Sinus
   a. Were polyps/tissue removed? _____

   _____

   b. What additional work was done to this sinus? _____

2. Sphenoid Sinus
   a. Were polyps/tissue removed? _____

   _____

3. Ethmoid Sinus
   a. Were polyps/tissue removed? _____

   _____

   b. Was this anterior, posterior, or both? _____

   _____

4. Inferior Turbinates
   a. Was there specific work done on this area? _____

   _____

5. What modifiers were appended extensively to the majority of CPT codes that reported the services provided in this case? _____

   _____

6. What does the diagnosis "pansinusitis" indicate? _____

   _____

20
Surgery Section (10004-69990)

Largest CPT Section

Each year CMS publishes a list of CPT surgery codes that are paid only as an inpatient procedure
- For example, 33300-33335, repair of wounds of the heart and great vessels, are inpatient procedures
  - Whereas 33285-33286, insertion or removal of cardiac event recorders, are paid as outpatient procedures
- Inpatient procedures reported with ICD-10-PCS codes
- Outpatient procedures reported with CPT surgery codes

Section Format

Divided by subspecialty, e.g., Integumentary, Cardiovascular

Notes and Guidelines

Throughout section
- Information varied and extensive
- "Must" reading
- Subsection notes apply to entire subsection
- Subheading notes apply to entire subheading
- Category notes apply to entire category
- Parenthetical information (Fig. 20.1)

Unlisted Procedure Codes

Used only when more specific code not found in Category I or Category III

Written report accompanies submission
Each unlisted code service paid on case-by-case basis

Separate Procedures

"(Separate procedure)" follows code description

Usually minor surgical procedure
Incidental to more major procedure:
- Breast biopsy before radical mastectomy would not be reported unless results of biopsy resulted in mastectomy, modifier-59 appended to biopsy code
- Appendectomy performed incidentally when other abdominal surgery is performed
Separate procedures reported when
- Only procedure performed

- With another procedure
  - On different site
  - Unrelated to major procedure

Major Guideline of Surgical Packages

Usually include
- Preoperative (before, preop)
- E/M service subsequent to decision for surgery but prior to surgery date
- Intraoperative (during, intraop)
- Postoperative (after—also known as global period, postop)
  - Post-anesthesia recovery (PAR)
  - Follow-up office visits
- Local/topical anesthesia and digital block
  To report these bundled services separately is "unbundling"
  Remember to use modifiers during global period for unrelated E/M, return to OR, etc.

Supplies

Supplies that are beyond those typically included in the procedure are reported separately
  Example: Report surgical tray with
- 99070 CPT, Medicine section
- A4550 HCPCS

Special Report

Submitting an unlisted service or one that is unusual, variable, or new may require a special report, as listed in Guidelines

Demonstrates medical necessity/appropriateness of service
Contains pertinent information describing service in terms of
- Nature
- Extent
- Need for procedure
- Time
- Effort
- Equipment necessary
  May also include complexity of symptoms, final diagnosis, physical findings, procedures, concurrent problems, and follow-up care

General Subsection (10004-10021)

Fine needle aspiration biopsies with or without (w/wo) imaging guidance

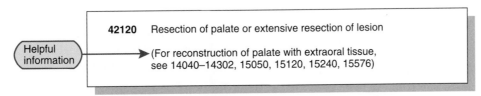

| Helpful information | **42120** Resection of palate or extensive resection of lesion |
| | (For reconstruction of palate with extraoral tissue, see 14040–14302, 15050, 15120, 15240, 15576) |

• **Figure 20.1** Parenthetical information in the CPT manual.

Pathology 88172, 88173, and 88177 are for evaluation of fine needle aspirate

Integumentary System Subsection (10040-19499)

Often used in all specialties of medicine

Not just surgeons or dermatologists; wide range of physicians
Subheadings of Integumentary Subsection
- Skin, Subcutaneous, and Accessory Structures
- Nails
- Pilonidal Cyst
- Introduction
- Repair (Closure)
- Destruction
- Breast

Skin, Subcutaneous, and Accessory Structures (10030-11646)

Introduction and Removal (10030-10036)

Report percutaneous image-guided fluid drainage of a catheter collection from soft tissue
- Example: Abscess, seroma, cyst, hematoma, or lymphocele
Reported once for each individual collection drained
Report codes 10035, 10036 for placement of soft tissue markers

Incision and Drainage (10040-10180)

I&D of abscess, carbuncle, boil, cyst, infection, hematoma, pilonidal cyst
- Lancing (cutting of skin)
- Aspiration (removal by puncturing lesion with a needle and withdrawing fluid)
Gauze or tube may be inserted for continued drainage

Excision—Debridement (11000-11047)

Dead tissue cut away and washed away with sterile saline

11000, 11001 Eczematous or infected skin
11004-11006 Debridement of infected area based on location and depth of necrotizing tissue (subcutaneous tissue, muscle, and fascia)
+11008 Removal of prosthetic material or mesh from abdominal wall
11010-11012 Foreign material with open fracture or dislocation
- Skin, subcutaneous tissue, muscle fascia, muscle, and bone
11042-11044 Subcutaneous tissue, muscle, bone

- Debridement partial thickness based on 20 square centimeters or less
11045-11047 Based on each additional 20 square centimeters

Paring or Cutting (11055-11057)

Removal by scraping or peeling (e.g., removal of corn or callus)
Codes indicate number: 1, 2-4, 4+

Biopsy (11102-11107)

Tangential, punch, incisional biopsies

Not all of lesion removed
- All lesion removed = excision
Do not use modifier -51
Codes indicate number: 1 or each additional
Tissue removed during excision, shaving, etc., and submitted to pathology is NOT reported separately as a biopsy
- Rather, it is included in the code for the excision

Skin Tag Removal (11200, 11201)

Benign lesions

Removed with scissors, blade, chemicals, electrosurgery, etc.
Do not use -51
- Codes indicate number: Up to and including 15 lesions and each additional 10 lesions or part thereof

Shaving of Lesions (11300-11313)

Removed by transverse incision or sliced horizontally

Based on
- Size (e.g., 1.1-2.0 cm)
- Location (e.g., arm, hand, nose)
Does not require suture closure
- Report most extensive lesion first with no modifier, then least extensive lesions with modifier -51

Benign/Malignant Lesions (11400-11646)

Codes divided: Benign or malignant

Physician assesses lesion as benign or malignant
Codes include local anesthesia and simple closure
Report each excised lesion separately
Lesion size
- Taken from physician's notes
- Includes greatest diameter plus narrowest margins of two sides (Fig. 20.2)
  Example: A benign lesion measuring 0.5 cm at widest point is removed with 0.5-cm margin at narrowest

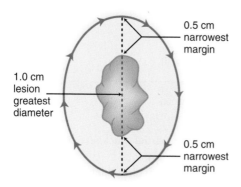

• **Figure 20.2** Calculating the size of a lesion.

point (each side, 0.5 + 0.5 = 1.0 cm). Reported as 1.5-cm lesion excision (11402)
- Do not take size from pathology report—storage solution shrinks tissue
- Margins (healthy tissue) are also taken for comparison with unhealthy tissue
- Re-excisions following initial excision of malignant lesion coded as excision of malignant lesion

All excised tissue pathologically examined
Codes 11400-11646 report excision of lesion
Destroyed lesions have no pathology samples
Example: Laser or chemical
Lesion closure
- Simple or subcutaneous closure included in removal
- Reported separately
  - Layered or intermediate, 12031-12057 (Repair—Intermediate)
  - Complex, 13100-13153 (Repair—Complex)

Nails (11719-11765)

Includes toes and fingers

Types of services
- Trimming, debridement, removal, biopsy, repair

Pilonidal Cyst (11770-11772)

Codes divided by
- Simple
- Extensive
- Complicated

Introduction (11900-11983)

Types of services
- Lesion injections (therapeutic or diagnostic), tattooing, tissue expansion, contraceptive insertion/removal, hormone implantation services, and insertion/removal of non-biodegradable drug delivery implant

Repair (Closure) (12001-13160)
Repair Factors in Wound Repair

As types of wounds vary, types of wound repair also vary

Length, complexity (simple, intermediate, complex), and site must be documented
- Length measured in centimeters
- Measured prior to closure

Types of Wound Repair

Simple. Superficial, epidermis, dermis, or subcutaneous tissue
- One-layer closure
- Dermabond closure
- Medicare report Dermabond closure with G0168

Intermediate. Layered closure of deeper layers of subcutaneous tissue and superficial fascia with skin closure
- Single-layer closure can be coded as intermediate if extensive debridement required

Complex. Greater than layered; may include multiple layers of tissue and fascia or extensive debridement

Example: Scar revision, complicated debridement, extensive undermining, stents, extensive retention sutures

Included in Wound Repair Codes

Simple ligation of vessels in an open wound
Simple exploration of nerves, blood vessels, and exposed tendons
Normal debridement
- Additional codes for debridement can be used when
  - Gross contamination requires prolonged cleaning
  - Appreciable amounts of devitalized/contaminated tissue are removed to expose healthy tissue
  - Debridement is provided without immediate primary closure

Grouping of Wound Repair

Add together lengths by
- **Complexity** of Wound
  - Simple, intermediate, complex
- **Location** of Wound
  - e.g., face, ears, eyelids, nose, lips
    1 inch = 2.54 cm
    - *Example:* **Same complexity, same codes description location:** Intermediate repairs of 2.9-cm laceration of leg and 1.1-cm laceration of buttocks. 2.9 + 1.1 = 4.0 cm (12032)
    - *Example:* **Different complexity:** Intermediate repair of 2.9-cm laceration of leg and simple repair of 1.1-cm laceration of buttocks. 2.9-cm intermediate repair (12032) and 1.1-cm simple repair (12001)
    - *Example:* **Same complexity, different code description locations:** Intermediate repair of 2.9-cm laceration of leg and intermediate repair of 1.1-cm laceration of nose. 2.9-cm intermediate repair of leg (12032) and 1.1-cm intermediate repair of nose (12051)

Do Not Group Wound Repairs That Are

Different complexities

Example: Simple repair and complex repair
Different locations as stated in the code description
Example: Simple repairs of scalp (12001) and nose (12011)

Adjacent Tissue Transfer, Flaps, and Grafts (14000-15778)

Information Needed to Code Graft

Type of graft—adjacent, free flap, etc.

Donor site (from)
Recipient site (to)
Any repair to donor site
Size of graft

Adjacent Tissue Transfer/Rearrangement (14000-14350)

Includes lesion excision and/or repair (e.g., Z-plasty, W-plasty, V-plasty, Y-plasty, rotation flap, advancement flap)

Codes based on size and location of graft
Primary defect results from excision of lesion
Secondary defect results from formation of flap
To select code, add the size of the primary and secondary defects together

Skin Replacement Surgery (15002-15431)

15002-15005 Site preparation based on size and site
15040-15261 Autografts/Tissue Cultured Autografts
- 15050-15431 Autograft codes by type and size
- 15271-15278 Skin substitute grafts
  Split-thickness: Epidermis and some dermis (Fig. 20.3)
  Full-thickness: Epidermis and all dermis

Allografts (15300-15431)

Bilaminate skin substitute
- Artificial skin, such as silicone-covered biodegradable collagen matrix
  Allograft: Donor graft
  Xenograft: Nonhuman donor
  Code is based on recipient site, not donor site

Flaps (15570-15776)

Some skin left attached to blood supply
- Keeps flap viable
- Donor site may be far from recipient site
- Flaps may be in stages
- Codes divided by location and size
- Formation of flap (15570-15576)
- Based on recipient location: Trunk, scalp, nose, etc.
  Transfer of flap (15650): Previously placed flap released from donor site
- Also known as walking or walk up of flap
- 15777 is an add-on code to report soft tissue reinforcement with biological implants

Muscle, Myocutaneous, or Fasciocutaneous Flaps (15733-15738)

- Based on recipient location; head and neck, trunk, upper or lower extremity

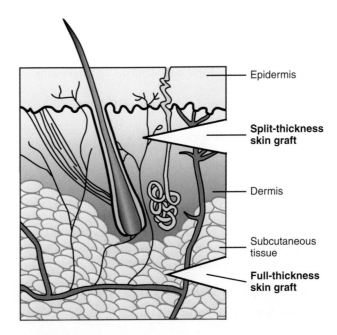

Epidermis

Split-thickness skin graft

Dermis

Subcutaneous tissue

Full-thickness skin graft

- **Figure 20.3** Split-thickness and full-thickness skin grafts.

- Repairs made with
  - Muscle
  - Muscle and skin
  - Fascia and skin
- Flaps rotated from donor to recipient site
- Includes closure donor site unless skin graft or local flaps are necessary

Other Procedures (15780-15879)

Many cosmetic procedures including:
- Dermabrasion
- Chemical peel
- Blepharoplasty
- Rhytidectomy
- Excessive skin excision

Pressure (Decubitus) Ulcers (15920-15999)

Excision and various closures
- Primary, skin flap, muscle, etc.
  Many codes "with ostectomy"
- Bone removal
  Locations
- Coccygeal (end of spine)
- Sacral (between hips)
- Ischial (lower hip)
- Trochanteric (outer hip)
  Site preparation only: 15936, 15937, 15946, 15956, or 15958
- Defect repair of donor site reported separately

Burns Local Treatment (16000-16036)

Codes for small, medium, and large
  Must calculate percentage of body burned
- <5% small
- 5% to 10% medium
- >10% large

Lund-Browder Classification Method (Fig. 20.4)
- Proportions of children differ from adults
- For instance, children's heads are larger
  Often require multiple debridements and redressing
  Based on
- Initial treatment of 1st-degree burn (16000)
- Size
  Report percent of burn and depth

Destruction (17000-17286)

Ablation (destruction) of tissue
- Laser, electrosurgery, cryosurgery, chemosurgery, etc.
- Benign/premalignant or malignant tissue
- Malignant tissue is based on location and size of lesion
- Benign/premalignant is based on the number of lesions removed/destroyed or size (sq cm)

Mohs Micrographic Surgery (17311-17315)

Surgeon acts as pathologist and surgeon

Removes one layer of lesion at a time
Continues until no malignant cells remain
Based on stages and number of specimens per stage indicated in medical record

Other Procedures (17340-17999)

Treatment of acne
- Cryotherapy
- Chemical exfoliation
- Electrolysis
- Unlisted procedures

Breast Procedures (19000-19499)

Divided based on procedure
- Incision
- Excision
- Introduction
- Mastectomy procedures
- Repair and/or Reconstruction

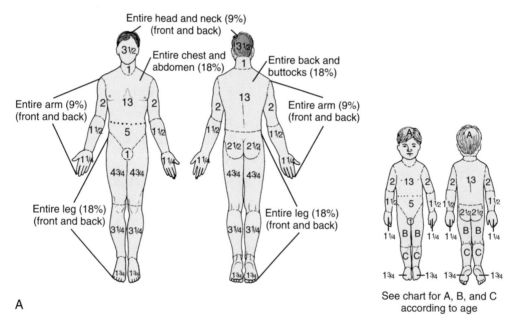

AGE	Birth–1 yr	1–4 yr	5–9 yr	10–14 yr	15 yr	Adult
Head	19	17	13	11	9	7
Neck	2					
Ant trunk	13					
Post trunk	13					
R buttock	2½					
L buttock	2½					
Genitalia	1					
R U arm	4					
L U arm	4					
R L arm	3					
L L arm	3					
R hand	2½	6½	8	8½	9	9½
L hand	2½	6½	8	8½	9	9½
R thigh	5½	5	5½	6	6½	7
L thigh	5½	5	5½	6	6½	7
R leg	5					
L leg	5					
R foot	3½					
L foot	3½					

B   BODY AREA

• **Figure 20.4** Lund-Browder Classification Method for estimating the extent of burns.

Use excision of lesion codes if entire lesion is removed during incisional biopsy

Use additional code for placement of radiological marker

Mastectomies based on extent of procedure

- Wide excision
- Removal of neoplasm, capsule, and surrounding margins
- Radical
- Wide excision and anatomical structure surrounding neoplasm

  Example: Muscle or fascia

- Conservative partial mastectomy in which lesion is removed with adequate margins (19301)
- Axillary dissection and partial mastectomy, 19302
- Radical and modified radical (19305, 19306, and 19307) based on extent
- Confirm whether pectoral muscles, axillary, or internal lymph nodes were removed
- 19307 most common and includes breast and axillary lymph node removal
- Code removal of lymph nodes separately unless included in code description
- Bilateral procedures, use -50

Biopsy/Removal of Lesion

Incisional biopsy: Incision made into lesion and small portion of lesion removed

Excisional biopsy: Entire lesion removed

Open incisional biopsy most complex (19101)

Percutaneous needle core biopsy without imaging guidance (19100)

- Same procedure with imaging guidance based on guidance method:
  - 19081, 19082, stereotactic
  - 19083, 19084, ultrasound
  - 19085, 19086, magnetic resonance

Complete, simple removal of a mass is reported with 19120

Lesion may be preoperatively marked with localization devices (clip, metallic pellet, wire, needle, radioactive seed) based on guidance method:

- 19281, 19282, mammographic
- 19283, 19284, stereotactic
- 19285, 19286, ultrasound
- 19287, 19288, magnetic resonance

PRACTICE EXERCISE 20.1   EXCISION, CHEEK LESION

OPERATIVE REPORT
LOCATION: Outpatient, Hospital
PATIENT: Mary Carbono
ATTENDING PHYSICIAN: Gary Sanchez, MD
SURGEON: Gary Sanchez, MD
PREOPERATIVE DIAGNOSIS: Right cheek lesion, unspecified behavior.
POSTOPERATIVE DIAGNOSIS: Right cheek lesion, unspecified behavior.
PROCEDURE PERFORMED: Excision of lesion, right cheek.
ANESTHESIA: General anesthetic by inhalational mask technique.
PROCEDURE: Following informed consent from the patient's mother, the patient was taken to the operating room and placed supine on the operating room table. The appropriate monitoring devices were placed on the patient, and general anesthesia was induced. It was maintained by inhalation mask technique. The right cheek was prepped and draped in a sterile fashion. The lesion, which was about 1.6 cm, somewhat raised, and erythematous, was injected at its base with 0.5 cc of 1% Xylocaine with 1:100,000 epinephrine. A #15-blade scalpel was used to perform a shave excision. No suture was placed. A sterile bandage was applied. The patient tolerated the procedure well. She was

allowed to recover from general anesthesia and was transferred to the recovery room in good condition.
Pathology Report Later Indicated: Benign lesion of cheek.

CPT Code(s): _____

_____

ICD-10-CM Code(s): _____

_____

Abstracting Questions

1. What method was used to excise the lesion? _____

_____

2. Does the pathologic status of the report affect CPT code assignment? _____

_____

3. Does the size and location of the lesion affect CPT code assignment? _____

_____

4. Does the pathologic status of the lesion affect the diagnosis code? _____

_____

PRACTICE EXERCISE 20.2   RIGHT BREAST WIDE EXCISION

OPERATIVE REPORT
LOCATION: Outpatient, Hospital
PATIENT: Jane Doe
ATTENDING PHYSICIAN: Gary Sanchez, MD
SURGEON: Gary Sanchez, MD
PREOPERATIVE DIAGNOSIS: Mass, right breast.
POSTOPERATIVE DIAGNOSIS: Mass, right breast.
OPERATIVE PROCEDURE: Right breast mass excision.
PROCEDURE: With the patient under general anesthesia, the breast and chest were prepped and draped in a sterile manner. An elliptical incision was made about the palpated mass, including the area around the nipple. This was excised

all the way down to the fascia of the breast and then submitted for frozen section. Frozen section revealed a carcinoma of the breast with what appeared to be a good margin all the way around it. We then maintained hemostasis with electrocautery and proceeded to close the breast tissue using 2–0 and 3–0 chromic. The skin was closed using 4–0 Vicryl in a subcuticular manner. Steri-Strips were applied. The patient tolerated the procedure well and was discharged from the operating room in stable condition.
Pathology Report Later Indicated: Primary, malignant neoplasm of the right breast nipple.

Continued

PRACTICE EXERCISE 20.2   RIGHT BREAST WIDE EXCISION—cont'd

CPT Code(s): _____

ICD-10-CM Code(s): _____

Abstracting Questions

1. Does the pathologic status of the lesion affect CPT code assignment? _____
_____

2. Does the size of the lesion affect CPT code assignment?
_____

3. Does the pathologic status of the lesion affect the diagnosis code? _____
_____

4. Does the location of the lesion affect the diagnosis code?
_____

5. Does the gender of the patient affect either code? _____
_____

PRACTICE EXERCISE 20.3   THENAR FLAP COVERAGE

OPERATIVE REPORT

Assign an external cause code to indicate how this injury occurred in addition to the diagnosis and service codes.
LOCATION: Outpatient, Hospital
PATIENT: Leslie May
ATTENDING PHYSICIAN: Gary Sanchez, MD
SURGEON: Gary Sanchez, MD
PREOPERATIVE DIAGNOSIS: Oblique volar amputation tip, right middle finger, while working on machinery.
POSTOPERATIVE DIAGNOSIS: Oblique volar amputation tip, right middle finger, while working on machinery.
PROCEDURE: Thenar flap coverage, tip, right middle finger.
ANESTHESIA: General.
PROCEDURE: The patient was brought to the operating room, and general anesthesia was induced. Right upper extremity was prepped with Betadine and draped in a sterile fashion. The limb was exsanguinated with a tourniquet inflated to 250 mm Hg for 45 minutes. Using 4× magnification loupes, we debrided the fingertip. It was a volar oblique amputation. However, there was loss of distal phalanx down to about half of the sterile nail matrix. We trimmed the nail plate back to the level of the bone, we debrided the wound, and it was quite clean. We then fabricated a thenar flap using a piece of paper glove as a template. We traced this out on the thenar eminence. We then incised this and elevated the flap with fatty tissue. The radialward digital nerve to the index finger was exposed, and we covered this over with muscle with 4–0 Vicryl suture. We next harvested a split-thickness skin graft from the ulnar aspect of the hand using the Davol dermatome. We then placed this graft in place and sutured it over the defect in the palm with 5–0 Vicryl suture. Tegaderm was then placed over the donor site on the ulnar aspect of the hand.

We then placed the finger down in the palm and then attached the flap with interrupted 5–0 nylon sutures. This covered the defect on the finger nicely. We next applied Xeroform over all wounds and applied wet cotton balls over the graft site to hold it in place, then placed as compression a hand bandage with fluffs, Kerlix, Kling, and plaster splints immobilizing the hand in an intrinsic plus position. The tourniquet was released, and good circulation returned to the hand.

The patient tolerated the procedure well. She went to the recovery room in excellent condition. She will be dismissed as an outpatient today with plans for follow-up back in the office in appropriately 2 weeks.

CPT Code(s): _____
_____

ICD-10-CM Code(s): _____
_____

Abstracting Questions

1. Was this an adjacent tissue transfer flap? _____
_____

2. Was the CPT code selection based on the recipient or donor site? _____
_____

3. Can the split-thickness skin graft for repair of the donor site be reported separately? _____
_____

4. What HCPCS modifier would be appropriate to append to the CPT code reported for the formation of the pedicle flap?
_____

5. Does the way in which the amputation occurred affect the diagnosis code selection? _____
_____

6. If the type of machinery used during the procedure were specified, what other type of diagnosis code would you have reported? _____

PRACTICE EXERCISE 20.4   LACERATION REPAIR

OPERATIVE REPORT

Assign an external cause code to indicate how the injury occurred.
LOCATION: Outpatient, Hospital
PATIENT: Rod Seim
ATTENDING PHYSICIAN: Gary Sanchez, MD
SURGEON: Gary Sanchez, MD
PREOPERATIVE DIAGNOSIS: Multiple simple lacerations, right middle finger due to arrow.

POSTOPERATIVE DIAGNOSIS: Multiple simple lacerations, right middle finger due to arrow.
PROCEDURE PERFORMED: Simple closure of lacerations to right middle finger.
ANESTHESIA: Ring block.
PROCEDURE: Ring block anesthesia was achieved with 1% Xylocaine without epinephrine. Once the ring block was successful, the patient was taken to the scrub sink and the finger gently scrubbed and thoroughly irrigated with water. Once the finger was cleansed, repair was performed. The

PRACTICE EXERCISE 20.4   LACERATION REPAIR—cont'd

patient had a small nick (1 cm) in the lateral band. This was tacked together with one 4–0 nylon suture. There was noted to be no dirt on the tendon after irrigating the finger. To minimize the risk for infection, it was elected to just loosely close this. The 5-cm, J-shaped wound was then closed with four 4–0 nylon sutures just to approximate the skin. Some fat at the edge of the volar wound was debrided with scissors, and some abrasion of the epidermis was also debrided with scissors. The volar wound was then closed with two 4–0 nylon sutures. Dressing and a TubeGauz dressing were then applied. The patient tolerated this well.

CPT Code(s): _____

_____

ICD-10-CM Code(s): _____

_____

Abstracting Questions

1. What type of repair was performed (simple, intermediate, complex)? _____

_____

2. Does the location on the body of the repair affect the choice of the CPT code assignment? _____

_____

3. Does the size of the repair affect the choice of CPT code? _____

4. The 7th character on the ICD-10-CM code indicates this was a/an _____ encounter.

5. Does the repair to the nick in the tendon affect the diagnosis coding? _____

_____

PRACTICE EXERCISE 20.5   MINIMAL DEBRIDEMENT

OPERATIVE REPORT

The patient is returned to the operating room during the postoperative period of a previous procedure.

LOCATION: Inpatient, Hospital
PATIENT: Pam Tieg
ATTENDING PHYSICIAN: Leslie Alanda, MD
SURGEON: Gary Sanchez, MD
PREOPERATIVE DIAGNOSES

1. Massive abdominal wound with multiple sites of fat necrosis and retroperitoneal tissue necrosis, predominantly fat.
2. Draining sinus, anterior abdominal wall.

POSTOPERATIVE DIAGNOSES

1. Massive abdominal wound with multiple sites of fat necrosis and retroperitoneal tissue necrosis, predominantly fat.
2. Draining sinus, anterior abdominal wall.

SURGICAL FINDINGS: There are about 10 sites of fat necrosis scattered throughout the anterior abdominal wall, but the posterior aspect of the wound (i.e., in the retroperitoneal space that is obliterated by the overhang of bowel) appeared to be clean as far as we could tell, and certainly there was no odor.

SURGICAL PROCEDURE

1. Minimal debridement of anterior abdominal wall wound.
2. Collection of specimen for amylase.

ANESTHESIA: General endotracheal.

PROCEDURE: The patient's abdomen was prepped with Betadine scrub and solution and draped in the routine sterile fashion. Multiple sites of fat necrosis were debrided, and one area of protrusion of the mesh was debrided. There was some clear fluid leaking from a sinus in the anterior abdominal wall, and we collected 2 cc of fluid from this and submitted it for amylase. The wound was then repacked with Kerlix-soaked dressings using 0.5% metronidazole, and fine mesh gauze was applied to the anterior abdominal wound. The patient seemed to tolerate the procedure well and left the area in good condition. We additionally did spray Hemaseel into a pocket in the retroperitoneal area where there was some bleeding that did not respond to cautery, and it was thought that this was more the nature of generalized oozing, and therefore the Hemaseel and packing were used for control.

CPT Code(s): _____

_____

ICD-10-CM Code(s): _____

_____

Abstracting Questions

1. Was the retroperitoneum re-explored? _____

_____

2. Does the return to the operating room require a modifier appended to the surgical procedure code? _____

Musculoskeletal System Subsection (20100-29999)

Subsection divided: Anatomic site, then service (e.g., excision)

Used extensively by orthopedic surgeons
 • Many codes commonly used by variety of physicians
Extensive notes
Most common

 • Fracture and dislocation treatments
 • "General" subheading
 • Arthroscopic procedures
 • Casting and strapping
Eponyms are "things" named after "people"

Example: Barr procedure is a tendon transfer of the lower leg (27690-27692), and Mitchell and Chevron or concentric type procedure is a distal metatarsal osteotomy (bunion correction) (28296)

- Procedures are often referred to with eponyms
- Check the index of the CPT manual for directions to eponym codes

Fracture Treatment

Type of treatment depends on type and severity of fracture

Diagnosis codes must support the procedure codes and document the medical necessity

Open: Surgically opened to view or remotely opened to place nail across fracture site
- Open reduction with internal fixation is ORIF

Closed: Not surgically opened

Percutaneous: Insertion of devices through skin or a remote site
- Percutaneous fracture treatment neither open nor closed

Treatment terms should not be confused with **types** of fractures:
- Open fracture: Fractured bone penetrates skin
- Closed fracture: Fractured bone does not penetrate skin

Traction

- Application of force to align bone
- Force applied by internal device (e.g., wire, pin) inserted into bone (skeletal fixation)
- Application of force by means of adhesion to skin (skin traction)

Manipulation

Use of force to return bone back to normal alignment by manual manipulation (reduction) or temporary traction
Codes often divided based on whether manipulation was or was not used

Dislocation

Bone displaced from normal joint position
Treatment: Return bone to normal joint location

Subheading "General"

Begins "Wound Exploration" (20100)

Depth: Difference between Integumentary and Musculoskeletal incision codes
Musculoskeletal used when underlying bone or muscle is involved or procedure is deep subcutaneous

Wound Exploration (20100-20103)

Traumatic penetrating wounds

Divided by wound location
Includes
- Enlargement
- Debridement

- Foreign body(ies) removal
- Ligation
- Repair of tissue and muscle

Use additional code for repair of major structures or blood vessels
Not used for integumentary repairs
- Unless the repair requires extension, enlargement, or exploration

Repair of major structure is reported instead when exploration leads to repair

Excision (20150-20251)

Biopsies for bone and muscle

Divided by
- Type of biopsy (bone/muscle)
- Depth
- Some by method

Can be percutaneous needle or excisional
Does not include tumor excision, which is coded separately
Biopsy with excision: Code only excision

Introduction or Removal (20500-20697)

Codes for
- Injections
- Aspirations
- Insertions
- Applications
- Removals
- Adjustments

Therapeutic sinus tract injection procedures
- Not nasal sinus
- Abscess or cyst with passage (sinus tract) to skin
- Antibiotic injected with use of radiographic guidance

Removal of foreign bodies lodged in muscle or tendon sheath
Integumentary removal codes for removal from skin
Injection into
- Tendon sheath
- Tendon origin
- Ligament
- Ganglion cyst
- Trigger points

Placement of needles or catheters into muscle and/or soft tissue
- For interstitial radioelement application

Arthrocentesis: Injection "and/or" aspiration of a joint
- Both aspiration and injection reported with one code (20600-20611)
- Codes based on joint size: Small, intermediate, major and with or without guidance
- Do not unbundle and report aspiration/injection with two codes

External Fixation

Device that holds bone in place

- Application, adjustment, removal under anesthesia
  Code fracture treatment and external fixation device (EFD)
- Unless treatment and fixation both included in fracture care code description
- Adjustment to (20693) and removal of (20694 [under anesthesia]) EFD are coded separately

Replantation (20802-20838)

Used to report reattachment of amputated limb
  Code by body area

Grafts (or Implants) (20900-20939)
Autogenous Grafts

Used to report harvesting through separate incision of
- Bone
- Cartilage
- Tendon
- Fascia lata
- Tissue
  Fascia lata grafts: From upper lateral thigh where fascia is thickest
  Some codes include obtaining grafting material (not coded separately)
  Some grafts are add-on codes for spine surgery only (20930-20938)

Other Procedures (20950-20999)

Monitoring interstitial fluid pressure (interstitial for compartment syndrome, etc.)
- Pressure increases due to increased accumulation of fluids, causing blood supply to be compromised
  Bone grafts identified by donor site
  Free osseocutaneous flaps: Bone grafts
- Taken along with skin and tissue overlying bone
  Electrical stimulation
- Used to speed bone healing
- Placement of stimulators externally or internally
- Ultrasound also used externally

Soft Tissue Tumors

Codes identify excision of soft tissue and subfascial (intramuscular) tumors
- Subcutaneous soft tissue tumors: Below skin but above deep fascia
- Fascial or subfascial soft tissue tumors: Within or below deep fascia (not bone)
- Soft tissue tumors: May involve resection from one or more layer (i.e., subcutaneous, subfascial)
  Example: 21011-21016 to report subcutaneous, subfascial, and soft tissue tumors

Arthrodesis

Fixation of joint (arthro = joint, desis = fusion)

- Bony structures of joint fused together to form one solid bone
- Fixation with pins, wires, rods, etc. to hold the joint immobile
  Often performed with other procedure such as fracture repair
- Arthrodesis of the spine is also called spinal fusion

Subsequent Subheadings

After General subheading, divided by anatomic location
- Anatomic subheadings divided by type procedure
  Example: Subheading "Head" divided by procedure
- Incision
- Excision
- Manipulation
- Head Prosthesis
- Introduction or Removal
- Repair, Revision, and/or Reconstruction
- Fracture and/or Dislocation
- Other Procedures

Spine and Spinal Instrumentation

Insertion of spinal instrumentation reported in addition to arthrodesis (fusion)

Many add-on codes reported in addition to definitive procedure
Spine (Vertebral Column), 22100-22899, divided by repair location (Fig. 20.5)
- Cervical (C1-C7)
  C1 = Atlas
  C2 = Axis
- Thoracic (T1-T12)
- Lumbar (L1-L5)
- Sacral (S1-S5)
- Coccyx (tailbone)
  Vertebral segment: Single complete vertebral bone with articular processes and laminae
  Vertebral interspace: Non-bony compartment between two vertebral bodies which contains the disc
  Single level = two vertebrae and the disc that separates them
  Percutaneous vertebroplasty
- Use of polymethylmethacrylate injected into the vertebral space
  - Polymethylmethacrylate is a type of bone cement/glue similar to texture of silicone
  - Adheres bone fragments together
  - Fills vertebral body defects

Types of Spinal Instrumentation
Segmental: Devices at each end of repair area + at least one other attachment
Nonsegmental: Devices at each end of defect only
Approach: Pay special attention to the approach used to perform the surgery
- Several different approaches to spine: Most common are anterior (front) and posterior (back)

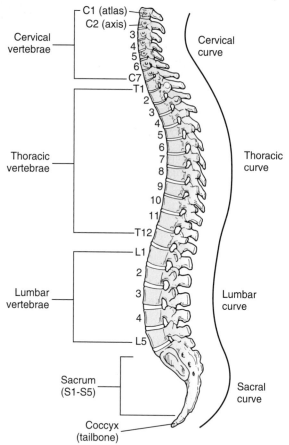

C1 (atlas)
C2 (axis)

Cervical vertebrae

3
4
5
6
C7

Cervical curve

T1
2
3
4
5
6
7
8
9
10
11
T12

Thoracic vertebrae

Thoracic curve

L1
2
3
4
L5

Lumbar vertebrae

Lumbar curve

Sacrum (S1-S5)

Sacral curve

Coccyx (tailbone)

• **Figure 20.5** The spinal cord is part of the central nervous system (CNS) and extends from the brain to the lower back.

- Most spinal instrumentation codes divided based on approach

Casts and Strapping (29000-29799)

Replacement procedure or initial placement to stabilize without additional restorative treatment

Example: Application of wrist splint or cast for wrist sprain
Initial fracture treatment includes placement and removal of first cast
- Subsequent cast applications coded separately
- Payers have strict individual reimbursement policies for subsequent casting

Application not coded when part of surgical procedure
Example: Application of wrist splint or cast for wrist sprain
Initial fracture treatment includes placement and removal of first cast
Elastic bandage application is not billed separately
Removal bundled into surgical procedure
Supplies reported separately

Endoscopy/Arthroscopy (29800-29999)

Surgical arthroscopy always includes diagnostic arthroscopy

Codes divided by joint
- Subdivided by procedure

Be aware of subterms and bundled procedures within code descriptions
Note: Parenthetical information following codes indicates codes to use if procedure was an open procedure

---

PRACTICE EXERCISE 20.6   STEROID INJECTION

LOCATION: Outpatient, Clinic
PATIENT: Kim Ortega
PRIMARY CARE PHYSICIAN: Frank Gaul, MD
SURGEON: Mohomad Almaz, MD
PROCEDURE PERFORMED: Steroid injection.
INDICATIONS: Left shoulder subacromial bursitis.
PROCEDURE: This procedure was done in the procedure area in the hospital.

After obtaining consent, area of the left shoulder was prepped in the usual fashion with Betadine; 6 cc of 1% lidocaine with 1 cc of Kenalog was injected without guidance in the left subacromial bursa without difficulty. The patient tolerated the procedure well without immediate complications. There was moderate relief of pain afterward.

The patient was advised to call me if she experiences any signs of infection, such as fever, chills, erythema, or swelling. She will call me in 3 days and tell me how she is doing.

CPT Code(s): _____

ICD-10-CM Code(s): _____
_____

Abstracting Questions

1. What is the medical term for inserting a needle into a joint?
_____
_____

2. Would the joint into which the needle is inserted affect CPT code assignment? _____
_____

PRACTICE EXERCISE 20.7   ARTHROPLASTY AND SPUR EXCISION

LOCATION: Outpatient, Hospital
PATIENT: Merry Hoffert
PRIMARY CARE PHYSICIAN: Frank Gaul, MD
SURGEON: Mohomad Almaz, MD
PREOPERATIVE DIAGNOSIS: Arthritis, secondary impingement, right ankle.

POSTOPERATIVE DIAGNOSES
1. Osteoarthritic change, grade 3/4 tibia, medial shoulder of the talus, right ankle.
2. Osteophytic spurring with secondary impingement, both hard and soft tissue anterior talotibial articulation, right ankle.

PRACTICE EXERCISE 20.7 ARTHROPLASTY AND SPUR EXCISION—cont'd

3. Impinging soft tissue entity, anterolateral aspect of the ankle.

PROCEDURES PERFORMED
1. Abrasion arthroplasty, right ankle.
2. Excision of osteoarthritic spurs of the anterior articular margin, distal tibia.

PROCEDURE: After a satisfactory level of general anesthesia and the patient in a supine position, the extremity was prepped and draped in a routine sterile manner. At this time we proceeded with the establishment of routine arthroscopic portals. We entered from an anteromedial direction with camera, anterolateral direction with camera, and anterolateral direction with in-cutting device. At this setting there was a proud prominence of secondary scar tissue formation. We proceeded with its resection at this time. There were also areas of secondary eburnation change diffusely of grade 2/3 about the lateral aspect of the talus and focally grade 3/4 changes about the medial shoulder of the talus and the tibia as they articulate. There was also the demonstration with dorsiflexion of secondary abutment of soft tissue and proud tibial spurring. At this setting, with use of mechanical in-cutting device, we reamed back the abutment of the diarticular tibia and also at this time proceeded with abrasion

chondroplasty and arthroplasty procedures where appropriate of the distal articular tibial plafond and the talus proper.

Medial and lateral recesses were evaluated at this time and were otherwise unremarkable. The posterior confines of the ankle other than the areas of graded arthritic change as noted above were otherwise unremarkable. With completion of this element of the procedure we simply proceeded with closure of portal sites. Both preprocedure and postprocedure arthroscopic photos were obtained for documentation purposes. The patient tolerated the procedure well and was transported to the recovery room in a stable manner.

CPT Code(s): _____

_____

ICD-10-CM Code(s): _____

_____

Abstracting Questions
1. What approach was used for this procedure? _____

2. Was the procedure limited or extensive? _____

_____

PRACTICE EXERCISE 20.8 FASCIAL SLING ARTHROPLASTY

LOCATION: Outpatient, Hospital
PATIENT: Becky Wellington
PRIMARY CARE PHYSICIAN: Ronald Green, MD
SURGEON: Mohomad Almaz, MD
PREOPERATIVE DIAGNOSIS: Degenerative arthritis carpometacarpal joint, left thumb.
POSTOPERATIVE DIAGNOSIS: Same as Preoperative.
PROCEDURES PERFORMED: Fascial sling arthroplasty, left thumb.
ANESTHESIA: General.

PROCEDURE: The patient was brought to the operating room and a general anesthetic was induced. The left upper extremity was prepped with Betadine and draped in a sterile fashion. The limb was exsanguinated and tourniquet inflated to 250 mm Hg for 40 minutes. With 4× magnification loupes, we made a Chevron incision at the base of the thumb metacarpal. Dissection was carried down to the CMC joints, preserving subcutaneous nerves and vessels. We made a longitudinal arthrotomy incision and exposed the trapezium. We then morselized the trapezium and slowly removed the pieces with the rongeur. We carefully removed the entire trapezium, preserving the underlying FCR tendon. There was eburnated bone at the base of the first metacarpal. We then placed a drill hole through the base of the first metacarpal from its dorsal surface to its volar ulnar base. We opened this up to accept the tendon transfer. We next harvested the flexor carpi radialis tendon through two incisions, a short 1-cm incision over the tendon at the distal wrist flexor crease and an incision parallel to this 10 cm up the forearm at the myotendinous junction, where the FCR was transected at the floor of the thumb. Both volar forearm wounds were then closed with 5–0 nylon suture.

We next transferred the FCR tendon through the hole at the base of the first metacarpal, which effectively slung the first metacarpal up to the second metacarpal. We then pinned this to the second metacarpal with a 0.045-inch Kirchner wire bent and cut off outside the skin. We next sutured the tendon to

the hole in the first metacarpal with 4–0 Vicryl sutures and packed bone graft into the hole to secure this. We then placed a 4–0 Vicryl suture in the floor of the wound, placed two Bunnell needles over the limbs of this, and then threaded the tendon onto this in an accordion fashion. We tied this Vicryl, pulled the tendon down into the defect, where the trapezium was excised, and filled this nicely. We then proceeded with capsular closure, imbrication of the capsule, and closed this with 4–0 Vicryl sutures. The appearance was excellent. We irrigated the wound with sterile saline and closed the skin with interrupted 5–0 nylon sutures. Next, we applied Xeroform, and a thumb spica compression hand bandage was then applied with plaster splints immobilizing the thumb. The tourniquet was released, and good circulation returned to the hand.

The patient tolerated the procedure well and went to the recovery room in excellent condition. She will be dismissed as an outpatient today with plans for follow-up back in the office in approximately 2 weeks.

DISCHARGE MEDICATION: Lorcet, 30 tablets.
Pathology Report: No specimen was sent.

CPT Code(s): _____

_____

ICD-10-CM Code(s): _____

_____

Abstracting Questions
1. On what area of the body was the arthroplasty performed?

_____

2. Was the tendon transfer bundled into the arthroplasty?

_____

3. Are modifiers reported with these procedures? _____

_____

PRACTICE EXERCISE 20.9   EXCISION BONE TUMOR

LOCATION: Outpatient, Hospital
PATIENT: Tyron Banks
PRIMARY CARE PHYSICIAN: Leslie Alanda, MD
SURGEON: Mohomad Almaz, MD
PREOPERATIVE DIAGNOSIS: Bone tumor, distal lateral right femur.
POSTOPERATIVE DIAGNOSIS: Same as Preoperative.
PROCEDURES PERFORMED: Excision bone tumor, distal right femur.
ANESTHESIA: General.

PROCEDURE: The patient was brought to the operating room and a general anesthetic was induced. Right lower extremity was prepped with Betadine and draped in a sterile fashion. The limb was exsanguinated, and tourniquet was inflated to 300 mm Hg for 25 minutes. Ioban drape was applied. A standard 4-inch longitudinal anterolateral incision was made beginning at the lateral patellar region and extending proximally. Dissection was carried down through the lateral parapatellar region and lateral parapatellar arthrotomy was performed. We entered down to the lateral femur where the tumor was palpable. This appeared to represent a chondroma on the lateral femur. We elevated the soft tissue and periosteum off of this and then used osteotomes to sharply excise this and gradually take this down to its base. It appeared to be bleeding normal bone, and at that point we did put bone wax on the bone. We then closed the periosteum with a running 0 Vicryl suture, then closed the fascia and joint with a running 0 Vicryl suture, and then closed the skin with a subcuticular 2–0 Vicryl suture and a running 4–0 Monocryl suture. Steri-Strips were applied with gauze dressing, Kling, ABD, Kerlix, and a Coban. The tourniquet was released, and good circulation returned to the leg.

The patient tolerated the procedure well. He will be dismissed as an outpatient today with plans for follow-up in the office in approximately 2 weeks.

DISCHARGE MEDICATIONS: Tylenol #3, 30 tablets.
Pathology Report Later Indicated: Benign neoplasm.

CPT Code(s): _____

_____

ICD-10-CM Code(s): _____

_____

Abstracting Questions

1. From what body part was the bone tumor excised? _____

_____

2. Was a graft required to repair the defect? _____

_____

3. Was any fixation required? _____

_____

4. What report is required to correctly assign a diagnosis to the excision? _____

_____

PRACTICE EXERCISE 20.10   EXCISION OF MASS, BURSA

LOCATION: Outpatient, Hospital
PATIENT: Brittany Lionel
PRIMARY CARE PHYSICIAN: Ronald Green, MD
SURGEON: Mohomad Almaz, MD
PREOPERATIVE DIAGNOSIS: Mass, left prepatellar bursa.
POSTOPERATIVE DIAGNOSIS: Same as Preoperative.
PROCEDURES PERFORMED: Excision of mass, left prepatellar bursa.
ANESTHESIA: Local infiltration with 1% Xylocaine, supplemented with IV sedation.

PROCEDURE: The patient was placed in the supine position on the operating room table. She pointed out the mass on the anterior aspect of her left knee, which was a very small mass, perhaps 2 or 3 mm in diameter. This bothers her when she kneels on her left knee, and she wanted it removed. We therefore marked it with a marking pen since it was not a large mass but was still nevertheless fairly easily palpable.

We then prepped her left knee with Betadine and draped it in a sterile fashion. She was given IV sedation. We then infiltrated the area around the mass with 1% Xylocaine. Once adequate anesthesia had been achieved, we exsanguinated the left leg with Esmarch bandage and inflated a tourniquet to 225 mm Hg. The total tourniquet time was about 6 minutes.

We created an incision in a longitudinal fashion directly over this mass and carried it down through the subcutaneous tissue. We very quickly found this mass, which was perhaps half the size of a pea (0.5 cm). It was fairly firm, and we sent it to pathology. It appears to be part of the left prepatellar bursa. We then excised some of the adjacent bursal tissue. We found this was located directly over the left patella and the patella was very visible underneath this mass. We then probed the area, looking for any other masses. We then thoroughly irrigated the area and closed the subcutaneous tissue with 2–0 Vicryl and the skin with 3–0 nylon suture. Pressure was applied to this area, and the tourniquet was released after 6 minutes of tourniquet time. We then applied a 4 × 4 dressing and an Ace wrap over this. She was then awakened and taken from the operating room in good condition, breathing spontaneously. The final sponge and needle counts were correct. She tolerated this procedure very well.

Pathology Report Later Indicated: Benign mass of left prepatellar bursa.

CPT Code(s): _____

_____

ICD-10-CM Code(s): _____

_____

Abstracting Questions

1. What was the body location of the tumor? _____

_____

2. What was the size of the mass? _____

_____

Respiratory System Subsection (30000-32999)

Anatomic site arrangement, such as:
- Nose
- Larynx
  Further subdivided by procedure, such as:
- Incision
- Excision

Endoscopy

Endoscopy in all subheadings except Nose
  Each preceded by "Notes"

Endoscopy Rule One

Code full extent of endoscopic procedure performed
  Example: Procedure begins at mouth and ends at bronchial tube
- Bronchial tube = full extent

Endoscopy Rule Two

Code correct approach
  Example: For removal:
- Interior lung lesion via endoscope inserted through mouth
- Exterior lung lesion via endoscope inserted through skin into chest
  Incorrect approach = incorrect code = incorrect or no reimbursement

Endoscopy Rule Three

Diagnostic endoscopy always included in surgical endoscopy
  Examples:
- Diagnostic bronchial endoscopy begins
- Identified foreign body
- Removed foreign body (surgical endoscopy)
- Only surgical endoscopy reported

Multiple Procedures

Frequent in respiratory coding
- **Watch for bundled services**
  Sequence primary procedure first, no modifier
  Sequence secondary procedures next, with -51
  Bilateral procedures often performed, use -50
  Format for reporting chosen by payer
  Example: Nasal lavage
- 31000 × 2
- 31000 and 31000-50
- 31000-50
- 31000-RT and 31000-LT

Nose (30000-30999)

Used extensively by otorhinolaryngologists (ear, nose, and throat [ENT] specialists)

Also used by wide variety of physicians in other specialties
Approach to nose
- External approach, use Integumentary System
- Internal approach, use Respiratory System

Incision (30000-30020)

Bundled into Incision codes are drain or gauze insertion and removal
  Supplies reported separately

Excision (30100-30160)

Contains intranasal biopsy codes

Polyp excision, coded by complexity
- Excision includes any method of destruction, even laser
- Use -50 (bilateral) for both sides
Turbinate excision and resection
- Three turbinates: Superior, middle, inferior
- Excision of inferior turbinate, 30130
- Excision of superior or middle turbinate, 30999
- Submucous resection of inferior turbinate, 30140
- Submucous resection of superior or middle turbinate, 30999

Introduction (30200-30220)

Common procedures
  Example: Injections to shrink nasal tissue or displacement therapy (saline flushes) to remove mucus
- Displacement therapy performed through nose

Removal of Foreign Body (30300-30320)

Distinguished by the site of removal, whether at office or hospital (requires general anesthesia)

Repair (30400-30630)

Many plastic procedures
- Rhinoplasty (reshaping nose internal and/or external)
- Septoplasty (rearrangement or repair of nasal septum)

Destruction (30801-30802)

Use of ablation (removing by cutting)

Used for removal of excess nasal mucosa or to reduce turbinate inflammation
Based on intramural or superficial extent of destruction
- **Intramural:** Deeper mucosa
- **Superficial:** Outer layer of mucosa

Other Procedures (30901-30999)

Control of nasal hemorrhage
- Packing
- Ligation
- Cauterization
- The packing may be anterior or posterior

Accessory Sinuses (31000-31299)

Subheadings include

- Incision (31000-31090)
- Excision (31200-31230)
- Endoscopy (31231-31297)
- Other Procedures (31299)

Codes for lavage (washing) of sinuses
- Cannula (hollow tube) placed into sinus
- Sterile saline solution flushed through

Procedures may involve multiple codes when multiple locations are accessed

Example: 31020, Sinusotomy, maxillary, can be coded with 31050 sinusotomy, sphenoid, and 31070 sinusotomy, frontal

Use -50 (bilateral) for both sides

Maxillary sinusotomy may use an external and intranasal approach to creating passage between sinus and nose
- Used to clear blocked or infected sinus
- Intranasal sinusotomy, 31020
- External sinusotomy, radical (such as Caldwell-Luc)

Access through mouth

Incision above eyetooth

Sinus is cleaned

New opening created or existing opening enlarged

Repair of fractures occurring during procedure may be coded separately if not included in code description

Larynx (31300-31599)
Excision (31300-31420)

Laryngotomy: Open surgical procedure to expose larynx
- For removal procedure (e.g., tumor)
  May be confused with Trachea/Bronchi codes for tracheostomy used to establish airflow

Introduction (31500-31502)

Used to establish, maintain, and protect air flow

Endotracheal intubation, establishment of airway

Based on planned (ventilation support) or emergency procedure

Endoscopy (31505-31579)

Uses terms *indirect* and *direct*
- **Indirect:** Tongue depressor with mirror used to view larynx
- **Direct:** Endoscopy passed into larynx; physician directly views vocal cords

Repair (31580-31592)

Several plastic procedures and fracture repairs

Laryngoplasty procedures based on purpose

Fracture code is open reduction code

Trachea and Bronchi (31600-31899)
Incision (31600-31614)

Most codes: Tracheostomy divided by
- Planned (ventilation support), based on age
- Emergency
  Divided by type
- Transtracheal or cricothyroid (location of incision)

Endoscopy (31615-31661)

Bronchoscope may be inserted into nose or mouth

Rigid endoscopy performed under general anesthesia

Flexible endoscopy usually performed under local or moderate (conscious) sedation

Bronchial Thermoplasty (31660, 31661)

Treatment for severe asthma in which radiofrequency is utilized to produce heat in the airways that results in reduction of the airway smooth muscles

Introduction (31717-31730)

Catheterization

Instillation

Aspiration

Tracheal tube placement

Excision, Repair (31750-31830)

Repairs of trachea and bronchi

Lungs and Pleura (32035-32999)
Incision (32035-32225)

Thoracotomy

Surgical opening of chest to expose to view.

Used for
- Biopsy
- Cyst
- Foreign body removal
- Cardiac massage, etc.

Excision/Removal (32310-32540)

Biopsy codes in both Excision and Incision categories
- Excisional biopsy with percutaneous needle
- Incisional biopsy with chest open
  Also services of pleurectomy, pneumocentesis, and lung removal
- **Segmentectomy:** 1 segment
- **Lobectomy:** 1 lobe
- **Bilobectomy:** 2 lobes
- **Total Pneumonectomy:** 1 lung

Thoracentesis

Needle inserted into pleural space for aspiration (withdrawal) of fluid and/or air (32554, 32555)

Introduction and Removal (32550-32557)

- Insertion of indwelling tunneled pleural catheter (removal 32552)
- Tube thoracostomy
- Placement of interstitial device(s) for radiation therapy guidance
- Thoracentesis and percutaneous pleural drainage

Destruction (32560-32562)

- Chemical pleurodesis
- Fibrinolysis, initial day, subsequent day

Cardiovascular System Subsection

CV coding may require codes from
- **Radiology:** Diagnostic studies
- **Medicine:** Nonsurgical and percutaneous
- **Surgery:** Open and percutaneous
  Both Medicine and Surgery sections contain invasive procedures

Cardiology Coding Terminology

Invasive: Enters body
- Incision
  Example: Opening chest for removal (e.g., tumor on heart)
- Percutaneous
  - Placement of catheter into artery or vein through the skin by means of wire threaded through needle and catheter slid over wire
  Example: PTCA (percutaneous transluminal coronary angioplasty) procedure
  Percutaneous—wire threaded through needle placed through skin into vessel and catheter placed over wire
- Cut down—small nick made into vessel under direct vision and catheter inserted
  Example: Catheter inserted into femoral or brachial artery
  Common catheters are:
- Broviac
- Hickman
- HydroCath
- Arrow multi-lumen
- Groshong
- Dual-lumen
- Triple-lumen
  Noninvasive: Procedures that do not break skin
  Example: Electrocardiogram
  Electrophysiology (EP): Study of electrical system of heart
  Example: Study of irregular heartbeat (arrhythmia)
- EP studies are in Medicine section, 93600-93662
- Electrophysiologic Operative Procedures are in Surgery section, 33250-33266

Nuclear Cardiology: Diagnostic and treatment specialty; uses radioactive substances to diagnose cardiac conditions
Example: Myocardial perfusion and cardiac blood pooling imaging studies

Cardiovascular in Surgery Section (33016-37799)

Codes for Procedures

Heart/Pericardium (33016-33999)
- Pacemakers, valve disorders
Arteries/Veins (34001-37799)

Heart/Pericardium (33016-33999)

Both percutaneous and open surgical
- Cardiologists often use percutaneous intervention; cardiovascular or thoracic surgeons often use open surgical procedures
  Extensive notes throughout
  Frequent changes with medical advances
  Examples of categories of Heart/Pericardium subheading
- Pericardium
- Cardiac Tumor
- Pacemaker or Implantable Defibrillator
  Examples of services
- Pericardiocentesis: Percutaneous withdrawal of fluid from pericardial space (pericarditis) (33016)
- Cardiac Tumor: Open surgical procedure for removal of tumor on heart (33130)

Pacemaker or Implantable Defibrillator (33202-33273)

Devices that assist heart in electrical function
- Differentiate between temporary and permanent devices
- Differentiate between one-chamber and dual-chamber devices
  Divided by where pacer placed, approach, and type of service
  Patient record indicates revision or replacement
- Pacemaker pulse generator is also called a battery
- Pacemaker leads are also called electrodes
  Usual follow-up 90 days (global period)

Placed
Atrium (single chamber)
- Pulse generator and one or more electrodes in atrium (single-chamber pacemaker)
Ventricle (single chamber)
- Pulse generator and one or more electrodes in ventricle (single-chamber pacemaker)
Both (dual chamber)
- Pulse generator and one electrode in right ventricle and one electrode in right atrium

- Biventricular, right ventricle, right atrium, and coronary sinus
- Pulse generator and one electrode in right ventricle, one electrode(s) may be placed in right atrium, and one electrode in the coronary sinus over the left ventricle

Approach
Epicardial: Open procedure to place electrodes on heart
Transvenous: Through vein to place in heart (endoscopic)

Type of Service
Initial placement or replacement of all or part of device
   Number of leads placed is important in code selection

Electrophysiologic Operative Procedures (33250-33266)
Surgeon repairs defect causing abnormal rhythm

Chest opened to full view
- Cardiopulmonary (CP) bypass usually used
Endoscopy procedure
- Without cardiopulmonary bypass
Codes based on reason for procedure and if CP bypass used

Subcutaneous Cardiac Rhythm Monitor (33285-33286)
Also known as cardiac event recorder or loop recorder
Placed using a small parasternal incision
Divided based on whether device is being inserted or removed

Cardiac Valves (33361-33478)
Divided by valve
- Aortic, mitral, tricuspid, pulmonary
   Subdivided by whether replacement, repair, resection, and use of bypass machine
   33361-33369 report transcatheter aortic valve replacement and implant

Coronary Artery Bypass Graft (CABG)
CABG performed for bypassing coronary arteries severely obstructed as in atherosclerosis or arteriosclerosis

Determine what was used in repair
- Vein (33510-33516)
- Artery (33533-33536)
- Both artery and vein (33517-33523 and 33533-33536)
Based on number of bypass grafts performed and if combined venous and arterial grafts are used
Example: Three venous grafts

Venous Grafting Only for Coronary Artery Bypass (33510-33516)
Based on number of grafts being replaced

Combined Arterial-Venous Grafting (33517-33530)
Divided based on number of grafts and whether initial procedure or reoperation

Procuring saphenous vein included, unless performed endoscopically
These codes are never used alone
- Arterial-Venous codes (33517-33523) report only **venous** graft portion of procedure
- Always used with Arterial Grafting codes (33533-33536)
Example: 3 vein grafts and 2 arterial grafts = 33519 and 33534
Open procurement of saphenous vein is included in procedure (not coded separately)
Code harvesting of saphenous vein graft separately when endoscopic video-assisted procurement is performed (33508)
Code harvesting separately for upper extremity or femoral vein

Arterial Grafting for Coronary Artery Bypass (33533-33548)
Divided based on number of grafts

Obtaining artery for grafting included in codes, except
- Procuring upper-extremity artery (e.g., radial artery), coded separately (35600)
   Several codes (33542-33548) for myocardial resection, repair of ventricular septal defect (VSD), and ventricular restoration

Endovascular Repair of Descending Thoracic Aorta (33880-33891)
Placement of an endovascular aortic prosthesis for repair of descending thoracic aorta
- Less invasive than traditional approach of chest or abdominal incision
   Synthetic aortic prosthesis placed via catheter
- Report fluoroscopic guidance separately 75956-75959
- Fluoroscopic guidance codes includes diagnostic imaging prior to placement and intraprocedurally
- Stent-graft (endoprosthesis) is deployed to reinforce weakened area

Extracorporeal Membrane Oxygenation and Extracorporeal Life Support Services (33946-33989)
Cardiac and/or respiratory support to the heart and/or lungs
- Provide cardiac and respiratory support for patients whose heart and lungs are diseased or damaged beyond function

Arteries and Veins Subheading (34001-37799)
Only for noncoronary vessels
- Divided based on whether artery or vein involved
   Example: Different codes for embolectomy, depending on artery or vein
- Catheters placed into vessels for monitoring, removal, repair
- Nonselective or selective catheter placement

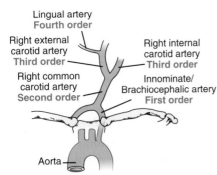

Lingual artery
Fourth order

Right external
carotid artery
Third order

Right internal
carotid artery
Third order

Right common
carotid artery
Second order

Innominate/
Brachiocephalic artery
First order

Aorta

• **Figure 20.6** Innominate/Brachiocephalic vascular family with first-, second-, third-, and fourth-order vessels.

- Nonselective: Direct placement without further manipulation
- Selective: Place and then manipulate into further order(s)
  Catheter Placement Example
- Nonselective: 36000 Introduction of needle into vein
- Selective: 36012 Placement of catheter into second-order venous system

Vascular Families Are Like a Tree

First-order (main) branch (tree trunk)
Second-order branch (tree limb)
Third-order branch (tree branch)
Innominate/Brachiocephalic vascular family (Fig. 20.6)
- Report farthest extent of catheter placement in a vascular family; labor intensity is increased with the extent of catheter placement

Embolectomy and Thrombectomy (34001-34490)

Embolus: Dislodged thrombus
Thrombus: Mass of material in vessel located in place of formation
- May be removed by dissection or balloon
Balloon: Threaded into vessel, inflated under mass, pulled out with mass
- Codes are divided by site of incision and whether artery or vein

Venous Reconstruction (34501-34530)

Types of Repairs
- Valve of the femoral vein
- Vena cava
- Saphenopopliteal vein anastomosis

Aneurysm

Aneurysm: Weakened arterial wall causing a bulge or ballooning
  Repair by removal, bypass, or coil placement
  Endovascular repair (34701-34848) from inside vessel
  Direct (35001-35152) from outside vessel

Endovascular Repair of Abdominal Aortic Aneurysm (34701-34706)

Reported separately; introduction of guideline and catheters

Other procedures performed at same time coded separately

Endovascular Repair of Iliac Aneurysm (34707-34708)

Extensive notes preceding codes—"must" reading
Includes introduction, positioning, and deployment of graft, stent and balloon angioplasty
Reported separately: Introduction of guidewire and catheters

Repair Arteriovenous Fistula (35180-35190)

Abnormal passage from artery or vein

Divided based on fistula type
- Congenital
- Acquired/traumatic
- By site
Repair methods
- Autogenous graft—fistula created artery to vein
- Non-auto fistula—biocompatible tube connecting artery to vein

Angioplasty

Divided as open or percutaneous and by vessel
- **Transluminal:** By way of vessel
- **Transluminal Angioplasty:** Catheter passed into vessel and a balloon is inflated to crush/flatten fatty deposits in vessel
  - Placement of eluting or non-eluting stents coded in addition to catheter placement
- Reported with codes 36902, 36905, 36907, and 37246-37249

Noncoronary Bypass Grafts (35500-35671)

Divided by
- Vein
- In-Situ Vein (veins repaired in their original place)
- Other Than Vein
Code by type of graft and vessels being used to bypass
Example: 35506 Bypass graft, with vein; carotid-subclavian
- Graft attached to carotid and to subclavian, bypassing defect of subclavian
Procurement of saphenous vein graft is included and not reported separately
Harvesting of upper-extremity vein (35500) or femoropopliteal vein (35572) is reported separately

Vascular Injection Procedures (36000-36598)

Divided into
- Intravenous
- Intra-arterial—Intra-aortic
- Venous
- Central venous access procedures
  Used for many procedures, including
- Local anesthesia
- Introduction of needle

- Injection of contrast material
- Preinjection and postinjection care related to injection procedure
  Example: Injection of opaque substance for venography (radiography of vein)

Central Venous Access (CVA) Procedures

Long-term use for medication/chemotherapy administration and short-term use for monitoring

Approach
- Central: jugular, subclavian, or femoral vein
- Peripheral: basilic or cephalic vein

Categories
1. Insertion
2. Repair
3. Replacement, partial or complete
4. Removal
5. Other central venous access procedure
6. Guidance for vascular access

Insertion (36555-36571)

Insertion of newly established venous access
- Tunneled under skin (e.g., Hickman, Broviac, Groshong)
- Nontunneled (e.g., Hohn catheter, triple lumen, PICC)
- Central (e.g., subclavian, internal jugular, femoral, inferior vena cava)
- Peripheral (basilic or cephalic vein)
  Codes divided by tunneled/nontunneled, with/without port, central/peripheral, and age

Repair (36575-36576)

Repair of malfunction without replacement with or without subcutaneous port or pump

Repair of central venous access device

No differentiation between age of patient or central/peripheral insertion

Replacement (Partial or Complete) (36578-36585)

Partial (36578) is replacement of catheter only

Complete (36580-36585) is replacement through same venous access site

Differentiated by tunneled/nontunneled, central/peripheral, and with or without subcutaneous port or pump

Removal (36589, 36590)

To be used for tunneled catheter

Removal of nontunneled catheter is not reported separately

Other Central Venous Access Procedures (36591-36598)

Collection of blood specimen

Declotting of catheter or access device by thrombolytic agent

Mechanical removal of obstructive material from around catheter or within lumen

Guidance for Vascular Access

77001, Fluoroscopic guidance for central venous access device placement, replacement, or removal
- Reported in addition to primary procedure

76937, Ultrasound guidance for vascular access
- Reported in addition to primary procedure

Transcatheter Procedures (37184-37218)

Arterial Mechanical Thrombectomy (37184-37186)
- Removal of thrombus by means of mechanical device
  From artery or arterial bypass graft

Venous Mechanical Thrombectomy (37187-37188)
- Removal of a thrombus by means of a mechanical device
  From vein

Arterial and venous mechanical thrombectomy may be performed as primary procedure or add-on
- Includes
  Introduction of device into thrombus
  Thrombus removal
  Injection of thrombolytic drug(s), if used
  Fluoroscopic and contrast guidance
  Follow-up angiography
- Report separately
  Diagnostic angiography
  Catheter placement(s)
  Diagnostic studies
  Pharmacologic thrombolytic infusion before or after (37211-37214, 75898)
  Other interventions

Other Procedures (37195-37218)

- Used to report a variety of transcatheter procedures
  Example: Transcatheter biopsy, therapy, infusion for thrombolysis or antispasmotic treatment of a vessel, retrieval of foreign object, occlusion or embolization, and intravascular stents

Endovascular Revascularization (Open or Percutaneous, Transcatheter) (37220-37235)

Lower extremity codes

Cardiovascular in Medicine Section (92920-93799)

Services can be
- Invasive or noninvasive
- Diagnostic or therapeutic
  Subheadings
- Therapeutic Services and Procedures
- Cardiovascular Monitoring Services
- Implantable, Insertable, and Wearable Cardiac Device Evaluations
- Cardiography
- Echocardiography
- Cardiac Catheterization

- Intracardiac Electrophysiologic Procedures/Studies
- Peripheral Arterial Disease Rehabilitation
- Noninvasive Physiologic Studies and Procedures
- Other Procedures

Therapeutic Services and Procedures (92920-92998)

Types of services
- Cardioversion
- Infusions
- Thrombolysis
- Catheter placement
  Codes divided by
- Method (e.g., balloon, blade)
- Location (e.g., aortic or mitral valve)
- Number (e.g., single or multiple vessels)

Intracoronary Brachytherapy (92974)

Uses radioactive substances to destroy re-stenosis of coronary vessel

Patients have had stent placed in coronary vessel

Stent "re-stenosis" (re-formation of plaque)

Add-on code

Cardiologist: Places guidewire and catheter

Radiation oncologist: Places radioactive elements

Cardiography (93000-93050)

Types of services
- Stress tests
- Holter monitor
- Electrocardiogram
  Separate codes for components of study, such as
- 93000 global
- 93005 tracing only
- 93010 interpretation and report only
  Codes report professional and/or technical components, so do not append -26 or -TC

Cardiovascular Monitoring Services (93224-93278)

Diagnostic procedures in-person or by means of remote technology to assess cardiovascular rhythm via ECG
- Holter monitors, 93224-93227
- Mobile telemetry, 93228, 93229
- Long-term continuous recorders, 93241-93248
- Event monitors, 93268-93272
  - Patient depresses a button on portable monitor when feeling a sensation (event), such as a flutter or dizziness
    Codes divided based on type of monitoring and time

Implantable, Insertable, and Wearable Cardiac Device Evaluations (93264, 93279-93298)

Diagnostic medical procedures for cardiac rhythm devices
- Devices are internal or external
- In-person or remote assessments
  Codes divided by

- Type of Service
  Implantation
  Interrogation
  Programming
- Devices such as:
  Implantable defibrillator
  Implantable loop recorder
- Number of leads or chambers
- Monitoring period must exceed 10 days
  Implantation procedures (93264, 93279-93291)
- Reported once per procedure

Interrogation device evaluation of implantable defibrillator (ICD) or pacemaker (93293-93296)
- ICDs may act as defibrillator or pacemaker
- Report interrogation or monitoring once per 90-day period

Interrogation device evaluation implantable cardiovascular monitor system (93297-93298)
- Report interrogation or monitoring once per 30-day period

Echocardiography (93303-93355)

Noninvasive Diagnostic Procedure

Ultrasound detects presence of cardiac or vascular disease

Codes divided by
- Approach
- Extent of study (e.g., limited, complete)
- Service provided (e.g., probe only, interpretation and report)

Cardiac Catheterization (93451-93572)

Used to identify valve disorders, abnormal blood flow

Many bundled services in catheterization codes
Examples:
- Introduction
- Positioning/Repositioning of catheter
- Pressure readings inside heart or vessels
- Blood samples
- Rest/Exercise studies
- Final evaluation and report
- Many codes are -51 exempt
- Many codes include moderate (conscious) sedation

Three Components of Coding Cardiac Catheterization

1. Placement of catheter
2. Injection
3. Imaging supervision, interpretation, and report
   Most codes have all three components in the code
   - Example: 93456 includes catheterization, injection, imaging
   Some codes require multiple codes
   - Example: 93531 reports catheterization for congenital cardiac anomalies, injection code (93563/93564) must be added

Intracardiac Electrophysiologic Procedures/Studies (93600-93662)

Services to diagnose and treat conditions of electrical system of heart
- Arrhythmic induction
- Mapping
- Ablation

EP System of Heart

Electrical conduction system
  Electrical recording codes divided based on location of recording device
  Example: Bundle of His or right ventricle
  Pacing: Temporary pacing to stabilize beating of heart
  Example: Intraventricular or intra-arterial pacing

Peripheral Arterial Disease (PAD) Rehabilitation (93668)

Rehabilitation sessions: 45-60 minutes
Use of motorized treadmill/track/bicycle to build patient's CV function
Supervised by exercise physiologist or nurse
If E/M is provided by physician, service is reported separately

Noninvasive Physiologic Studies and Procedures (93701-93790)

Category contains codes for services such as
- **Plethysmography:** Recordings of changes in size of body part when blood passes through it
- **Electronic Analysis:** Checks electronic function of devices, such as pacemakers
- **Ambulatory Blood Pressure Monitoring:** Outpatient basis over 24-hour period
- **Thermograms:** Visual recordings of body temperature

Other Procedures (93797-93799)

Codes 93797 and 93798 report professional outpatient cardiac rehabilitation services, per session
- With or without ECG monitoring

Cardiovascular in Radiology Section (75557-75774)

Radiology section, Heart (75557-75574) and Aorta/Arteries (75600-75774) subsections

Prior to 1992, Radiology section contained codes for entire CV procedures
Major revision to CV radiology codes 1992
Divided complete procedures into two components: technical and professional
Example: Angiography
- Technical component angiography—remains in Radiology section

- Professional component injection—moved to Surgery section
Complete angiography requires radiology code and surgery code
Reflects common practice of cardiologist's performing injection and radiologist's performing angiography

Contrast Material

Often radiologic procedures use contrast material to improve image

Many codes have contrast material bundled into service
- "with contrast" or "with or without contrast"
Only injected contrast qualifies as "with contrast"
Contrast not included in description but used in procedure:
  Code contrast material and injection separately
- Specify site where service is received to differentiate between global (total), technical, and professional components of the procedure
Non-hospital-based (not employed by hospital) physician usually performs procedure in hospital outpatient department: Use -26 to report only professional component

---

EXAMPLE

Component Coding

Two physicians (cardiologist and radiologist from same facility) perform angiography of third-order brachiocephalic artery with contrast
- Cardiologist places catheter (36217), Surgery section
- Radiologist performs angiography (75710), Radiology section
- Supply of contrast material (99070), Medicine section

Hemic and Lymphatic System Subsection (38100-38999)

Divisions

- Spleen
- General
- Lymph Nodes and Lymphatic Channels

Spleen Subheading (38100-38200)

Spleen easily ruptured, causing massive and potentially lethal hemorrhage

Excision:
- Splenectomy: Total or partial/open or laparoscopic
Often done as part of more major procedure
- Bundled into major procedure
- Repair
- Laparoscopy

General (38204-38243)

Bone Marrow

Codes divided based on

- Preservation
- Preparation
- Purification
- Aspiration
- Biopsy
- Harvesting
- Transplantation

Hematopoietic Progenitor Cell (HPC)

Obtained from bone marrow, peripheral blood apheresis, umbilical cord blood

Types of Cells

Allogenic: Same species (38240)
Autologous: Patient's own (38241)

Lymph Nodes and Lymphatic Channels Subheading (38300-38999)

Two types of lymphadenectomies:

1. **Limited:** Pelvic and para-aortic lymph nodes only for neoplasm staging
2. **Radical:** Aortic and/or splenic lymph nodes and surrounding tissue for neoplasm staging

    Often bundled into more major procedure (e.g., prostatectomy)

    Do not unbundle and report lymphadenectomy separately

Mediastinum and Diaphragm Subsection (39000-39499)

Incision codes for foreign body removal, biopsy, or drainage
    Excision codes for removal of cyst or tumor

Diaphragm (39501-39599)

Only two categories: Repair and Other Procedures
    Includes hernia and laceration repairs

PRACTICE EXERCISE 20.11 ANGIOGRAM

Assign the codes for the catheterizations only.

RADIOLOGY REPORT
LOCATION: Inpatient, Hospital
PATIENT: Joy Gigel
ORDERING PHYSICIAN: John Hodgson, MD
ATTENDING/ADMIT PHYSICIAN: Frank Gaul, MD
RADIOLOGIST: Morton Monson, MD
PERSONAL PHYSICIAN: Frank Gaul, MD
EXAMINATION: Carotid/cerebral angiogram.
CLINICAL SYMPTOMS: Intracranial bleed.

CAROTID/CEREBRAL ANGIOGRAM: The patient is a 54-year-old female who was found to have an intracranial bleed. Carotid/cerebral angiogram was requested by Dr. Hodgson, neurosurgery.

APPROACH: Right common femoral artery.

VESSELS INJECTED

1. Proximal thoracic aorta.
2. Right common carotid artery.
3. Right internal carotid artery.
4. Left common carotid artery.
5. Left vertebral artery.

FOLLOW-UP: Dr. Hodgson.

Prior to the start of the study, the procedure was explained to the patient's husband by Dr. Hodgson, including risks, complications, and alternatives. The patient's husband understood and consented to the exam. This study was performed on an emergency basis.

The patient was prepped and draped in the usual sterile fashion. Utilizing single wall technique following administration of local anesthesia (1% lidocaine), a #5 French flush catheter was introduced into the right common femoral artery through a vascular sheath, and the tip was advanced into the proximal thoracic aorta. Contrast was injected, and sequential digital subtraction angiography films were obtained.

The flush catheter was then exchanged for a #4 French Osborne catheter for select evaluation of both common carotid arteries, as well as the right internal carotid artery and the left vertebral artery. Again, contrast was injected, and multiple views of the carotid bifurcations and cerebral vessels were obtained.

On arch injection, there is no significant stenosis at the origin of the great vessels. There is an antegrade flow in both vertebral arteries. Please note that the right vertebral artery is somewhat smaller when compared to the left.

On evaluation of the carotid bifurcations, there is no evidence of narrowing or irregularity.

On evaluation of cerebral vessels, there is no evidence of aneurysm, extravasation, or arteriovenous malformation. Please note that there is marked medial and superior displacement of the vessels in the right middle cerebral artery distribution. There is also midline shift of all the cerebral structures of the left as well as midline shift to the left of the anterior cerebral arteries. These findings are consistent with the patient's intraparenchymal bleed predominantly in the right temporal lobe seen on CT study from an outside institution.

The patient tolerated the procedure well. The puncture site was closed with sutures utilizing the Perclose device. There was no evidence of bleeding, hematoma, or change in peripheral pulses at the termination of the study.

IMPRESSION: Carotid/cerebral angiogram with multiple findings as described above.

Dr. Hodgson was present during this examination.

CPT Code(s): _____

ICD-10-CM Code(s): _____

_____

Continued

PRACTICE EXERCISE 20.11 ANGIOGRAM—cont'd

Abstracting Questions

1. What CPT Appendix could you reference to understand how to code the procedure performed in the report? _____
   _____

2. What vessels were evaluated? _____
   _____

3. Are right and left HCPCS modifiers appended to the catheter insertion codes? _____
   _____

4. Are both the right common carotid and right internal carotid reported? _____
   _____

5. Is the left common carotid reported? _____

6. Is the left vertebral artery reported? _____
   _____

7. Why does the proximal thoracic aorta not get reported?
   _____

PRACTICE EXERCISE 20.12 DIALYSIS CATHETER REPLACEMENT

LOCATION: Outpatient, Hospital
PATIENT: Sally Perez
ATTENDING PHYSICIAN: George Orbitz, MD
SURGEON: George Orbitz, MD
PREOPERATIVE DIAGNOSIS: ESRD.
POSTOPERATIVE DIAGNOSIS: ESRD.
PROCEDURE PERFORMED: Dialysis catheter replacement.
ANESTHESIA: Local.

   DESCRIPTION OF PROCEDURE: After obtaining consent, the 46-year-old patient was put in the Trendelenburg position. The area of the right IJ vein where the catheter was placed was prepped in the usual fashion. A guidewire was advanced without difficulty. The old dialysis catheter was taken out. Tip was sent for culture. A new 11.5 French 13.5-cm temporary dialysis catheter was advanced through the right IJ vein over the guidewire using the Seldinger technique without difficulty. Both ports had good blood return. Both ports were flushed with saline and heparin. The catheter was secured to the skin. The patient tolerated the procedure well without immediate complications.

CPT Code(s): _____
_____

ICD-10-CM Code(s): _____
_____

Abstracting Questions

1. Was the catheter placement venous or arterial? _____
   _____

2. Was this an open or percutaneous insertion? _____
   _____

3. Was the catheter a central or peripheral insertion? _____
   _____

4. Was this reported as an insertion or a replacement? _____
   _____

5. What was the principal reason for the encounter? _____
   _____

PRACTICE EXERCISE 20.13 CATHETER PLACEMENT

Report the services, diagnosis(es), and any sedation provided to this patient by the interventional radiologist.
LOCATION: Outpatient, Hospital
PATIENT: John Cane
PRIMARY CARE PHYSICIAN: Rapheal White, MD
INTERVENTIONAL RADIOLOGIST: Edward Riddle, MD
EXAMINATION: Right IVJ Port-a-Cath placement.
CLINICAL SYMPTOMS: Primary lung cancer. Access required for chemotherapy.

   PORT-A-CATH PLACEMENT: Informed consent was obtained from this 26-year-old patient. The right neck and infraclavicular region were prepped and draped in the usual sterile fashion. Skin and subcutaneous tissues were infiltrated with 1% lidocaine with epinephrine. Under ultrasound guidance, access was obtained into the right jugular vein, and over a 0.035 J-tip guidewire the needle was exchanged for a 10 French peel-away sheath. A subcutaneous pocket was created in the right infraclavicular region using blunt dissection. A #9.6 French Bard single-lumen Port-a-Cath was placed into the pocket and a subcutaneous tunnel created from the pocket to the right IJV puncture site. The #9.6 French catheter was advanced through the tunnel and placed through the peel-away sheath. The sheath was removed. Under fluoroscopic

observation the distal tip of the catheter was positioned in the right atrium. The pocket was closed using subcutaneous interrupted sutures with 4–0 Vicryl and a subcuticular stitch with 4–0 Vicryl. The right neck incision site was closed using vertical mattress suture technique with 3–0 Ethilon.

   Patient received conscious sedation for 45 minutes. The patient's pulse oximeter and vital signs were monitored throughout the exam. There were no complications. The patient tolerated the procedure well and left the radiology department in stable condition.

   A single digital spot radiograph obtained demonstrates the single-lumen port placed via a right IJV approach with the distal tip of the catheter in the right atrium.

CPT Code(s): _____
_____

ICD-10-CM Code(s): _____
_____

Abstracting Questions

1. Was the catheter inserted by the radiologist? _____
   _____

PRACTICE EXERCISE 20.13   CATHETER PLACEMENT—cont'd

2. Was the catheter inserted into the venous or arterial system? _____

3. Was the catheter inserted centrally or peripherally? _____

4. Was the catheter tunneled? _____

5. Was a subcutaneous port/pump inserted? _____

6. Does the age of the patient affect code assignment? _____

7. What were the two types of guidance used? _____

8. The catheter inserted was used for access for what purpose? _____

PRACTICE EXERCISE 20.14   AORTOGRAM

LOCATION: Outpatient, Hospital
PATIENT: Theodore Lambert
PRIMARY CARE PHYSICIAN: Ronald Green, MD
INTERVENTIONAL RADIOLOGIST: Edward Riddle, MD
EXAMINATION: Arch aortogram with bilateral carotid and cerebral arteriograms.
CLINICAL SYMPTOMS: Previous stroke; carotid artery stenosis.

AORTOGRAPHIC TECHNIQUE: Informed consent was obtained. The right groin was prepped and draped in the usual sterile fashion. Skin and subcutaneous tissues were infiltrated with 1% lidocaine. Access was obtained of the right common femoral artery, and over a 0.035 Bentson guidewire the needle was exchanged for a 5 French sheath. Over the guidewire a #5 French Pigtail catheter was threaded to the aortic arch and angiography was performed in the LAO projection during mechanical injection of contrast through the catheter. The catheter was exchanged for a #5 French H1H catheter. The right vertebral artery was selectively catheterized using the H1H and a 0.035 angled Glidewire. Posterior fossa arteriogram was performed during hand injection of contrast through the catheter. This was performed in AP and lateral projections.

The right common carotid artery was selectively catheterized using the Glidewire and H1H catheter. Right carotid arteriogram was performed in three projections during mechanical injection of contrast through the catheter. AP and lateral cerebral arteriography on the right was performed during mechanical injection of contrast through the catheter.

The left common carotid artery was selectively catheterized using the Glidewire and H1H. Left carotid arteriogram was performed during hand injection of contrast through the catheter. Cerebral arteriogram was performed on the left during hand injection of contrast through the catheter.

Catheter and sheath were removed. Hemostasis was obtained using a 6 French AngioSeal device. The patient received conscious sedation. His pulse oximeter and vital signs were monitored throughout the exam. There were no complications. He tolerated the procedure well and left the radiology department in stable condition.

ARCH AORTOGRAM: The arch is unremarkable. Origins of the great vessels are normal in caliber with no stenosis seen. Subclavian arteries are patent. Bilateral vertebral arteries are patent. Left common carotid artery is small in caliber and indicates that the left internal carotid artery is completely occluded.

POSTERIOR FOSSA ARTERIOGRAM: Visualized distal right vertebral artery is patent. Basilar artery is unremarkable, as are the bilateral posterior cerebral arteries. No aneurysm is seen. No anterior cerebral arterial circulation is noted on this posterior fossa injection.

RIGHT CAROTID ARTERIOGRAM: Calcified atheromatous disease of the carotid bulb and proximal internal carotid artery is noted. There is approximately 30-40% diameter narrowing of the carotid bulb, with no significant stenosis seen involving the proximal internal carotid artery. There is a 90-95% diameter narrowing of the proximal external carotid artery.

LEFT CAROTID ARTERIOGRAM: The common carotid artery is small in caliber, with the distal common carotid artery demonstrating a high-grade stenosis with a "string sign." The internal carotid artery is completely occluded.

RIGHT CEREBRAL ARTERIOGRAM: The distal internal carotid artery and the intracranial internal carotid artery are widely patent. The right anterior and middle cerebral artery and their distribution are unremarkable, with no stenosis seen. No hypervascular or hypovascular mass is present. No aneurysm is seen. The left anterior and middle cerebral arterial supply is provided via a patent anterior communicating artery. No abnormalities are seen on the left anterior or middle cerebral arterial supply.

LEFT CEREBRAL ARTERIOGRAM: As discussed above, the left cerebral anterior circulation is provided from the right cerebral anterior circulation. There is no intracranial supply on the left seen via external carotid branches. No reconstitution of the left internal carotid artery is seen.

IMPRESSION
1. Negative arch aortogram with a small-caliber left common carotid artery.
2. Negative posterior fossa arteriogram.
3. 30-40% diameter narrowing of the carotid bulb on the right, with no significant stenosis of the right internal carotid artery seen.
4. Complete occlusion of the left internal carotid artery.
5. The left anterior and middle cerebral arteries receive their supply via patent anterior communicating artery from the right anterior arterial circulation.

CPT Code(s): _____

ICD-10-CM Code(s): _____

Abstracting Questions

1. What does LAO stand for? _____

2. In the Left Carotid Arteriogram section of the report, the radiologist refers to a "string sign." What is a string sign? _____

PRACTICE EXERCISE 20.15 EXTREMITY ANGIOGRAM

LOCATION: Outpatient, Hospital
PATIENT: George Ball
PRIMARY CARE PHYSICIAN: Ronald Green, MD
SURGEON: Gary Sanchez, MD
INTERVENTIONAL RADIOLOGIST: Edward Riddle, MD
EXAMINATION: Right lower extremity angiogram and thrombolysis.
CLINICAL SYMPTOMS: Cold right foot.

RIGHT LOWER EXTREMITY ANGIOGRAM AND THROMBOLYSIS: This 62-year-old male presented a month ago with ischemic changes below the knee of the right lower extremity. Some years earlier, the patient had a femoral-popliteal Gore-Tex graft placed. At the time of the angiogram a month ago, there was clot of virtually all the arteries commencing in the distal external iliac artery. We saw very few collateralizations extending into the right lower extremity. Subsequent lytic procedure cleared the Gore-Tex graft and the popliteal artery, but there was then very hard material in the distal popliteal artery that was resistant to the tPA lysis. Subsequently, the patient was taken to the operating room by Dr. Sanchez, where he placed a vein graft from the proximal third of the Gore-Tex graft and inserted it into the posterior tibial artery. The patient then did very well. He now presents acutely with ischemic changes of the right foot.

The patient is on heparin and had been taking Plavix and aspirin as an outpatient. The present procedure was performed via the left femoral artery with single-wall micropuncture entry and placement of a #5 French sheath. A #5 French Omni Flush catheter was then positioned into the right external iliac artery for examination of the right lower extremity.

There is a patency of the right external iliac artery to the junction with the common femoral artery. The common femoral artery is virtually occluded. One or two proximal branches are arising from the artery. The superficial femoral artery and the Gore-Tex graft are occluded. There was also no visualization of the saphenous vein graft. Some collaterals from the deep femoral artery can be visualized at the level of the knee. Although these are scant, they are certainly more than we appreciated when the patient initially arrived here last month.

Utilizing a long Glidewire, I obtained access into the Gore-Tex graft. While traversing the Gore-Text graft, I kept the curve of the wire pointed anteromedially, hoping that we might enter the vein graft. I was able to extend the Glidewire all the way to the knee. Subsequently, a Mewissen catheter with 15 cm of holes was placed proximally with the most proximal hole in the beginning of the clot in the common femoral artery. Coaxially, a Katzen wire with 12 cm of holes was positioned into the graft. tPA was then commenced through both catheters. The patient was medicated with intravenous Versed and fentanyl. He will return to the angiographic suite in the morning.

IMPRESSION: Complete occlusion of the patient's superficial femoral artery, Gore-Tex femoral-popliteal graft, and saphenous graft that extends from the Gore-Tex graft to the posterior tibial artery. Coaxial system has been appropriately placed and tPA lysis started.

CPT Code(s): _____

ICD-10-CM Code(s): _____

_____

Abstracting Question

1. The furthest extent of this selective catheterization was to the _____ artery and to this order? _____

_____

_____

Digestive System Subsection (40490-49999)

Divided by anatomic site from mouth to anus + organs that aid digestive process

Example: Liver and gallbladder
Many bundled procedures

Endoscopy

Diagnostic procedure always bundled into surgical endoscopic
 Code to furthest extent of procedure

Endoscopy Terminology

Notes define specific terminology
 Code descriptions are specific regarding
- Technique and depth of scope
- Esophagoscopy: Esophagus only
- Esophagogastroscopy: Esophagus and past diaphragm
- Esophagogastroduodenoscopy: Esophagus and beyond pyloric channel

- Proctosigmoidoscopy: Rectum and sigmoid colon (6-25 cm)
- Sigmoidoscopy: Entire rectum, sigmoid colon, and may include part of descending colon (26-60 cm)
- Colonoscopy: Entire colon, rectum to cecum, and may include terminal ileum (greater than 60 cm)

Laparoscopy and Endoscopy

Some subheadings have both laparoscopy (outside) and endoscopy (inside) procedures
 Example: Subheading Esophagus
- Endoscopy views inside
- Laparoscopy—scope inserted through umbilicus; views from outside

Hemorrhoidectomy and Fistulectomy Codes (46200-46320)

Divided by
- Location
  - Internal
  - External

- Complexity
  - Simple: No repair procedure involved
  - Complex: Includes repair procedure and fissurectomy
- Anatomy
  - Subcutaneous: No muscle involvement
  - Submuscular: Sphincter muscle
- Complex fistulectomy involves excision/incision of multiple fistulas

Hernia Codes (49491-49659)

Divided by
- Type of hernia
  Example: Inguinal, femoral
- Initial or subsequent repair
- Age of patient determines code choice
- Clinical presentation
  - **Strangulated:** Blood supply cut off
  - **Incarcerated:** Cannot be returned to cavity (not reducible)
    Additional code is used for implantation of mesh or prosthesis for incisional or ventral hernias only
- Open or laparoscopic surgical approaches

PRACTICE EXERCISE 20.16 OROGASTRIC TUBE PLACEMENT

OPERATIVE REPORT
The intraoperative KUB was provided by the radiologist, and you are only reporting the services of Dr. Friendly.
LOCATION: Outpatient, Hospital
PATIENT: Otto Garth
ATTENDING/ADMIT PHYSICIAN: Alma Naraquist, MD
SURGEON: Larry P. Friendly, MD
INDICATION: Feeding, patient with gastroparesis.
  PROCEDURE: The patient was placed in the sitting position and then tilted to the right with a wedge. CORFLO was placed at the level of 19 cm without any complications. KUB was then done demonstrating the tip of the CORFLO in the third portion of the duodenum. After confirmation of postpyloric position of the CORFLO, the patient was started on UltraCal at 10 cc/hour.
CPT Code(s): _____

_____

ICD-10-CM Code(s): _____

Abstracting Questions

1. What does KUB stand for? _____

_____

2. What type of tube is a CORFLO? _____

_____

PRACTICE EXERCISE 20.17   GASTROJEJUNOSTOMY PLACEMENT

Because this is an interventional radiologist performing the procedure, report both the procedure and the radiology services.
RADIOLOGY REPORT
LOCATION: Outpatient, Hospital
PATIENT: Betty Frye
ORDERING PHYSICIAN: Ronald Green, MD
ATTENDING/ADMIT PHYSICIAN: Ronald Green, MD
INTERVENTIONAL RADIOLOGIST: Monica Hamilton, MD
EXAMINATION: Gastrojejunostomy placement.
CLINICAL SYMPTOMS: Malnutrition needing nutritional support.
  INDICATION: The patient is a 69-year-old female requiring tube feeding. Placement of a #14 French Shetty gastrojejunostomy catheter was requested by Dr. Green for nutritional support.
  Prior to the start of the study, the procedure was explained to the patient, including the risks, complications, and alternatives. The patient understood and consented to the procedure.
  PERCUTANEOUS GASTROJEJUNOSTOMY PLACEMENT: The patient was prepped and draped in the usual sterile fashion. Using ultrasound guidance, we localized the edge of the liver. Through a previously placed nasogastric tube, the stomach was distended with air.
  Using fluoroscopic guidance following administration of local anesthesia (1% lidocaine), we performed gastropexy utilizing four Medi-Tech T-tacks at the mid- to distal aspect of the stomach.

  Using multiple wires and catheters, an extra-stiff guidewire was ultimately placed with the tip in the proximal jejunum. Following multiple dilatations, a #14 French Shetty gastrojejunostomy catheter was placed with the tip in the proximal jejunum. A small amount of contrast was administered, which revealed adequate placement. There is no evidence of extravasation or other significant abnormalities.
  The patient tolerated the procedure well. There was no evidence of bleeding at the termination of the study.
  IMPRESSION: Placement of a #14 French Shetty gastrojejunostomy catheter with the tip in the proximal jejunum, as described above.

CPT Code(s): _____

_____

ICD-10-CM Code(s): _____

_____

Abstracting Questions

1. What was the approach for insertion of the gastrostomy tube? _____

_____

2. Was the ultrasonic guidance separately reported? _____

_____

3. Was the radiology service to check placement separately reported? _____

_____

PRACTICE EXERCISE 20.18   CYSTOTOMY

OPERATIVE REPORT

Dr. Martinez operated on this patient yesterday. The patient presents to the emergency department with an acute abdomen. You are to report only Dr. Martinez's services.

LOCATION: Inpatient, Hospital
PATIENT: Patti Bryan
ATTENDING PHYSICIAN: Gary Sanchez, MD
SURGEONS: Paula Smithson, MD, and Andy Martinez, MD

PREOPERATIVE DIAGNOSES
1. Acute abdomen.
2. Hematuria with suspected bladder injury.

POSTOPERATIVE DIAGNOSES
1. Iatrogenic cystotomy with urine extravasation into the peritoneal cavity.
2. Peritonitis.
3. Extensive intestinal adhesions.

PROCEDURES PERFORMED
1. Exploratory laparotomy.
2. Closure of cystotomy.
3. Extensive intestinal adhesiolysis.

SURGICAL INDICATIONS: This patient is a 32-year-old female who had undergone a Hasson laparoscopy that I performed yesterday. She presented to the emergency department last night with abdominal pain and findings of an acute abdomen. She also had a leukopenia. She was not running a fever. She was noted on insertion of the catheter into the bladder to have some grossly bloody urine.

OPERATIVE FINDINGS: There was less than 1-cm laceration in the dome of the bladder that was extravasating through the bladder. There was a large amount of urine in the peritoneal cavity and some slightly foul-smelling purulent fluid as well. This looked relatively murky and was just not plain urine. There were multiple intestinal adhesions, mostly involving the small bowel. No perforation of the bowel could be detected. The appendix was normal.

OPERATIVE DESCRIPTION: After induction of general anesthesia with patient in the supine position, the abdomen was prepped and draped. The abdomen was opened through a midline hypogastric incision excising her old scar on the way

in. The above findings were noted initially, and Dr. Smithson was able to isolate the small bladder dome laceration. This was smaller than one would expect if a 5-mm laparoscopic trocar had gone through the bladder. I believe that the edge of the bladder probably was nicked. Dr. Smithson will dictate her note concerning the cystotomy repair. We then ran the bowel in its entirety from the ligament of Treitz on down to the ileocecal junction. There were multiple interloop adhesions, which were lysed by Dr. Smithson. She will dictate her note separately. Some omental adhesions were also lysed. After copious irrigation of the abdominal cavity, we then irrigated with heparinized lactated Ringer's and left some of the Ringer's in the abdomen. The peritoneum was closed with a running 2–0 Vicryl. The fascia was closed with interrupted figure-of-eight 0 Vicryl, and the skin closed with staples. Blood loss estimation was 100 cc. The patient received 3000 cc of lactated Ringer's during the case.

Specimens to pathology were cultures of the peritoneal fluid. A Foley catheter was changed at the end of the case. The patient was returned to the recovery room in stable condition.

CPT Code(s): _____

_____

ICD-10-CM Code(s): _____

_____

Abstracting Questions

1. What procedures were performed during this operative session? _____
_____

2. Which procedure did Dr. Martinez perform? _____
_____

3. Were any modifiers required for the two surgeons involved in the same session, and if so, which modifier? _____
_____

PRACTICE EXERCISE 20.19   SMALL-BOWEL ANASTOMOSIS

OPERATIVE REPORT

LOCATION: Inpatient, Hospital
PATIENT: Dona Kelly
ATTENDING PHYSICIAN: Ronald Green, MD
SURGEON: Daniel G. Olanka, MD
PREOPERATIVE DIAGNOSIS: Multiple intestinal fistulas.
POSTOPERATIVE DIAGNOSIS: Multiple intestinal fistulas.

PROCEDURE PERFORMED: Excision of abdominal wall and small bowel with primary anastomosis of small bowel.

PRELIMINARY NOTE: This patient is well known to us. She has had multiple abdominal procedures to try to repair a very large abdominal wall hernia. She is outside the postoperative period of the hernia repair. She basically has no abdominal cavity left, and all her intestine resides outside the abdomen. There is such a drag on her abdominal wall that she has developed fistulas at the base of where the bowel rests against the mesh, and these have become unmanageable in the home setting. On this basis, we take this very high-risk patient to the operating room, with appropriate counseling for the family about the dire consequences.

OPERATIVE NOTE: With the patient under general anesthesia, the abdomen was prepped and draped in a sterile manner. A long incision was made above the area of the

fistulas, and we began to work our way down onto the mesh. Unfortunately, we entered the bowel at multiple points and had multiple enterotomies into the small bowel *(small intestine)* and colon *(large intestine)*. Finally we got everything freed up and were able to resect some of the abdominal wall that had adherent small bowel to it *(this indicates that part of the small intestine was removed)*. We were able to repair all of the enterostomies and a right colotomy using two layers of suture, an inner layer of Vicryl, and an outer layer of silk. We then copiously irrigated the abdominal field and used some large retention-type sutures to bring the wound together for partial closure. It is our hopes that the bowel that remains is viable *(this indicates that part of the bowel was removed)*. This procedure took substantially greater time than typically would be required. *(This statement indicates -22 may be assigned.)* We measured it at approximately 200 cm of length of her small bowel, and we are hopeful that this will be enough for her to nourish adequately.

CPT Code(s): _____

_____

ICD-10-CM Code(s): _____

_____

PRACTICE EXERCISE 20.19   SMALL-BOWEL ANASTOMOSIS—cont'd

Abstracting Questions

1. Was a portion of the large or small intestine removed?_____

_____

2. What statement indicates that modifier -22 would be appended to the CPT code? _____

_____

PRACTICE EXERCISE 20.20   PYLOROPLASTY

OPERATIVE REPORT

Report only Dr. White's surgical services. Note in this case that the surgeon began the procedure as a percutaneous liver biopsy, but because the patient could not hold his breath long enough for the biopsy to be obtained, Dr. White decided to discontinue the percutaneous biopsy and take the patient directly to the operating room for an open procedure. Two surgeons (co-surgeons) are performing this case. Dr. Sanchez, in his operative report, states that the patient was turned to a lateral position, prepped, and draped and the chest was opened to expose the esophagus. The distal esophagus was mobilized under direct vision and divided above the diseased segment. The distal esophagus and the attached proximal stomach were removed. The remaining stomach was pulled into the chest and connected to the stump of the proximal esophagus. Drains were placed and a chest tube inserted and the incision was closed.

LOCATION: Inpatient, Hospital

PATIENT: Ted Boyd

ATTENDING PHYSICIAN: Larry Friendly, MD

PRIMARY CARE PHYSICIAN: Ronald Green, MD

SURGEONS: Loren White, MD, and Gary Sanchez, MD

PREOPERATIVE DIAGNOSIS: Barrett's esophagus with severe dysplasia, possible carcinoma.

POSTOPERATIVE DIAGNOSIS: Barrett's esophagus with severe dysplasia, possible carcinoma, hemangioma liver.

PROCEDURES PERFORMED

1. Exploratory laparotomy.
2. Biopsy of liver lesion.
3. Immobilization of stomach with pyloroplasty.
4. Placement of feeding tube.

PRELIMINARY NOTE: This patient is a 63-year-old man who has been referred by Dr. Green for a bleeding esophageal lesion. This was seen and scoped, and the patient was markedly anemic. Biopsies showed it to be severe dysplasia with possible cancer present. He has had a rather extensive workup including complete cardiac workup. CT of the abdomen showed some lesions within the liver, which we tried to have biopsied percutaneously, but the patient could not hold his breath well enough and the lesions were too close to the diaphragm, so we do not have a tissue diagnosis on these. After all this workup we are taking the patient to the operating room for exploration. Assuming that he does not have disease metastatic to the liver, we will proceed with an esophagogastrectomy in the Ivor-Lewis technique. The abdominal portion of the procedure, which I am dictating, will be done by myself, and then Dr. Sanchez will do the chest portion of the procedure.

OPERATIVE NOTE: With the patient under general anesthesia, the abdomen was prepped and draped in a sterile manner. Midline incision was made from the xiphoid to below the pubis. Sharp dissection was carried down into the peritoneal cavity, and hemostasis was maintained with electrocautery. We began by exploring the abdominal cavity. The liver was carefully palpated. The area that had been identified on CT was at the very apex of the right lobe of the liver, we could feel this area; it did not have a thickened feel to it but was more consistent with an area of hemangioma. There was a small secondary lesion on the undersurface of the right

lobe. A **wedge biopsy** of this was taken and it did return a diagnosis of hemangioma. The rest of the liver appeared normal, and I thought that we did not need to proceed with anything further. We thus began with mobilization of the stomach, taking down the greater curvature vessels, preserving the gastroepiploica. We carried our dissection all the way up into the hiatal hernia, preserving the blood supply to the spleen and not injuring it. We were then able to detach the left gastric artery such that the stomach was tethered on its other vasculature but appeared completely viable. All these vessels were taken down with clamps and ligatures of 2–0 silk. We then circumferentially went around the esophagus and carried our dissection all the way back toward the pylorus. We then had the entire stomach freed up from pylorus all the way up to the diaphragm. *(The esophagus has been mobilized where it passes through the diaphragm and the stomach has been totally freed up so that when the chest is opened Dr. Sanchez will perform the remaining part of the surgery.)* The stomach appeared viable with reasonable circulation. A Heineke-Mikulicz **pyloroplasty** was then performed opening the pylorus in one direction and closing it in another using interrupted 3–0 silk sutures to complete the pyloroplasty. With this accomplished, we then picked up the **jejunum** approximated 40 or 50 cm beyond the ligament of Treitz and placed a red rubber **feeding tube** using a Witzel technique; this was a number 18-2. This was attached to the skin and brought out through a separate stab incision. The abdominal cavity was then checked for hemostasis and everything appeared to be intact. We then closed the incision using running 0–loop nylon. We closed the skin with staples. A sterile dressing was applied. With all this completed, the patient remained in the operating room and will be positioned by Dr. Sanchez for the thoracic portion of the procedure.

Pathology Report Later Indicated: Hemangioma.

CPT Code(s): _____

_____

ICD-10-CM Code(s): _____

_____

Abstracting Questions

1. Can the discontinued percutaneous liver biopsy be reported? _____

_____

2. If reporting the percutaneous liver biopsy, what modifier(s) is/are required? _____

_____

3. Was the wedge biopsy reported? _____

4. Dr. White performed an immobilization and what other procedure? _____

_____

5. Was the Barrett's and hemangioma reported separately?

_____

Urinary System Subsection (50010-53899)

Anatomic division
- Kidney
- Ureter
- Bladder
- Urethra
  Further divided by procedure such as:
- Incision
- Excision
- Introduction
- Repair
- Laparoscopy
- Endoscopy

Kidney Subheading (50010-50593)

Endoscopy codes are for procedure performed through previously established stoma or incision

Caution: Codes may be unilateral or bilateral

Introduction Category (50382-50435)

Codes divided by renal pelvis catheter procedures or other introduction procedures

Renal pelvis catheters further divided; internally dwelling or externally accessible

Catheters for drainage and injections and for radiography

Aspirations

Insertion of guidewires

Tube changes

Usually reported with radiology component

Ureter Subheading (50600-50980)

Caution: Codes may be unilateral or bilateral
  Divided by type of procedure
- Incision
- Excision
- Introduction
- Repair
- Laparoscopy
- Endoscopy

Bladder Subheading (51020-52700)

Includes codes for
- Incision
- Removal
- Excision
- Introduction
- Urodymics
- Repair
- Laparoscopy
- Endoscopy

- Cystoscopy
- Urethroscopy
- Cystourethroscopy
- Transurethral surgery
  Vesical Neck and Prostate
  Many bundled codes
  Example: Urethral dilation is included with insertion of cystoscope
  Read all descriptions carefully

Urodynamics (51725-51798)

Procedures relate to motion and flow of urine
  Used to diagnose urine flow obstructions
  Bundled: All instruments, equipment, fluids, gases, probes, catheters, technician's fees, medications, gloves, trays, tubing, and other sterile supplies

Vesical Neck and Prostate (52400-52700)

Contains codes for transurethral resection of the prostate (TURP)

Example: 52601 reports a complete transurethral electrosurgical resection of the prostate and includes vasectomy, meatotomy, cystourethroscopy, urethral calibration and/or dilation, internal urethrotomy, and control of any postoperative bleeding

Other approaches are reported with 55801-55845

Example: 55801 reports a removal of the prostate gland (prostatectomy) through an incision in the perineum and includes vasectomy, meatotomy, urethral calibration and/or dilation, internal urethrotomy, and control of any postoperative bleeding

Male Genital System Subsection (54000-55899)

Penis
Testis
Epididymis
Tunica Vaginalis
Scrotum
Vas Deferens
Spermatic Cord
Seminal Vesicles
Prostate

Biopsy Codes

Located in anatomical subheading to which the codes refer

Example: Biopsy codes in subheadings
- Epididymis (Excision)
Example: 54800, needle biopsy of epididymis
- Testis (Excision)
Example: 54500, needle biopsy of testis

Penis (54000-54450)

Incision codes (54000-54015) differ from Integumentary System codes
- Penis incision codes assigned for deeper structures

Destruction (54050-54065)

Codes divided by
- Extent: Simple or extensive
- Method of destruction, e.g., chemical, cryosurgery
  Extensive destruction can be by any method

Excision (54100-54164)

Commonly used codes for biopsy and circumcision

Introduction (54200-54250)

Many procedures for corpora cavernosa (spongy bodies of penis)
- Injection procedures for Peyronie disease (toughening of corpora cavernosa)
- Treatments for erectile dysfunction (ED)

Repair (54300-54440)

Many plastic repairs
  Some repairs are staged (more than one procedure)
- Stage indicated in code description

Reproductive System Procedures (55920)

Code 55920 reports the placement of catheters/needles into pelvic organs/genitalia
  For subsequent interstitial radioelement application

Intersex Surgery Subsection (55970-55980)

Only 2 codes within subsection
1. Male to female
2. Female to male
   Complicated procedures completed over extended period of time
   Performed by multiple physicians with extensive specialized training

Female Genital System Subsection (56405-58999)

Anatomic division: From vulva to ovaries
- Many bundled services

Vulva, Perineum, and Introitus (56405-56821)

Skene's gland reported with Urinary System, Incision or Excision codes
- Group of small mucous glands, lower end of urethra
  - Paraurethral duct

Incision (56405-56442)

I&D of abscess of vulva, perineal area, or Bartholin's gland

Marsupialization (56440)

Cyst incised
Drained
Edges sutured to sides to keep cyst open, creating a pouch-like repair

Destruction (56501, 56515)

Lesions destroyed by variety of methods
- Destruction = Eradication (not to be confused with excision; excision is removal)
  Divided by simple or extensive destruction
- Complexity based on physician's judgment
- Stated in medical record
  Destruction has no pathology report

Excision (56605-56740)

Biopsy includes
- Local anesthetic
- Biopsy
- Simple closure
  Code based on number of lesions biopsied

Vulvectomy

Surgical removal of portion of vulva (56620-56640)

Based on extent and size of area removed
Extent
- Simple: Skin and superficial subcutaneous tissues
- Radical: Skin and deep subcutaneous tissues
Size
- Partial: <80% vulvar area
- Complete: >80% vulvar area
Extent and size indicated in operative report

Repair (56800-56810)

Includes plastic repair

Read notes following category
- If repair procedure for wound of genitalia, use Integumentary System code

Endoscopy (56820-56821)

By means of a colposcope with or without biopsy(ies)

Vagina (57000-57426)

Codes divided based on service, e.g., incision, excision

Introduction (57150-57180)

Includes vaginal irrigation, insertion of devices, diaphragm, cervical caps
  Report device inserted separately

- 99070 or HCPCS National Level II codes, such as A4261 (cervical cap)

Repair (57200-57335)

For nonobstetric repairs
- Obstetric repairs, report Maternity Care and Delivery codes

Manipulation (57400-57415)

Dilation: Speculum inserted into vagina, which is enlarged by dilator

Endoscopy/Laparoscopy (57420-57426)

Colposcopy codes based on purpose
- e.g., biopsy, diagnostic
  Includes code for laparoscopic approach for repair of paravaginal defect

Cervix Uteri (57452-57800)

Cervix uteri, narrow lower end of uterus
  Services include endoscopy, excision, repair, manipulation

Excision (57500-57558)

Conization codes
  Conization: Removal of cone of tissue from cervix
  LEEP (loop electrocautery excision procedure) technology may be used for conizations or loop electrode biopsies

Corpus Uteri (58100-58579)

Many complex procedures
- Often very similar wording in code descriptions
- Requires careful reading and specific documentation in the medical record

Excision (58100-58294)

Dilation and curettage (D&C, 58120) of nonobstetric uterus
- After dilation, curette used to scrape uterus
- Coded according to circumstances: Obstetrical or nonobstetrical
  Do not report postpartum hemorrhage service with 58120
- Report 59160—Maternity and Delivery code
  Many hysterectomy codes
- Based on approach (vaginal, abdominal), extent (uterus, fallopian tubes, etc.), and weight of uterus
  Often secondary procedures performed with hysterectomy
  Do not report secondary, related minor procedures separately

Introduction (58300-58356)

Common procedures
- e.g., insertion of an IUD
  Report supply of device separately
  Specialized services

- e.g., artificial insemination procedures
  Used to report physician component of service
  Component coding
- Necessary with catheter procedures for hysterosonography
- Notes following codes indicate radiology guidance component codes

Laparoscopy/Hysteroscopy (58541-58579)

Laparoscopic approach for:
- Removal of myomas
- Radical hysterectomy
- Supracervical and laparoscopic vaginal hysterectomies
  Codes divided by tissue removed and weight of uterus
- Hysteroscopy codes divided on procedure performed (e.g., lysis of uterine adhesions, endometrial ablation)

Oviduct/Ovary (58600-58770)

Oviduct: Fallopian tube
  Incision category contains tubal ligations
- When during same hospitalization as cesarean delivery, tubal ligation is reported with code +58611

Laparoscopy (58660-58679)

Through abdominal wall
  Codes in the laparoscopy and hysteroscopy section are divided by procedure performed (e.g., lysis of adhesions, removal adnexal structures)
  Caution: If only diagnostic laparoscopy
- Do not report Female Genital System codes
- Report 49320, Digestive System
  Many codes can be reported separately with appropriate modifiers
  Example: 58660 Laparoscopy, surgical, with lysis of adhesions, can be reported with any of the indented codes that follow 58660 (58661-58673)

Ovary (58800-58960)

Two categories only: Incision and Excision

Incision: Primarily for drainage of cysts and abscesses
- Divided by surgical approach
Excision: Biopsy, wedge resection, and oophorectomy

In Vitro Fertilization (58970-58976)

Specialized codes used by physicians trained in fertilization procedures
- Codes divided by type of procedure and method used

Maternity Care and Delivery Subsection (59000-59899)

Divided by service, such as:
- Antepartum and Fetal Invasive Services

Amniocentesis
Fetal non-stress test
Fetal monitoring during labor
- Type of delivery
Vaginal delivery
C-section
Delivery after previous C-section
- Abortion

Gestation

Fetal gestation: Approximately 266 days (40 weeks)
EDD: Estimated Date of Delivery
- 280 days from last menstrual period (LMP)

Trimesters

First, LMP to less than 14 weeks 0 days
Second, 14 weeks 0 days to less than 28 weeks 0 days
Third, 28 weeks 0 days until deliver

Global Package and Delivery

Uncomplicated maternity care includes
- Antepartum care = Before delivery
- Delivery
- Postpartum care = After delivery

Antepartum Care Includes

Initial and subsequent H&P (history and physical)

Blood pressures
Weight
Routine chemical urinalysis
Fetal heart tones
Monthly visits to 28 weeks
Twice-a-month visits, weeks 29 to 36
Weekly visits from week 37 to delivery
Listed in notes preceding 59000
- Services not related to antepartum care are reported separately

Example: Pregnant female with complaint of suspicious mole on left shoulder
- Visits OB/GYN physician, who provides antepartum care
- Service regarding mole, not antepartum care, requires good documentation in the maternity record and a specific diagnosis relative to the treatment provided

Delivery Includes

Admission to hospital with admitting H&P

Management of uncomplicated labor
Vaginal or cesarean section delivery
- Complications coded separately
- Listed in notes preceding 59000

Postpartum Care Includes

Normal follow-up care for 6 weeks after delivery
- Hospital visits, office visits
- Listed in notes preceding 59000

Antepartum and Fetal Invasive Services (59000-59076)

Amniocentesis: Insertion of needle into pregnant uterus, withdrawal of fluid (59000, 59001)
- Ultrasound guidance with 59000 (76946)
- Ultrasound guidance included with 59001
- Component coding often part of services in subheading

Fetal services: Include stress tests, blood sampling, monitoring, and therapeutic procedures

Excision (59100-59160)

Postpartum curettage: Removes remaining pieces of placenta or clotted blood (59160)
Nonobstetric curettage: 58120 (Corpus Uteri, Excision)

Introduction (59200)

Insertion of cervical dilator: Used to prepare and soften the cervix for an abortive procedure or delivery (for abortive procedure, see 59855)
Cervical ripening agents may be introduced to prepare cervix
- Separate procedure and not reported when part of more major procedure

Repair (59300-59350)

Only for repairs during pregnancy
Repairs done as a result of delivery or during pregnancy
Episiotomy or vaginal repair by other than attending physician
Suture closure (cerclage) of cervix or repair of uterus (hysterorrhaphy)

Routine Global Obstetric Care

Includes antepartum care, delivery, and postpartum care
59400, Vaginal delivery
59510, Cesarean delivery
59610, Vaginal delivery after previous cesarean delivery (VBAC)
59618, Cesarean delivery following attempted vaginal delivery after previous cesarean delivery

Note: Take care when assigning diagnosis codes for normal versus complicated delivery. ICD-10-CM states specific guidelines for a normal delivery.

Episiotomies and Use of Forceps

Included in delivery
 Not reported separately

Physician Provides Only Portion of Global Routine Care, Delivery

59409, Vaginal delivery only
59514, Cesarean delivery only
59612, Vaginal delivery only, after previous cesarean delivery
59620, Cesarean delivery only, following attempted vaginal delivery after previous cesarean delivery

Delivery of Twins

Payers differ on reporting format

- -22 (Unusual Procedural Services)
- -51 (Multiple Procedures)

Abortion Services (59812-59857)

Spontaneous: Happens naturally (for a complete spontaneous abortion, report with a code from the E/M section [99202-99233])
Incomplete: Requires medical intervention
Induced: Intentional termination of pregnancy
Missed: Fetus dies naturally but does not abort during first 22 weeks of gestation
Septic: Abortion with infection
Medical intervention
- Dilation and curettage or evacuation (suction removal)
- Intra-amniotic injections (saline or urea)
- Vaginal suppositories (prostaglandin)

PRACTICE EXERCISE 20.21 RENAL TUMOR EXCISION

LOCATION: Inpatient, Hospital
PATIENT: Brian Eberhoft
ATTENDING PHYSICIAN: Leslie Alanda, MD
SURGEON: Ira Avila, MD
PREOPERATIVE DIAGNOSIS: Right renal tumor.
POSTOPERATIVE DIAGNOSIS: Complex right renal cyst (acquired).
PROCEDURE PERFORMED: Right renal exploration; de-roofing of right renal cyst.
ANESTHESIA: General.
CLINICAL NOTE: Mr. Eberhoft is a 78-year-old gentleman found to have an enlarging right complex renal mass. This does not enhance but has irregular boundaries and has increased in size over the past year. It is located on the medial posterior part of the right kidney adjacent to the renal hilum. Options were discussed with the patient, and he elected to proceed with exploration and possible partial nephrectomy or radical nephrectomy depending on findings.
PROCEDURE: The patient was given a general endotracheal anesthetic as well as an epidural for intraoperative and postoperative analgesia. An incision was made over the tip of the 10th rib and the tip of the 10th rib excised. A small hole in the pleura was created, which was closed at the end of the case.

The patient has very poor fascial structures and very poor superficial muscle development. The peritoneal space was entered and the kidney identified. The Omni retractor was used for exposure. The ascending color was reflected off of Gerota's fascia. The duodenum had made a large turn over top of the renal hilum, and the duodenum was kocherized carefully. The renal vein and renal artery were identified, isolated, and surrounded with vessel loops.

The kidney was mobilized. The adrenal was quite superficial within Gerota's fascia, and the fascia was accidentally torn during the mobilization of the kidney. This was controlled with hemoclips. There was a large perinephric fat pad that was mobilized with the kidney initially, and then Gerota's fascia opened posteriorly. The area in question was identified. The patient had some reaction around the area, but this was not significant. There was a lot of fat adherent to the kidney that was dissected off the posterior region around the renal hilum to identify the mass. The mass

appeared to be cystic in origin. A total of 3 cc of cyst fluid was aspirated from this and sent for cytology.

The cyst room was then opened. There was only a very small part of the cyst visible at the renal surface. Inspection of the cyst wall showed it to be smooth without masses. A small vessel was seen coursing inferiorly. This was cauterized. The renal pelvis was identified and Jelco catheter placed, and 5 cc of methylene blue–stained saline was injected through this to ensure that there was no communication with the cyst cavity and the renal pelvis. There was none.

The entire cyst wall was then cauterized. It was packed with Surgicel. Surgicel was also placed over the adrenal gland to help ensure hemostasis. Hemostasis was ensured. Vessel loops were removed. The kidney was then returned to renal fossa. A 10-mm Jackson-Pratt drain was left through a left lower quadrant stab wound and was placed adjacent to the de-roofed renal cyst.

The peritoneum was inspected, and there was no other abnormality identified on laparotomy.

The abdominal wall was then closed with three layers of 1 Vicryl. The skin was closed with surgical clips. A dressing was applied. Abdominal binder was applied. Prior to beginning closure of the abdominal wall, the rent in the pleura was closed with 3–0 Vicryl. Air was removed using a red rubber catheter in the usual fashion.

Sponge and needle counter were reported correct. The patient had a Foley catheter placed intraoperatively, and he had good urine output throughout the case. Estimated blood loss was 300 cc. He was transferred to the recovery room in good condition.

CPT Code(s): _____

_____

ICD-10-CM Code(s): _____

_____

Abstracting Questions

1. Was this procedure reported as an excision, even though the cyst was drained and the cyst wall retained? _____

_____

PRACTICE EXERCISE 20.21   RENAL TUMOR EXCISION—cont'd

2. Was de-roofing of renal cyst the same as an excision?

_____

3. Did the accidental tear of the fascia require a separate, reportable repair? _____

_____

4. Was a modifier reported? _____

_____

5. Was the diagnosis for an acquired or congenital renal cyst?

_____

PRACTICE EXERCISE 20.22   RENAL MASS

LOCATION: Inpatient, Hospital
PATIENT: Myra Grossman
ATTENDING PHYSICIAN: Ronald Green, MD
SURGEON: Ira Avila, MD
PREOPERATIVE DIAGNOSIS: Right renal mass.
POSTOPERATIVE DIAGNOSIS: Right renal cyst (acquired).
PROCEDURE PERFORMED: Laparoscopic exploration of kidneys, de-roofing, and biopsy of right renal mass.
ANESTHESIA: General.

SURGICAL INDICATIONS: This is a 20-year-old female who has a complex right renal cyst. She has been evaluated and worked up by Dr. Green. Options have been discussed, and she has elected to proceed with the exploration.

PROCEDURE: The patient was prepped and draped in the right flank position. A Foley catheter was placed. An incision was made. A retroperitoneal laparoscopic approach was used to approach the kidney, the cyst isolated, vessels identified and surrounded with vessel loops. The cyst was then aspirated and contents sent for cytology. The roof was ablated free and the base biopsied. There was some bleeding from the bases, which was controlled with 3–0 Chromic suture ligature. 3–0 Chromic sutures were used to close the cyst defect. A 10-mm flat Jackson-Pratt drain was left through a separate stab wound and sutured to the skin. The wound was closed with Vicryl and skin with clips. The patient tolerated the procedure well and was transferred to the recovery room in good condition. Estimated blood loss was 100 cc.

Pathology Report Later Indicated: Both pathology and cytology reports demonstrating benign cyst.

CPT Code(s): _____

_____

ICD-10-CM Code(s): _____

_____

Abstracting Question

1. What surgical approach was used for this procedure?

_____

PRACTICE EXERCISE 20.23   ABDOMINAL HYSTERECTOMY

OPERATIVE REPORT
LOCATION: Inpatient, Hospital
PATIENT: Maggie Brock
ATTENDING PHYSICIAN: Andy Martinez, MD
SURGEON: Andy Martinez, MD
PREOPERATIVE DIAGNOSES
1. Chronic menorrhagia.
2. Uterine fibroids.
POSTOPERATIVE DIAGNOSES
1. Chronic menorrhagia.
2. Uterine fibroids.

PROCEDURE PERFORMED: Total abdominal hysterectomy and bilateral salpingo-oophorectomy.

ANESTHESIA: General endotracheal.

SURGICAL INDICATION: This patient is a 48-year-old multiparous female who had had problems with chronic menorrhagia, unsuccessfully treated with hormone manipulation. She had known fibroids as well. Endometrial biopsy preoperatively was benign.

OPERATIVE FINDINGS: The uterus was about 10- to 12-week size with multiple leiomyomas. There was a functional-appearing cyst on the left ovary that contained some clear fluid. The right ovary was normal. The appendix was retrocecal but otherwise unremarkable.

OPERATIVE DESCRIPTION: After induction of general anesthesia, the patient was in the supine position. The abdomen and vagina were prepped, and Foley catheter placed; the patient was then draped. The abdomen was opened through a midline hypogastric incision, excising the old skin scar on the way in. Bowel was then packed out of the pelvis and a self-retaining Balfour retractor was placed. The uterus was elevated with clamps at the cornual areas. The left round ligament was clamped, divided, suture ligated with 0 Vicryl. All sutures were 0 Vicryl unless otherwise indicated. The peritoneal lateral to the left infundibulopelvic ligament was opened with Metzenbaum scissors, isolated in the left ovarian vasculature. This pedicle was isolated, clamped, divided, and doubly ligated. An identical procedure was carried out in the structures on the right side. The anterior and posterior leaves of the broad ligament were taken down with Metzenbaum scissors. There was some abnormal scarring and retraction of the bladder flap on the left side due to her prior cesarean sections. We then skeletonized the uterine artery pedicles on either side. The uterine artery pedicles were clamped with curved Rogers clamps, cut, and suture ligated. The cardinal ligaments and paracervical tissue were taken with two bites of straight Heaney-Ballantine clamps and suture ligated. The vaginal angle was then clamped with curved Rogers clamps, cut and held. The anterior vagina was opened with scalpel; then the upper vagina was incised circumferentially with right-angled scissors. The uterus was then removed and handed off. The vaginal angles were sutured with 0 Vicryl, and the vaginal cuff was closed with a series of interrupted figure-of-eight 0 Vicryl sutures. There was a small bleeding area on one of the cardinal ligament pedicles on the left side. This was isolated with an Allis clamp and secured with a

Continued

PRACTICE EXERCISE 20.23 ABDOMINAL HYSTERECTOMY—cont'd

suture ligature. Sponges were then removed. Sponge and needle counts were correct. The abdominal fascia was closed with interrupted 0 Ethibond sutures and the skin with staples. Blood loss estimation by anesthesia was 250 cc. Specimen to pathology: Uterus, tubes, and ovaries. Final sponge and needle counts were correct.

CPT Code(s): _____

ICD-10-CM Code(s): _____

Abstracting Questions

1. What factors affect CPT code assignment for the abdominal hysterectomy? _____
   _____

2. What factors affect the diagnosis code selection for the uterine leiomyoma? _____
   _____

3. What is another name for leiomyoma? _____
   _____

PRACTICE EXERCISE 20.24 CESAREAN SECTION

OPERATIVE REPORT

The physician who performs the cesarean section will also provide the postpartum care in this case.

LOCATION: Inpatient, Hospital
PATIENT: Joan Tisdale
ATTENDING PHYSICIAN: Andy Martinez, MD
SURGEON: Andy Martinez, MD
PREOPERATIVE DIAGNOSES
1. Intrauterine pregnancy at 31 weeks and 6 days.
2. Abruptio placentae.

POSTOPERATIVE DIAGNOSES
1. Intrauterine pregnancy at 31 weeks and 6 days.
2. Abruptio placentae.

PROCEDURE PERFORMED: Primary low transverse cervical cesarean section.
ANESTHESIA: General endotracheal.

SURGICAL INDICATIONS: The patient is a 31-year-old woman, gravida 4, para 3, at 31 weeks 6 days by menstrual dates, who was transferred on an emergency basis because of uterine bleeding. She had an apparent abruption on ultrasound, and the vagina was filled with blood clot. For these reasons, she was taken to surgery for an emergency cesarean section.

OPERATIVE FINDINGS: The infant is female, born at 2007 hours, weighing 2125 grams (4 lb 10 ounces), with Apgar scores of 8 at 1 minute and 9 at 5 minutes. There was a lot of blood in the uterine cavity and some adherent clot to the placenta, estimated to be less than 10% abruption. The tubes and ovaries were normal.

PROCEDURE: The abdomen was prepped and draped. A Foley catheter was in. The patient was then given a general endotracheal anesthetic, and the abdomen was opened through a Pfannenstiel incision. Bladder flap was opened transversely with scissors, and bladder was dissected downward bluntly with a hand. A small incision was made in the myometrium of the lower uterine segment, and then entry into the uterus was accomplished bluntly with a Kelly clamp. Low transverse incision was made with bandage scissors. The infant was delivered without undue difficulty. The infant's mouth

and nose were suctioned with a bulb syringe, the cord was clamped and cut, and the infant was handed to Dr. Ortez and the ICN staff. A segment of the cord was taken for cord blood gases, and the placenta was then delivered manually. Inspection of the uterine incision revealed there was a brisk bleeder near the left corner of the incision, and this was oversewn initially and the first layer was a running locked 0 Vicryl. The second layer was a running horizontal Lembert 0 Vicryl. The pelvis was irrigated with saline. The uterine incision was inspected, and there was a small amount of oozing from the incision, which was controlled with a single figure-of-eight 0 Vicryl suture. When hemostasis was adequate and lap sponges were correct, attention was directed toward closure. The peritoneum was loosely approximated in the midline with a couple of mattress sutures of 2–0 Vicryl. A medium Hemovac drain was placed subfascially to exit below the right side of the incision. The fascia was closed with running 0 Vicryl using two strands, one from either side to the middle and tied independently. The skin was closed with staples and the drain sutured to the skin with silk. Estimated blood loss was 1200-1500 cc.

Specimen to pathology was placenta. Final sponge and needle counts were correct.

CPT Code(s): _____

ICD-10-CM Code(s): _____

Abstracting Questions

1. What factor in this case determines the appropriate C-section code? _____
   _____

2. In addition to the placental abruption, what other two diagnoses must be reported? _____
   and _____

PRACTICE EXERCISE 20.25 LABIAL EXCISION

OPERATIVE REPORT
LOCATION: Inpatient, Hospital
PATIENT: Mary Brown
ATTENDING PHYSICIAN: Andy Martinez, MD
SURGEON: Andy Martinez, MD
PREOPERATIVE DIAGNOSIS: Vulvar intraepithelial neoplasia III of the right labia.
POSTOPERATIVE DIAGNOSIS: Vulvar intraepithelial neoplasia III of the right labia.
PROCEDURE PERFORMED: Radical excision, right labia.
PREAMBLE: The patient is a 47-year-old woman who presented with a right labial lesion. This was biopsied and reported as being VIN-III; invasion cannot be ruled out. The decision was therefore made to proceed with radical excision of the right vulva.
PROCEDURE: The patient was taken to the operating room and general anesthetic was administered. The patient was then prepped and draped in the usual manner in lithotomy position, and the bladder was emptied with a straight catheter. The vulva was then inspected. On the right labia majora at approximately the 11 o'clock position, there was a multifocal lesion present. A marking pen was then used to mark out an elliptical incision leaving a 1-cm border on all sides. The skin ellipse was then excised using the knife. Bleeders were cauterized with electrocautery. A running locked suture of 2-0

Vicryl was then placed in the deeper tissues. The skin was finally reapproximated with 4-0 Vicryl in an interrupted fashion. Good hemostasis was thereby achieved. The patient tolerated this procedure well. There were no complications. Estimated blood loss was 75 cc.

Pathology Report Later Indicated: Neoplasia III, carcinoma in situ.

CPT Code(s): _____

ICD-10-CM Code(s): _____

Abstracting Questions

1. In what area of the female genital anatomy is the labia located? _____

2. CPT code assignment was affected by the extent (partial/complete) and what other factor? _____

3. Define "in situ." _____

Endocrine System Subsection (60000-60699)

Nine glands in endocrine system; only four included in subsection
1. Thyroid
2. Parathyroid
3. Thymus
4. Adrenal

Pituitary and Pineal
See Nervous System subsection

Pancreas
Digestive System

Ovaries and Testes
Respective genital systems

Divided into two subheadings
- Thyroid Gland
- Parathyroid, Thymus, Adrenal Glands, Pancreas, and Carotid Body

Carotid Body
Refers to area adjacent to the bifurcation of the carotid artery
  Can be site of tumors

Thyroid Gland, Excision Category (60100-60281)

- **Lobectomy:** Partial or subtotal (something less than total)

- **Thyroidectomy:** Total (all) Thyroid, 1 gland with 2 lobes

Nervous System Subsection (61000-64999)

Divided anatomically
- Skull, Meninges, and Brain
- Spine and Spinal Cord
- Extracranial Nerves, Peripheral Nerves, and Autonomic Nervous System

Skull, Meninges, and Brain (61000-62258)
Category Examples:
Injection, Drainage, or Aspiration
  Twist Drills, Burr Hole(s), or Trephine

Conditions That Require Openings Into Brain to Relieve Pressure
Insert monitoring devices
Place tubing
Inject contrast material

Craniectomy or Craniotomy (61304-61576)
Craniectomy involves removal of portion of skull, at operative site, performed emergently to prevent herniation of brain into the brainstem

Craniotomy—bone flap is replaced after surgery
Codes divided by site and condition for which procedure is performed

Surgery of Skull Base (61580-61619)

Skull base: Area at base of cranium
- Lesion removal from this area very complex

Surgery of Skull Base Terminology

Approach procedure used to gain exposure of lesion

Definitive procedure is what is done to lesion

Repair/reconstruction procedure reported separately only if extensive repair

Approach procedure and definitive procedure coded separately

Example: Removal of an intradural lesion using middle cranial fossa approach
- 61590 approach procedure, middle cranial fossa and
- 61608 definitive procedure of intradural resection of lesion

Cerebrospinal Fluid (CSF) Shunt Category (62180-62258)

Performed to drain fluid

Codes describe, e.g.:
- Placement of devices
- Reprogramming
- Replacement
- Removal of shunting devices

Spine and Spinal Cord (62263-63746)

Codes divided by condition and approach

Often used are
- Unilateral or bilateral procedures (-50)
- Multiple procedures (-51)
- Radiologic supervision and fluoroscopic guidance coded separately

Includes codes for
- Myelography injections 62302-62305
  - Spinal or steroid anesthetic injections 62320-62326
  - Intrathecal or epidural catheter placement/implantation 62350-62355

Extracranial Nerves, Peripheral Nerves, and Autonomic Nervous System (64400-64999), Introduction/Injection of Anesthetic Agent (Nerve Block), Diagnostic or Therapeutic Category (64400-64530)

Includes codes for
- Nerve blocks 64486-64489, 64505-64530
  - Bundled when used as anesthesia for procedure
- Paravertebral facet joint injections 64490-64495, diagnostic or therapeutic
- Epidural injections 64479-64484
  - Used to provide pain relief
  - As compared with an epidural catheter placement used for anesthetic purposes

Eye and Ocular Adnexa Subsection (65091-68899)

Terminology extremely important
- Code descriptions often vary only slightly
  Understanding of eye anatomy is necessary for proper coding in this subsection
  Codes divided anatomically, e.g.,
- Eyeball
- Anterior segment
- Posterior segment
- Ocular adnexa
- Conjunctiva
  Some codes specifically for previous surgery
  Example: Insertion of ocular implant, secondary (65130)
  Much bundling
  Example: Subheading Posterior Segment, Prophylaxis category notes indicate:
- "The following descriptors (67141, 67145) are intended to include all sessions in a defined treatment period."

Cataracts

Method used depends on type of cataract and surgeon preference

Nuclear cataract: Most common, center of lens (nucleus), due to aging process

Cortical cataract: Forms in cortex of lens and extends outward; frequent in diabetics

Subcapsular cataract: Forms at back of lens, increased rate in diabetics, those who take steroid medications, certain genetic factors, and eye trauma

Removal and Lens Replacement (66830-66986)

- Extracapsular cataract extraction (ECCE)
  Patient retains posterior outer shell of the lens
  Soft cortex and rest of shell is removed in multiple pieces
  Posterior shell helps prevent vitreous prolapse
- Intracapsular cataract extraction (ICCE) is total removal
  Removes lens and capsule in one piece
- Phacoemulsification
  Small incision into eye and introduction of probe
  High-frequency waves fragment cataract (extracapsular); then suctioned out
  Lens placed through same small incision

Eyelids (67700-67999)

Blepharotomy (67700)
- Incision into eyelid for drainage of abscess
  Blepharoplasty
- Repair of eyelid
- Codes in Integumentary System (15820-15823), report removal of excess skin
- Codes in Eye and Ocular Adnexa (67916, 67917, 67923, 67924), report muscle repairs and slings
  Selection of code depends on technique used to repair eyelid
- Blepharoplasty codes with specific techniques, 67901-67908

Auditory System Subsection (69000-69979)

Codes divided by
- External Ear (69000-69399)
- Middle Ear (69420-69799)
- Inner Ear (69801-69949)
- Temporal Bone, Middle Fossa Approach (69950-69979)
  Understanding of ear anatomy is necessary for proper coding in this subsection
  External, middle, and inner ear further divided by procedure, such as
- Incision
- Excision
- Removal
- Repair
  Myringotomy and tympanostomy
- Eustachian tube connects middle ear to back of throat for drainage
- Fluid collects in middle ear when tube does not function properly

- Prevents air from entering middle ear and pressure builds
- Surgical intervention
  Myringotomy (incision into tympanic membrane)
  Tympanostomy (placement of PE [pressure equalization] tube)

Operating Microscope Subsection (+69990)

Employed with procedures using microsurgical techniques

Code in addition to primary procedure performed
Do not report separately when primary procedure description includes microsurgical techniques
Example: 15758 Free fascial flap with microvascular anastomosis
Note that following 15758 is the statement:
- "(Do not report code 69990 in addition to code 15758)" indicating to the coder not to report the use of the operating microscope separately
Do not report 69990 when magnifying loupes are used

PRACTICE EXERCISE 20.26   INTRACEREBRAL HEMATOMA

OPERATIVE REPORT
LOCATION: Inpatient, Hospital
PATIENT: Suzy Kunklemann
ATTENDING PHYSICIAN: Gary Sanchez, MD
SURGEON: Gary Sanchez, MD
PREOPERATIVE DIAGNOSIS: Intracerebral hematoma (nontraumatic), right temporal lobe.
POSTOPERATIVE DIAGNOSIS: Intracerebral hematoma (nontraumatic), right temporal lobe.
PROCEDURE PERFORMED: Osteoplastic craniotomy, right temporal area; evacuation of intracerebral hematoma.
ANESTHESIA: General.
PROCEDURE: Under general anesthesia, the patient's head was placed in the Mayfield pins. The right frontal temporoparietal area was prepped and draped in the usual manner. A linear incision was made extending from the midline of the temporal fossa up to the midportion of the scalp. The skin was incised. The temporalis muscle was separated and divided off the bone. I did a craniotomy here the size of a half-dollar and made a burr hole. I utilized the craniotome to elevate the bone flap, and this was a free bone flap. This was then removed. We placed the Weitlaners into the wound and then incised the dura in a cruciate fashion over the temporal lobe. I then entered the middle temple gyrus and irrigated much of the clot from the temporal and posterior parietal areas, and evacuated the clot from the area. This took copious irrigation. We used cotton balls for hemostasis. I did this

numerous times until all the bleeders were coagulated. I then lined the cystic cavity with Gelfoam and coagulated the edges of the raw brain. I closed the dura with 4–0 Vicryl. This was closed in a watertight fashion. I used 2–0 Vicryl to elevate the dura to the bone flap with Wurzburg plates, two of them, utilizing plates and screws. I then closed the scalp in one layer using 0 Vicryl on the temporalis muscle and fascia, and the skin was approximated with 2–0 nylon interrupted mattress sutures. Dressing was applied, and the patient was on the ventilator and discharged to the surgical intensive care unit.

CPT Code(s): _____

_____

ICD-10-CM Code(s): _____

Abstracting Questions

1. Was the procedure performed a surgical craniotomy?

_____

2. Does the area of the skull being opened affect the code?

_____

3. What was the purpose of the procedure? _____

_____

4. Does the purpose of the procedure affect the CPT code?

_____

PRACTICE EXERCISE 20.27   PARIETAL BURR HOLES

OPERATIVE REPORT
LOCATION: Inpatient, Hospital
PATIENT: Reed Scaleni
ATTENDING PHYSICIAN: Gary Sanchez, MD
SURGEON: Gary Sanchez, MD
PREOPERATIVE DIAGNOSIS: Subacute subdural hematoma (nontraumatic), right side.

POSTOPERATIVE DIAGNOSIS: Subacute subdural hematoma (nontraumatic), right side.
PROCEDURE PERFORMED: Burr hole times two, right frontal and right posterior parietal.
ANESTHESIA: General.
PROCEDURE: Under general anesthesia, the patient's head was prepped and draped in the usual manner. The

Continued

PRACTICE EXERCISE 20.27   PARIETAL BURR HOLES—cont'd

incision was made. Straight line linear incisions over the frontal and posterior parietal areas were made on the right side. Retractors were placed. Burr holes remained. The dura was visualized. The bony edges were waxed with beeswax. The dura was incised, both the frontal and the parietal holes. Serosanguineous fluid and clouded blood exuded. I cleaned it out until the supernatant was clear. The brain was found to be pulsating beneath. We then placed two medium-size Penrose drains and closed the galea with 2–0 Vicryl. The skin was approximated with surgical staples, and the Penrose drains were anchored with sutures. A dressing was applied. The patient was discharged to the PAR.

CPT Code(s): _____

_____

ICD-10-CM Code(s): _____

_____

Abstracting Questions

1. What determines the code assignment for burr holes of the skull? _____

_____

2. Does the location of the hematoma being drained/aspirated make a difference in the CPT code assignment? _____

_____

3. Was this CPT code reported twice for the two burr holes? _____

4. Was a modifier reported to indicate which side of the skull was drilled? _____

_____

PRACTICE EXERCISE 20.28   CARPAL TUNNEL

OPERATIVE REPORT
LOCATION: Outpatient, Hospital
PATIENT: Judy Burns
ATTENDING PHYSICIAN: Gary Sanchez, MD
SURGEON: Gary Sanchez, MD
PREOPERATIVE DIAGNOSIS: Left carpal tunnel syndrome.
POSTOPERATIVE DIAGNOSIS: Left carpal tunnel syndrome.
PROCEDURE PERFORMED: Carpal tunnel released, left wrist.
ANESTHESIA: Regional.
   PROCEDURE: After a satisfactory level of regional anesthesia, the extremity was addressed once it had been sterilely prepped and draped. Throughout the procedure the patient needed some focal augmentation for sharp pain characteristics at the level of the skin most distally about the skin wound. Sharp dissection was conducted down to the palmaris fascia. We identified the deep transverse ligament. In a blunt manner, we undermined this, and with use of a Freer interposing between deep transverse carpal ligament and the medial nerve, sharply dissected over the Freer, releasing the

impinging structures about the carpal canal. The probe palpation, the tendinous structures, and the floor of the carpal canal were otherwise unremarkable. She has at this time an exiting thenar motor branch, which was not obscured. There is an hourglass deformity of the median nerve as noted. At completion of this the wound was irrigated, followed by closure of the dermal planes and application of a splint. The patient tolerated the procedure well and was transported to the recovery room in a stable manner.

CPT Code(s): _____

_____

ICD-10-CM Code(s): _____

_____

Abstracting Question

1. Release of the carpal tunnel has what effect on the median nerve? _____

_____

PRACTICE EXERCISE 20.29   REPAIR OF PSEUDOMENINGOCELE

OPERATIVE REPORT
   This patient is returned to the operating room during the postoperative period for a decompression laminectomy performed by the same physician who now performs the pseudomeningocele repair.
LOCATION: Inpatient, Hospital
PATIENT: Debbie Smith
ATTENDING PHYSICIAN: Gary Sanchez, MD
SURGEON: Gary Sanchez, MD
PREOPERATIVE DIAGNOSIS: Pseudomeningocele.
POSTOPERATIVE DIAGNOSIS: Pseudomeningocele.
PROCEDURE PERFORMED: Repair of pseudomeningocele at the L4-5 level just to the left of the midline.
   PROCEDURE: The patient was taken to the operating room and underwent placement of a spinal drain by the anesthesiologist. She then underwent induction of a general endotracheal anesthesia. She was flipped to the prone position

and was thoroughly prepped and draped. The previous incision was reopened and was extended approximately 1 inch both superiorly and inferiorly. A large amount of spinal fluid came forth. There was a well-epithelialized membrane underneath the subcutaneous tissue extending deep to the muscle. This was excised as much as possible. I first dissected the paraspinal muscles laterally on each side along the L2 vertebra. I identified epithelial lining consistent with a pseudomeningocele. I saw a small leak and thought that I saw spinal fluid coming from the small defect. I gave a Valsalva maneuver, but it was not crystal clear whether this was spinal fluid or merely epidural blood. Anyway, I packed this off with Surgicel, placed a small fat graft, and secured it with a 4–0 Nurolon. I then used the FloSeal and Duragen to seal off the defect. I began reapproximating the muscle when I then noticed that there was spinal fluid again coming from the inferior portion of the incision. I exposed the lamina of L5

PRACTICE EXERCISE 20.29 REPAIR OF PSEUDOMENINGOCELE—cont'd

bilaterally and placed a retractor. I then noticed that there was a dural defect just to the left of the midline between the L4 and L5 laminae. I did a partial hemilaminectomy of L5 on the left side and was able to place three separate 4–0 Nurolon sutures through the dural defect. Care was taken to depress the nerve within the dural sac with a #4 Penfield. I then directly repaired the dura and did not see any further spinal fluid leakage with a Valsalva maneuver. I then used some FloSeal and strategically placed pieces of Surgicel to cover the defect. I then placed a small piece of Duragen on top of this as well. I irrigated with copious amounts of saline. I then closed the muscle in the deep fascia with interrupted 2–0 Vicryls, which were very closely approximated. I then used interrupted 2–0 Vicryl to close the subcutaneous tissue. The skin was closed with a running 4–0 nylon interlocking stitch. A sterile dressing was placed.

The patient tolerated the procedure well without apparent complications. The spinal drain was sutured in by me at the end of the procedure. She was taken to the recovery room in stable condition. Sponge, instrument, and needle counts were correct times two.

CPT Code(s): _____

ICD-10-CM Code(s): _____

Abstracting Questions

1. Repair of the pseudomeningocele is repair of what? _____

2. What procedure was performed to clear the approach for the repair of the dura tear? _____

3. Does the pseudomeningocele make a difference in the CPT code assignment? _____

4. What modifiers are required? _____

PRACTICE EXERCISE 20.30 LAMINECTOMY WITH FORAMINOTOMY

OPERATIVE REPORT
LOCATION: Inpatient, Hospital
PATIENT: Karen Origami
ATTENDING PHYSICIAN: Gary Sanchez, MD
SURGEON: Gary Sanchez, MD
PREOPERATIVE DIAGNOSIS: Severe spinal stenosis from L3 through L5.
POSTOPERATIVE DIAGNOSIS: Severe spinal stenosis from L3 through L5 without neurogenic claudications.
PROCEDURES PERFORMED
1. Bilateral L3 laminectomy with foraminotomy.
2. Bilateral L4 laminectomy with foraminotomy.
3. Bilateral L5 laminectomy with foraminotomy.
INDICATION: This patient is a 79-year-old female who presented with severe neurogenic claudication, left greater than right. Workup included an MRI scan, which showed severe spinal stenosis from L3 through L5. After discussion of the options, she elected to undergo surgery. She was informed that this was an elective surgery and was not life or limb threatening. The risks of the procedure were thoroughly discussed, and the patient consented to proceed.
PROCEDURE: The patient was taken to the operating room and underwent induction after general endotracheal anesthesia in the supine position. She was then flipped to the prone position on the operating room table and the knees were flexed. The lower lumbar spine was thoroughly prepped and draped, and a vertical midline skin incision was made from the L3 to the S1 spinous processes. The skin was infiltrated with local anesthetic prior to making the incision. Using the monopolar cautery, I identified the spinous processes of L2 through S1 bilaterally. Then using the periosteal elevator, I retracted the paraspinal muscles laterally bilaterally. Deep retractors were placed. At this point, I used the handheld rongeur and removed the spinous processes of L4 and L3. An intraoperative x-ray was done to verify the location. At this, the L5 spinous process was then removed. I then alternated between the rongeurs and the high-speed burr, and drilled down the medial facets and the lamina of L5, L4, and L3. I then began using the Kerrison and removed the inferior lamina of L5 and proceeded from a caudal to cephalad direction. I alternated between the high-speed drill and the Kerrison

rongeurs and eventually removed the lamina and the medial facets bilaterally of L3 through L5. There was noted to be very severe compression of the thecal sac at the L4-5 level as there was a grade 1 spondylolisthesis at that level. There was also noted to be severe spinal stenosis at the L3-4 level. After an adequate decompression, I made sure that the decompression extended laterally out to the exiting nerve roots on each side bilaterally. The nerve roots were particularly tight at the L4-5 level, where the spondylolisthesis was located. At no time was there a dural tear or spinal fluid leak. I irrigated with copious amounts of saline. Bleeding bone edges were waxed. The gutters were lined with Surgicel, and a piece of Gelfoam was placed over the exposed dura. I irrigated again. I closed the wound in layers with interrupted 0 and 2–0 Vicryl. Skin was closed with a running 3–0 Vicryl subcuticular stitch. Benzoin and one-half-inch Steri-Strips and a sterile dressing were placed.

The patient tolerated the procedure well without apparent complication. She will go to the recovery room after the surgery. Sponge, instrument, and needle counts were correct.

CPT Code(s): _____

ICD-10-CM Code(s): _____

Abstracting Questions

1. In addition to the laminectomy with foraminotomy, what other procedure was performed? _____

2. Which vertebrae were addressed? _____

3. How many codes are necessary to report all three vertebrae? _____

4. What modifiers are required? _____

21

Radiology Section (70010-79999)

Radiology: Branch of medicine that uses radiant energy to diagnose and treat patients

Specialist in radiology: Radiologist (doctor of medicine)

Radiology Subsections

1. Diagnostic Radiology
2. Diagnostic Ultrasound
3. Radiologic Guidance
4. Breast, Mammography
5. Bone/Joint Studies
6. Radiation Oncology
7. Nuclear Medicine

Procedures

Fluoroscopy views inside of body, projects onto television screen

Live images by which physician can view function, structure, and defects or anomalies within an organ

Example: 71047, 76000 chest x-ray with fluoroscopy

Magnetic Resonance Imaging (MRI)

Example: 72148 MRI of spinal canal

Tomography or Computed Axial Tomography (CAT or CT Scan)

Example: 70450 tomographic scan of head or brain

Planes of Body (Fig. 21.1)

Position and Projection

Position = method of positioning patients for examination

Projection path = pathway traveled by x-ray beam

Component Coding

Three component terms
1. Professional
2. Technical
3. Global

Professional Component

Physician portion of service, includes
- Supervision of technician
- Interpretation of results, including written report

Technical Component
- Technologist's services
- Equipment, film, and supplies

Global Procedure

Both professional and technical portions of radiology service

Component Modifiers

If only professional component of radiology service provided: add modifier -26

If only technical component provided: add modifier -TC
- -TC HCPCS modifier used with CPT and HCPCS codes

If both professional and technical components of radiology service are provided by physician who owns equipment and facility, pays technician and supplies (global), no modifier is needed

Example: Chest x-ray
- Professional component: 71048-26 (supervision and final report)
- Technical component: 71048-TC (technician, supplies, equipment)
- Global procedure: 71048 (both professional and technical)

Third-party payers usually reimburse
- 40% professional component
- 60% technical component
- 100% global procedure

Contrast Material

Statement "with contrast" indicates injection service included in code

Oral or rectal contrast does not qualify for "with contrast"

Notes indicate codes for components

Example: 75801, Lymphangiography, parenthetical note above code indicates: "For injection procedure for lymphatic system, use 38790"

Interventional Radiologist

Combination radiologist and surgeon

Provides total procedure for cystography with contrast

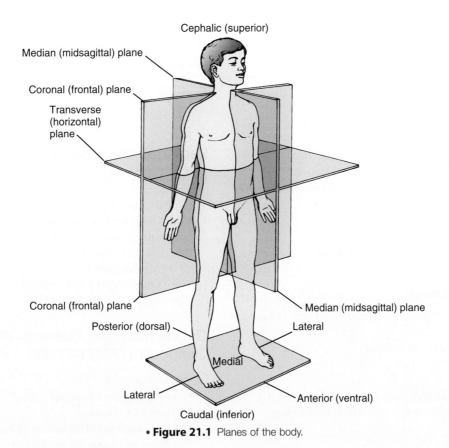

Cephalic (superior)

Median (midsagittal) plane

Coronal (frontal) plane

Transverse
(horizontal)
plane

Coronal (frontal) plane

Median (midsagittal) plane

Posterior (dorsal)

Lateral

Medial

Lateral

Anterior (ventral)

Caudal (inferior)

• **Figure 21.1** Planes of the body.

- Report 74430, x-ray portion
- 51600 for injection procedure
- Plus code for supply of contrast material (e.g., 99070)

Diagnostic Radiology Subsection (70010-76499)

Most standard radiographic procedures
 Codes often divided by whether contrast material used
 Codes further divided by number of views
 Example: 71048, Chest x-ray, 4 views or more
 Used to:
 - Diagnose disease
 - Monitor disease process—progression or remission
 - Therapeutic procedures (guidance)

Diagnostic Procedures Include

X-ray
Computerized axial tomography (CAT or CT scan)
Magnetic resonance imaging (MRI)
Angiography
 Fluoroscopy
 3D rendering

Computed Axial Tomography (CAT or CT)

X-ray image taken in sections
 Computer reconstructs and enhances image

Magnetic Resonance Imaging (MRI)

Uses magnetic fields to produce an image displayed on computer screen
 Codes of same area (e.g., spine) divided by whether or not contrast material used

Angiography

Used to view vessel obstructions
 Dye injected into vessel
 Radiologist uses angiography to diagnose vascular conditions
 Example:
 - Malformation
 - Stroke (cerebrovascular accident, CVA)
 - Myocardial infarction (MI)

NOTE

Remember

If fewer than total number of views specified in code provided: Report -52, Reduced Service

Diagnostic Ultrasound Subsection (76506-76999)

Uses high-frequency sound waves to image anatomic structures
Nine subheadings of Diagnostic Ultrasound
Primarily based on anatomy

A-Mode (A = Amplitude)

Technique used to map structure outline in one-dimensional image

M-Mode (M = Motion)

Technique used to display one-dimensional movement of structure

B-Scan (B = Brightness)

Technique used to display two-dimensional movement of tissues and organs
Known as gray scale ultrasound

Real-Time Scan

Technique used to display both structure and motion with time of organ and tissues in a two-dimensional image

Extent of Study

Codes often divided on extent of study
Example: Extent of scan as follows
- **Complete:** Scans entire body or body region
- **Limited:** Scans part of body, e.g., one organ
- **Follow-up/repeat:** Limited study of part of body that was scanned previously

Three Locations for Ultrasound Services

76506-76999: Radiology codes for diagnostic ultrasound services
93875-93990: Medicine codes for non-invasive vascular studies
93303-93355: Medicine codes for echocardiography

Radiologic Guidance Subsection (77001-77022)

Guidance
- Fluoroscopic
- Computed tomography
- Magnetic resonance imaging
- Other

Breast Mammography Subsection (77046-77063)

Example: Computer-aided detection and screening
Some codes specify unilateral/bilateral

Bone/Joint Studies Subsection (77071-77086)

Example: Bone density, bone mineral density, and joint survey

Radiation Oncology Subsection (77261-77799)

Therapeutic use of radiation
Codes both professional and technical services
Subheadings divided based on treatment
Initial consultation, prior to decision to treat, reported with E/M code
- **Outpatient:** 99241-99245
- **Inpatient:** 99251-99255

Clinical Treatment Planning—Professional Component (77261-77299)

Includes
- Interpretation of special testing
- Tumor localization
- Determination of treatment volume
- Choice of treatment method
- Determination of number of treatment ports
- Selection of treatment devices
- Other necessary procedures
  Clinical Treatment Planning consists of
- Planning
- Simulation

Three Levels of Planning (77261-77263)

1. **Simple:** One treatment area, one port, or one set of parallel ports
2. **Intermediate:** Three or more ports, two separate treatment areas, multiple blocking
3. **Complex:** Complex blocking, custom shielding blocks, tangential ports, special wedges, 3+ treatment areas, special beams

Simulation (77280-77293)

Determining placement of treatment areas/ports for radiation treatment
Does not include administration of radiation

Definitions of Simulation
1. **Simple:** 1 treatment area with 1 port or pair of ports
2. **Intermediate:** 3+ ports, 2 separate treatment areas, multiple blocking
3. **Complex:** Tangential ports, 3+ treatment areas, complex blocking
4. **Computer-generated 3D:** reconstruction of volume of tumor and critical structures

Medical Radiation, Physics, Dosimetry, Treatment Devices, and Special Services (77295, 77300-77370)

Decision making services of physicians
- Treatment types
- Dose calculation and placement (dosimetry)
- Development of treatment device

Stereotactic Radiation Treatment Delivery (77371-77373)

Delivers large radiation dose to specific tumor sites
- Computer(s) map location
- Radiation delivered to one or more sites

Radiation and Neutron Beam Treatment Delivery (77401-77525)

Technical component of actual delivery of radiation

Information Needed to Code Radiation Treatment Delivery

Amount of radiation delivered
  Type of radiation—electron (most common), neutron, or proton
  Number of
  - Areas treated (single, two, three, or more)
  - Ports involved (single, three or more, tangential)
  - Blocks used (none, multiple, custom)

Reporting Radiation Treatment Management (77427-77499)

Professional (physician) portion of services, including
- Review port films
- Review dosimetry, dose delivery, treatment parameters
- Treatment set-up
- Patient examination for medical E/M

Report in units of five fractions, unless last 3-4 fractions are at the end of the treatment; then you can count the last 3-4 as an additional fraction

Hyperthermia (77600-77615)

Use of heat by means of ultrasound, probes, microwave, etc.
  Treatment delivered at three levels:
  - External (superficial and deep)
  - Interstitial
  - Intracavitary
Used in addition to radiation therapy or chemotherapy
Includes three months follow-up after procedure

Clinical Brachytherapy (77750-77799)

Placement of radioactive material into or around site of tumor
- Intracavitary (within body cavity)
- Interstitial (within tissues)

Source

Radioactive element delivers radiation dose over time
  Example: Seeds, ribbons, or capsules
  - **Ribbons:** Seeds embedded on tape and inserted into tissue
  - Tape is cut to desired length, thereby controlling amount of radiation

Clinical Brachytherapy Codes Divided Based on

Number of sources applied
- Simple 1-4
- Intermediate 5-10
- Complex 11+

Nuclear Medicine Subsection (78012-79999)

Placement of radioactive material into body and measurement of emissions
  Used for both diagnosis and treatment
  Codes divided primarily on organ system
  - Except "Therapeutic," which is for radiopharmaceutical therapies

PRACTICE EXERCISE 21.1 CRANIAL CT

RADIOLOGY REPORT
LOCATION: Inpatient, Hospital
PATIENT: Bill Arnold
ORDERING PHYSICIAN: Timothy L. Pleasant, MD
ATTENDING/ADMIT PHYSICIAN: Timothy L. Pleasant, MD
RADIOLOGIST: Morton Monson, MD
PERSONAL PHYSICIAN: Ronald Green, MD
EXAMINATION: Cranial CT.
CLINICAL SYMPTOMS: Altered mental status.
TECHNIQUE: Axial noncontrast CT scan of the head.
   INTERPRETATION: There is diffuse mild enlargement of the sulci and ventricles. Periventricular diminished density is present bilaterally and is prominent near the trigones of the lateral ventricles. There is a 1-mm high-density area seen on image 10 in the left posterior temporal occipital region.
   In the posterior fossa the fourth ventricle is normal in position. Mildly prominent cerebellar folia are present.
   No abnormalities of the orbits, paranasal sinuses, or temporal bone can be seen.
   There is a small amount of calcification in the paraclinoid and carotid arteries.
CONCLUSIONS
   1. Mild diffuse cerebral atrophy.

2. Periventricular changes consistent with age-related ischemic change.
3. Tiny calcification in the left posterior temporal occipital region. Finding is nonspecific and could reflect previous granulomatous calcification, intraluminal calcification, Pantopaque, or calcification in a lesion. Recommend clinical correlation and cranial MRI if appropriate.
4. Vascular calcifications are present.
CPT Code(s): _____

ICD-10-CM Code(s): _____

Abstracting Questions

1. What was the clinical symptom that prompted this CT?
_____

2. Sulci were referred to in the Interpretation section. What are sulci? _____
_____

PRACTICE EXERCISE 21.2 GALLBLADDER ULTRASOUND

RADIOLOGY REPORT
LOCATION: Outpatient, Hospital
PATIENT: Dan Diel
ORDERING PHYSICIAN: Daniel G. Olanka, MD
ATTENDING/ADMIT PHYSICIAN: Daniel G. Olanka, MD
RADIOLOGIST: Morton Monson, MD
PERSONAL PHYSICIAN: Ronald Green, MD
EXAMINATION: Gallbladder ultrasound.
CLINICAL SYMPTOMS: Increased bilirubin.
   GALLBLADDER ULTRASOUND: Examination was technically difficult with some limitations due to overlying leads. Large right pleural effusion identified. Gallbladder is visualized. No obvious gallstones or gallbladder wall thickening. Only short portions of the common hepatic duct and common bile duct are visualized. Common hepatic duct measures 3.6 mm, and common bile duct measures 5.2 mm. These values are within normal limits. There is limited assessment of the liver, which is grossly unremarkable.
   IMPRESSION: Gallbladder ultrasound with limitations as discussed above. Grossly unremarkable sonographic appearance of the gallbladder. No obvious dilatation of the common duct. Large right pleural effusion identified.

CPT Code(s): _____

ICD-10-CM Code(s): _____

Abstracting Questions

1. What subcategory within Radiology in the CPT was referenced for assignment of a code for this case? _____
_____

2. What body area was evaluated? _____
_____

3. What code range in the CPT was reviewed to select the ultrasound code? _____
_____

4. What modifier was appended to the CPT code? _____
_____

PRACTICE EXERCISE 21.3 STRESS TEST

RADIOLOGY REPORT
LOCATION: Outpatient, Hospital
PATIENT: Harry Stein
ORDERING PHYSICIAN: James Noonar, MD
ATTENDING/ADMIT PHYSICIAN: James Noonar, MD
RADIOLOGIST: Morton Monson, MD
PERSONAL PHYSICIAN: Ronald Green, MD
   EXAMINATION: Adenosine stress test and resting Myoview, left ventricle, with estimate of left ventricular ejection fraction.

CLINICAL SYMPTOMS: Chest pain.
   ADENOSINE STRESS AND RESTING MYOVIEW EVALUATION, LEFT VENTRICLE, WITH ESTIMATE OF LEFT VENTRICULAR EJECTION FRACTION: Clinical information states chest pain. This is a patient with known coronary artery disease. The patient has had prior replacement of aortic and mitral valve 3 to 4 years ago by history. The patient has a previous Cardiolite scan from December 24 two years ago that showed "fixed posterior/inferior wall perfusion defect extending into the cardiac apex." On September 12 of

PRACTICE EXERCISE 21.3   STRESS TEST—cont'd

this year, the patient was given adenosine challenge under the supervision of Dr. Dawson, who will report on that portion of the evaluation. On September 12, the patient was injected with 27.2 mCi of technetium-99m–tagged tetrofosmin. Views of the left ventricle were then acquired with a SPECT nuclear medicine camera and reformatted into the standard projections. On September 13, the patient was returned to the nuclear medicine department for resting or redistribution scan and injected with 26.2 mCi of technetium-99m–tagged tetrofosmin. Again, views of the left ventricle were acquired with the SPECT nuclear medicine camera and reformatted into standard projections. Comparison of the stress and resting images shows no area to suggest perfusion defect. Nothing to suggest ischemia or infarct is seen. All segments of the left ventricle are perfused.

IMPRESSION

1. Adenosine challenge as the stress. That will be reported by Dr. Dawson.

2. Normal adenosine stress and resting Myoview evaluation, left ventricle. No region suggesting ischemia or infarct.
   ADDENDUM: Previously described fixed perfusion defect involving posterior/inferior wall and apex is no longer seen.
   Left ventricular ejection fraction estimated at 66%. This is normal. Normal is 50% or greater.
   CPT Code(s): _____

ICD-10-CM Code(s): _____

Abstracting Questions

1. Does use of the SPECT camera affect code assignment? _____

2. Were the left ventricular perfusion and ejection fractions reported separately? _____

PRACTICE EXERCISE 21.4   HEAD ULTRASOUND

LOCATION: Inpatient, Hospital
PATIENT: Jason Whittle
ATTENDING PHYSICIAN: Rolando Ortez, MD
CLINICAL SYMPTOMS: Premature, weight 1800 grams.

HEAD ULTRASOUND: Sonographic evaluation of the newborn brain was performed through the anterior fontanel. The study was performed in the coronal and sagittal planes. There is a hyperechoic area seen within the right subependymal region. This measures 0.6 × 0.4 × 0.5 cm. I suspect this is a subependymal hemorrhage. There is also an area within the left intraparenchymal region measuring 0.9 × 1.0 × 1.4 cm. This is a hyperechoic area, which may represent an intraparenchymal hemorrhage on the left parietal/occipital region. There is also question of a small septum cavum pellucidum. This is difficult to state for certain, however.

CONCLUSION

1. What appears to be a right subependymal hemorrhage, as discussed above.
2. Hyperechoic area within the left intraparenchymal region. It may also represent a focal area of hemorrhage measuring 1 cm in greatest diameter.

3. Question of small septum cavum pellucidum as a congenital variation. This is very questionable and difficult to assess for the patient's age. The ventricles themselves do not appear to be grossly dilated.
   CPT Code(s): _____

ICD-10-CM Code(s): _____

Abstracting Questions

1. In what CPT section was the code to report this service located? _____

2. In what CPT category of codes was the code to report this service located? _____

PRACTICE EXERCISE 21.5   NEONATAL CYSTOURETHROGRAM

LOCATION: Inpatient, Hospital
PATIENT: Crystal Morgan
ATTENDING PHYSICIAN: Rolando Ortez, MD
RADIOLOGIST: Morton Monson, MD
CLINICAL SYMPTOMS: Congenital hydronephrosis.

VOIDING URETHROCYSTOGRAPHY: The study is technically limited due to the infant's inability to cooperate. The urinary bladder was filled to presumed capacity before spontaneous voiding. The bladder capacity is estimated at 25 cc. No immediate, delayed, or voiding reflux is demonstrated.

IMPRESSION: No definite vesicoureteral reflux demonstrated.

CPT Code(s): _____

ICD-10-CM Code(s): _____

Abstracting Questions

1. Was this an acquired or congenital condition? _____

2. What type of evaluation was performed? _____

22

Pathology and Laboratory Section (80047-89398, 0001U-0138U)

- Organ or Disease-Oriented Panels
- Drug Assay
- Therapeutic Drug Assays
- Evocative/Suppression Testing
- Consultations (Clinical Pathology)
- Urinalysis
- Molecular Pathology
- Multianalyte Assays with Algorithmic Analyses
- Chemistry
- Hematology and Coagulation
- Immunology
- Transfusion Medicine
- Microbiology
- Anatomic Pathology
- Cytopathology
- Cytogenetic Studies
- Surgical Pathology
- In Vivo (Transcutaneous) Laboratory Procedures
- Other Procedures
- Reproductive Medicine Procedures

Pathology and Laboratory

Codes for laboratory test only
Specimen collection coded separately
Example: Venous blood draw reported with 36415 (Surgery section)

Facility Indicators

Allow additional tests without physician written order
Example: Urinalysis positive for bacteria, built-in indicator for culture

Pathology/Laboratory Caution

Report second or subsequent tests without -51, multiple procedures

Organ or Disease-Oriented Panels (80047-80081)

Groups of tests often ordered together

Examples:
- Basic Metabolic Panel
- General Health Panel
- Electrolyte Panel

Rules of Panels

All tests must have been conducted

Do not use -52, Reduced Service
Additional tests, over those in panel, reported separately
If all tests in panel not done
- List each test separately
- Do not use panel code

Drug Assay

Presumptive Drug Class Screening (80305-80307)

Identifies presence or absence of drug
Chromatography procedure in which single or multiple drugs identified
- Reports thin layer chromatography procedure(s)
- Screening(s) is presumptive
Code by method performed
Example:
- Chemical analyzers = 80307
- Read by instrument = 80306
Does not identify amount of drug present
- Only presence or absence

Therapeutic Drug Assays (80150-80299)

Reports the presence and amount (quantitative)
Material examined can be from any source

Drugs listed by generic names
Example: Amitriptyline, generic name for brand name Elavil

Evocative/Suppression Testing (80400-80439)

Measures stimulating (evocative) or suppressing agents

Codes report only technical component of service
Additional services reported
  • Supplies and/or drugs used in testing (99070 or HCPCS code)
E/M code reported for physician monitoring of test

Consultations (Clinical Pathology) (80500, 80502)

At request of physician
  Additional information about specimen
  Consultant prepares written report

Levels

Limited without review of medical record
  Comprehensive with review of medical record

More Consultation Codes (88321-88334)

Surgical Pathology
Used when pathologist either
  • Reviews slides, material, or reports
  • Provides consultation during surgery
Reported by number of specimens

Urinalysis (81000-81099)
Tests on Urine

Method of test
  • e.g., tablet, reagent, or dipstick
Reason for test
  • e.g., pregnancy
Constituents being tested for
  • e.g., bilirubin, glucose

Equipment Used

Automated or nonautomated
With or without microscope

Molecular Pathology (81105-81408, 81479)

  • 81105-81383 are Tier 1 procedures that report molecular assay
    • More common gene procedures
    • Example, breast cancer gene—81162 (BRCA1 or BRCA2)
  • 81400-81408, 81479 are Tier 2 procedures to report less commonly performed analyses

Multianalyte Assays With Algorithmic Analyses (81490-81599)

Analyses that use the results of various measures and patient information to predict probabilities in a numeric form
  CPT notes and Appendix O provide further detail

Chemistry (82009-84999)

Specific tests on any bodily substances
  • Urine
  • Blood
  • Breath
  • Feces
  • Sputum
    Most are for quantitative (amount of) screenings only
    Few report qualitative (presence of) screenings
    Samples from different sources reported separately, e.g., blood, feces
    Samples taken different times of day reported separately

Hematology and Coagulation (85002-85999)

Laboratory procedures on blood

Example:
  • Complete blood count (CBC)
  • White blood cell count (WBC)
Codes divided based on method of
  • Blood draw
  • Test being conducted

Immunology (86000-86849)

Identifying immune system conditions caused by antibodies and antigens
  Example: Hepatitis C antibody screening

Tissue Typing (86805-86849)

Compatibility test on tissue
  • Match donor to recipient
  • Measure/monitor cytotoxic reactions

Transfusion Medicine (86850-86999)

Blood bank codes
Tests performed on blood or blood products
Identifies
  • Collection
  • Processing
  • Typing

Microbiology (87003-87999)
Study of Microorganisms

Identification of organism
Sensitivities of organism to antibiotics

Anatomic Pathology (88000-88099)

Postmortem examinations

- Autopsies

  Reports only physician service

  Codes divided on extent of exam and type of examination—gross versus gross and microscopic

  Example: Gross examination without central nervous system (88000)

Cytopathology (88104-88199)

Identifies cellular changes

Common laboratory procedures, e.g., Pap smear

Codes divided by

- Type of procedure
- Technique used

Cytogenetic Studies (88230-88299)

Branch of genetics concerned with cellular abnormalities and pathologic conditions

  Example: Chromosomes

Surgical Pathology (88300-88399)

Pathology Terminology

Specimen sample of tissue of suspect area

- Basis of reporting determined by number of labeled specimens

  Block: Frozen piece of specimen

  Section is a slice of frozen block

Evaluation of Specimens to Determine Disease Pathology

Tissue removed during procedures undergoes pathology evaluation

Operative report usually coded after pathology report received

Pathology reports usually coded with operative report

Unit of measure (88300-88309), specimen

- 2 separately identifiable anus tags, each examined, 88304 × 2
- 1 anus tag examined in 2 different areas of tag, 88304

Types of Pathologic Examination

Microscopic: With microscope

Gross: Without microscope

- 88300, only gross exam code
- Other codes are gross and microscopic

Six Levels of Surgical Pathology

Based on specimen examined, e.g., breast, prostate, lung, and reason for evaluation, e.g., radical procedure for suspected carcinoma

  Levels divided on complexity of examination

Example:

  88305, Colon, Biopsy

  88307, Colon, Segmental Resection, Other than for Tumor

  88309, Colon, Total Resection

Level I

Specimen can be accurately diagnosed without microscopic examination

Level II

Gross and microscopic examination is performed on the specimen

Levels III, IV, V, and VI

Include gross and microscopic examination and additional ascending levels of physician work (increasing difficulty)

  Based upon method of or need for removal

  Same anatomical site can be listed in each level

  Additional service codes 88311-88399 are not included in codes 88300-88309

  Example: Special stains (88312)

PRACTICE EXERCISE 22.1 L3-4 DISC

LOCATION: Outpatient, Hospital
PATIENT: Corrine Wilson
ATTENDING PHYSICIAN: Timothy Pleasant, MD
SURGEON: Timothy Pleasant, MD
PATHOLOGIST: Grey Lonewolf, MD
CLINICAL HISTORY: Lumbar disc L3-4 herniation.
SPECIMEN RECEIVED: L3-4 disc.
  GROSS DESCRIPTION: The specimen is labeled with the patient's name and "lumbar disc L3-4" and consists of fibrillary pink-tan tissue fragments. Representative section in one cassette.
  MICROSCOPIC DIAGNOSIS: Fragments of fibrocartilage, consistent with herniated disc L3-4.
CPT Code(s): _____
_____

ICD-10-CM Code(s): _____
_____

Abstracting Questions

1. How would the code for this service be referenced in the CPT index? _____
_____

2. Was the examination gross, microscopic, or both? _____
_____

3. What was the level of surgical pathology? _____

4. Does the pathologic status of the tissue affect the diagnosis code? _____
_____

PRACTICE EXERCISE 22.2 UTERUS, BILATERAL TUBES, AND OVARIES

LOCATION: Outpatient, Hospital
PATIENT: Tina Highdorn
ATTENDING PHYSICIAN: Ira Avila, MD
SURGEON: Ira Avila, MD
PATHOLOGIST: Grey Lonewolf, MD
CLINICAL HISTORY: Menorrhagia.
SPECIMEN RECEIVED: Uterus, bilateral tubes, and ovaries.
  GROSS DESCRIPTION: The specimen is labeled with the patient's name and "uterus, bilateral tubes, and ovaries" and consists of 370 gm; this includes the complete uterus with tubes and ovaries. The uterus measures 14 cm in length × 10 cm in fundal diameter. The specimen is distorted by several bulging areas on the surface. The cervix is transverse. The endometrium is up to 0.3 cm thick and composed of pale tan color. Cut section of the myometrium reveals multiple whirling masses, up to 3 cm in diameter, consisting of white whirling tissue. The fallopian tubes have been surgically divided. The left ovary measures 5 × 4 cm and contains a central cystic structure with smooth lining. A section of the left tube and ovary is placed in cassette labeled 7. The right ovary measures 3 × 2 × 1.5 cm and is composed of wrinkled tan tissue. A section of the right tube and ovary is placed in cassette labeled 8.
  MICROSCOPIC DIAGNOSIS: Sections of cervix show squamous metaplasia. Sections of endometrium show tubular glands lined by pseudostratified columnar epithelium. Small nests of endometrial glands and stroma are noted in the superficial myometrium. Sections of myometrium show masses, consisting of interdigitating bands of smooth muscle. Section of left fallopian tube is unremarkable. Section of left

ovary shows a follicle cyst. Sections of right fallopian tube are unremarkable. Section of right ovary shows physiologic structures.
  DIAGNOSIS
  Complete uterus, tubes, and ovaries showing:
1. Squamous metaplasia, cervix.
2. Proliferating endometrium.
3. Adenomyosis, uterus.
4. Multiple intramural leiomyomata.
5. Status post surgical division of fallopian tubes.
6. Follicle cyst, left ovary.
  CPT Code(s): _____
_____

  ICD-10-CM Code(s): _____
_____

Abstracting Questions

1. When you reference "Metaplasia, cervix" in the Index of the ICD-10-CM, you are referred to what code? _____
_____

2. The clinical history was menorrhagia. What is menorrhagia?
_____
_____

3. Why was it not correct to report menorrhagia as the diagnosis? _____
_____

PRACTICE EXERCISE 22.3 PLACENTA

LOCATION: Inpatient, Hospital
PATIENT: Cindy Kretchenhoff
ATTENDING PHYSICIAN: Ira Avila, MD
SURGEON: Ira Avila, MD
PATHOLOGIST: Grey Lonewolf, MD
CLINICAL HISTORY: 31 weeks, 6 days' gestation, possible placental abruption.
SPECIMEN RECEIVED: Placenta.

  GROSS DESCRIPTION: Submitted in formalin, labeled with the patient's name, and "placenta" is 600 gm. Discoid placenta measuring 18 × 17 × 3 cm, with three centrally attached vessels and 5 cm long umbilical cord. The umbilical cord shows no knots or gross abnormalities (cassette 1). The membranes are tan and opaque and show no significant exudates, nodules, or green discoloration (cassette 2). The fetal surface of placenta shows a normal vascular pattern. The maternal surface features multiple intact cotyledons. No

Continued

PRACTICE EXERCISE 22.3 PLACENTA—cont'd

significant adherent blood clot or cotyledon compression is seen. Sectioning reveals dark red to purple spongy parenchyma without significant scarlike areas or masses. Representative sections of central and peripheral placenta are submitted in cassettes 3 and 4, respectively (two separate specimens, placenta and umbilical cord).

MICROSCOPIC DIAGNOSIS: Sections are umbilical cord showing three vessels. No significant inflammatory infiltrates are seen. Sections of membranes feature intact chorionic and amnionic membranes. Focal mild neutrophilic infiltrates are identified within chorionic membranes. Sections of placenta show multiple chorionic villi with villous architecture consistent with 32 weeks' gestational age. Villous vascularity is within normal limits. There is mild intervillous fibrin deposition. No significant large vessels lesions are seen. Minimal neutrophilic infiltrates are present within the fibrin beneath the chorionic plate.

DIAGNOSIS: Placenta, delivery; early third-trimester placenta, membranes, and umbilical cord showing mild early placentitis.

COMMENTS: While no gross pathologic changes of placental abruption are seen, acute abruption may not be accompanied by demonstrable placental changes at the time of pathologic examination.

CPT Code(s): _____

_____

ICD-10-CM Code(s): _____

_____

Abstracting Questions

1. How many specimens were examined? _____

   _____

2. According to the notes in the CPT manual before 88300, the unit of services for codes 88300 through 88309 is the what? _____

3. Also in the notes of the CPT manual before 88300, a specimen is defined as tissue(s) submitted for individual and separate attention, requiring individual examination and pathologic _____

   _____.

PRACTICE EXERCISE 22.4 CERVICAL DISC

LOCATION: Outpatient, Hospital
PATIENT: Sally Reagon
ATTENDING PHYSICIAN: Timothy Pleasant, MD
SURGEON: Timothy Pleasant, MD
PATHOLOGIST: Grey Lonewolf, MD
CLINICAL HISTORY: Severe cervical spinal stenosis.
SPECIMEN RECEIVED: Cervical disc.
GROSS DESCRIPTION: The specimen is labeled with the patient's name and "cervical disc" and consists of approximately 5 grams of tan fibrous fragments.
MICROSCOPIC DIAGNOSIS: Sections show disc tissue.
DIAGNOSIS: Disc tissue (cervical).

CPT Code(s): _____

_____

ICD-10-CM Code(s): _____

_____

Abstracting Question

1. What statement in the code description for 88304 identifies cervical disc pathological examination? _____

   _____

PRACTICE EXERCISE 22.5 CEREBRAL HEMATOMA

LOCATION: Inpatient, Hospital
PATIENT: Daniel Smithson
ATTENDING PHYSICIAN: Timothy Pleasant, MD
SURGEON: Timothy Pleasant, MD
PATHOLOGIST: Grey Lonewolf, MD
CLINICAL HISTORY: Nontraumatic cerebral bleeding.
SPECIMEN RECEIVED: Cerebral hematoma.
GROSS DESCRIPTION: Submitted in formalin and labeled with the patient's name and "cerebral hematoma" are fragments of reddish brown blood clot measuring approximately 4.5 × 3.5 × 1.5 cm in aggregate. Representative fragments are submitted in one cassette.
MICROSCOPIC DIAGNOSIS: Sections show fragments of fresh blood clot and a single fragment of brain parenchyma featuring intact cortex and underlying white matter and mild-to-moderate edema. No neoplasm is identified.
DIAGNOSIS: Cerebral hematoma, evacuation: Recent blood clot and benign brain parenchyma.

CPT Code(s): _____

_____

ICD-10-CM Code(s): _____

_____

Abstracting Question

1. How many cassettes were submitted? _____

   _____

23
Medicine Section (90281-99607)

Most procedures noninvasive (not entering body)

Contains invasive procedures
Example: 92973, Percutaneous thrombectomy
Many specialized tests
Example: Audiology and biofeedback
Special lightning bolt icon (⚡)
- Indicates substances pending FDA (Food and Drug Administration) approval

Immunizations

Often used
Two types of immunizations
- Active and passive
Correct coding includes
- Supply injected
- Administration of injection

Active—Bacteria or Virus

Bacteria that cause disease made nontoxic (toxoid)
- Injected to build immunity
  Small dose active virus injected (vaccine)
- Injected to build immunity
  Example: Poliovirus

Passive Immunization

Does not cause immune response
    Contains antibodies against certain diseases—immune globulins

Immune Globulins (90281-90399)

Identifies immune globulin product
    Example: Botulism antitoxin
    Report administration separately

Immune Globulin Codes Divided by

Type
e.g., rabies, hepatitis B

Method
e.g., intramuscular, intravenous, subcutaneous

Dose
e.g., full dose, minidose

Immunization Administration (90460-90474)

Administration (giving of substance)
- Reported in addition to substance given
- 90460, 90461 Patients through age 18 when counseled regarding immunization
- 90471-90474
- 90471, +90472 = Percutaneous, intradermal, subcutaneous, or intramuscular injection
- 90473, +90474 = Oral or intranasal

Methods of Administration

- Percutaneous
- Intradermal
- Subcutaneous
- Intramuscular
- Intranasal
- Oral

Report Administration for Each Dose— Single or Combination

Example: 10-year-old patient receives 3 separate injections
- 90471 administration tetanus
- 90472 administration rubella
- 90472 administration diphtheria
  OR depending on payer:
- 90471 administration tetanus
- 90472 × 2 administration rubella and diphtheria

Vaccines, Toxoids (Vaccine Product Codes) (90476-90749)

Many codes age or dosage specific
Example: 90702, Diphtheria and tetanus toxoids absorbed (DT), younger than 7 years
Codes for products for single diseases
Example: 90713, Poliovirus vaccine, inactivated (IPV)
Codes for combination diseases

Example: 90700, diphtheria, tetanus toxoids, and acellular pertussis (DTaP)

Some vaccines given on schedule

Example: 90633, 2-dose hepatitis A vaccine

- 1st dose, 1st visit
- 2nd dose, 2nd visit

Caution: There Are Multiple Diphtheria Codes

- 90696-90723 diphtheria and diphtheria with other substances

    Example: 90698, diphtheria, tetanus toxoids, and acellular pertussis (synthetic form of pertussis) (DTaP), *Haemophilus influenzae* type b (HiB), and inactivated poliovirus (IPV) for IM use

---

> **NOTE**
>
> **Remember**
>
> Third-party payers do not usually require modifier -51 used with Vaccine/Toxoid codes
>
> Rather, depending on payer, list each code multiple times or use times (x) symbol and indicate number

---

Important Reporting Rule

If vaccine administered during an office visit that was not related to the E/M

- Report E/M service (with modifier -25) + vaccine + administration

    Office visit for vaccine only: Report only vaccine and the administration (no E/M service)

Routine Vaccinations

Influenza

Substance (vaccine) 90653-90668 and 90685-90688

- G0008 HCPCS National Level II for Medicare patients
- 90471/90472

Pneumococcal

Substance (vaccine) 90732

Administration

- G0009 HCPCS National Level II for Medicare
- 90471/90472 administration

Psychiatry (90785-90899)

Psychiatric Diagnostic Evaluation

Involved assessment to identify patient diagnosis and develop treatment plan

Codes for evaluation (90791) and evaluation with medical service (90792)

Psychotherapy

Therapeutic treatment of psychological disorder or behavior

Service reported with codes 90832-90838

- Time-based codes
    - 90832, 90833 (16-37 minutes), 90834, 90836 (38-52 minutes), 90837, 90838 (53 minutes or more)
- Codes subdivided based on if psychotherapy provided in addition to a primary procedure
- Provided to patient only

Other Psychotherapy

- Crisis psychotherapy provides treatment for a patient experiencing a reaction to a more specific event or situation (90839, 90840)

    Codes 90845-90853 report services for
- Psychoanalysis
- Family, multiple-family, and group psychotherapy

Biofeedback (90901, 90912-90913)

Used to help patients gain control over body processes

Example: Elevated BP (blood pressure) or manage chronic pain

Patient training in biofeedback by professional

- Continues on own

Services often part psychophysiologic (mind/body) therapy

90912 reports initial 15 minutes, 90913 add-on code reports each additional 15 minutes

Dialysis (90935-90999)

Cleanses blood

- Temporary (non-ESRD [end-stage renal disease])
- Permanent (ESRD)

Two parts to report ESRD dialysis services

- Physician service
- Hemodialysis procedure

Hemodialysis Service (90935-90940)

Hemodialysis is the procedure

Used for ESRD and non-ESRD

Billed per day for inpatients receiving hemodialysis and also for outpatient non-ESRD

Includes all physician E/M services related to procedure

- Use modifier -25 if separate E/M service provided

Miscellaneous Dialysis Procedures (90945-90947)

Describes other dialysis procedures

Example: Peritoneal dialysis in which toxins are passively absorbed into dialysis fluid

Services billed on per-day basis for inpatient ESRD patients

ESRD Physician Services (90951-90970)

Include

- Establishment of dialyzing cycle
- Physician services
- E/M outpatient dialysis visits
- Telephone calls
- Patient management during dialysis

Reported Per Month: 90951-90966

Month is defined as 30 days

Less than full month of service 90967-90970 per day

Codes divided by age and number of encounters

Codes are used to report outpatient dialysis services for ESRD patients

Other Diagnosis Procedures (90989-90999)

Patients can receive training in self-dialysis (90989, 90993)

Codes divided by complete or partial training program

Gastroenterology (91010-91299)

For tests and treatments of esophagus, stomach, and intestine

Codes usually reported with E/M or consultation service code

- **Caution:** Many bundled services

Ophthalmology (92002-92499)

Contains E/M "eye" codes

Definitions for new and established patients same as for E/M section

Codes are for bilateral services

- If only one eye, use modifier -52 (reduced service)

Special Ophthalmologic Services (92015-92287)

For special evaluations of visual system

Goes beyond those usually provided in evaluation

May be reported in addition to basic visual service

Special Otorhinolaryngologic Services (92502-92700)

Special treatments and diagnostic services

Example: Nasal function tests (rhinomanometry) or audiometric tests

All hearing tests bilateral unless one ear indicated in description

Cardiovascular in Medicine Section (See pg. 182 for Details)

Services can be

- Invasive or noninvasive
- Diagnostic or therapeutic

Subheadings

- Therapeutic Services and Procedures
- Cardiography
- Cardiovascular Monitoring Services
- Implantable, Insertable, and Wearable Cardiac Device Evaluations
- Echocardiography
- Cardiac Catheterization
- Intracardiac Electrophysiologic Procedures/Studies
- Peripheral Arterial Disease Rehabilitation

- Noninvasive Physiologic Studies and Procedures
- Other Procedures
- Other Vascular Studies

Home and Outpatient International Normalized Ratio (INR) Monitoring Services, 93792 and 93793

- Anticoagulants such as warfarin
  - Thins the blood
- By physician or another qualified health care professional
- Provided in home or outpatient setting
  - 93792 reports training
  - 93793 reports management, billed once per day

Noninvasive Vascular Diagnostic Studies (93880-93998)

Vascular codes for procedures on noncoronary veins and arteries

Include

- Patient care
- Supervision and interpretation (S&I)
- Copy of results

Pulmonary (94002-94799)

For ventilation management therapies and diagnostic tests

Includes procedure and interpretation of test results

- Additional E/M service reported separately

Allergy and Clinical Immunology (95004-95199)

Divided into three subheadings

1. Allergy Testing (95004-95070)
2. Ingestion Challenge Testing (95076-95079)
3. Allergen Immunotherapy (95115-95199)

Allergy Testing (95004-95070)

Sensitivity testing using various types of tests with type and number of tests based on physician's judgment

Example: Percutaneous, intracutaneous, inhalation

Example: Extracts, venoms, biologics, and foods

Medical record will indicate

- Number and type of tests
- Method testing

Ingestion Challenge Testing (95076, 95079)

- Sensitivity to food, drugs, and other substances
- 95076 initial 120 minutes; 95079 each additional 60 minutes
- Services less than 60 minutes, report E/M code

Allergen Immunotherapy (95115-95199)

Codes divided into three types of services:

1. Injection only
2. Prescription and injection

3. Provision of antigen (substance) only
Physician service bundled into immunotherapy codes
If separate E/M service provided, report separately

Neurology and Neuromuscular Procedures (95700-96020)

Contains codes to report tests, such as
- Sleep tests
- Muscle tests (electromyography)
- Range-of-motion measurements
- Electroencephalogram (EEG)
- Electromyography (EMG)
- Analysis and programming of neurostimulators
- Motion analysis
- Functional brain mapping
Many bundled services
Services usually provided in addition to E/M service

Medical Genetics and Genetic Counseling Services (96040)

Trained genetic counselors assess risk of genetic defects in offspring

Includes
- Pedigree construction
- Obtaining structured genetic history
- Analysis of risk
- Counseling

Central Nervous System (CNS) Assessments/ Tests (96105-96146)

Used to report
- Psychological tests
- Speech/Language assessments
- Developmental progress assessments
- Thinking/Reasoning examinations
Standardized cognitive performance testing
Codes based on per-hour basis/first hour, each additional 30 minutes
- Includes written report of results

Health Behavior Assessment and Intervention (96156-96171)

- Identify psychological behavior, emotional, cognitive, or social factors important to treatment or management of physical health problems

Hydration, Therapeutic, Prophylactic, Diagnostic Injections and Infusions, and Chemotherapy and Other Highly Complex Drug or Highly Complex Biologic Agent Administration (96360-96549)

Infusion: Therapeutic procedure to introduce fluid into body

Hydration: Infusion for purpose of rehydration; includes prepackaged fluid

Injection: Subcutaneous (Sub-Q, SC), intramuscular (IM), intra-arterial (IA), and intravenous (IV)

Codes report the physician work related to the infusion, hydration, or injection
- Affirmation of treatment plan
- Direct supervision of staff
- Significant, separately identifiable E/M is reported with -25

Codes include
- Local anesthesia
- Intravenous start
- Access to indwelling intravenous catheter or port
- Flush at conclusion
- Standard tubing, syringes, and supplies

Multiple drug administrations in same session are reported separately

Use only one initial code to report multiple infusions or injections or combinations
For the physician, assign initial code based on primary reason for encounter
The secondary infusion/injection is reported with a subsequent or concurrent code, unless the protocol requires two separate IV sites
Example: If three different agents were administered in the same session, report one initial code and two additional sequential codes
Determination of initial code is based on primary reason for encounter
Some codes are time based, so medical documentation must indicate time infusion begins and ends
Time is defined as the actual time used to administer the drug/substance

Hydration (96360, 96361)

IV infusion for hydration and includes prepackaged fluid/ electrolytes
- 96360 IV infusion for hydration up to 1 hour
- 96361 IV infusion for hydration, each additional hour
  - Report for hydration intervals greater than 30 minutes beyond 1 hour
  - Start infusion time over if a different bag is started
  - Do not report hydration codes when the fluid is used to administer a drug (incidental hydration)
  - Do not report hydration codes for infusion of <30 minutes

Therapeutic, Prophylactic, and Diagnostic Injections and Infusions (Excludes Chemotherapy and Other Highly Complex Drug or Highly Complex Biologic Agent Administration) (96365-96379)

Types of drug administration
- Therapeutic
- Prophylactic
- Diagnostic

Codes divided by administration method
- Subcutaneous
- Intramuscular
- Intra-arterial
- Intravenous push
  A push is defined as when a health care professional is needed to administer the drug/substance and monitor the patient for an infusion that takes 15 minutes or less to administer
  Also report the substance administered
  96365-96368 report therapeutic, prophylactic, or diagnostic IV infusions, other than hydration and chemotherapy
- Typically require direct physician supervision
- Special consideration for preparing, dosing, or disposing
- Trained staff who administer infusion
- Monitoring of vital signs during infusion

Chemotherapy and Other Highly Complex Drug or Highly Complex Biologic Agent Administration (96401-96549)

Represents only preparation and administration of chemotherapy
- If separate E/M service provided, report E/M code + -25
  Report all drugs/substances separately
  Codes are not limited to patients with diagnosis of cancer
  Codes also include infusion of antineoplastic agents, monoclonal antibody agents, and biological response modifiers for treatment of noncancer diagnoses
  Chemical can be administered (injected) into
- Lesion
- Vein
- Tissue
- Muscle
- Artery
- Cavity
- Nerve
  Intravenously injected chemicals: Two methods of delivery of chemical
1. IV push quickly delivers substance/medication into vein (15 minutes or less)
2. IV infusion delivers over longer period of time
   Codes often divided by time the infusion/injection procedure takes
   Example: 96413 chemotherapy administration, intravenous, infusion up to 1 hour
   Report the initial code that represents the main reason why the patient was being treated, even though it might not be the first drug/substance infused
   Example: Patient received 1 hour of hydration first, then 2 hours of chemotherapy intravenously. Code the initial chemotherapy infusion 96413 for the first hour of chemo, 96415 for the second hour, then code 96360 for the hydration
   Special supplies (e.g., special needles) reported separately using 99070 or HCPCS National Level II code
   Report any intra-arterial catheter placement with 36620-36640
   Injections with chemotherapy

- Report separately any analgesic or antiemetic (for vomiting)
- Given before or after chemotherapy

> **NOTE**
> Use code J0881 to report injection of darbepoetin alfa and J0885 to report injection of epoetin alfa

Photodynamic Therapy (96567-96574)

Used in addition to bronchoscopy or endoscopy codes
Injected agent remains in premalignant cells longer than normal cells
- After agent dissipates from normal cells, patient exposed to laser light
- Agent absorbs light
- Light produces oxygen and premalignant cells destroyed

Special Dermatologic Procedures (96900-96999)

Usually specialized procedures provided on consultation basis
- Separate E/M consultation code would then be appropriate
  Treatment of skin conditions:
  Actinotherapy—with ultraviolet light
  Photochemotherapy—with light-sensitive chemicals and light rays

Physical Medicine & Rehabilitation (97010-97799)

Used by physicians and therapists to report a variety of services

Treatments

Traction
Modalities
Electrical stimulation (used to help heal fractures)
Therapeutic procedures
Gait training
Functional activities

Patient Training

Codes often have time components
Example: 97761 reports prosthetic training, extremity(ies), initial encounter, each 15 minutes

Active Wound Care Management (97597-97610)

Debridement

Debridement without anesthesia with removal of devitalized tissue by different techniques, such as water pressure, sharp selective debridement with scissors, scalpel, and forceps
97597 and 97598 include total surface area of all wounds

Codes based on centimeters treated

Nonselective debridement (97602): Healthy tissue removed along with necrotic tissue, with wet-to-moist dressings, enzymatic or abrasive methods

Negative pressure wound therapy (NPWT) (97605, 97606)

- Vacuuming of drainage and tissue from wound
  - Then negative pressure draws the edges of the wound together
- Application of topical medications/ointments
- Assessment of wound
- Directions to patient on continued care of wound
- Each code for ongoing care reported on per-session basis

Osteopathic and Chiropractic Services (98925-98943)

Both inpatient and outpatient settings
Physician services bundled into codes
Codes divided by body area

Education and Training for Patient Self-Management (98960-98962)

- Use of standardized curriculum for education to individual or group for management of illness

Non–Face-to-Face Nonphysician Services (98966-98972)

Reports nonphysician E/M services using telephone/Internet
Established patient, family member of the patient, or a guardian
98966-98968 telephone E/M services

98970-98972 online digital E/M services
To report physician services, see 99441-99443

Special Services, Procedures, and Reports (99000-99082)

Handling and conveyance of laboratory specimens
- 99000-99002
  Postoperative follow-up visits included in surgical package
- 99024
  Office visits after posted hours or in locations other than office
- 99050-99060
  Supplies and materials
- 99070
  Hospital mandated on-call services
- 99026, 99027

Moderate (Conscious) Sedation (99151-99157)

Type of sedation in which the patient can respond to verbal commands
When sedation is provided by same physician performing procedure, report with 99151-99153
- Second physician provides sedation, report with 99155-99157
  Included in service is:
- Patient assessment
- IV establishment
- Administration of agent
- Maintenance of sedation
- Monitoring of vital signs
- Recovery
  Codes divided based on patient age (under 5, 5 and over) and time (15 minutes and each 15 minutes over)

PRACTICE EXERCISE 23.1 CARDIAC CATHETERIZATION

CARDIAC CATHETERIZATION REPORT
LOCATION: Inpatient, Hospital
PATIENT: Wade Land
REFERRING PHYSICIAN: James Noonar, MD
CARDIOLOGIST: Marvin Elhart, MD
INDICATION: Unstable angina.
PROCEDURE: Right iliofemoral angiography, left heart catheterization, selective coronary angiography, and left ventriculography.
COMPLICATIONS: None.
   RESULTS: Hemodynamics: The left ventricular pressure before the LV gram was 133/7 with an LVEDP of 11. After the LV gram it was 130/8 with an LVEDP of 12. The aortic pressure on pullback was 130/59.
   Left Ventriculography: Showed that the left ventricle is normal in size. It was hard to assess segmental wall motion because of the frequency of PVCs; however, the overall left ventricular systolic function was normal. There might be some distal anterior wall hypokinesis.
   Selective Coronary Angiography
1. Right coronary artery: This was a medium-size dominant artery that has mild diffuse atherosclerotic changes. After the PDA there was about 30% narrowing.

2. Left main coronary artery: This has 80-90% eccentric narrowing in the midportion.
3. Left circumflex artery: This was a medium-size artery that has mild atherosclerotic changes proximally. It gave rise to a medium-size bifurcating first obtuse marginal that has 99% proximal narrowing. The inferior of the two branches, which was a smaller size artery, has 90% proximal narrowing.
4. Left anterior descending coronary artery: This was a medium-size artery that has mild diffuse atherosclerotic changes. The first diagonal was a small artery that had 90% proximal narrowing. The second diagonal was a larger artery that has about 60% narrowing in the midportion. Immediately after that diagonal, the left anterior descending artery has about 50% narrowing. There was moderate diffuse disease after that. Please note that the visualization of the diagonals and the left anterior descending artery was rather limited as we tried not to inject in a strong way into the left main.
CONCLUSION
1. Normal overall left ventricular systolic function.
2. Severe left main disease.
3. Severe left circumflex and first diagonal disease.

PRACTICE EXERCISE 23.1 CARDIAC CATHETERIZATION—cont'd

RECOMMENDATIONS
1. Maximum medical treatment.
2. Intra-aortic balloon pump.
3. Consult CT surgery to evaluate the patient for bypass surgery.

CPT Code(s): _____

_____

ICD-10-CM Code(s): _____

_____

Abstracting Questions

1. What are the three categories bundled into the code reported for cardiac catheterization? _____

_____

2. What was the approach for this procedure? _____

_____

3. Was a modifier required on the catheterization code, and if a modifier was required, which one would it be? _____

_____

4. For what two procedures were injections provided?

_____

PRACTICE EXERCISE 23.2 SAPHENOUS VEIN MAPPING

RADIOLOGY REPORT
LOCATION: Outpatient, Hospital
PATIENT: Mirta Hubert
ORDERING PHYSICIAN: James Noonar, MD
ATTENDING/ADMIT PHYSICIAN: James Noonar, MD
RADIOLOGIST: Morton Monson, MD
PERSONAL PHYSICIAN: Alma Naraquist, MD
EXAMINATION: Saphenous vein mapping.

CLINICAL SYMPTOMS: Pre-coronary artery bypass graft; atherosclerotic heart disease of native coronary arteries, chest pain.

FINDINGS: The left greater saphenous vein was mapped from midthigh through the proximal calf. Measurements above the knee were 1.0 × 0.92 cm, at the knee 0.73 × 0.73 cm, and below the knee 0.54 × 0.54 cm. The multiple branches encountered were not evaluated.

CPT Code(s): _____

_____

ICD-10-CM Code(s): _____

_____

Abstracting Question

1. What type of scan was used for mapping of vessels?

_____

PRACTICE EXERCISE 23.3 VENOUS ULTRASOUND

RADIOLOGY REPORT
LOCATION: Inpatient, Hospital
PATIENT: Dave James
ORDERING PHYS ICIAN: Frank Gaul, MD
ATTENDING/ADMIT PHYSICIAN: Frank Gaul, MD
RADIOLOGIST: Morton Monson, MD
PERSONAL PHYSICIAN: Frank Gaul, MD
EXAMINATION: Bilateral lower extremity venous ultrasound.
CLINICAL SYMPTOMS: Leg pain and swelling. Rule out deep venous thrombosis.

FINDINGS: This examination was somewhat limited as a result of the patient being recently out of surgery and unable to be moved at all. As visualized, both the right and the left common femoral, superficial femoral, popliteal, and posterior tibial veins are fully compressible and demonstrate the presence of normal spontaneous, phasic, and augmented flow.

IMPRESSION: No evidence for deep venous thrombosis is seen within either of the lower extremities. Please see above comments.

CPT Code(s): _____

_____

ICD-10-CM Code(S): _____

_____

Abstracting Question

1. What is a deep venous thrombosis? _____

_____

PRACTICE EXERCISE 23.4
EXTREMITIES ULTRASOUND

RADIOLOGY REPORT
LOCATION: Outpatient, Hospital
PATIENT: Eric Tayes
ORDERING PHYSICIAN: Frank Gaul, MD
ATTENDING/ADMIT PHYSICIAN: Frank Gaul, MD
RADIOLOGIST: Morton Monson, MD
EXAMINATION: Ultrasound of both lower extremities; abdomen ultrasound.
CLINICAL SYMPTOMS: Lower extremity swelling, difficulty breathing.
FINDINGS: Ultrasound examination of the deep venous system of both lower extremities is negative. No evidence of deep venous thrombosis in either lower extremity. The posterior tibial, greater saphenous, and popliteal through the femoral veins are patent and negative for thrombus bilaterally. Normal phasicity.

Abdomen Ultrasound: Diffusely coarsened echotexture of the liver with some nodularity consistent with fatty infiltration. Cirrhotic configuration of the liver. Small calcified granuloma in the spleen. The spleen is otherwise negative. There is ascites in all four quadrants. No bile duct dilatation. No gallbladder wall thickening or cholelithiasis. Small amount of fluid adjacent to the gallbladder is likely related to the ascites. The pancreas is obscured by bowel gas. The abdominal aorta is of normal caliber. The right kidney measures approximately 9 cm in length and shows no evidence of hydronephrosis, calculi, or mass. The left kidney measures approximately 9.9 cm in length and shows no evidence of hydronephrosis, calculi, or mass.

CPT Code(s): _____

_____

ICD-10-CM Code(s): _____

_____

Abstracting Questions

1. How was the scan for the abdomen different from the scan for the extremities? _____

_____

2. How would the "cirrhotic configuration of the liver" diagnosis be reported? _____

_____

PRACTICE EXERCISE 23.5
RENAL DIALYSIS PROGRESS NOTE

RENAL DIALYSIS PROGRESS NOTE
LOCATION: Outpatient, Clinic
PATIENT: Jyl Couts
PHYSICIAN: Ira Avila, MD
The 45-year-old patient presents today for regular monthly visit. She has been slightly tired. She denies any shortness of breath or chest pain. No constipation. The patient complains of some weakness in her legs when she walks to the grocery store.

PHYSICAL EXAMINATION: Her blood pressure at home has been in the 130s/80s. On exam today, her weight is 152.5 pounds. Regular heart rate at 79 per minute. The lungs are clear bilaterally without crackles. No edema in the extremities. Catheter condition is good, and the exit site is clean and dry. No evidence of infection.
IMPRESSION/PLAN
1. The patient is on CAPD, two bag sizes of 1.5% and 2.5%; doing well with that.
2. She is on 4000 units of EPO once a week due to anemia due to end-stage renal disease with hemoglobin of 12. We will continue that at this time.
3. The patient has possibility of claudication. She has history of an aneurysm, which was measured at 6.1 cm on a CT scan done in the transverse section. We will obtain an ultrasound to follow up on her abdominal aortic aneurysm and do ABIs on the lower extremities.
4. The patient requested a handicap permit, and I will hold that for now until we do her studies.
The patient seems to agree with the plan.

CPT Code(s): _____

_____

ICD-10-CM Code(s): _____

_____

Abstracting Questions

1. Does the type of dialysis the patient receives affect code selection? _____

_____

2. What is end-stage renal disease? _____

_____

24
HCPCS Coding

Developed by Centers for Medicare and Medicaid Services (CMS)
- Formerly HCFA
  HCPCS developed in 1983
  CPT did not contain all codes necessary for Medicare services reporting

One of Two Levels of Codes

1. Level I, CPT
2. Level II, HCPCS, also known as national codes

Phased-out Level III, Local Codes

Developed by Medicare and other carriers for use at local level
Varied by locale
Discontinued October 2002 due to HIPAA code set regulations
Some codes incorporated into HCPCS Level I and Level II

Level II, National Codes

Codes for wide variety of providers
- Physicians
- Dentists
- Orthodontists
  Codes for wide variety of services
- Specific drugs
- Durable medical equipment (DME)
- Ambulance services

Code book published every January, but codes are added and deleted throughout the year and providers are notified through carrier bulletins

Format

Begins with letter, followed by four digits

Example: E0605, Vaporizer, room type
Each letter represents group codes
Example: "J" codes used to report drugs, J0585, onabotulinumtoxinA, 1 unit

Temporary Codes

Certain letters indicate temporary codes
Example: K0552, Supplies for external drug infusion pump
- K codes are temporary codes

HCPCS National Level II Index

Directs coder to specific codes
Do not code directly from index
Reference main portion of text before assigning code
Alphabetical order

Table of Drugs

Listed by generic name, not brand name

PART 5

ICD-10-CM and ICD-10-PCS Coding

25
ICD-10-CM Overview

Introduction

Morbidity (illness)
Mortality (death)
CM = Clinical Modification
PCS = Procedural Coding System
Provides continuity of data
World Health Organization's ICD-10 used globally
The United States develops ICD-10-CM and ICD-10-PCS
   version

Uses of ICD-10-CM

Facilitate payment of health services
Evaluate patients' use of health services
Fiscal entities track health care costs
Research
   • Health care quality
   • Future needs
   • Newer cancer center built if patient use warrants
   • Predict health care trends
   • Plan for future health care needs

ICD-10-CM on CMS-1500 (Fig. 25.1)

Diagnoses establish medical necessity
Services and diagnoses must correlate
CMS-1500 example (Fig. 25.1)

Ethics

Documentation must support diagnosis and match procedures or service performed
Example:
   • Services provided

• Diagnosis justifies services
   If in doubt, check it out; don't make assumptions
   Your job: Translate documentation into ICD-10-CM
      codes

Format

Diseases, Tabular List
Diseases, Alphabetic Index

Diseases, Tabular List

Contains alphanumeric codes with descriptions
   A00-Z99 diagnosis codes describe condition
   22 chapters

Diseases, Alphabetic Index

Appears first in book
Refers coder to alphanumeric code in Volume 1
Never code directly from Index!

Placeholder

Character "X" is used as a placeholder for future expansion
   Example: T36-T50 range of codes, "X" is placeholder
      • T35.5X1A: Poisoning by, tetracyclines, intentional
         self-harm, initial encounter

7th Character

Certain categories have 7th character
   Example: T36-T50 range of codes, "A" is 7th character
      to report initial encounter
      • T36.4X2A: Poisoning by tetracyclines, intentional
         self-harm, initial encounter

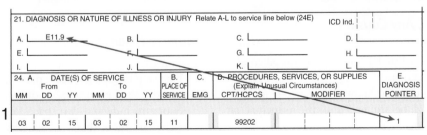

• **Figure 25.1** Diagnosis code and service must correlate.

Abbreviations

Symbols, abbreviations, punctuation, and notations
  NEC: Not elsewhere classifiable
  - No more-specific code exists
  - Means "other specified"
  NOS: Not otherwise specified
  - Unspecified in documentation

Punctuation

[ ] Brackets

Tabular:
- Enclose synonyms, alternative wording, or explanatory phrases
- Helpful, additional information
- Can affect code
- Located in Tabular List A00-Z99

Index: Brackets enclose manifestation codes

( ) Parentheses

Located in Tabular List and Index
- Contain enclosed nonessential modifiers
  Does not affect code

: Colon

Located in Tabular
  Completes statement with one or more modifiers
  Bold type
  Codes and code titles in Tabular

Italicized Type

Located in Tabular
  see
  Located in Index
  see also, see condition, *see also* condition, *omit code*

Includes, Excludes, Use Additional Code

Includes: Conditions included in code
Excludes1: Condition not coded here
Excludes2: Not included here code but may be an additional code, when documented
Use additional code: Assignment of other code(s) as necessary

And/With

And: Means "and/or"
  With: One condition with (in addition to) another condition; "associated with" or "due to"

Code, if Applicable, Any Causal Condition First

May be principal or first-listed diagnosis if no causal condition applicable or known
- If the causal condition is known, then a code for that condition should be sequenced as the principal or first-listed code diagnosis

Alphabetic Index

Nonessential modifiers: Have no effect on code selection
- Enclosed in parentheses
- Clarify diagnosis
  Example: **Ileus** (bowel) (colon) (inhibitory) (intestine) K56.7

Terms

Main terms (bold typeface)
  Subterms
  - Indented two spaces to right
  - Not bold

Cross References in the Index

Directs you: *see, see also, use*
- "*see*" directs you to specific term, must be reference
  Example: Pelade—*see* Alopecia, areata
- "*see also*" directs you to another term for more information, may also be reference
  Example: Pneumopericarditis—*see also* Pericarditis
- "*see* condition" directs you to specific information about assignment of the code
  Example: Vesicourethrorectal—*see* condition
- "*see also* condition" directs you to specific information about assignment of the code
  Example: Abdomen, abdominal—*see also* condition
- "*use*" directs you to the appropriate entry

Notes

Define terms
  Give further coding instructions
  Example: Tabular H00-H59
  - Note: Use an external cause code following the code for the eye condition, if applicable, to identify the cause of the eye condition

Eponyms

Disease or syndromes named for person
  Example: Goldberg-Maxwell syndrome E34.51

Etiology and Manifestation of Disease

Etiology = cause of disease
  Manifestation = symptom
  Combination codes = etiology and manifestation in one code
  Example: E11.341 Type 2 diabetes mellitus with severe nonprolifererative diabetic retinopathy with macular edema

Index to Diseases

Largest part
  First step in coding, locate main term in Index by condition, sign, symptom, or disease—not body area
  Subterms indented two spaces to right
  May have more than one subterm

Table of Neoplasms

Table of Neoplasms (illustrated in Fig. 25.2)
- Located after the Z Index entries

Table of Drugs and Chemicals

Located after the Index of Diseases

Contains classification of drugs and substances to identify poisoning, adverse effects, and underdosing
- Adverse effect occurs when substance is taken correctly but patient has a negative reaction to substance

Condition code for drug found under "Adverse Effect" column
- Poisoning occurs when substance is incorrectly taken

Example: Amoxicillin prescribed for bronchitis causes rash (adverse effect); or rather than one tablet of prescribed amoxicillin, patient takes four tablets and nausea results (poisoning)

Drug name placed alphabetically on left under heading "Substance" (Fig. 25.3)

First column: "Poisoning, Accidental (Unintentional)" lists code for substance involved if not related to an adverse effect

	Malignant Primary	Malignant Secondary	Ca in situ	Benign	Uncertain Behavior	Unspecified Behavior
appendix	C18.1	C78.5	D01.0	D12.1	D37.3	D49.0
arachnoid	C70.9	C79.49	—	D32.9	D42.9	D49.7
cerebral	C70.0	C79.32	—	D32.0	D42.0	D49.7
spinal	C70.1	C79.49	—	D32.1	D42.1	D49.7
areola	C50.0-●	C79.81	D05.-●	D24.-●	D48.6-●	D49.3
arm NEC	C76.4-●	C79.89	D04.6-●	D36.7	D48.7	D49.89

• **Figure 25.2** Table of Neoplasms.

Substance	External Cause (T-Code)					
	Poisoning, Accidental (Unintentional)	Poisoning, Intentional Self-Harm	Poisoning, Assault	Poisoning, Undetermined	Adverse Effect	Underdosing
Acetylsalicylic acid (salts)	T39.011	T39.012	T39.013	T39.014	T39.015	T39.016
enteric coated	T39.011	T39.012	T39.013	T39.014	T39.015	T39.016
Acetylsulfamethoxypyridazine	T37.0X1	T37.0X2	T37.0X3	T37.0X4	T37.0X5	T37.0X6
Achromycin	T36.4X1	T36.4X2	T36.4X3	T36.4X4	T36.4X5	T36.4X6
ophthalmic preparation	T49.5X1	T49.5X2	T49.5X3	T49.5X4	T49.5X5	T49.5X6
topical NEC	T49.0X1	T49.0X2	T49.0X3	T49.0X4	T49.0X5	T49.0X6
Aciclovir	T37.5X1	T37.5X2	T37.5X3	T37.5X4	T37.5X5	T37.5X6
Acid (corrosive) NEC	T54.2X1	T54.2X2	T54.2X3	T54.2X4	—	—
Acidifying agent NEC	T50.901	T50.902	T50.903	T50.904	T50.905	T50.906
Acipimox	T46.6X1	T46.6X2	T46.6X3	T46.6X4	T46.6X5	T46.6X6
Acitretin	T50.991	T50.992	T50.993	T50.994	T50.995	T50.996
Aclarubicin	T45.1X1	T45.1X2	T45.1X3	T45.1X4	T45.1X5	T45.1X6

• **Figure 25.3** Table of Drugs and Chemicals.

External cause codes identify how poisoning occurred (V, W, X, Y codes)

Table Headings

Poisoning, Accidental (Unintentional)
Poisoning, Intentional Self-Harm
Poisoning, Assault
Poisoning, Undetermined
Adverse Effect
Underdosing (never a primary or first-listed code)

V, W, X, Y Codes

External Causes of Injuries and Poisonings
    Provides additional information about the nature of the injury/poisoning, locality, activity, and status codes
    Never principal (inpatient) or first-listed/primary (outpatient) diagnosis
    Separate Index to External Causes
    Located after Table of Drugs and Chemicals
- Alphabetical listing with main terms in bold
- Subterms indented two spaces to right under main term

A Word of Caution About the Alphabetic Index

Some words in Index do not appear in Tabular—saves space
    Exact word may not be in code description in Tabular
- Usually found in Alphabetic Index
- Must locate term in Index and then locate in Tabular
- Additional coding instructions found in Tabular

Tabular List

Major Division

Classification of Diseases and Injuries
- 22 chapters

Classification of Diseases and Injuries

Main portion of ICD-10-CM
    Codes from A00-Z99
    Most chapters are body systems
    Example:
- Digestive System
- Respiratory System

Divisions of Classification of Diseases and Injuries

Blocks: A group of related conditions
    Category: Represents single disease/condition
    Subcategory: More specific to etiology, anatomical site and severity
    7th character requirement
        Available for select codes in Chapters 13, 15, 18, 19, 20
    Assign to highest level of specificity, based on documentation
- If 4th to 7th characters exist, do not report a code with fewer characters

> **NOTE**
>
> **Remember**
>
> Assign to highest level of specificity, based on documentation

26

Using ICD-10-CM

ICD-10-CM Official Guidelines for Coding and Reporting (OGCR) developed by Cooperating Parties
- American Hospital Association (AHA)
- American Health Information Management Association (AHIMA)
- Centers for Medicare and Medicaid Services (CMS)
- National Center for Health Statistics (NCHS)

General Guidelines

Appendix A of this text contains Evolve Resources to link to the ICD-10-CM OGCR
    You must know and follow Guidelines when assigning diagnoses codes
- All certification examinations adhere to the OGCR
    In ICD-10-CM the chapter instructions take precedence over the OGCR
- As you review this ICD-10-CM material, locate the information in the OGCR
- In this way, you will become familiar with the location of OGCR content to be able to quickly reference the OGCR during the examination

Steps to Diagnosis Coding

Identify MAIN term(s) in diagnosis
Locate MAIN term(s) in Index
Review subterms
Follow cross-reference instructions (e.g., *see*, *see also*)
Verify code(s) in Tabular

Remember

Read Tabular notes
    Code to highest specificity
    NEVER CODE FROM INDEX!
    A dot/dash (./-) after a code means additional character(s) required

OGCR Section I.A.9. Other (NEC) and Unspecified (NOS)

NEC = Not elsewhere classifiable
- More specific code does NOT exist
    NOS = Not otherwise specified (means "unspecified")

- Available information NOT specific enough
- Use ONLY if more specific code NOT available

OGCR Section I.B.2. Level of Detail in Coding

Assign diagnosis to highest level of specificity
    Do NOT use 3-character code if there is 4-character code
    Do NOT use 4-character code if there is 5, 6, or 7 character available

OGCR Section I.B.8. Acute and Chronic Conditions

Exists alone or together
    May be separate or combination codes
    If two codes, code acute first
    Example: Acute (K85.9) and chronic (K86.1) pancreatitis
    Combination code: Both acute and chronic conditions in one code
    Example: K80.46 Calculus of bile duct with acute and chronic cholecystitis without obstruction

OGCR Section I.B.9. Combination Code

Always use combination code to classify two diagnoses or diagnosis with associated complication
    Example: Rubella encephalitis B06.01

OGCR Section I.B.7. Multiple Coding for Single Condition

Etiology (cause)
Manifestation (symptom)
- brackets [ ]
    Example: Disease, heart, amyloid E85.4 [I43]

OGCR Section I.B.11. Impending or Threatened Condition

Code any condition described as impending or threatened
- Code the symptoms

OGCR Section I.B.13. Laterality

For bilateral sites, the final character identifies laterality
- Right, left, unspecified
  - M93.271 Osteochondritis dissecans, right ankle and joints of right foot

- M93.272 Osteochondritis dissecans, left ankle and joints of left foot
- If no bilateral code is available and condition is bilateral, assign separate codes for left and right

OGCR Section I.B.14. Documentation by Clinicians Other than Patient's Provider

Code assignment based on medical documentation by patient's provider

Exceptions:

- BMI documentation may be from health care provider other than physician, such as dietitian
- Depth of nonpressure ulcers
- Nurse often documents pressure ulcer stages
- Emergency medical technician often documents the coma scale
- NIH stroke scale (NIHSS)

Associated diagnosis must be documented by patient's provider

BMI is assigned as secondary diagnosis (categories **Z55-Z65**) only

Selection of Primary/First-Listed Diagnosis

Condition for encounter
Documented
Responsible for services provided
Also list coexisting condition(s) or comorbidity(ies)

OGCR Section II.H. Uncertain Diagnosis

If diagnosis states
- Probable
- Suspected
- Likely
- Questionable
- Possible
- Rule Out
    Do not code condition. Code the symptoms
    Example: "Cough and fever, probably pneumonia"
    Code cough and fever; do NOT code pneumonia

Diagnosis and Services

Diagnosis and procedure MUST correlate
Medical necessity established
No correlation = No reimbursement

OGCR Section I.A.7. Punctuation

Codes in Brackets
Never sequence as first-listed diagnosis
Always sequence in order listed in Index
Example: Chorioretinitis, in (due to) histoplasmosis B39.9 [H32]
- Code first histoplasmosis (B39.9), then chorioretinitis (H32)

OGCR Section II.B. Two or More Interrelated Conditions

When two or more interrelated conditions exist and either could be the principal or first-listed diagnosis, either is sequenced first
Example: Patient with mitral valve stenosis and coronary artery disease (two interrelated conditions)
- Either can be principal diagnosis and sequenced first
- Resource intensiveness affects choice

OGCR Section II.C. Two or More Equal Diagnoses

Either can be sequenced first
Example: Diagnosis of viral gastroenteritis and dehydration

Late Effects (Sequela)

Location in the OGCR: Section I.B.10.
Late effect residual of (remaining from) previous illness/injury
- e.g., Burn that leaves scar
Residual coded first (scar)
Cause (burn) coded second
Late effect codes are not in a separate chapter; rather, throughout Tabular
Reference the term "Late, effect(s)" in the Index; you are directed to "*see* Sequelae"
There is no time limit on developing a residual
There may be more than one residual
Example: Patient has a stroke (I63.9) and develops paralysis on right dominant side (hemiparesis, I69.951) and loss of ability to communicate (aphasia, I69.920)

27

ICD-10-CM Chapters 1-10

Chapter 1, Certain Infectious and Parasitic Diseases

Divided based on etiology (cause of disease)
Many combination codes
Example: B37.0 candidiasis stomatitis infection of mouth, which reports both the organism and condition with one code

Multiple Codes

Sequencing must be considered.
- UTI due to Escherichia coli
  - N39.0 (UTI) etiology
  - B96.2- (E. coli) organism (in this order)

OGCR Section I.C.1.A. Human Immunodeficiency Virus

Code HIV or HIV-related illness ONLY if stated as confirmed in diagnostic statement
- B20 HIV or HIV-related illness
- Z21 Asymptomatic HIV status
- R75 Inconclusive HIV serology

Previously Diagnosed HIV-Related Illness

Code prior diagnosis HIV-related disease B20 (HIV)
NEVER assign these patients to:
- Z21 (Asymptomatic) or
- R75 (Nonspecific serologic evidence of HIV)

Sequencing

- HIV-related condition code:
  B20 HIV followed by all reported HIV-related conditions
- Unrelated condition for patient with HIV:
  Code unrelated condition(s) followed by B20, then all reported HIV-related conditions

HIV and Pregnancy

This is an exception to HIV sequencing
  During pregnancy, childbirth, or puerperium, code:
- O98.7- (Other specified infections and parasitic diseases)
- Followed by B20 (HIV) and then all code(s) for HIV-related illness(es)

Asymptomatic HIV during pregnancy, childbirth, or puerperium
- O98.7– (Other specified infections and parasitic diseases)
- Z21 (Asymptomatic HIV infection status)
- Reporting asymptomatic HIV varies by state
  - Check the state's reporting laws

Inconclusive Laboratory Test for HIV

R75 (Inconclusive serologic test for HIV)
- Reporting inconclusive laboratory HIV tests varies by state
  - Check the state's reporting laws

HIV Screening

Code Z11.4 (Screening for human immunodeficiency virus [HIV])
- Patient in high-risk group for HIV
- Z72.89 (Other problems related to lifestyle)
  Patients returning for HIV screening results = Z71.7 (HIV counseling)

Caution

Incorrectly applying these HIV coding rules can cause patient hardship
  Insurance claims for patients with HIV usually need patient's written agreement to disclosure

OGCR Section I.C.1.d. Sepsis, Severe Sepsis, and Septic Shock

Sepsis: Assign systemic infection code as first-listed diagnosis when sepsis is present
- Assign a sepsis code as secondary when sepsis develops during encounter
  Septicemia/Sepsis: Usually an A41.9 septicemia code and a R65.- SIRS code (in this order)
- Code the organ system dysfunction by the SIRS (e.g., J96.9, respiratory failure followed by R65.2-)
  Septic Shock: Organ dysfunction associated with severe sepsis
- Code underlying systemic infection (e.g., A41.9) followed by the SIRS code with septic shock (R65.21)

Chapter 2, Neoplasms

Two steps for coding neoplasms
- Incorrectly applying these neoplasm codes can also cause patient hardship
  1. Index: Locate histologic type of neoplasm (e.g., sarcoma, melanoma); review all instructions
  2. Locate code identified (usually in Neoplasm Table in Index) by body site

Neoplasm Table divided into columns:
- Malignant (Primary)
- Malignant (Secondary)
- Ca in situ
- Benign
- Uncertain
- Unspecified Behavior

  Example: Pathology report confirmed diagnosis stated in operative report of primary malignant neoplasm of the bladder neck.
- ICD-10-CM, Neoplasm Table, bladder, neck, under Malignant, Primary column, C67.5
- Reference in the Tabular to ensure accurate assignment. Coded as primary site unless specified as secondary site (metastasis)

Bone	Meninges	Brain
Peritoneum	Diaphragm	Pleura
Heart	Retroperitoneum	Liver
Lymph nodes	Spinal cord	Mediastinum

Unknown status of neoplasm is always reported with D49.9

OGCR Section I.C.2. Neoplasms

Treatment directed at malignancy: Neoplasm is principal/first-listed diagnosis
- Except for chemotherapy, immunotherapy, or radiotherapy:
  - Therapy (treatment), listed first (Z51.–)
  - Neoplasm, listed second
    Chemotherapy: Z51.11
    Radiotherapy: Z51.0
    Immunotherapy: Z51.12

First-Listed Diagnosis, Neoplasms

Surgical removal of neoplasm and subsequent chemotherapy or radiotherapy
- Code malignancy as principal/first-listed diagnosis
  Surgery to determine extent of malignancy
- Code malignancy as principal/first-listed diagnosis

History and Secondary Metastasis of Neoplasms

Report category Z85, "Personal history of malignant neoplasm," if:
- Neoplasm was previously destroyed, AND
- No longer being treated
  If patient receives treatment for secondary neoplasm (metastasis)

- Secondary neoplasm is principal/first-listed diagnosis
- Even though primary is known

Anemia and Complications With/of Neoplasm

Patient treated for anemia due to neoplasm, code in this order:
- Neoplasm
- D63.0 Anemia in neoplastic disease

Patient treated for dehydration due to neoplasm or therapy, code in this order:
- Dehydration
- Neoplasm

Anemia associated with therapy:
- Adverse effect code
- Anemia
  Neoplasm
  Patient admitted to repair complication of surgery for an intestinal malignancy
- Complication, principal/first-listed diagnosis
- Complication is reason for encounter
- Malignancy, secondary diagnosis

Z Codes and Neoplasms

Patient receiving chemotherapy or radiotherapy after removal of neoplasm code:
- Therapy
- Active neoplasm
  Do NOT report H/O (history of) neoplasm

Chapter 3, Diseases of the Blood and Blood-Forming Organs and Certain Disorders Involving the Immune Mechanism

Includes anemia, blood disorders, coagulation defects
    Often used code: Anemia
    Many different types of anemia:
- Hereditary hemolytic (D58.9)
- Iron deficiency (D50.9)
- Acquired hemolytic (D59.9)
- Aplastic (D61.9)
- Other specified (D64.89)
- Unspecified (D64.9)

Multiple coding often necessary
Identify underlying disease condition

Chapter 4, Endocrine, Nutritional, and Metabolic Diseases

Disorders of Other Endocrine Glands

Diabetes Mellitus (E10 or E11) coded frequently
- Combination codes include DM type and complication of affected body system
  Example:
- E11.39 reports Type 2 diabetes mellitus with other diabetic ophthalmic complications

- Often requires two codes
- Z79.4 used in addition to diabetes code to report long-term use of insulin

  Temporary insulin use not coded to Z79.4; only long-term

  If type not indicated, report type 2

  Type 1 diabetic is one who is insulin-dependent

  Patient with type 2 diabetes may receive insulin for periods when diabetes is uncontrolled

Other Metabolic and Immunity Disorders Section

Disorders such as gout and dehydration

Disorders often have many names

- E05.00 Thyrotoxicosis with diffuse goiter also known as
  - Basedow's disease
  - Graves' disease
  - Hyperthyroidism with goiter

Chapter 5, Mental, Behavioral, and Neurodevelopmental Disorders

Includes codes for:

- Personality disorders
- Stress disorders
- Neuroses
- Psychoses
- Sexual dysfunction, etc.

  Pain disorders related to psychological factors

- Assign F45.42 for pain disorder with related psychological factors (see note following G89, acute or chronic pain)

  Mental and behavioral disorders due to psychoactive substance use

- In remission, F10-F19 with -11, -21
- Psychoactive substance use, abuse, and dependence, one code assigned based on hierarchy (see OGCR, Section I.C.5.b.2.)

Chapter 6, Diseases of Nervous System

Central Nervous System

  Peripheral Nervous System

Pain—Category G89

Acute or chronic pain not elsewhere classified due to:

- Acute pain due to trauma G89.11
- Acute post-thoracotomy pain G89.12
- Central pain syndrome G89.0
- Other acute postoperative pain G89.18
- Neoplasm related pain (acute) (chronic) G89.3
- Chronic pain due to trauma G89.21
- Chronic post-thoracotomy pain G89.22
- Other chronic postprocedural pain G89.28
- Chronic pain syndrome G89.4

  Principal/Primary diagnosis

- When definitive diagnosis not established
- Pain management is reason for encounter/admission

Chapter 7, Diseases of Eye and Adnexa

Does not contain all the eye and adnexa codes

  Example: Traumatic injury to eye and orbit of eye, S05.-

  Hordeolum, infection of sebaceous gland of eyelid (stye)

  Reported on location and type

  Example: Externum, report H00.01- or internum, report H00.02-

  Chalazion, infection of eyelid that forms mass

  Reported based on location

  Entropion = turning inward of eyelid (H02.0–)

  Ectropion = turning outward of eyelid (H02.1–)

  Lacrimal System, category H04

  Reported based on right, left, bilateral, unspecified

Chapter 8, Diseases of Ear and Mastoid Process

Excludes2 indicates other categories for reporting other ear conditions

  Examples: Endocrine, nutritional and metabolic disease (E00-E89)

  H60-H95 reports diseases of:

- External ear
- Middle ear
- Inner ear
- Mastoid
- Other
- Surgical complications NEC

Chapter 9, Diseases of Circulatory System

OGCR Section I.C.9.a. Hypertension

Assign hypertension (arterial, benign, essential, malignant, primary, systemic) to I10

OGCR Section I.C.9.a.1. Hypertension with Heart Disease

Category I11

- Any condition in I50.- or I51.4-I51.7, I51.89, I51.9 due to hypertension
- Use additional code(s) to specify type(s) of heart failure (I50.-)

OGCR Section I.C.9.a.2. Hypertensive Chronic Kidney Disease

Cause-and-effect relationship assumed in chronic kidney failure with hypertension

  Category I12 Hypertensive chronic kidney disease

- Includes any condition in N18.- due to hypertension chronic kidney disease

Use additional code to identify stage of chronic kidney disease N18.1-N18.4, N18.9

OGCR Section I.C.9.a.3. Hypertensive Heart and Chronic Kidney Disease

Assign category I13 when both hypertensive chronic kidney disease and hypertensive heart disease stated in diagnosis

Assume cause-and-effect relationship
Includes any condition in I11.- with any condition in I12.- cardiorenal disease; cardiovascular renal disease
* Use additional code from category I50 to identify type of heart failure
* Use additional code to identify stage of chronic kidney disease (N18.1-N18.4, N18.9)

OGCR Section I.C.9.a.4. Hypertensive Cerebrovascular Disease for Secondary Pulmonary Hypertension

Use additional code to identify presence of hypertension (I10-I15)
Code:
* Cerebrovascular disease (I60-I69)
* Type of hypertension (I10-I15)

OGCR Section I.C.9.a.5. Hypertensive Retinopathy

Code:
* Hypertensive retinopathy (H35.0-)
* Type of hypertension (I10-I15)
The sequencing is based on the reason for the encounter.

OGCR Section I.C.9.a.6. Hypertension, Secondary

Hypertension caused by an underlying condition
Code:
* Underlying condition
* Type of hypertension (I15)

OGCR Section I.C.9.a.7. Hypertension, Transient

Transient hypertension: Temporary elevation of BP
Do NOT assign I10-I15, Hypertensive disease
* Hypertension diagnosis NOT established
* Assign either:
  * R03.0, Elevated blood pressure
  * O13.-, Gestational hypertension without significant proteinuria (pregnancy induced)
  * O14.-, Pre-eclampsia, for transient hypertension of pregnancy with significant proteinuria

OGCR Section I.C.9.a.8. Hypertension, Controlled

Hypertension controlled by therapy
* Assign appropriate code from categories I10-I15

OGCR Section I.C.9.a.9. Hypertension, Uncontrolled

Untreated hypertension
Uncontrolled hypertension
Assign appropriate code from categories I10-I15

OGCR Section I.C.9.a.10. Hypertensive Crisis

Documented hypertensive urgency, hypertensive emergency, or unspecified hypertensive crisis
Assign code from category I16
Code also any identified hypertensive disease (I10-I15)
Sequencing based on reason for encounter

OGCR Section I.C.9.a.10. Pulmonary Hypertension

Assign code from category I27
Code also associated condition/adverse effect for secondary pulmonary hypertension
Sequencing based on reason for encounter

Chapter 10, Diseases of Respiratory System

Watch for "Use additional code to identify infectious organism"
* Some codes include the specific organism and do not need an additional code
* Respiratory Failure Sequencing
  If the respiratory failure is due to an acute condition, such as MI [myocardial infarction] or acute exacerbation of a chronic condition, such as COPD [chronic obstructive pulmonary disease], sequence the acute condition first
  Example: MI (acute condition) and respiratory failure
* Sequence MI (I21.9) first and respiratory failure (J96.0) second
  If the respiratory failure (acute condition) is due to a chronic nonrespiratory condition (such as myasthenia gravis), sequence the respiratory failure first
  Example: Acute respiratory failure (acute) and myasthenia gravis (chronic)
* Sequence acute respiratory failure (J96.0) first and myasthenia gravis (G70.00) second

Acute Respiratory Infection Section

Frequently assigned codes, such as:
* Common cold (J01.-)
* Sore throat (J02, acute pharyngitis)
* Acute tonsillitis (J03)
* Acute bronchitis (J20-J21), chronic bronchitis (J41-J42)
* Acute upper respiratory infection (J06.9)
* Influenza (J09-J10)
* Pneumonia (J12-J18)
  Read OGCR Section I.C.10.a., or Chapter 10 for specifics on coding COPD and asthma

28

ICD-10-CM Chapters 11-14

Chapter 11, Diseases of Digestive System

Mouth to anus and accessory organs

Extensive subcategories
Cholelithiasis (K80)
Commonly assigned codes
- Ulcers (K25-K28)
  - Gastric (K25)
  - Duodenal (K26)
  - Peptic (K27)
  - Gastrojejunal (K28)
  - Hernias (K40-K46)

Chapter 12, Diseases of Skin and Subcutaneous Tissue

Skin

Epidermis
Dermis
Subcutaneous tissue
Infectious skin/Subcutaneous tissue
Scar tissue

Accessory Organs

Sweat glands
  Sebaceous glands
  Nails
  Hair and hair follicles
  Other
  Example: Cellulitis of right finger due to *Staphylococcus*, report:
  - Cellulitis L03.011
  - Staphylococcus aureus B95.61

Chapter 13, Diseases of Musculoskeletal System and Connective Tissue

Bone
  Bursa
  Cartilage

Fascia
Ligaments
Muscle
Synovia
Tendons

Sections

Infectious arthropathies (joint disease)
  Inflammatory polyarthropathies
  Osteoarthritis
  Other joint disorders
  Dentofacial anomalies
  Systemic connective tissue disorders
  Deforming dorsopathies
  Spondylopathies
  Other dorsopathies
  Disorders of muscle
  Disorders of synovium and tendons
  Other soft tissue disorders
  Disorders of bone density and structure
  Other osteopathies
  Chondropathies
  Other disorders of the musculoskeletal system and connective tissue

Intraoperative and postprocedural complications and disorders of musculoskeletal system, not elsewhere classified
  Biomechanical lesions, not elsewhere classified

Chapter 14, Diseases of Genitourinary System

Commonly assigned codes:
- Urinary tract infection (N39.0)
- Inflammatory diseases of prostate (N41)
- Inflammatory disease of female pelvic organs (N70-N77)
  Stages of chronic kidney disease
- Stage 1: Blood flow through kidney increases, kidney enlarges (N18.1)
- Stage 2: (mild) Small amounts of blood protein (albumin) leak into urine (microalbuminuria) (N18.2)

- Stage 3: (moderate) Albumin and other protein losses increase. Patient may develop high blood pressure and kidney loses ability to filter waste (N18.30)
- Stage 4: (severe) Large amounts of urine pass through kidney; blood pressure increases (N18.4)
- Stage 5: Ability to filter waste nearly stops (N18.5)

- End-stage renal failure (N18.6)
  When documentation indicates chronic renal disease (CKD) and ESRD, report ESRD
- Unspecified (N19)
  Status post–kidney transplant, assign Z94.0
- Patient may still have CKD

29

ICD-10-CM Chapters 15-22

Chapter 15, Pregnancy, Childbirth, and the Puerperium

Used only on the **maternal** record
- Admission for pregnancy, complication
- Obstetric complication = first-listed diagnosis
  Chapter 15 codes take precedence over codes from other chapters unless the documentation indicates the condition being treated is not affecting the management of the pregnancy

  The majority of codes in Chapter 15 have a final character indicating the trimester of pregnancy

  7 characters are required on specified codes in Chapter 15

OGCR Section I.C.15.a. General Rules

Not all encounters are pregnancy-related

Example: Pregnant woman, broken ankle; report:
- Broken ankle
- Z33.1 Pregnant state incidental

Must be documented in medical record that condition being treated is not affecting pregnancy
- If NOT documented, assume condition is affecting pregnancy

Trimesters

Trimesters are counted from the first day of the last menstrual period
- 1st trimester: Less than 14 weeks 0 days
- 2nd trimester: 14 weeks 0 days to less than 28 weeks 0 days
- 3rd trimester: 28 weeks 0 days until delivery

OGCR Section I.C.15.b.1. Complications of Pregnancy, Childbirth, and the Puerperium

Chapter 15 codes (O00-O9A)
- Assigned only to mother's medical record
- Not assigned to newborn medical record
  Episodes when no delivery occurs
- Principal diagnosis should correspond to the principal complication of the pregnancy which necessitated the encounter.

OGCR Section I.C.15.b.4, When a delivery occurs
OGCR Section I.C.15.b.5, Outcome of delivery code (Z37) when delivered

OGCR Section I.C.15.b.1.-2. Selection of Principal or First-listed Diagnosis

Routine prenatal visits, no complications:
- Z34, Supervision, normal pregnancy
  Prenatal outpatient visits for high-risk pregnancies
- O09, Supervision of high-risk pregnancy

OGCR Section I.C.15.n.1.-3. Normal Delivery

Normal delivery includes:
- Vaginal delivery
- Minimal or no assistance
- With or without episiotomy
- No fetal manipulation or instrumentation
- Full-term, single, liveborn infant

Postpartum Period

After delivery and continues for 6 weeks

Peripartum Period

Defined as the last month of pregnancy to five months postpartum

Abortions

No identifiable fetus
  500 grams or less
  Less than 22 weeks' gestation
  Codes O00-O08

Abortions With Liveborn Fetus

Attempted abortion results in liveborn fetus
- Category O60 (Early onset of delivery) appropriately Assign Z37 (Outcome of delivery)
  Attempted abortion code also assigned

Chapter 16, Certain Conditions Originating in the Perinatal Period

Birth through 28 days following birth

Conditions Originating in Perinatal Period (P00-P96)
- Perinatal period through 28th day following birth
- Codes can be used after 28th day, if documented that condition originated during perinatal period

Chapter 16 codes are ONLY for use on the newborn record

Assign Z38.– as first-listed diagnosis according to type of birth

Use of Codes Z00

Z00.11 Newborn health examination
    Suspected of having an abnormal condition
    Infant 28 days or less
    Excludes1 health check for child over 28 days old (Z00.12-)

Coding Additional Diagnosis

Code conditions that require
- Treatment
- Further investigation
- Additional resource
    Prolonged length of stay (LOS)
    Implications for future care
    Insignificant conditions, signs, symptoms
- Resolve with no treatment
- Need no code
- EVEN IF documented

Prematurity and Fetal Growth Retardation

Codes from categories
- P05 (Slow fetal growth and fetal malnutrition) and
- P07 (Disorders relating to short gestation and low birthweight NEC)
    Not assigned solely on birthweight or gestational age
    Use physician's assessment of maturity
    Use additional code for weeks of gestation (P07.30, P07.31, P07.32)

Chapter 17, Congenital Malformations, Deformations, and Chromosomal Abnormalities

When a malformation/deformation/or chromosomal abnormality does not have a unique code assignment, assign additional code(s) for any manifestations that may be present.

Codes from Chapter 17 may be used throughout the life of the patient. If a congenital malformation or deformity has been corrected, a personal history code should be used to identify the history of the malformation or deformity.

Chapter 18, Symptoms, Signs, and Abnormal Clinical and Laboratory Findings, Not Elsewhere Classified

Do NOT code a sign or symptom if
- Definitive diagnosis made (symptoms are part of disease)

Used only if no specific diagnosis made
One category requires 7 characters (Coma, R40.2-)

Chapter 19, Injury, Poisoning, and Certain Other Consequences of External Causes

Block Examples

- S00-S09 Injuries to the head
- S10-S19 Injuries to the neck
- S20-S29 Injuries to the thorax
- S30-S39 Injuries to the abdomen, lower back, lumbar spine, pelvis, and external genitals
- S40-S49 Injuries to the shoulder and upper arm
- S50-S59 Injuries to the elbow and forearm
- S60-S69 Injuries to the wrist, hand, and fingers
- S70-S79 Injuries to the hip and thigh
- S80-S89 Injuries to the knee and lower leg
- S90-S99 Injuries to the ankle and foot

When Coding Injuries

- Assign separate codes for each injury unless a combination code is provided, in which case the combination code is assigned
- Multiple injury codes are provided in ICD-10-CM but should not be assigned unless information for a more specific code is not available
- Traumatic injury codes (S00-T14.9) are not assigned for normal, healing surgical wounds or to identify complications of surgical wounds
- Most categories in Chapter 19 have 7th character extensions that are required for each applicable code

Most categories in this chapter have three extensions (with the exception of fractures):

A, initial encounter
D, subsequent encounter
S, sequela

External Cause Codes: Index and Tabular

V, W, X, Y, Z code Index located following the Table of Drugs and Chemicals
    Directly before the Tabular
    Not in the Index to Disease and Injuries
    Codes V, W, X, Y are located in Chapter 20 in the Tabular

Chapter 20, External Causes of Morbidity

Adverse effects of correct medication correctly given and correctly taken

Provide supplemental information
Identify
- Cause of an injury or poisoning
- Intent (unintentional or intentional)
- Place it occurred
- Activity

Chapter 20, General Code Guidelines

Use with any code in Volume 1 in the range of A00.0-T88.9, Z00-Z99

7th character required on most codes to describe the initial encounter, subsequent encounter, or sequela (late effect)

Assign as many external cause codes as necessary
Certain external cause codes are combination codes
Initial encounter
- Use external cause code, if applicable

Table of Drugs and Chemicals

Follows the Neoplasm Table in Index
Alphabetic listing with codes
Do NOT code directly from Table
Always reference Tabular

Late Effects of External Cause

Should be used with late effect of a previous injury/poisoning
Should NOT be used with related current injury code
Report using the external cause code with the 7th character extension "S" for Sequela
These codes should be used with any report of a late effect or sequel resulting from a previous injury

Signs and Symptoms and Definitive Diagnosis

Do NOT code a sign/symptom if definitive diagnosis made
- Symptoms are part of disease
Use only if no specific diagnosis is made

Burns/Corrosions Classified

According to extent of body surface involved
Burn site NOT specified
Additional data required
Burn—heat
Corrosion—chemical

Category

Category T31.- = % body surface involved and % body surface involved in 3rd-degree burns
Lund-Browder Classification Method applies
Burn Example: 3rd-degree burn of abdomen (10%) and 2nd-degree burn of left thigh (5%) by hot water, initial encounter
- T21.32XA Burn, abdomen, 3rd degree
- T24.212A Burn, thigh, left, 2nd degree
- T31.11 15% total burn area and 10% 3rd degree
- X12.XXXA Burn by hot liquid

Debridement of Wound, Infection, or Burn

Excisional debridement
- Cut away
- Performed by physician or other health care provider
Nonexcisional procedure

- Shaved or scraped
- Performed by physician or nonphysician

Coding for Multiple Injuries

Separate code for each injury
Most serious injury first

Vessel and Nerve Damage

Code primary injury first
- Use additional code if nerve damage minor
Primary injury = Nerve damage
- Code nerve damage first

Multiple Fractures

Same coding principles as multiple injuries
Code multiple fractures by site
Sequenced by severity

Fractures

Not indicated as closed or open = closed
Same bone fractured AND dislocated:
- Code fracture ONLY (highest level of injury)
- Laterality

Chapter 21, Factors Influencing Health Status and Contact With Health Services

Z Codes

Located after Y99.9 in Tabular
Three characters before decimal (e.g., Z11.8)
Main terms: Contraception, counseling, dialysis, status, examination

Uses of Z Codes

Not sick BUT receives health care (e.g., vaccination)
Services for known disease/injury (e.g., chemotherapy)
A circumstance/problem that influences patient's health BUT NOT current illness/injury
Example: Organ transplant status
Example: Birth status and outcome of delivery (newborn)

Special Note About "History of"

Index to Disease, MAIN term "History"
Entries between "family" and "visual loss Z82.1" = "family history of"
Entries after "family" and after "visual loss Z86.69" = "personal history of"
Draw a line in the Index of your ICD-10-CM coding manual to indicate end of "family history" entries and beginning of "personal history" entries

History Z Codes

Section I.C.21. of the OGCR contains specific guidelines that identify how Z codes can be listed (first, first/additional, additional only)

Categories in Tabular

Z85	Personal history of malignant neoplasm
Z86.59	Personal history of mental and behavioral disorder
Z87.89	Personal history of other specified conditions

Except: Z87.39 Personal history of arthritis, and Z87.79 Personal history of congenital malformations. These conditions are life-long so are not true history codes

Z88	Allergy status to medicinal agents
Z91.89	Other personal risk factors presenting hazards to health
Z80	Family history of primary malignant neoplasm

Z82.8	Family history of certain other disabilities and chronic diseases
Z84.89	Family history of other specified conditions

Chapter 22, Codes for Special Purposes

New ICD-10-CM chapter for 2021
Includes two codes at this time

U07.0	Vaping-related disorder (see Section I.C.10.e., Vaping-related disorders)
U07.1	COVID-19 (see Section I.C.1.g.1., COVID-19 infection)

30
Outpatient Coding

OGCR Section IV, Diagnostic Coding and Reporting Guidelines for Outpatient Services

Part of ICD-10-CM OGCR, Section IV

Guideline A

Use term first-listed diagnosis for outpatient settings

Outpatient surgery: If procedure is not performed due to contraindications, report the reason for the surgery as first-listed diagnosis

Observation stay: Report medical condition as first-listed diagnosis

Patient admitted for outpatient surgery develops complications requiring admission to observation, report reason for admission, followed by codes for complications

Guideline B

Use codes A00.0-T88.9, Z00-Z99 to report diagnosis, symptoms, conditions, problems, complaints, or other reason(s) for visit

Guideline C

Accurate reporting of ICD-10-CM diagnosis codes, documentation should include patient's condition, specific diagnosis(es), symptoms, problems, or reason for encounter

Guideline D

Codes that describe symptoms and signs (rather than diagnoses) are acceptable for outpatient coding

Guideline E

Encounters for circumstances other than a disease or injury are reported with Z00-Z99

Guideline F

Level of detail in coding ICD-10-CM: code to highest number of characters available

Guideline G

First-listed diagnosis is the diagnosis, condition, problem, or other reason for encounter/visit

Guideline H

Uncertain diagnoses are not reported in outpatient settings

Report the condition that is the reason for the encounter, such as symptoms, signs, abnormal test results

Guideline I

Chronic diseases are treated on an ongoing basis

Report the disease each time the disease is treated or managed

Guideline J

Code all documented conditions that coexist

Do not code conditions that were previously treated and no longer exist

Guideline K

Patients receiving diagnostic services only, the first-listed code is the diagnosis, condition, problem, or other reason for encounter that is chiefly responsible for services

Routine laboratory/radiology tests

- When no signs, symptoms, or diagnoses are available, report Z01.89
- When test is to evaluate sign, symptom, or diagnosis, report both the V code and a code to report the reason for the test

  Report any confirmed or definitive diagnosis(es) documented in the test result interpretation
- Do not code signs and symptoms as additional diagnoses

Guideline L

Patients receiving therapeutic services only, sequence first the diagnosis, condition, problem, or reason for encounter chiefly responsible for service

- Report other diagnosis(es), such as chronic conditions, as secondary diagnosis(es)

Guideline M

Patients receiving preoperative evaluations only

- Report a code from subcategory Z01.81 as first-listed diagnosis

- Report condition that prompted surgery as secondary diagnosis
- Code also any findings related to preoperative evaluation

Guideline N

Ambulatory surgery: Report the diagnosis for which the surgery was performed

Report the postoperative diagnosis if different from preoperative diagnosis

Guideline O

See OGCR, Section I.C.15

Routine prenatal visits, no complications:
- Z34, Supervision, normal first pregnancy

Prenatal outpatient visits for high-risk pregnancies
- O09, Supervision of high-risk pregnancy

Guideline P

Encounters for general medical examinations, with or without abnormal findings, report Z00.0-

If examination results in abnormal finding, report as first-listed diagnosis a code for general medical examination with abnormal findings
- Secondary code to report the abnormal finding

Guideline Q

Encounters for routine health screening, see OGCR, Section I.C.21

31

ICD-10-PCS, Reporting Inpatient Procedures

Appendix A of this text contains Evolve Resources to link to ICD-10-PCS OGCR
90% of codes refer to surgical procedures
10% refer to diagnostic and therapeutic procedures

- Codes assigned by hospitals to report facility services provided to inpatients
- Procedures done in physician's office or outpatient ASC are coded using CPT/HCPCS codes
- Surgeon uses CPT to report services to inpatients

Table of Contents

Contains the Sections of the ICD-10-PCS coding system
    Appendix A of the manual contains the definitions used within the system

Alphabetic Index

Index terms in bold
- Subterms not in bold
Alphabetical arrangement as illustrated in Fig. 31.1
Cross-reference feature is "*see*"
    Example: Inferior tarsal plate
    see Eyelid, Lower, Right
    see Eyelid, Lower, Left
Never code directly from Index.

Tabular List

Tables of Sections
    Usually subdivided by:
- Body System
- Operation
- Body Part
- Approach
- Device
- Qualifier

Tables of Characters to Be Assigned (Illustrated in Fig. 31.2)

All PCS codes have 7 characters.
Fig. 31.3 illustrates a PCS coding grid.
Fig. 31.4 illustrates an example of building code 00160J6 from the grid

Index

Use Index to locate code by means of alphabetic lookup
    Index based on root operation terms with subentries based on:
- Body System
- Body Part
- Operation
- Device

Guidelines

ICD-10-PCS has separate Official Guidelines for Coding and Reporting

---

A

Abdominal aortic plexus *use* Abdominal Sympathetic Nerve
Abdominal esophagus *use* Esophagus, Lower
Abdominohysterectomy *see* Resection, Uterus ØUT9
Abdominoplasty
    see Alteration, Abdominal Wall, ØWØF
    see Repair, Abdominal Wall, ØWQF
    see Supplement, Abdominal Wall, ØWUF
Abductor hallucis muscle
    use Foot Muscle, Right
    use Foot Muscle, Left

- **Figure 31.1** ICD-10-PCS Tables.

SECTIONS

Ø	Medical and Surgical
1	Obstetrics
2	Placement
3	Administration
4	Measurement and Monitoring
5	Extracorporeal Assistance and Performance
6	Extracorporeal Therapies
7	Osteopathic
8	Other Procedures
9	Chiropractic
B	Imaging
C	Nuclear Medicine
D	Radiation Therapy
F	Physical Rehabilitation and Diagnostic Audiology
G	Mental Health
H	Substance Abuse Treatment

• **Figure 31.2** Sections of ICD-10-PCS.

www.cms.gov/Medicare/Coding/ICD10/Downloads/2021-ICD-10-PCS-Guidelines.pdf or http://evolve.elsevier.com/Buck/examreview

Bundling

Included in all surgical procedures
- Opening and closing of surgical site
- Approach, except where approach differs from code description
  Example: Microscopic approach used instead of described approach
- Do not unbundle and code these separately
- If closure takes place during separate surgical procedure, closure can be coded separately

> **NOTE**
>
> **Remember**
>
> ICD-10-CM and ICD-10-PCS are required for the CCS certification examination.

SECTION: Ø MEDICAL AND SURGICAL
BODY SYSTEM: Ø CENTRAL NERVOUS SYSTEM AND CRANIAL NERVES
OPERATION: 1 **BYPASS:** Altering the route of passage of the contents of a tubular body part

Body Part	Approach	Device	Qualifier
6 Cerebral Ventricle	Ø Open 3 Percutaneous 4 Percutaneous Endoscopic	7 Autologous Tissue Substitute J Synthetic Substitute K Nonautologous Tissue Substitute	Ø Nasopharynx 1 Mastoid Sinus 2 Atrium 3 Blood Vessel 4 Pleural Cavity 5 Intestine 6 Peritoneal Cavity 7 Urinary Tract 8 Bone Marrow A Subgaleal Space B Cerebral Cisterns
6 Cerebral Ventricle	Ø Open 3 Percutaneous 4 Percutaneous Endoscopic	Z No Device	B Cerebral Cisterns
U Spinal Canal	Ø Open 3 Percutaneous 4 Percutaneous Endoscopic	7 Autologous Tissue Substitute J Synthetic Substitute K Nonautologous Tissue Substitute	2 Atrium 4 Pleural Cavity 6 Peritoneal Cavity 7 Urinary Tract 9 Fallopian Tube

• **Figure 31.3** ICD-10-PCS Table.

0 = Medical and Surgical section	First = section of medical service
0 = Central Nervous System	Second = body system
1 = Bypass	Third = type of operation
6 = Cerebral Ventricle	Fourth = body part
0 = Open	Fifth = approach
J = Synthetic Substitute	Sixth = device
6 = Peritoneal Cavity	Seventh = qualifier

• **Figure 31.4** Building code 00160J6.

PART 6

Physician-based Examinations

32

Physician-based Examinations

NOTE

Disclaimer

Every effort has been made to ensure that the content of the practice exams in Part 6 and on the companion Evolve website resemble the format and content of current certification examinations. However, the examinations may be revised at any time, and it is your responsibility to review all certification information published by the certifying organization.

You have three opportunities to practice taking each physician-based examination:

- Pre-Examination (before study)
- Post-Examination (after study)
- Final Examination (at the end of your complete program of study)

For the purposes of this text, two physician-based practice exam formats have been developed so you can focus on the exam format that most closely resembles the certification exam you've chosen to take:

- Physician Exam (Format A)
  Pre-/Post-Examination and Final Examination (150 multiple-choice questions each)
- Physician Exam (Format B)
  Pre-/Post-Examination and Final Examination (97 multiple-choice questions and 8 case scenarios each)

You should have the following manuals:

- 2021 ICD-10-CM (*International Classification of Diseases, 10th Revision, Clinical Modification*)
- 2020 HCPCS (*Healthcare Common Procedure Coding System*)
- 2021 CPT (*Current Procedural Terminology*)

No other reference material, other than a medical dictionary for Physician Exam (Format B), is allowed for any of the practice examinations.

- For all Pre-Examinations, Post-Examinations, and Final Examinations, you will need a computer, Internet access,

and the three coding references (ICD-10-CM, HCPCS, CPT).

- For the Physician Exam (Format A): Final Examination, you will also need paper, pencils, and an eraser.
- Each organization's certification examination has different scoring requirements, but as you take the examinations with this text, you should strive for 80% to 90% on the Post-Examination and 70% as a minimum on the Final Examination.

NOTE

To enable the learner to calculate an examination score, minimums have been identified as "passing" within this text; however, this may or may not be the percentage identified by the certifying organization as a "passing" grade. It is your responsibility to review all certification information published by the certifying organization.

NOTE

It is expected that the examiner is able to assign key components when reporting evaluation and management services. See updated E/M questions for examples of the new format. All categories of codes (I, II, and III) are potentially on the examination.

Pre-Examination and Post-Examination

The Pre-Examination is located on the companion Evolve website. The purpose of the Pre-Examination is only to assess your beginning level of knowledge and skill—your starting place. Based on your scores, you can tailor your study to target your weakest areas and increase your scores. Take the Pre-Examination before you begin your studies.

Your score will automatically be calculated for you. A passing score for the examinations in this text requires 70%.

The practice examinations program on Evolve will calculate and retain your scoring information.

Immediately on completion of your study, you should complete the Post-Examination on Evolve. After you are finished, the program will automatically compare your Pre-Examination scores with your Post-Examination scores and will store your results. By comparing the results of the Pre-Examination and the Post-Examination (the same examination will be taken twice), the program illustrates the improvements you have achieved or the areas that you will need to practice more on before taking the Final Examination.

Rationales for each question are available for review after you complete the Post-Examination. Study the questions for which you did not choose the right response. Did you misread the question, did you not know the material well enough to answer correctly, or did you run out of time? Knowing why you missed a question is an important step toward improving your skill level.

Ideally, you should complete each examination in one sitting; if time does not allow, spread the examination times over several periods. There are no time extensions during an actual examination setting, and learning how to judge the amount of time you should spend on each question is an important part of this learning experience to prepare you for the real certification examination.

Final Examination

If you scored well on all areas of the Post-Examination (80% or higher), you are ready to move on to the Final

Examination, located in Part 6 of the text for Physician Exam (Format A), and on the companion Evolve site for Physician Exam (Format B).

For Physician Exam (Format A), there is an answer sheet on which to place your answers; it is located directly before the examination. Remove your answer sheet from this text, and enter your answer for each of the 150 questions using paper and pencil.

Once you have completed the answer sheet, go to the electronic program on Evolve to enter your answers on the electronic score sheet. The electronic program will then provide you with the answers and compare your scores to illustrate your improvement.

A passing score for the Final Examination is the same as for the Pre/Post-Examination—70%.

If you did not attain a minimum score on each section, you should develop a plan to restudy those particular areas where the examination indicates you are having difficulties. There are rationales for each question in the Final Examination, and you should review that information as well as material in the text. You can take any of the practice examinations again after your additional study.

Physician Exam (Format A) FINAL EXAMINATION ANSWER SHEET

Medical Terminology

1. Ⓐ Ⓑ Ⓒ Ⓓ
2. Ⓐ Ⓑ Ⓒ Ⓓ
3. Ⓐ Ⓑ Ⓒ Ⓓ
4. Ⓐ Ⓑ Ⓒ Ⓓ
5. Ⓐ Ⓑ Ⓒ Ⓓ
6. Ⓐ Ⓑ Ⓒ Ⓓ
7. Ⓐ Ⓑ Ⓒ Ⓓ
8. Ⓐ Ⓑ Ⓒ Ⓓ

Anatomy

9. Ⓐ Ⓑ Ⓒ Ⓓ
10. Ⓐ Ⓑ Ⓒ Ⓓ
11. Ⓐ Ⓑ Ⓒ Ⓓ
12. Ⓐ Ⓑ Ⓒ Ⓓ
13. Ⓐ Ⓑ Ⓒ Ⓓ
14. Ⓐ Ⓑ Ⓒ Ⓓ
15. Ⓐ Ⓑ Ⓒ Ⓓ
16. Ⓐ Ⓑ Ⓒ Ⓓ

ICD-10-CM/Diagnosis

17. Ⓐ Ⓑ Ⓒ Ⓓ
18. Ⓐ Ⓑ Ⓒ Ⓓ
19. Ⓐ Ⓑ Ⓒ Ⓓ
20. Ⓐ Ⓑ Ⓒ Ⓓ
21. Ⓐ Ⓑ Ⓒ Ⓓ
22. Ⓐ Ⓑ Ⓒ Ⓓ
23. Ⓐ Ⓑ Ⓒ Ⓓ
24. Ⓐ Ⓑ Ⓒ Ⓓ
25. Ⓐ Ⓑ Ⓒ Ⓓ
26. Ⓐ Ⓑ Ⓒ Ⓓ

HCPCS Level II

27. Ⓐ Ⓑ Ⓒ Ⓓ
28. Ⓐ Ⓑ Ⓒ Ⓓ
29. Ⓐ Ⓑ Ⓒ Ⓓ
30. Ⓐ Ⓑ Ⓒ Ⓓ
31. Ⓐ Ⓑ Ⓒ Ⓓ
32. Ⓐ Ⓑ Ⓒ Ⓓ

Compliance and Regulatory

33. Ⓐ Ⓑ Ⓒ Ⓓ
34. Ⓐ Ⓑ Ⓒ Ⓓ
35. Ⓐ Ⓑ Ⓒ Ⓓ
36. Ⓐ Ⓑ Ⓒ Ⓓ
37. Ⓐ Ⓑ Ⓒ Ⓓ

Coding Guidelines

38. Ⓐ Ⓑ Ⓒ Ⓓ
39. Ⓐ Ⓑ Ⓒ Ⓓ
40. Ⓐ Ⓑ Ⓒ Ⓓ
41. Ⓐ Ⓑ Ⓒ Ⓓ
42. Ⓐ Ⓑ Ⓒ Ⓓ
43. Ⓐ Ⓑ Ⓒ Ⓓ

10000 Integumentary System

44. Ⓐ Ⓑ Ⓒ Ⓓ
45. Ⓐ Ⓑ Ⓒ Ⓓ
46. Ⓐ Ⓑ Ⓒ Ⓓ
47. Ⓐ Ⓑ Ⓒ Ⓓ
48. Ⓐ Ⓑ Ⓒ Ⓓ
49. Ⓐ Ⓑ Ⓒ Ⓓ
50. Ⓐ Ⓑ Ⓒ Ⓓ
51. Ⓐ Ⓑ Ⓒ Ⓓ
52. Ⓐ Ⓑ Ⓒ Ⓓ
53. Ⓐ Ⓑ Ⓒ Ⓓ

20000 Musculoskeletal System

54. Ⓐ Ⓑ Ⓒ Ⓓ
55. Ⓐ Ⓑ Ⓒ Ⓓ
56. Ⓐ Ⓑ Ⓒ Ⓓ
57. Ⓐ Ⓑ Ⓒ Ⓓ
58. Ⓐ Ⓑ Ⓒ Ⓓ
59. Ⓐ Ⓑ Ⓒ Ⓓ
60. Ⓐ Ⓑ Ⓒ Ⓓ
61. Ⓐ Ⓑ Ⓒ Ⓓ
62. Ⓐ Ⓑ Ⓒ Ⓓ
63. Ⓐ Ⓑ Ⓒ Ⓓ

30000 Respiratory and Cardiovascular System

64. Ⓐ Ⓑ Ⓒ Ⓓ
65. Ⓐ Ⓑ Ⓒ Ⓓ
66. Ⓐ Ⓑ Ⓒ Ⓓ
67. Ⓐ Ⓑ Ⓒ Ⓓ
68. Ⓐ Ⓑ Ⓒ Ⓓ
69. Ⓐ Ⓑ Ⓒ Ⓓ
70. Ⓐ Ⓑ Ⓒ Ⓓ
71. Ⓐ Ⓑ Ⓒ Ⓓ
72. Ⓐ Ⓑ Ⓒ Ⓓ
73. Ⓐ Ⓑ Ⓒ Ⓓ

40000 Digestive System

74. Ⓐ Ⓑ Ⓒ Ⓓ
75. Ⓐ Ⓑ Ⓒ Ⓓ
76. Ⓐ Ⓑ Ⓒ Ⓓ
77. Ⓐ Ⓑ Ⓒ Ⓓ
78. Ⓐ Ⓑ Ⓒ Ⓓ
79. Ⓐ Ⓑ Ⓒ Ⓓ
80. Ⓐ Ⓑ Ⓒ Ⓓ
81. Ⓐ Ⓑ Ⓒ Ⓓ
82. Ⓐ Ⓑ Ⓒ Ⓓ
83. Ⓐ Ⓑ Ⓒ Ⓓ

50000 Urinary, Male Genital System, Female Genital System, and Maternity Care and Delivery

84. Ⓐ Ⓑ Ⓒ Ⓓ
85. Ⓐ Ⓑ Ⓒ Ⓓ
86. Ⓐ Ⓑ Ⓒ Ⓓ
87. Ⓐ Ⓑ Ⓒ Ⓓ
88. Ⓐ Ⓑ Ⓒ Ⓓ
89. Ⓐ Ⓑ Ⓒ Ⓓ
90. Ⓐ Ⓑ Ⓒ Ⓓ
91. Ⓐ Ⓑ Ⓒ Ⓓ
92. Ⓐ Ⓑ Ⓒ Ⓓ
93. Ⓐ Ⓑ Ⓒ Ⓓ

60000 Endocrine System, Hemic and Lymphatic System, Nervous System, Eye and Ocular Adnexa, Auditory System

94. Ⓐ Ⓑ Ⓒ Ⓓ
95. Ⓐ Ⓑ Ⓒ Ⓓ
96. Ⓐ Ⓑ Ⓒ Ⓓ
97. Ⓐ Ⓑ Ⓒ Ⓓ
98. Ⓐ Ⓑ Ⓒ Ⓓ
99. Ⓐ Ⓑ Ⓒ Ⓓ
100. Ⓐ Ⓑ Ⓒ Ⓓ
101. Ⓐ Ⓑ Ⓒ Ⓓ
102. Ⓐ Ⓑ Ⓒ Ⓓ
103. Ⓐ Ⓑ Ⓒ Ⓓ

Evaluation and Management (E/M)

104. Ⓐ Ⓑ Ⓒ Ⓓ
105. Ⓐ Ⓑ Ⓒ Ⓓ
106. Ⓐ Ⓑ Ⓒ Ⓓ
107. Ⓐ Ⓑ Ⓒ Ⓓ
108. Ⓐ Ⓑ Ⓒ Ⓓ
109. Ⓐ Ⓑ Ⓒ Ⓓ
110. Ⓐ Ⓑ Ⓒ Ⓓ
111. Ⓐ Ⓑ Ⓒ Ⓓ
112. Ⓐ Ⓑ Ⓒ Ⓓ
113. Ⓐ Ⓑ Ⓒ Ⓓ

Anesthesia

114. Ⓐ Ⓑ Ⓒ Ⓓ
115. Ⓐ Ⓑ Ⓒ Ⓓ
116. Ⓐ Ⓑ Ⓒ Ⓓ
117. Ⓐ Ⓑ Ⓒ Ⓓ
118. Ⓐ Ⓑ Ⓒ Ⓓ
119. Ⓐ Ⓑ Ⓒ Ⓓ
120. Ⓐ Ⓑ Ⓒ Ⓓ
121. Ⓐ Ⓑ Ⓒ Ⓓ

70000 Radiology

122. Ⓐ Ⓑ Ⓒ Ⓓ
123. Ⓐ Ⓑ Ⓒ Ⓓ
124. Ⓐ Ⓑ Ⓒ Ⓓ
125. Ⓐ Ⓑ Ⓒ Ⓓ
126. Ⓐ Ⓑ Ⓒ Ⓓ
127. Ⓐ Ⓑ Ⓒ Ⓓ
128. Ⓐ Ⓑ Ⓒ Ⓓ
129. Ⓐ Ⓑ Ⓒ Ⓓ
130. Ⓐ Ⓑ Ⓒ Ⓓ

80000 Laboratory / Pathology

131. Ⓐ Ⓑ Ⓒ Ⓓ
132. Ⓐ Ⓑ Ⓒ Ⓓ
133. Ⓐ Ⓑ Ⓒ Ⓓ
134. Ⓐ Ⓑ Ⓒ Ⓓ
135. Ⓐ Ⓑ Ⓒ Ⓓ
136. Ⓐ Ⓑ Ⓒ Ⓓ
137. Ⓐ Ⓑ Ⓒ Ⓓ
138. Ⓐ Ⓑ Ⓒ Ⓓ
139. Ⓐ Ⓑ Ⓒ Ⓓ
140. Ⓐ Ⓑ Ⓒ Ⓓ

90000 Medicine

141. Ⓐ Ⓑ Ⓒ Ⓓ
142. Ⓐ Ⓑ Ⓒ Ⓓ
143. Ⓐ Ⓑ Ⓒ Ⓓ
144. Ⓐ Ⓑ Ⓒ Ⓓ
145. Ⓐ Ⓑ Ⓒ Ⓓ
146. Ⓐ Ⓑ Ⓒ Ⓓ
147. Ⓐ Ⓑ Ⓒ Ⓓ
148. Ⓐ Ⓑ Ⓒ Ⓓ
149. Ⓐ Ⓑ Ⓒ Ⓓ
150. Ⓐ Ⓑ Ⓒ Ⓓ

Physician Exam (Format A)—Final Examination

Direction: Report only the professional component unless specifically directed to do otherwise within the question.

Subject Area: Medical Terminology

1. This term means the surgical removal of the fallopian tube:
   - A. ligation
   - B. hysterectomy
   - C. salpingostomy
   - D. salpingectomy

2. This combining form means thirst:
   - A. dips/o
   - B. acr/o
   - C. cortic/o
   - D. somat/o

3. This term is also known as a homograft:
   - A. autograft
   - B. allograft
   - C. xenograft
   - D. zenograft

4. Which of the following terms means taste?
   - A. Meissner
   - B. Pacinian
   - C. gustatory
   - D. astrocytes

5. This suffix means removal:
   - A. -penia
   - B. -ectomy
   - C. -itis
   - D. -pexy

6. Which of the following terms does NOT describe a receptor of the body?
   - A. mechanoreceptor
   - B. proprioceptor
   - C. thermoreceptor
   - D. endoreceptor

7. This term means abnormal thickening of the skin:
   - A. ductus
   - B. dermatofibroma
   - C. dermatitis
   - D. pachyderma

8. The term that defines the relaxation phase of the heartbeat is:
   - A. systole
   - B. sinoatrial
   - C. diastole
   - D. septa

Subject Area: Anatomy

9. This is the first portion of the small intestine:
   - A. jejunum
   - B. ileum
   - C. duodenum
   - D. cecum

10. This is a part of the inner ear:
    - A. vestibule
    - B. malleus
    - C. incus
    - D. stapes

11. This is the area behind the cornea:
    - A. anterior chamber
    - B. choroid layer
    - C. ciliary body
    - D. fundus

12. Which of the following is a covering of the chamber walls of the heart?
    - A. endocardium
    - B. myocardium
    - C. pericardium
    - D. epicardium

13. The shaft of a long bone:
    - A. diaphysis
    - B. epiphysis
    - C. metaphysis
    - D. periosteum

14. The act of turning upward, such as the hand turned palm upward:
    - A. supination
    - B. adduction
    - C. pronation
    - D. circumduction

15. The middle layer of the skin, also known as the corium or true skin:
    - A. epidermis
    - B. stratum corneum
    - C. dermis
    - D. subcutaneous

16. This is the collarbone:
    - A. patella
    - B. tibia
    - C. scapula
    - D. clavicle

Subject Area: ICD-10-CM

17. Three-week-old female with obstructive apnea.
    - A. P28.3
    - B. P28.4
    - C. R06.81
    - D. G47.33

18. Mild intellectual disabilities due to congenital iodine-deficiency hypothyroidism.
    - A. E00.9, F70
    - B. E01.8, F70
    - C. E03.0, F78
    - D. F70, E00.9

19. Admission for hemodialysis because of acute renal failure.
    A. Z49.01, N17.9
    B. N19, Z49.01
    C. N17.9, Z99.2
    D. Z99.2, N17.9
20. Glomerulonephritis due to viral hepatitis.
    A. N05, B19
    B. B19, N00.9
    C. N05.9, B19.9
    D. B19.9, N05.9
21. Initial encounter to repair a laceration of the left hand.
    A. S61.412A
    B. S61.402A, Y93.9
    C. S61.421A
    D. S61.412A, Y93.9
22. Mr. Hallberger is 62 and has multiple problems. I am examining him in the intensive critical care unit. I understand he has fluid overload with acute renal failure and was started on ultrafiltration by the nephrologist on duty. He has an abnormal chest x-ray. He has preexisting type II diabetes mellitus and sepsis. We are left with a patient now who is still sedated and on a ventilator because of acute respiratory failure. Code the diagnoses only.
    A. A42.7, N18.9, J96.00, R60.9, E11.29, R84.9
    B. A42.7, R18.8, J96.00, N17.0, E11.4, R91.8
    C. A41.9, B17.0, J96.00, E11.9, E86.9, R91.8, 99223
    D. A41.9, N17.9, J96.00, E11.9, R91.8
23. Bloody stool.
    A. P54.1
    B. R19.5
    C. K92.1
    D. K62.5
24. A lethargic patient presents with vomiting and severe cramping and the physician determines during the initial encounter that the condition was caused by the ingestion of five tablets of Tylenol with codeine and half a bottle of whiskey.
    A. T40.2X4, T39.1X4, T51.0X4, R53.83, R11.10, R10.9
    B. T40.2X4A, T39.1X4A, R53.82, R11.10, R10.9
    C. T40.2X4A, T39.1X4A, T51.0X4A, R53.83, R11.11, R10.9
    D. T40.2X4A, T39.1X4A, T51.0X4A, R53.83, R11.10, R10.9
25. Initial encounter to treat a fracture of the right patella with abrasion.
    A. S82.001A, S80.211A
    B. S82.001A
    C. S80.211A, S82.001B
    D. S82.001B
26. Sarcoidosis with cardiomyopathy.
    A. D86.89
    B. D86.85
    C. D86.89, I42.9
    D. D85.85, I42.9

Subject Area: HCPCS

27. A patient is issued a 22-inch seat cushion for his wheelchair.
    A. E2601
    B. E0950
    C. E0190
    D. E2602
28. A patient with chronic lumbar pain previously purchased a TENS and now needs replacement batteries.
    A. E1592
    B. A5082
    C. A4772
    D. A4630
29. A patient presents for trimming of 10 dystrophic toenails.
    A. G0127 × 2, L60.3
    B. G0127, G0127 × 9, L60.0
    C. G0127, L60.3
    D. G0127 × 5, G0127 × 5, Q84.6
30. A patient with chronic obstructive pulmonary disease is issued a medically necessary nebulizer with a compressor and humidifier for extensive use with oxygen delivery.
    A. E0570, E0550
    B. E0555, E0571
    C. E0580, E0550
    D. E0575, E0550
31. Which HCPCS modifier indicates the great toe of the right foot?
    A. T1
    B. T3
    C. T4
    D. T5

Subject Area: Practice Management

32. This program was developed by CMS to promote national correct coding methods and to control inappropriate payment of Part B claims and hospital outpatient claims.
    A. NCCI
    B. NFS
    C. HIPAA
    D. MA-PA
33. What is an NPI?
    A. National Payer Incentive
    B. National Provider Identification
    C. National Provider Index
    D. National Payer Identification
34. The RBRVS is a
    A. payment reform implemented in 1992
    B. listing of the customary charge for services
    C. payment list that indicates the prevailing charge in a locality
    D. listing of the physician's individual charges for a service

35. Which of the following is NOT considered fraud or abuse?
    A. Lack of documentation of medical necessity for services reported
    B. Accepting a $20 gift card from a shoe repair representative for each Medicare patient referred to his store
    C. Referring patients to a radiology center in which your physician is a partner
    D. Going to lunch with a pharmaceutical representative

36. This document is a notification to the patient in advance of services rendered that Medicare probably will not pay for those services, in addition to providing the estimated cost for which the patient will be responsible.
    A. Waiver of Liability
    B. Coordination of Benefits
    C. Advanced Beneficiary Notice
    D. UPIN

37. This entity develops and publishes an annual plan that outlines the Medicare monitoring program.
    A. MAC
    B. FI
    C. OIG
    D. CMS

Subject Area: Coding Guidelines

38. Which punctuation mark between codes in the index of the CPT manual indicates a range of codes is available?
    A. period
    B. comma
    C. semicolon
    D. hyphen

39. Which of the following most accurately describes the designation "(Separate procedure)." The procedure is:
    A. Integral to another procedure.
    B. Reported if it is the only procedure performed.
    C. Reported if the procedure is unrelated to a more major procedure performed at the same time at a different site.
    D. All of the above

40. Specific coding guidelines in the CPT manual are located in:
    A. the index.
    B. the introduction.
    C. the beginning of each section.
    D. Appendix A.

41. The symbol that indicates an add-on code in the CPT manual is:
    A. ▲
    B. ●
    C. +
    D. ▶ ◀

42. When you see the symbol ⊘ next to a code in the CPT manual, you know that:
    A. the code is a new code.
    B. the code contains new or revised text.
    C. the code is a modifier −51 exempt code.
    D. FDA approval is pending.

43. The term that indicates this is the type of code for which the full code description can be known only if the common part of the code (the description preceding the semicolon) of a preceding entry is referenced:
    A. stand-alone
    B. indented
    C. independent
    D. add-on

Subject Area: 10000 Integumentary System

44. **OPERATIVE REPORT**
    OPERATIVE PROCEDURE: Excision of back lesion.
    INDICATIONS FOR SURGERY: The patient has an enlarging lesion on the upper midback.
    FINDINGS AT SURGERY: There was a 5-cm, upper midback lesion.
    OPERATIVE PROCEDURE: With the patient prone, the back was prepped and draped in the usual sterile fashion. The skin and underlying tissues were anesthetized with 30 mL of 1% lidocaine with epinephrine. Through a 5-cm transverse skin incision, the lesion was excised. Hemostasis was ensured. The incision was closed using 3-0 Vicryl for the deep layers and running 3-0 Prolene subcuticular stitch with Steri-Strips for the skin.

    The patient was returned to the same-day surgery center in stable postoperative condition. All sponge, needle, and instrument counts were correct. Estimated blood loss is 0 mL.
    PATHOLOGY REPORT LATER INDICATED: Dermatofibroma, skin of back. Assign code(s) for the physician service only.
    A. 11406, 12002, D23.5
    B. 11424, D21.6
    C. 11406, 12032, D23.5
    D. 11606, D04.5

45. What CPT and ICD-10-CM codes would be used to code a subsequent encounter in which a split-thickness skin graft, both thighs to the abdomen, measuring 45 × 21 cm is performed on a patient who has third-degree burns of the abdomen? Documentation stated 20% of the body surface was burned, with 9% third degree. The patient also sustained second-degree burns of the upper back.
    A. 15100 × 2, T21.32XD, T21.24XD, T31.0
    B. 15100, 15101 × 9, T21.32XD, T21.23XD, T31.20
    C. 15100, 15101-51 × 9, T21.32XA, T21.23XA, T31.20
    D. 15100, 15101 × 8, T21.32XD, T21.23XD

46. EMERGENCY DEPARTMENT REPORT CHIEF COMPLAINT: Nasal bridge laceration.

SUBJECTIVE: The patient is a 74-year-old male who presents to the emergency department with a laceration to the bridge of his nose. He fell in the bathroom tonight. He recalls the incident. He just sort of lost his balance. He denies any vertigo. He denies any chest pain or shortness of breath. He denies any head pain or neck pain. There was no loss of consciousness. He slipped on a wet floor in the bathroom and lost his balance; that is how it happened. He has not had any blood from the nose or mouth.

PAST MEDICAL HISTORY:

1. Parkinson's
2. Back pain
3. Constipation

MEDICATIONS: See the patient record for a complete list of medications.

ALLERGIES: NKDA.

REVIEW OF SYSTEMS: Per HPI. Otherwise, negative.

PHYSICAL EXAMINATION: The exam showed a 74-year-old male in no acute distress. Examination of the HEAD showed no obvious trauma other than the bridge of the nose, where there is approximately a 1.5- to 2-cm laceration. He had no bony tenderness under this. Pupils were equal, round, and reactive. EARS and NOSE: OROPHARYNX was unremarkable. NECK was soft and supple. HEART was regular. LUNGS were clear but slightly diminished in the bases.

PROCEDURE: The wound was draped in a sterile fashion and anesthetized with 1% Xylocaine with sodium bicarbonate. It was cleansed with sterile saline and then repaired using interrupted 6-0 Ethilon sutures (Dr. Barney Teller, first-year resident, assisted with the suturing).

ASSESSMENT: Nasal bridge laceration, status post-fall.

PLAN: Keep clean. Sutures out in 5 to 7 days. Watch for signs of infection.

A. 12051, S01.21XA, W01.10XA
B. 12011, S01.21XA, W01.10XA
C. 12011, S01.20XA, W01.10XA
D. 12011, 11000, S01.20XA, S01.20XS

47. The patient is brought to surgery for repair of an accidentally inflicted open wound of the left thigh, the total extent measuring approximately 40 × 35 cm.

DESCRIPTION OF PROCEDURE: The legs were prepped with Betadine scrub and solution and then draped in a routine sterile fashion. Split-thickness skin grafts measuring about a 10,000th-inch thick were taken from both thighs, meshed with a 3:1 ratio mesher, and stapled to the wounds. The donor sites were dressed with scarlet red, and the recipient sites were dressed with Xeroform, Kerlix fluffs, and Kerlix roll, and a few ABD pads were used for absorption.

Estimated blood loss was negligible. The patient tolerated the procedure well and left surgery in good condition.

A. 15120, 15121 × 12, S71.132A
B. 15100, 15101, 11010, S71.132A
C. 15220, 15221 × 13, S71.102A
D. 15100, 15101 × 13, S71.102A

48. What CPT and ICD-10-CM codes would be used to code the destruction by cryosurgery of a malignant lesion on the skin of the female genitalia measuring 1.6 cm?

A. 17272, C51.9
B. 11602, C57.9
C. 11420, C79.82
D. 11622, C51.9

49. SAME-DAY SURGERY

DIAGNOSIS: Inverted nipple with mammary duct ectasia, left.

OPERATION: Excision of mass deep to left nipple. With the patient under general anesthesia, a circumareolar incision was made with sharp dissection and carried down into the breast tissue. The nipple complex was raised up using a small retractor. We gently dissected underneath to free up the nipple entirely. Once this was done, we had the nipple fully unfolded, and there was some evident mammary duct ectasia. An area 3 × 4 cm was excised using electrocautery. Hemostasis was maintained with the electrocautery, and then the breast tissue deep to the nipple was reconstructed using sutures of 3-0 chromic. Subcutaneous tissue was closed using 3-0 chromic, and then the skin was closed using 4-0 Vicryl. Steri-Strips were applied. The patient tolerated the procedure well and was returned to the recovery area in stable condition. At the end of the procedure, all sponges and instruments were accounted for.

A. 19120-RT, N60.42
B. 11404-LT, N62
C. 19112, N60.42
D. 19120-LT, N60.42

50. This patient returns today for palliative care to her feet. Her toenails have become elongated and thickened, and she is unable to trim them on her own. She states that she has had no problems and no acute signs of any infection or otherwise to her feet. She returns today strictly for trimming of her toenails.

EXAMINATION: Her pedal pulses are palpable bilaterally. The nails are mycotic, 1 through 4 on the left, and 1 through 3 on the right.

ASSESSMENT: Onychomycosis, 1 through 4 on the left and 1 through 3 on the right.

PLAN: Mild debridement of mycotic nails × 7. This patient is to return to the clinic in 3 to 4 months for follow-up palliative care.

A. 11721 × 7, B35.9
B. 99212, 11721, B35.1
C. 11719, B35.1
D. 11721, B35.1

51. OPERATIVE REPORT

With the patient having had a wire localization performed by radiology, she was taken to the operating room and, under local anesthesia of the left breast, was prepped and draped in a sterile manner. A breast line incision was made through the entry point of the wire, and a core of tissue surrounding the wire (approximately 1 × 2 cm) was removed using electrocautery for hemostasis. The specimen, including the wire, was then submitted to radiology, and the presence of the lesion within the specimen was confirmed. The wound was checked for hemostasis, and this was maintained with electrocautery. The breast tissue was reapproximated using 2-0 and 3-0 chromic. The skin was closed using 4-0 Vicryl in a subcuticular manner. Steri-Strips were applied. The patient tolerated the procedure well and was discharged from the operating room in stable condition. At the end of the procedure, all sponges and instruments were accounted for.

Pathology report later indicated: Benign tissue, breast.

A. 11602-LT, N64
B. 11400-LT, C50.912
C. 19125-LT, D24.2
D. 19125-LT, D24.1

52. What CPT and ICD-10-CM codes would be assigned to report an initial encounter for treatment of a 40 sq cm debridement of an open anterior abdominal laceration, including subcutaneous tissue and muscle, with grit and rubble? The patient fell while speed walking and landed on a sharp rock, injuring the epigastric region of the abdomen.

A. 11000, S31.129A, W01.118A, W45.8A, Y93.01A
B. 11010, S31.622A, W18.39, W45.8
C. 11042, 11045, S31.142A
D. 11043, 11046, S31.122A, W01.118A, W45.8XXA, Y93.01

53. What code(s) is used by the radiologist when performing ultrasound preoperative placement of a needle localization wire of a single lesion of the breast? The patient was diagnosed with adenocarcinoma of the upper outer quadrant of the right breast, primary site.

A. 19285-RT, 19125-RT, C50.511
B. 19125-RT, C50.411
C. 19285-RT, C50.411
D. 19286-RT, C50.511

Subject Area: 20000 Musculoskeletal System

54. A small incision was made over the left proximal tibia, and a traction pin was inserted through the bone to the opposite side. Weights were then affixed to the pins to stabilize the closed tibial fracture temporarily until fracture repair could be performed. Assign codes for the physician service.

A. 20650-LT, S82.102A
B. 20663-LT, S82.162A
C. 20690-LT, S82.302A
D. 20692-LT, S82.302A

55. OPERATIVE REPORT

PREOPERATIVE DIAGNOSIS: Left thigh abscess.
PROCEDURE PERFORMED: Incision and drainage of left thigh abscess.
OPERATIVE NOTE: With the patient under general anesthesia, he was placed in the lithotomy position. The area around the anus was carefully inspected, and we saw no evidence of communication with the perirectal space. This appears to have risen in the crease at the top of the leg, extending from the posterior buttocks region up toward the side of the base of the penis. In any event, the area was prepped and draped in a sterile manner. Then we incised the area in fluctuation. We obtained a lot of very foul-smelling, almost stool-like material (it was not stool, but it was brown and very foul-smelling material). This was not the typical pus one sees with a *Staphylococcus aureus*–type infection. The incision was widened to allow us to probe the cavity fully. Again, I could see no evidence of communication to the rectum, but there was extension down the thigh and extension up into the groin crease. The fascia was darkened from the purulent material. I opened some of the fascia to make sure the underlying muscle was viable. This appeared viable. No gas was present. There was nothing to suggest a necrotizing fasciitis. The patient did have a very extensive inflammation within this abscess cavity. The abscess cavity was irrigated with peroxide and saline and packed with gauze vaginal packing. The patient tolerated the procedure well and was discharged from the operating room in stable condition.

A. 26990-LT, L02.416A
B. 27301-LT, L02.416
C. 27301-LT, L02.416A
D. 27025-LT, L02.416

56. OPERATIVE REPORT

PREOPERATIVE DIAGNOSIS: Compound fracture, left humerus, with possible loss of left radial pulse.
PROCEDURE PERFORMED: Open reduction internal fixation, left compound humerus fracture.
PROCEDURE: While under a general anesthetic, the patient's left arm was prepped with Betadine and draped in sterile fashion. We then created a longitudinal incision over the anterolateral aspect of his left arm and carried the dissection through the subcutaneous tissue. We attempted to identify the lateral intermuscular septum and progressed to the fracture site, which was actually fairly easy to do because there was some significant tearing and rupturing of the biceps and brachialis muscles. These were partial ruptures, but the bone was relatively easy to expose through this. We then identified the fracture site and thoroughly irrigated it with several liters of saline. We also noted that the radial nerve was easily visible, crossing along the posterolateral aspect of the fracture site. It

was intact. We carefully detected it throughout the remainder of the procedure. We then were able to strip the periosteum away from the lateral side of the shaft of the humerus both proximally and distally from the fracture site. We did this just enough to apply a 6-hole plate, which we eventually held in place with six cortical screws. We did attempt to compress the fracture site. Due to some comminution, the fracture was not quite anatomically aligned, but certainly it was felt to be very acceptable.

Once we had applied the plate, we then checked the radial pulse with a Doppler. We found that the radial pulse was present using the Doppler, but not with palpation. We then applied Xeroform dressings to the wounds and the incision. After padding the arm thoroughly, we applied a long-arm splint with the elbow flexed about 75 degrees. He tolerated the procedure well, and the radial pulse was again present on Doppler examination at the end of the procedure.

A. 24515-RT, S42.352A
B. 24500-LT, S42.392B
C. 24515-LT, S42.352B
D. 24505-LT, S42.352B

57. John, an 84-year-old male, tripped while on his morning walk. He stated he was thinking about something else when he inadvertently tripped over the sidewalk curb and fell to his knees. X-ray indicated a fracture of his right patella. With the patient under general anesthesia, the area was opened and extensively irrigated. The left aspect of the patella was severely fragmented, and a portion of the patella was subsequently removed. The remaining patella fragments were wired. The surrounding tissue was repaired, thoroughly irrigated, and closed in the usual manner.

A. 27524-RT, S82.001A, W10.1XXA
B. 27520-RT, S82.001A, W10.1XXA
C. 27524-RT, S82.099A, W19.XXXA
D. 27524-RT, S82.001A, W19.XXXA

58. Libby was thrown from a horse while riding along the side of the road; a truck that honked the horn as it passed her startled her horse. The horse reared up and Libby was thrown to the ground. The medial condyle of her left tibia was fractured and required insertion of multiple pins to stabilize the defect area. A Monticelli multiplane external fixation system was then attached to the pins. Code the placement of the fixation device and diagnosis(es) only.

A. 20661-LT, S82.142A, V80.018A
B. 20692-LT, S82.132A, V80.010A
C. 20692-LT, S82.142A, V80.018A
D. 20690-LT, S82.132A, S82.142A

59. Maryann received a blow to her right tibial shaft while moving a large stuffed chair up a flight of stairs when the person in front of the chair slipped and released his hold on the chair. The full weight of the chair was pushed against her. When she was unable to hold the chair in place, both she and the chair fell to the landing a dozen steps below. The chair tipped on its side and landed on her tibia. On x-ray, the right tibia shaft was fractured in three places. Screws and pins were placed through the skin to secure the fracture sites.

A. 27750-RT, S82.291A, W20.8XXA
B. 27756-RT, S82.291A, W19.XXXA
C. 27756-RT, S82.201A, W20.8XXA
D. 27750-RT, S82.201A, W20.8XXA

60. The physician applies a Minerva-type fiberglass body cast from the hips to the shoulders and to the head. Before application, a stockinette is stretched over the patient's torso, and further padding of the bony areas with felt padding was done. The patient was diagnosed with Morquio-Brailsford kyphosis. Assign codes for the physician service only.

A. 29040, E76.219, M49.80
B. 29710, M40.10
C. 29010, M49.80, E76.219
D. 29000, M41.20, E76.219

61. Mary tells her physician that she has been having pain in her left wrist for several weeks. The physician examines the area and palpates a ganglion cyst of the tendon sheath. He marks the injection sites, sterilizes the area, and injects corticosteroid into two areas of the left wrist.

A. 20550-LT × 2, M67.422
B. 20551-LT, M67.432A
C. 20551-LT × 2, M67.422A
D. 20612-LT, M67.432

62. Darin was a passenger in an automobile rollover accident and was not wearing a seat belt at the time. He was thrown from the automobile and was pinned under the rear of the overturned vehicle. He sustained craniofacial separation, Le Fort III fracture that required complicated internal and external fixation using an open approach to repair the extensive damage. A halo device was used to hold the head immobile.

A. 21435, 20661
B. 21435
C. 21432
D. 21436, 20661

63. Carl Ostrick, a 21-year-old male, slipped on a patch of ice on his sidewalk while shoveling snow. When he fell, his left hand was wedged under his body and his second carpometacarpal joint was dislocated. After manipulating the joint back into normal alignment, the surgeon on the following day fixed the dislocation by placing a wire through the skin at the tip of the finger and on through the carpometacarpal joint to maintain alignment. Code the subsequent procedure and diagnoses.

A. 26608-F1, S63.052A, W00.0XXA
B. 26650-FA, S63.042D, W19.XXXD
C. 26706-LT, S63.002D, W00.0XXD
D. 26676-LT, S63.052D, W00.0XXD

Subject Area: 30000 Respiratory System and
Cardiovascular System

64. OPERATIVE PROCEDURE

PREOPERATIVE DIAGNOSIS: 68-year-old male in a coma.

POSTOPERATIVE DIAGNOSIS: 68-year-old male in a coma.

PROCEDURE PERFORMED: Placement of a triple lumen central line in right subclavian vein.

With the usual Betadine scrub to the right subclavian vein area and with a second attempt, the subclavian vein was cannulated and the wire was threaded. The first time the wire did not thread right, and so the attempt was aborted to make sure we had good identification of structures. Once the wire was in place, the needle was removed and a tissue dilator was pushed into position over the wire. Once that was removed, the central lumen catheter was pushed into position at 17 cm and the wire removed. All three ports were flushed. The catheter was sewn into position, and a dressing applied.

A. 36011, R40.20X0
B. 36011, R40.20
C. 36556, R40.20X0
D. 36556, R40.20

65. What CPT and ICD-10-CM codes report a percutaneous insertion of a dual-chamber pacemaker by means of the subclavian vein? The diagnosis is sick sinus syndrome, tachy-brady.

A. 33249, I47.1, I49.5
B. 33217, I49.5
C. 33208, I49.5
D. 33240, I44.0, I47.1

66. OPERATIVE REPORT

PREOPERATIVE DIAGNOSIS: Atelectasis of the left lower lobe.

PROCEDURE PERFORMED: Fiberoptic bronchoscopy with brushings and cell washings.

PROCEDURE: The patient was already sedated, on a ventilator, and intubated; so his bronchoscopy was done through the ET tube. It was passed easily down to the carina. About 2 to 2.5 cm above the carina, we could see the trachea, which appeared good, as was the carina. In the right lung, all segments were patent and entered, and no masses were seen. The left lung, however, had petechial ecchymotic areas scattered throughout the airways. The tissue was friable and swollen, but no mucous plugs were noted, and all the airways were open, just somewhat swollen. No abnormal secretions were noted at all. Brushings were taken as well as washings, including some with Mucomyst to see whether we could get some distal mucous plug, but nothing really significant was returned. The specimens were sent to appropriate cytological and bacteriological studies. The patient tolerated the procedure fairly well.

A. 31622, 31623-51, J98.11
B. 31623, P28.0
C. 31623-LT, J98.11
D. 31624, P28.0

67. OPERATIVE REPORT

PREOPERATIVE DIAGNOSIS:
1. Hypoxia.
2. Pneumothorax.

POSTOPERATIVE DIAGNOSIS:
1. Hypoxia.
2. Pneumothorax.

PROCEDURE: Chest tube placement.

DESCRIPTION OF PROCEDURE: The patient was previously sedated with Versed and paralyzed with Nimbex. Lidocaine was used to numb the incision area in the midlateral left chest at about nipple level. After the lidocaine, an incision was made, and we bluntly dissected to the area of the pleural space, making sure we were superior to the rib. On entrance to the pleural space, there was immediate release of air noted. An 18-gauge chest tube was subsequently placed and sutured to the skin. There were no complications for the procedure, and blood loss was minimal.

DISPOSITION: Follow-up, single-view, chest x-ray showed significant resolution of the pneumothorax except for a small apical pneumothorax that was noted. Code only the operative procedure and diagnosis(es).

A. 32556, R09.02, J93.9
B. 32551, 71045, R09.02, J93.9
C. 32551, J93.9, R09.02
D. 32556, R09.02, J93.0

68. OPERATIVE REPORT

PREOPERATIVE DIAGNOSIS: Atherosclerotic heart disease.

POSTOPERATIVE DIAGNOSIS: Atherosclerotic heart disease.

OPERATIVE PROCEDURE: Coronary bypass grafts × 2 with a single graft from the aorta to the distal left anterior descending and from the aorta to the distal right coronary artery.

PROCEDURE: The patient was brought to the operating room and placed in a supine position. Under general intubation anesthesia, the anterior chest and legs were prepped and draped in the usual manner. A segment of greater saphenous vein was harvested from the left thigh, utilizing the endoscopic vein harvesting technique, and prepared for grafting. The sternum was opened in the usual fashion, and the left internal mammary artery was taken down and prepared for grafting. The flow through the internal mammary artery was very poor. The patient did have a 25-mm difference in arterial pressure between the right and left arms, the right arm being higher. The left internal mammary artery was therefore not used. The pericardium was incised sharply and a pericardial well created. The patient was systemically heparinized and placed on bicaval to aortic cardiopulmonary bypass with the stump in the main pulmonary artery for cardiac decompression. The patient was cooled to 26°C, and on fibrillation an aortic cross-clamp was applied and potassium-rich cold crystalline cardioplegic solution was administered through the aortic root with satisfactory cardiac arrest. Subsequent doses were given down the vein grafts as the anastomoses were completed and via the coronary sinus in a retrograde fashion. Attention was directed to the right coronary artery. The end of the greater saphenous vein was then anastomosed with 7-0 continuous Prolene distally. The remaining graft material was then grafted to the left anterior descending at the junction of the middle and distal third. The aortic cross-clamp was removed after 149 minutes with spontaneous cardioversion. The usual maneuvers to remove air from the left heart were then carried out using transesophageal echocardiographic technique. After all the air was removed and the patient had returned to a satisfactory temperature, he was weaned from cardiopulmonary bypass after 213 minutes utilizing 5 g per kilogram per minute of dopamine. The chest was closed in the usual fashion. A sterile compression dressing was applied, and the patient returned to the surgical intensive care unit in satisfactory condition.

A. 33511, 33517, I70.91
B. 33511, 33508, I25.10
C. 33534, 33508, I25.709
D. 33511, 33517, I25.10

69. **OPERATIVE REPORT:** The patient is in for a bone marrow biopsy. The patient was sterilized by standard procedure. Bone marrow core biopsies were obtained from the left posterior iliac crest with minimal discomfort. At the end of the procedure, the patient denied discomfort, without evidence of complications. The patient has diffuse, large B-cell malignant lymphoma. Assign codes for the physician service only.

A. 20225, C83.00
B. 38221, C83.30
C. 38230, C83.00
D. 38220, C83.30

70. Patient is a 40-year-old male who was involved in a motor vehicle crash. He is having some pulmonary insufficiency.

PROCEDURE: Bronchoscope was inserted through the accessory point on the end of the ET tube and was then advanced through the ET tube. The ET tube came pretty close to the carina. We selectively intubated the right mainstem bronchus with the bronchoscope. There were some secretions here, and these were aspirated. We then advanced this selectively into first the lower and then the middle and upper lobes. Secretions were present, more so in the middle and lower lobes. No mucous plug was identified. We then went into the left mainstem and looked at the upper and lower lobes. There was really not much in the way of secretions present. We did inject some saline and aspirated this out. We then removed the bronchoscope and put the patient back on the supplemental O_2. We waited a few minutes. The oxygen level actually stayed pretty good during this time. We then reinserted the bronchoscope and went down to the right side again. We aspirated out all secretions and made sure everything was clear. We then removed the bronchoscope and pulled back on the ET tube about 1.5 cm. We then again placed the patient on supplemental oxygenation.

FINDINGS: No mucous plug was identified. Secretions were found mainly in the right lung and were aspirated. The left side looked pretty clear.

A. 31646, J80, V49.9XXA
B. 32654, J98.4, V49.9
C. 31645-50, J80, V49.9XXA
D. 31645-RT, J80, V49.9XXA

71. This 52-year-old male has undergone several attempts at extubation, all of which failed. He also has morbid obesity and significant subcutaneous fat in his neck. The patient is now admitted for a flap tracheostomy and cervical lipectomy. The cervical lipectomy is necessary for adequate exposure and access to the trachea and also to secure tracheotomy tube placement. Assign code(s) for the physician service only.

A. 31610, 15839-51
B. 31610
C. 31610, 15838
D. 31603, 15839-51

72. Connie was brought to the operating room for repair of an acute, traumatic diaphragmatic hernia.

A. 39540, K44.9
B. 39503, K44.0
C. 39541, K44.9
D. 39540, Q79.0

73. This patient returns to the operating room for placement of an additional chest tube for an anterior pneumothorax due to a contusion lung injury. The same physician had just placed a chest tube 4 days earlier.

A. 32551, S27.0XXD
B. 32554, S27.329D
C. 32551-58, S27.329D
D. 32551, S25.419D

Subject Area: 40000 Digestive System

74. What CPT code would you use if the physician performs a pyloroplasty and vagotomy in the same surgical session?

A. 43865
B. 50400
C. 43635
D. 43640

75. This 43-year-old female comes in with a peritonsillar abscess. The patient is brought to same-day surgery and given general anesthetic. On examination of the peritonsillar abscess, an incision was made and fluid was drained. The area was examined again, saline was applied, and then the area was packed with gauze. The patient tolerated the procedure well.
    A. 42825, J36
    B. 42700, J36
    C. 42825, J35.01
    D. 42700, J36.00

76. **OPERATIVE REPORT**
    PREOPERATIVE DIAGNOSIS: Abdominal pain.
    POSTOPERATIVE DIAGNOSIS: Normal endoscopy.
    PROCEDURE: The flexible video therapeutic endoscope was passed without difficulty into the oropharynx. The gastroesophageal junction was seen at 40 cm. Inspection of the esophagus revealed no erythema, ulceration, varices, or other mucosal abnormalities. The stomach was entered and the endoscope advanced to the second duodenum. Inspection of the second duodenum, first duodenum, duodenal bulb, and pylorus revealed no abnormalities. Retroflexion revealed no lesions along the curvature. Inspection of the antrum, body, and fundus of the stomach revealed no abnormalities. The patient tolerated the procedure well. The patient complained of abdominal pain and weight loss.
    A. 45378, R10.9, R63.4
    B. 43235, R10.9, R63.4
    C. 49320, R63.0, R10.9
    D. 43255, E66.01, R10.32

77. This 70-year-old male is brought to the operating room for a biopsy of the pancreas. A wedge biopsy is taken and sent to pathology. The report comes back immediately, indicating that primary malignant cells were present in the specimen. The decision is made to perform a total pancreatectomy. Code the operative procedure(s) and diagnosis only.
    A. 48100, C78.89
    B. 48155, C25.8
    C. 48155, 48100-51, C25.9
    D. 48155, 48100-51, 88309, C25.9

78. This patient is taken to the operating room from the intensive care unit (ICU). The area of the stoma appears to be necrotic, and on this basis the surgeon indicates that the patient has been taken back to the operating room. The stoma was originally created 4 months ago by her previous surgeon.
    PROCEDURE PERFORMED: Revision ileostomy stoma.
    OPERATIVE NOTE: With the patient moved onto the operating table, the abdomen was prepped and draped. The segment of bowel that was serving as the ileostomy was freed up. Going in through this large open wound, we were able to identify which segment

of bowel this was. We resected the end of the bowel that was necrotic and freed up enough of the distal small bowel so that we could bring it out through a new stoma that was placed lateral to the original stoma. The stoma was created, the bowel was brought out, and the mucosa was sewn onto the skin. With this accomplished, we appeared to have a viable stoma. The patient tolerated this procedure and was returned to the ICU in stable condition.
    A. 44310, K94.00
    B. 45136, L03.311
    C. 44314, K94.13
    D. 44312, K94.03

79. This patient is brought back to the operating room during the postoperative period by the same physician to repair an esophagogastrostomy leak, transthoracic approach, done 2 days ago. The patient is status post-esophagectomy for esophageal cancer and is still undergoing chemotherapy. Code the procedure and the diagnosis for the complication.
    A. 43320-78, C15.9
    B. 43340-78, Z85.01
    C. 43341, K94.33, D49.0
    D. 43415-78, K94.33, C15.9

80. The patient was taken to the operating room for a repair of a strangulated inguinal hernia. This hernia was previously repaired 4 months ago.
    A. 49521, K40.31
    B. 49520, K40.00
    C. 49492, K40.90
    D. 49521-78, K40.31

81. The physician is using an abdominal approach to perform a proctopexy combined with a sigmoid resection; the patient was diagnosed with colon cancer, primary site sigmoid flexure of the colon.
    A. 45540, C18.7
    B. 45541, C18.9
    C. 45550, C18.7
    D. 45347, C19

82. What code would you use to report a rigid proctosigmoidoscopy with removal of two nonadenomatous polyps of the rectum by snare technique?
    A. 45320, K62.1
    B. 45388, D12.8
    C. 45309 × 2, K62.1
    D. 45315, K62.1

83. **OPERATIVE REPORT**
    PREOPERATIVE DIAGNOSIS: Leaking from intestinal anastomosis.
    POSTOPERATIVE DIAGNOSIS: Leaking from intestinal anastomosis.
    PROCEDURE PERFORMED: Proximal ileostomy for diversion of colon. Oversew of right colonic fistula.
    OPERATIVE NOTE: This patient was taken back to the operating room from the intensive care unit. She was having acute signs of leakage from an anastomosis

I performed 3 days previously. We took down some of the sutures holding the wound together. We basically exposed all of this patient's intestine. It was evident that she was leaking from the small bowel as well as from the right colon. I thought the only thing we could do would be to repair the right colon. This was done in two layers, and then we freed up enough bowel to try to make an ileostomy proximal to the area of leakage. We were able to do this with great difficulty, and there was only a small amount of bowel to be brought out. We brought this out as an ileostomy stoma, realizing that it was of questionable viability and that it should be watched closely. With that accomplished, we then packed the wound and returned the patient to the intensive care unit.

 A. 44310, K91.89
 B. 44310-78, K91.89, T85.638A
 C. 45136, K91.89
 D. 45136-78, K91.89

Subject Area: 50000 Urinary, Male Genital System, Female Genital System, and Maternity Care and Delivery

84. This patient is a 35-year-old at 36 weeks' gestation. She presents in spontaneous labor. Because of her prior cesarean section, she is taken to the operating room to have a repeat lower-segment transverse cesarean section performed. The patient also desires sterilization, so a bilateral tubal ligation will also be performed. A single, liveborn infant was the outcome of the delivery.
 A. 59510, 58600-51, Z30.2, Z3A.36
 B. 59620, 58615-51, O60.14X0, Z37.0, Z38.01, Z3A.36
 C. 59514, 58605-51, Z37.0, Z3A.36
 D. 59514, 58611, O34.211, O60.14X0, Z37.0, Z30.2, Z3A.36

85. The pediatric physician takes this newborn male to the nursery to perform a clamp circumcision with regional block.
 A. 54160, N47.0
 B. 54150, Z41.2
 C. 54160, Z41.2
 D. 54150, N47.0

86. **OPERATIVE REPORT**
 PREOPERATIVE DIAGNOSIS: Possible recurrent transitional cell carcinoma of the bladder.
 POSTOPERATIVE DIAGNOSIS: No evidence of recurrence.
 PROCEDURE PERFORMED: Cystoscopy with multiple bladder biopsies.
 PROCEDURE NOTE: The patient was given a general mask anesthetic, prepped, and draped in the lithotomy position. The 21-French cystoscope was passed into the bladder. There was a hyperemic area on the posterior wall of the bladder, and a biopsy was taken. Random biopsies of the bladder were also performed. This area was fulgurated. A total of 7 sq cm of bladder was fulgurated. A catheter was left at the end of the procedure. The patient tolerated the procedure well and was transferred to the recovery room in good condition. The pathology report indicated no evidence of recurrence.
 A. 52224, N32.89, Z85.51
 B. 51020, 52204, Z80.52
 C. 52234, Z85.51
 D. 52224 × 4, D41.4

87. This 1-year-old boy has a midshaft hypospadias with a very mild degree of chordee. He also has a persistent right hydrocele. The surgeon brought the boy to surgery to perform a right hydrocele repair and one-stage repair of hypospadias with preputial onlay flap.
 A. 54322, 55040, Q54.1, N43.3, Q54.4
 B. 54322, 55041-51, Q54.1, N43.3
 C. 54324, 55060-51, Q54.1, N43.3
 D. 54324, 55060, Q54.1, N43.3, Q54.4

88. This gentleman has worsening bilateral hydronephrosis. He did not have much of a post-void residual on bladder scan. He is taken to the operating room to have a bilateral cystoscopy and retrograde pyelogram. The results come back as gross prostatic hyperplasia with urinary retention as the cause of the hydronephrosis.
 A. 52005, N40.0
 B. 52000, N13.39, N40.1
 C. 52005, N40.0, N13.39
 D. 52000-50, N13.39, N40.1

89. This patient is a 42-year-old female who has been having prolonged and heavy bleeding during menstruation.
 SURGICAL FINDINGS: On pelvic exam under anesthesia, the uterus was normal size and firm. The examination revealed no masses. She had a few small endometrial polyps in the lower uterine segment.
 DESCRIPTION OF PROCEDURE: After induction of general anesthesia, the patient was placed in the dorsolithotomy position, after which the perineum and vagina were prepped, the bladder straight catheterized, and the patient draped. After bimanual exam was performed, a weighted speculum was placed in the vagina and the anterior lip of the cervix was grasped with a single tooth tenaculum. An endocervical curettage was then done with a Kevorkian curet. The uterus was then sounded to 8.5 cm. The endocervical canal was dilated to 7 mm with Hegar dilators. A 5.5-mm Olympus hysteroscope was introduced using a distention medium. The cavity was systematically inspected, and the preceding findings noted. The hysteroscope was withdrawn and the cervix further dilated to 10 mm. Polyp forceps was introduced, and a few small polyps were removed. These were sent separately to the lab. Sharp endometrial curettage was then done. The hysteroscope was then reinserted, and the polyps had essentially been removed. The patient tolerated the procedure well and returned to the recovery room in stable condition. Pathology confirmed benign endometrial polyps.

    A. 58558, 57460-51, N92.0, N84.0
    B. 58558, N92.0, N84.0
    C. 58558, 57558-51, N92.0, N84.0
    D. 58558, N92.1, D49.59

90. OPERATIVE REPORT

PREOPERATIVE DIAGNOSIS: Missed abortion with fetal demise, 11 weeks.

POSTOPERATIVE DIAGNOSIS: Missed abortion with fetal demise, 11 weeks.

PROCEDURE: Suction D&C.

The patient was prepped and draped in a lithotomy position under general mask anesthesia, and the bladder was straight catheterized; a weighted speculum was placed in the vagina. The anterior lip of the cervix was grasped with a single-tooth tenaculum. The uterus was then sounded to a depth of 8 cm. The cervical os was then serially dilated to allow passage of a size 10 curved suction curette. A size 10 curved suction curette was then used to evacuate the intrauterine contents. Sharp curette was used to gently palpate the uterine wall with negative return of tissue, and the suction curette was again used with negative return of tissue. The tenaculum was removed from the cervix. The speculum was removed from the vagina. All sponges and needles were accounted for at completion of the procedure. The patient left the operating room in apparent good condition having tolerated the procedure well.

    A. 59812, O03.9, Z3A.11
    B. 59812, O07.39, Z3A.11
    C. 59820, O02.1, Z3A.11
    D. 59856, O02.1, Z3A.11

91. OPERATIVE REPORT

PREOPERATIVE DIAGNOSIS: Right ureteral stricture.

POSTOPERATIVE DIAGNOSIS: Right ureteral stricture.

PROCEDURE PERFORMED: Cystoscopy, right ureteral stent change.

PROCEDURE NOTE: The patient was placed in the lithotomy position after receiving IV sedation. He was prepped and draped in the lithotomy position. The 21-French cystoscope was passed into the bladder, and urine was collected for culture. Inspection of the bladder demonstrated findings consistent with radiation cystitis, which has been previously diagnosed. There is no frank neoplasia. The right ureteral stent was grasped and removed through the urethral meatus; under fluoroscopic control, a guidewire was advanced up the stent, and the stent was exchanged for a 7-French 26-cm stent under fluoroscopic control in the usual fashion. The patient tolerated the procedure well.

    A. 51702-LT, N13.5
    B. 52005-RT, N30.90
    C. 52332-RT, N30.90
    D. 52332-RT, N13.5

92. This 41-year-old female presented with a right labial lesion. A biopsy was taken and the results were reported as VIN III, cannot rule out invasion. The decision was therefore made to proceed with wide local excision of the right vulva.

PROCEDURE: The patient was taken to the operating room and general anesthesia was administered. The patient was then prepped and draped in the usual manner in lithotomy position, and the bladder was emptied with a straight catheter. The vulva was then inspected. On the right labium minora at approximately the 11 o'clock position, there was a multifocal lesion. A marking pen was then used to mark out an elliptical incision, leaving a 1-cm border on all sides. The skin ellipse was then excised using a knife. Bleeders were cauterized with electrocautery. A running locked suture of 2-0 Vicryl was then placed in the deeper tissue. The skin was finally reapproximated with 4-0 Vicryl in an interrupted fashion. Good hemostasis was thereby achieved. The patient tolerated this procedure well. There were no complications.

    A. 56605, C51.9
    B. 56625, D07.1
    C. 56620, D07.1
    D. 11620, C51.9

93. This 32-year-old female presents with an ectopic pregnancy without intrauterine pregnancy. The physician elects to remove the entire left fallopian tube with the products of conception laparoscopically.

    A. 59120, O00.90
    B. 59151, O00.90
    C. 58943, O00.102
    D. 59120, O00.80

Subject Area: 60000 Endocrine System, Hemic and Lymphatic System, Nervous System, Eye and Ocular Adnexa, Auditory System

94. OPERATIVE REPORT

PREOPERATIVE DIAGNOSIS: FUO.

PROCEDURE PERFORMED: Lumbar puncture.

DESCRIPTION OF PROCEDURE: The patient was placed in the lateral decubitus position with the left side up. The legs and hips were flexed into the fetal position. The lumbosacral area was sterilely prepped. It was then numbed with 1% Xylocaine. I then placed a 22-gauge spinal needle on the first pass into the intrathecal space between the L4 and L5 spinous processes. The fluid was minimally xanthochromic. I sent the fluid for cell count for differential, protein, glucose, Gram stain, and culture. The patient tolerated the procedure well without apparent complication. The needle was removed at the end of the procedure. The area was cleansed, and a Band-Aid was placed.

    A. 62272, R68.12
    B. 62268, R50.9
    C. 62272, R60.9, R50.9
    D. 62270, R50.9

95. OPERATIVE REPORT

PREOPERATIVE DIAGNOSIS: Paralytic ectropion, left lower eye.

PROCEDURE PERFORMED: Medial tarsorrhaphy, left lower eye.

In the operating room, after intravenous sedation, the patient was given a total of about 0.5 mL of local infiltrative anesthetic. The skin surfaces on the medial area of the lid, medial to the punctum, were denuded. A bolster had been prepared and double 5-0 silk suture was passed through the bolster, which was passed through the inferior skin and raw lid margin, then through the superior margin, and out through the skin. A superior bolster was then applied. The puncta were probed with wire instrument and found not to be obstructed. The suture was then fully tied and trimmed. Bacitracin ointment was placed on the surface of the skin. The patient left the operating room in stable condition, without complications, having tolerated the procedure well.

A. 67875-LT, H02.155
B. 67710-LT, H02.135
C. 67882-LT, H02.109
D. 67880-LT, H02.155

96. Marginal laceration involving the left lower eyelid and laceration of the left upper eyelid involving the tarsus. Both required full-thickness repair. Also, there were multiple stellate lacerations above the left eye, totaling 24.2 cm and requiring full-thickness layered repair. Assign code(s) for the physician service only.

A. 67935-E2, 12017
B. 67930-E2, 13152-51, 13153
C. 67935-E2, 67935-E1-51, 12056-51
D. 67935-E2, 12017-51

97. This 66-year-old male has been diagnosed with a senile cataract of the posterior subcapsular and is scheduled for a cataract extraction by phacoemulsification of the right eye. The physician has taken the patient to the operating room to perform a posterior subcapsular cataract extraction with IOL placement, diffuse of the right eye.

A. 66982-RT, H25.031
B. 66984-RT, H25.041
C. 66983-RT, H25.031
D. 66830-RT, H25.041

98. OPERATIVE REPORT

PREOPERATIVE DIAGNOSIS: Brain tumor versus abscess.

PROCEDURE: Craniotomy.

DESCRIPTION OF PROCEDURE: Under general anesthesia, the patient's head was prepped and draped in the usual manner. It was placed in Mayfield pins. We then proceeded with a craniotomy. An inverted U-shaped incision was made over the posterior right occipital area. The flap was turned down. Three burr holes were made. Having done this, I then localized the tumor through the burr holes and dura. We then made an incision in the dura in an inverted U-shaped fashion. The cortex looked a little swollen but normal. We then used the localizer to locate the cavity. I separated the gyrus and got right into the cavity and saw pus, which was removed. Cultures were taken and sent for pathology report, which came back later describing the presence of clusters of gram-positive cocci, confirming that this was an abscess. We cleaned out the abscessed cavity using irrigation and suction. The bed of the abscessed cavity was cauterized. Then a small piece of Gelfoam was used for hemostasis. Satisfied that it was dry, I closed the dura. I approximated the scalp. A dressing was applied. The patient was discharged to the recovery room.

A. 61154, G06.0
B. 61154, D49.6
C. 61320, G06.0, B96.89
D. 61150, D49.6

99. This patient is in for a recurrent herniated disc at L5-S1 on the left. The procedure performed is a repeat laminotomy and foraminotomy at the L5-S1 interspace.

A. 63030-LT, M51.27
B. 63030-LT, M51.07
C. 63042-LT, M51.07
D. 63042-LT, M51.27

100. OPERATIVE REPORT

PREOPERATIVE DIAGNOSIS: Herniated disc L4-5 on the left.

PROCEDURE PERFORMED: Laminotomy, foraminotomy, removal of herniated disc L4-5 on the left.

PROCEDURE: Under general anesthesia, the patient was placed in the prone position and the back was prepped and draped in the usual manner. An incision was made in the skin extending through subcutaneous tissue. Lumbodorsal fascia was divided. The erector spinae muscles were bluntly dissected from the lamina of L4-5 on the left. The interspace was localized. I then performed a generous laminotomy and foraminotomy here, and retracted on the nerve root. It was obvious there was a herniated disc. I removed it, entered the space, and removed degenerating material, satisfied that I had decompressed the root well. There were free fragments lying around beneath the nerve root. We removed all of these. I was able to pass a hockey stick down the foramen across the midline, satisfied I had taken out the large fragments from the interspace at L4-5, and decompressed it well. I irrigated the wound well, put a Hemovac drain in the wound, and then closed the wound in layers using double-knotted 0 chromic on the lumbodorsal fascia with Vicryl 2-0 plain, in the subcutaneous tissue, and surgical staples on the skin. A dressing was applied. The patient was discharged to the recovery room.

A. 63030-LT, M51.26
B. 63012-LT, M51.46
C. 63047-LT, M51.9
D. 63047-LT, 63048-LT, M51.26

101. This patient came in with an obstructed ventriculo-peritoneal shunt. The procedure performed was to be a revision of shunt. After inspecting the shunt system, the entire cerebrospinal fluid shunt system was removed and a similar replacement shunt system was placed. Patient has normal pressure hydrocephalus (NPH).

  A. 62180, T85.890A, G91.0
  B. 62258, T85.890A, G91.2
  C. 62256, T85.890A, G91.1
  D. 62190, T85.890A, G91.2

102. Twist drill hole for a left frontal ventricular puncture for implanting catheter, layered repair of 8-cm scalp laceration, and repair of multiple facial and eyelid lacerations with an approximate total length of 12 cm. Assign code(s) for the physician service only.

  A. 61020, 12015-51
  B. 61107, 12034-51, 12015-51
  C. 61215, 12015-51
  D. 61107, 12034-51

103. What CPT and ICD-10-CM codes would you assign to report the removal of 30% of the left thyroid lobe, with isthmusectomy? The diagnosis was benign growth of the thyroid.

  A. 60210, D34
  B. 60220, D44.0
  C. 60212, D49.7
  D. 60225, D34, D49.7

Subject Area: Evaluation and Management (E/M)

104. Dr. Black admits a patient with an 8-day history of a low-grade fever, tachycardia, tachypnea, and possible radiologic evidence of basal consolidation of the lung and limited pleural effusion on the left side, per patient as seen at outside clinic several days prior. The patient has also been experiencing swelling of the extremities. The pulse is rapid and thready, as checked by patient on her own during the past couple days. A complete ROS of constitutional factors, ophthalmologic, otolaryngologic, cardiovascular, respiratory, gastrointestinal, genitourinary, musculoskeletal, integumentary, neurologic, psychiatric, endocrine, hematologic, lymphatic, allergic, and immunologic was performed and negative except for the symptoms described above. Past history includes tachycardia and pneumonia. Family history includes heart disease, hypertension, and high cholesterol in both parents. The patient drinks only occasionally and quit smoking 4 years ago. The comprehensive examination was performed and diminished bowel sounds were noted. The physician orders laboratory tests and radiographic studies, including a follow-up chest x-ray as he considers the extensive diagnostic options and the medical decision-making complexity is high for this patient.

  A. 99233, R00.0, R50.9, R06.82, J90, R19.15, Z87.891
  B. 99233, R00.0, I47.9, R06.82, J18.1, J90

  C. 99223, R00.0, R50.9, R06.82
  D. 99223, R50.9, R00.0, R06.82, J90, R19.15, Z87.891, Z82.49

105. Bill, a retired U.S. Air Force pilot, was on observation status 12 hours to assess the outcome of a fall from the back of a parked pickup truck into a gravel pit. History of Present Illness: The patient is a 42-year-old gentleman who works at the local garden shop. He explained that yesterday he fell from his pickup truck as he was loading gravel for a landscaping project. He lost his footing when attempting to climb from the pickup bed and fell approximately 4 feet and landed on a rock that was protruding from the ground 4 inches, striking his head on the rock. He did not lose consciousness, but was dizzy. He subsequently developed a throbbing headache (8/10) and swelling at the point of impact. The duration of the dizziness was approximately 10 minutes. The headache persisted for 26 hours after the fall. He did take ibuprofen without significant improvement in the pain level. Review of Systems: Constitutional, eyes, ears, nose, throat, lungs, cardiovascular, gastrointestinal, skin, neurologic, lymphatic, and immunologic negative except for HPI statements. PFSH: He is married and has 2 children. He has been working at the garden shop for 4 years. He currently smokes one pack of cigarettes a day and has smoked for 10 years. His father died of heart disease when he was 52. He has one brother with ankylosing spondylitis and one sister who is healthy as far as he knows. His mother died when he was 14 years old. He is currently on no prescribed medications. A comprehensive exam is documented and rendered. The medical decision making is of low complexity.

  The physician discharged Bill from observation that same day after 10 hours, after determining that no further monitoring of his condition was necessary. The physician provided a detailed examination and indicated that the medical decision making was of a low complexity.

  A. 99218, R51.9, W17.89XA
  B. 99234, Z04.2, W17.89XA, Y93.H2
  C. 99217, Z04.2, W17.89XA
  D. 99234, 99217, R51.9, W17.89A

106. A gynecologist admits an established patient, a 35-year-old female with dysfunctional uterine bleeding, after seeing her in the clinic that day. During the course of the history, the physician notes that the patient has a history of infrequent periods of heavy flow. She has had irregular heavy periods and intermittent spotting for 4 years. The patient has been on a 3-month course of oral contraceptives for symptoms with no relief. The patient states that she has occasional headaches. A complete ROS was performed, consisting of constitutional factors, ophthalmologic, otolaryngologic, cardiovascular, respiratory, gastrointestinal, genitourinary, musculoskeletal, integumentary, neurologic, psychiatric, endocrine, hematologic, lymphatic, allergic, and immunologic which were all negative, except for the symptoms described above. The family history is positive for endometrial cancer, with mother, two aunts, and two sisters who had endometrial cancer. The patient has a personal history of cervical and endometrial polyp removal 3 years prior to admission. The patients states that she does not smoke and only drinks socially. As a part of the comprehensive examination, the physician notes the patient has a large amount of blood in the vault and an enlarged uterus. The prolonged hemorrhaging has resulted in a very thin and friable endometrial lining. The physician orders the patient to be started on intravenous Premarin and orders a full laboratory workup. The medical decision making is of moderate complexity.

A. 99215, 99222, Z87.42, Z80.49
B. 99222, N93.8, Z87.42, Z80.49
C. 99215, 99222, N92.5, Z87.42, Z80.49
D. 99222, N92.1, Z80.49

107. Karra Hendricks, a 37-year-old female, is an established patient who presents to the office with right lower quadrant abdominal pain with fever. The patient states she has had the pain for 3 days. She has taken Tylenol for her fever with some relief. The patient does have occasional diarrhea and headaches. She smokes approximately 5-10 cigarettes a day and drinks socially. The physician performs an examination. The medical decision making is noted to be of a moderate complexity.

A. 99203, R10.31
B. 99215, R10.32, R50.9
C. 99214, R10.31, R50.9
D. 99221, R10.33, R50.9

108. A neurological consultation in the emergency department of the local hospital is requested by the ED physician for a 25-year-old male with suspected closed head trauma. The neurologist saw the patient in the ED. The patient had a loss of consciousness this morning after receiving a blow to the head in a basketball game. He presents to the emergency department with a headache, dizziness, and confusion. During the course of the history, the patient relates that he has been very irritable, confused, and has had a bit of nausea since the incident. All other systems reviewed and are negative: Constitutional, ophthalmologic, otolaryngologic, cardiovascular, respiratory, genitourinary, musculoskeletal, integumentary, psychiatric, endocrine, hematologic, lymphatic, allergic, and immunologic. The patient states that he does have a history of headaches and that both parents have hypertension, also a grandfather with heart disease. He also states that he does drink beer on the weekends and does not smoke. Physical examination reveals the patient to be unsteady and exhibiting difficulty in concentration when stating months in reverse. The pupils dilate unequally (anisocoria). The physician continues with a complete comprehensive examination involving an extensive review of neurological function. The neurologist orders a stat CT and MRI. The physician suspects a subdural hematoma or an epidural hematoma and the medical decision-making complexity is high. The neurologist admits the patient to the hospital. Assign codes for the neurologist's services only.

A. 99285, R41.82, R42, R51.9, W22.8XXA, Y93.67
B. 99253, R51.9, R41.82, R42, W22.8XXA, Y93.67
C. 99255, H57.02, R51.9, R41.0, R42, W22.8XXA, Y93.67
D. 99245, R51.9, R41.82, R42, W22.8XXA, Y93.67

109. Dr. Stephanopolis makes subsequent hospital visits to Salanda Ortez, who has been in the hospital for primary viral pneumonia. She was experiencing severe dyspnea, rales, fever, and chest pain for over a week. The patient states that this morning she had nausea and her heart was racing while she was experiencing some dyspnea and SOB. The chest radiography showed patchy bilateral infiltrates and basilar streaking. Sputum microbiology was positive for a secondary bacterial pneumonia. An expanded problem-focused physical examination was performed. The medical decision making complexity was moderate. The patient was given intravenous antibiotic as treatment for the bacterial pneumonia.

A. 99233, R06.02, R50.9, R07.9
B. 99232, J15.9, J12.9
C. 99221, R06.02, R50.9, R07.9
D. 99234, J15.8

110. An obstetrician is requested by Dr. A to provide an office consultation to a 23-year-old female with first-trimester bleeding. The patient presents with a history of brownish discharge and occasional pinkish discharge. During the history, the patient relates that she has had suprapubic pain in the past week and cramping. She states her pain is 8/10. She has felt nausea and has vomited on three occasions. On one occasion, the nausea was accompanied by dizziness and vertigo. All other systems are negative at this time and included: Constitutional factors, ophthalmologic, otolaryngologic, cardiovascular, respiratory, musculoskeletal, integumentary, neurologic, psychiatric, endocrine, hematologic, lymphatic, allergic, and immunologic. The PFSH included patient history of tonsillectomy with family history of breast cancer on her mother's side. The patient does not smoke or drink. The physician conducts a comprehensive examination focused on the chief complaint and related systems. The uterus is found to be soft and involuted. There is cervical motion tenderness and significant abdominal tenderness on palpation. A left pelvic mass is palpated in the left quadrant. The physician orders a pelvic ultrasound, a complete CBC, and differential. Considering the range of possible diagnoses, the medical decision-making complexity is high.

A. 99255, O03.4, R19.00
B. 99242, O20.0, R19.00
C. 99245, O20.9, R19.04
D. 99245, O46.90, R19.04

111. Dr. Martin admits a 65-year-old female patient to the hospital to rule out acute pericarditis following a severe viral infection. The patient has complained of retrosternal, sharp, intermittent pain of 2 days' duration that is reduced by sitting up and leaning forward, accompanied by tachypnea. ROS: She does not currently have chest pain but is complaining of shortness of breath. She states that her legs and feet have been swollen of late. She reports no change in her vision or her hearing, and she has not had a rash. No dyspnea stated. PFSH: She states that she has had an echocardiogram in the past when she complained of chest tightness and her family physician gave her some medication, but she is not certain what it was. She has three adult children, all healthy. Her husband is deceased. She does not smoke or consume alcohol. Her father died at age 69 from congestive heart failure, and her mother died of influenza at 70. Refer to the admission form for a list of current medications. The examination was detailed. The medical decision making was of high complexity.
A. 99236, R07.2, R06.82, R06.02
B. 99223, I30.9, I50.9
C. 99245, I30.9, I50.9
D. 99221, R07.2, R06.82, R06.02

112. A 57-year-old male was sent by his family physician to a urologist for an office consultation due to hematuria. The patient has had bright red blood in his urine sporadically for the past 3 weeks. His family physician gave him a dose of antibiotic therapy for urinary tract infection; however, the symptom still persists. The patient states that he does experience some lower back discomfort when urinating, with no fever, chills, or nausea. The patient is currently taking Lotrel 10/20 for his hypertension, which is stable at this time, and has allergies to Sulfa. The urologist performs a detailed history and physical examination. The urologist recommends a cystoscopy to be scheduled for the following day and discusses the procedure and risks with the patient. The urologist also contacted the family physician with the recommendations and is requested to proceed with the cystoscopy and any further follow-up required. The medical decision making is of moderate complexity. A report was sent to attending physician. Report only the office service.
A. 99243, R31.0, M54.5
B. 99244-57, 52000, R31.9, M54.5
C. 99253, R31.9, M54.5
D. 99221, R31.0, M54.5

113. A 56-year-old established male patient presents to his family physician for a preventive checkup at the local outpatient clinic. The physician conducts a multisystem history and physical examination, and the checkup takes 45 minutes.
A. 99214, Z02.71
B. 99403, Z02.1
C. 99386, Z00.00
D. 99396, Z00.00

Subject Area: Anesthesia

114. Which HCPCS modifier indicates an anesthesia service in which the anesthesiologist medically directs one CRNA?
A. QX
B. QY
C. QZ
D. QK

115. This is the anesthesia formula:
A. B + M + P
B. B + P + M
C. B + T + M
D. B + T + N

116. Anesthesia service for a needle biopsy of the pleura, 32400.
A. 00528
B. 00500
C. 00520
D. 00522

117. If the anesthesia service were provided to a patient who had severe systemic disease, what would the physical status modifier be?
A. P1
B. P2
C. P3
D. P4

118. This type of anesthesia is also known as a nerve block.
A. Local
B. Epidural
C. Regional
D. MAC

119. The anesthesiologist provides anesthesia services for a kidney harvest from a living donor for transplant.
A. 00868
B. 01990
C. 00860
D. 00862

120. Anesthesia service includes the following care:
A. Preoperative, intraoperative
B. Preoperative, intraoperative, postoperative
C. Intraoperative, postoperative
D. Preoperative, postoperative

121. What qualifying circumstances code would be used to identify the administration of anesthesia that is complicated by an emergency condition?
A. 99100
B. 99116
C. 99135
D. 99140

Subject Area: 70000 Radiology

122. EXAMINATION OF: Right hip.

DIAGNOSIS: Primary unilateral osteoarthritis right hip.

ONE-VIEW RIGHT HIP: A single frontal view is obtained of the right hip. No previous studies are available for comparison. Right hip arthroplasty is seen. Alignment appears grossly unremarkable on this single view. There are skin staples present. Air is seen in the soft tissues, likely due to recent surgery. There appear to be two drains present. The tip of one overlies the soft tissues superolateral to the greater trochanter. The second one is more inferior. The tip overlies the right proximal femoral prosthesis.

IMPRESSION: Single view of the right hip with findings consistent with recent right total hip arthroplasty.

A. 72100, M16

B. 73501-RT, M16.11

C. 72100-26, M16.1

D. 73501-26-RT, M16.11, Z96.641

123. EXAMINATION OF: Cervical spine.

CLINICAL SYMPTOMS: Herniated disc.

FINDINGS: A single spot fluoroscopic film from the operating room is submitted for interpretation. The cervical spine is not well demonstrated above the level of the inferior aspect of C6. There is a metallic surgical plate seen anterior to the cervical spine. The cephalic portion of the plate is at the level of C6 at its superior endplate. That extends in an inferior direction, presumably anterior to C7; however, there is not adequate visualization of C7 to confirm location. Density overlies the C6-7 intervertebral disc space, suggesting the presence of a bone plug in this area; however, again visualization is not adequate in this area. Further evaluation with plain radiographs is recommended.

A. 72100-26, M51.26

B. 72020-26, M50.20

C. 72100-52-26, M50.20

D. 72020-52-26, M51.26

124. This patient undergoes a gallbladder sonogram due to epigastric pain. The report indicates that the visualized portions of the liver are normal. No free fluid noted within Morison's pouch. The gallbladder is identified and is empty. No evidence of wall thickening or surrounding fluid is seen. There is no ductal dilatation. The common hepatic duct and common bile duct measure 0.4 and 0.8 cm, respectively. The common bile duct measurement is at the upper limits of normal.

A. 76700-26, R10.84

B. 76705-26, R10.13

C. 76775-26, R10.33

D. 76705, R10.84

125. EXAMINATION OF: Chest.

CLINICAL SYMPTOMS: Pneumonia.

PA AND LATERAL CHEST X-RAY.

CONCLUSION: Ventilation within the lung fields has improved compared with previous study.

A. 71046-26, J15.8

B. 71034, J15.8

C. 71046-26, J18.9

D. 71046, J18.9

126. EXAMINATION OF: Abdomen and pelvis.

CLINICAL SYMPTOMS: Ascites.

CT OF ABDOMEN AND PELVIS: Technique: CT of the abdomen and pelvis was performed without oral or IV contrast material per physician request. No previous CT scans for comparison.

FINDINGS: No ascites. Moderate-sized pleural effusion on the right.

A. 74160-26, R18.8

B. 74176-26, J90

C. 74150, J90

D. 74160, R18.8

127. Report the professional component of the following service: This 68-year-old male is seen in Radiation Oncology Department for prostate cancer. The oncologist performs a complex clinical treatment planning, approves a dosimetry calculation, manages a complex isodose plan, and orders treatment devices, which include blocks, special shields, and wedges. He also performs treatment management. The patient had 5 days of radiation treatments for 2 weeks, a total of 10 days of treatment.

A. 77263, 77300-26, 77307-26, 77334, C61

B. 77300, 77307, 77334, 77427 × 2, C61

C. 77263, 77300-26, 77307-26, 77334-26, 77427 × 2, C61

D. 77263, 77427 × 2, C61

128. This 69-year-old female is in for a magnetic resonance examination of the brain because of new seizure activity. After imaging without contrast, contrast was administered and further sequences were performed. Examination results indicated no apparent neoplasm or vascular malformation.

A. 70543-26, R56.00

B. 70543-26, R56.9

C. 70553-26, R56.9

D. 70553, G40.909

129. EXAMINATION OF: Brain.

CLINICAL FINDING: Acute onset, severe headache.

COMPUTED TOMOGRAPHY OF THE BRAIN was performed without contrast material.

FINDINGS: There is blood within the third ventricle. The lateral ventricles show mild dilatation with small amounts of blood.

IMPRESSION: Acute nontraumatic subarachnoid hemorrhage.

A. 70460-26, R51.9

B. 70250, R51.9

C. 70450-26, I60.9

D. 70450-26, R51.9

130. This patient is suffering from primary lung cancer and is in for a follow-up diagnostic CT scan of the thorax with contrast material. Code the physician component only.
    A. 71250-26, C78.00
    B. 71260, C34.90
    C. 71260-26, C34.90
    D. 71270-26, D49.1

Subject Area: 80000 Pathology and Laboratory

131. This 69-year-old female presents to the laboratory after her physician ordered quantitative and qualitative assays for troponin to assist in the diagnosis of her chief complaint of acute onset of chest pain.
    A. 84484, 80299, R07.2
    B. 84512, 84484, 80299, R07.89
    C. 84484, 84512, R07.9
    D. 84484, 84512, R07.89

132. **Report the global service.**
    CLINICAL HISTORY: Mass, left atrium.
    SPECIMEN RECEIVED: Left atrium.
    GROSS DESCRIPTION: The specimen is labeled with patient's name and "left atrial myxoma" and consists of a 4 × 4 × 2-cm ovoid mass with a partially calcified hemorrhagic white-tan tissue.
    INTRAOPERATIVE FROZEN SECTION DIAGNOSIS: Myxoma
    MICROSCOPIC DESCRIPTION: Sections show a well-circumscribed mass consisting of fibromyxoid tissue showing numerous vascular channels. Areas of superficial ulceration and chronic inflammatory infiltrate are noted. Areas of calcification are also present.
    DIAGNOSIS: Myxoma, benign, left atrium.
    A. 88305, D49.89
    B. 88307-26, 88331-26, D15.1
    C. 88307, 88331-26, D15.1
    D. 88305, D15.1

133. This 34-year-old established female patient is in for her yearly physical and lab. The physician orders a comprehensive metabolic panel, hemogram automated and manual differential WBC count (CBC), and a thyroid-stimulating hormone. Code the lab only.
    A. 99395, 80050
    B. 80050-52
    C. 80069, 80050
    D. 80050

134. **CLINICAL HISTORY:** Necrotic soleus muscle, right leg.
    SPECIMEN RECEIVED: Soleus muscle, right leg.
    GROSS DESCRIPTION: Submitted in formalin, labeled with the patient's name and "soleus muscle right leg," are multiple irregular fragments of tan, gray, brown soft tissue measuring 8 × 8 × 2.5 cm in aggregate. Multiple representative fragments are submitted in four cassettes.
    MICROSCOPIC DESCRIPTION: The slides show multiple sections of skeletal muscle showing severe

coagulative and liquefactive necrosis. Patchy neutrophilic infiltrates are present within the necrotic tissue.
    DIAGNOSIS: Soft tissue, soleus muscle, right leg debridement; necrosis and patchy acute inflammation, skeletal muscle—infective myositis.
    A. 88305-26, M60.003
    B. 88304-26, M60.061
    C. 88307-26, I96
    D. 88304-26, M62.561

135. This patient is in for a kidney biopsy (50200) because a mass was identified by ultrasound. The specimen is sent to pathology for gross and microscopic examination. Report the technical and professional components for this service. The results are pending.
    A. 88305-26, N28.89
    B. 88307-26, N28.9
    C. 88307, N28.89
    D. 88305, N28.89

136. This patient presented to the laboratory yesterday to have blood drawn for a creatine measurement. The results came back at higher than normal levels; therefore, the patient was asked to return to the laboratory today for a repeat creatine blood test before the nephrologist is consulted. Report the second day of test only.
    A. 82540 × 2, R79.89
    B. 82550, R79.89
    C. 82550, R94.4
    D. 82540, R79.89

137. Code a pregnancy test, urine.
    A. 84702
    B. 84703
    C. 81025
    D. 84702 × 2

138. This is a patient with atrial fibrillation who comes to the clinic laboratory routinely for a total digoxin level. This test was performed today.
    A. 80162, 80102, I50.9
    B. 81001, Z51.81, Z79.899, I49.01
    C. 80162, Z51.81, Z79.899, I48.91
    D. 80162, I48.91

139. What CPT code would you use to report a bilirubin, total (transcutaneous)?
    A. 82252
    B. 82247
    C. 82248
    D. 88720

140. **CLINICAL HISTORY:** Boil, left groin.
    SPECIMEN RECEIVED: Necrotic fascia left groin and leg (anterior and posterior).
    GROSS DESCRIPTION: The specimen is labeled with the patient's name and "fascia left groin and leg" and consists of multiple segments of skin and soft tissue measuring up to 30 cm in greatest dimension. The skin is unremarkable, with the soft tissue being hemorrhagic and friable and foul smelling.

MICROSCOPIC DESCRIPTION: Sections of skin and soft tissue show coagulative necrosis with neutrophilic exudates.

DIAGNOSIS: Skin and soft tissue, left groin and leg, anterior and posterior showing coagulative necrosis and acute inflammation.

A. 88304, L02.92
B. 88305-26, I96
C. 88304-26, I96, L02.224
D. 88305, L03.314

Subject Area: 90000 Medicine

141. What CPT code would be used to code the technical aspect of an evaluation of swallowing by video recording using a flexible endoscope?
A. 92611
B. 92612
C. 92610
D. 92613

142. The patient presented for a spontaneous nystagmus test that included gaze, fixation, and recording and used vertical electrodes. Assign code(s) for the physician service only.
A. 92541
B. 92547
C. 92541, 92544, 92547
D. 92541, 92547

143. How would you report a screening hearing test in which no abnormalities are reported?
A. 92551, Z13.5
B. 92555, Z01.10
C. 92553, Z01.10
D. 92620, Z13.5

144. This 40-year-old patient who is a type II diabetic is seen in an inpatient setting for psychotherapy. The doctor spends 50 minutes face-to-face with the patient. The patient is seen for depression.
A. 90834, F32.9, E11.69
B. 90832, F32.9, E11.69
C. 90834, F32.9, E11.9
D. 90832, F32.9, E11.9

145. A patient presents for a pleural cavity chemotherapy session with 10 mg doxorubicin HCl that requires a thoracentesis to be performed.
A. 96446, J9000
B. 96440, 32554, J9000
C. 96440, J9000
D. 96446, 32554, J9000

146. What CPT code would be used to report a home visit to care for the mechanical ventilation of a respiratory patient?
A. 99503
B. 99504
C. 99505
D. 99509

147. Which code would be used to report an EEG (electroencephalogram) provided during carotid surgery?

A. 95816
B. 95819
C. 95822
D. 95955

148. **INDICATION:** Pulmonary hypertension secondary to newly diagnosed acute myocardial infarction.

PROCEDURE PERFORMED: Insertion of Swan-Ganz catheter.

DESCRIPTION OF PROCEDURE: The right internal jugular and subclavian area was prepped with antiseptic solution. Sterile drapes were applied. Under usual sterile precautions, the right internal jugular vein was cannulated. A 9-French introducer was inserted, and a 7-French Swan-Ganz catheter was inserted without difficulty. Right atrial pressures were 2 to 3, right ventricular pressures 24/0, and pulmonary artery 26/9 with a wedge pressure of 5. This is a Trendelenburg position. The patient tolerated the procedure well.

A. 93451, 93503-51, I21.9
B. 93454, I27.20
C. 93503, 93452, I27.20
D. 93503, I27.20, I21.9

149. **DIALYSIS INPATIENT NOTE:** This 24-year-old male patient is on continuous ambulatory peritoneal dialysis (CAPD) using 1.5% dialysate. He drains more than 600 mL. He is tolerating dialysis well. He continues to have some abdominal pain, but his abdomen is not distended. He has some diarrhea. His abdomen does not look like acute abdomen. His vitals, other than blood pressure in the 190s over 100s, are fine. He is afebrile.

At this time, I will continue with 1.5% dialysate. Because of diarrhea, I am going to check stool for white cells, culture. Next we will see what the primary physician says today. His HIDA scan was normal. The patient suffers from ESRD and has had 6 encounters this month. Code this service.

A. 90947, 90960, N18.6, R19.7, Z99.2
B. 90945, N18.6, R19.7, Z99.2
C. 90960, N18.6, Z99.2
D. 90945, N18.6

150. **DIAGNOSIS:** Atrial flutter.

PROCEDURE PERFORMED: Electrical cardioversion.

DESCRIPTION OF PROCEDURE: The patient was sedated with a total of 5 mg of Versed and morphine. She was cardioverted with 50 joules into sinus tachycardia. The patient was given a 20-mg Cardizem IV push. Her heart rate went down to the 110s, and she was definitely in sinus tachycardia.

CONCLUSION: Successful electrical cardioversion of atrial flutter into sinus tachycardia.

A. 92961, I49.1
B. 92960, I48.92
C. 92960, 92973, I48.92
D. 92960, R00.0

PART **7**

Facility-based Examinations

33
Facility-based Examinations

You have three opportunities to practice taking a facility-based examination:

- Pre-Examination (before study)
- Post-Examination (after study)
- Final Examination (at the end of your complete program of study)

For the purposes of this text, the facility-based practice exam is labelled "Facility Exam (Format C)." It includes a Pre-/Post-Examination and Final Examination, each with 97 multiple-choice questions and 8 case scenarios.

You should have the following manuals:

- 2021 ICD-10-CM, (*International Classification of Diseases, 10th Revision, Clinical Modification*)
- 2021 ICD-10-PCS (*International Classification of Disease, 10th Revision, Procedure Coding System*)
- 2020 HCPCS (*Healthcare Common Procedure Coding System*)
- On the certification examination, HCPCS questions are on the theory portion of the examination, not on the practical portion of the examination
- 2021 CPT (*Current Procedural Terminology*)

No other reference material, other than a medical dictionary, is allowed for any of the examinations.

- For the Pre-, Post-, and Final Examinations, you will need a computer, Internet access, and the four coding references (ICD-10-CM, ICD-10-PCS, HCPCS, CPT).
- Each organization's certification examination has different scoring requirements, but as you take these examinations, you should strive for 80% to 90% on the Post-Examination and 70% as a minimum on the Final Examination.

Pre-Examination and Post-Examination

The Pre-Examination is located on the companion Evolve website. The purpose of the Pre-Examination is only to assess your beginning level of knowledge and skill—your starting place. Based on your scores, you can tailor your study to target your weakest areas and increase your scores. Take this examination before you begin your studies.

Your score will automatically be calculated for you. A passing score for the examinations in this text requires 70%.

The practice examinations program on Evolve will calculate and retain your scoring information.

Immediately on completion of your study, you should complete the Post-Examination on Evolve. After you are finished, the program will automatically compare your Pre-Examination scores with your Post-Examination scores, and will store your results. By comparing the results of the Pre-Examination and the Post-Examination (the same examination will be taken twice), the program illustrates the improvements you have achieved or the areas that you will need to practice more on before taking the Final Examination.

Rationales for each question are available for review after you complete the Post-Examination. Study the questions for which you did not choose the right response. Did you misread the question, did you not know the material well enough to answer correctly, or did you run out of time? Knowing why you missed a question is an important step to improving your skill level.

Ideally, you should complete each examination in one sitting; if time does not allow, spread the examination times over several periods. There are no time extensions in an actual examination setting, and learning how to judge the amount of time you spend on each question is an important part of this learning experience to prepare you for the real certification examination.

Final Examination

If you scored well on all areas of the Post-Examination (80% or higher), you are ready to move on to the Final Examination, which is also on the companion Evolve website. Once you have completed the Final Examination, the program will compare all your scores to illustrate your improvement.

A passing score for the Final Examination is the same as for the Pre-/Post-Examination—70%.

If you did not attain a minimum score on each section, you should develop a plan to restudy those particular areas where the examination indicates you are having difficulties. There are rationales for each question in the Final Examination, and you should review that information as well as material in the text. You can take any of the practice examinations again after your additional study.

Figure Credits

1-1 ©Elsevier Collection

1-2 ©Elsevier Collection

4-4 ©Elsevier Collection

7-3 From Kumar V, Abbas AK, Aster JC: *Robbins and Cotran Pathologic Basis of Disease*, ed 9, Philadelphia, 2015, Saunders.

8-3 ©Elsevier Collection

8-7 From Damjanov I: *Pathology for the Health Professions*, ed 5, St. Louis, 2017, Elsevier.

8-8 From Kissane JM, editor: *Anderson's Pathology*, ed 9, St. Louis, 1990, Mosby.

11-1 ©Elsevier Collection

11-2 From Canale ST, Beaty JH: *Campbell's Operative Orthopaedics*, ed 11, Philadelphia, 2008, Mosby.

11-3 From Patton KT, Thibodeau GA: *Anatomy & Physiology*, ed 8, St. Louis, 2013, Mosby.

13-2 From Yanoff M, Duker J, editors: *Ophthalmology*, ed 4, St. Louis, 2014, Saunders.

14-1 Courtesy U.S. Department of Health and Human Services, Centers for Medicare and Medicaid Services.

14-2 From *Federal Register*, September 30, 2019, Vol. 84, No. 189, Rules and Regulations.

14-3 Courtesy U.S. Department of Health and Human Services, Centers for Medicare and Medicaid Services.

15-1 From *Federal Register*, September 30, 2019, Vol. 84, No. 189, Rules and Regulations.

15-2 From *Final 2020 APC Grouping of HCPCS Codes* (website): www.cms.gov/apps/ama/license.asp?file=/Medicare/Medicare-Fee-for-Service-Payment/HospitalOutpatientPPS/Downloads/2020-OPPS-APC-Offset-File.zip

15-3 From *Payment Status Indicators for the Hospital Outpatient Prospective Payment System Addendum* (website): https://www.cms.gov/Medicare/Medicare-Fee-for-Service-Payment/HospitalOutpatientPPS/Downloads/CMS1506FC_Addendum_D1.pdf

15-4 Modified from *Final APC Payment Rate and Co-Insurance Amount* (website): https://www.cms.gov/medicaremedicare-fee-service-paymenthospitaloutpatientppsaddendum-and-addendum-b-updates/january-2020-correction

15-5 From *Final 2020 Drugs and Biologicals with Pass-Through Status* (website): https://www.cms.gov/Medicare/Medicare-Fee-for-Service-Payment/HospitalOutpatientPPS/passthrough_payment

15-6 From *ICD-10-CM/PCS MS-DRG v37.0 Definitions Manual* (website): https://www.cms.gov/icd10m/version37-fullcode-cms/fullcode_cms/P0001.html

15-7 From *ICD-10-CM/PCS MS-DRG v37.0 Definitions Manual* (website): https://www.cms.gov/icd10m/version37-fullcode-cms/fullcode_cms/P0299.html

15-8 From *ICD-10-CM/PCS MS-DRG v37.0 Definitions Manual* (website): https://www.cms.gov/icd10m/version37-fullcode-cms/fullcode_cms/P0003.html

15-9 From *ICD-10-CM/PCS MS-DRG v37.0 Definitions Manual* (website): https://www.cms.gov/icd10m/version37-fullcode-cms/fullcode_cms/P0038.html

15-10 From *ICD-10-CM/PCS MS-DRG v37.0 Definitions Manual* (website): https://www.cms.gov/icd10m/version37-fullcode-cms/fullcode_cms/P0048.html

15-11 From *ICD-10-CM/PCS MS-DRG v37.0 Definitions Manual* (website): https://www.cms.gov/icd10m/version37-fullcode-cms/fullcode_cms/P0004.html

16-1 Courtesy U.S. Department of Health and Human Services, Centers for Medicare and Medicaid Services.

17-3 Courtesy U.S. Department of Health and Human Services, Centers for Medicare and Medicaid Services.

19-1 Courtesy U.S. Department of Health and Human Services, Centers for Medicare and Medicaid Services.

20-4 From Roberts JR, Custalow CB, Thomsen TW: *Roberts and Hedges' Clinical Procedures in Emergency Medicine and Acute Care*, ed 7, Philadelphia, 2019, Elsevier.

25-2 From Elsevier: *Buck's 2021 ICD-10-CM for Hospitals*, St. Louis, 2021, Elsevier.

25-3 From Elsevier: Buck's 2021 ICD-10-CM for Hospitals, St. Louis, 2021, Elsevier.

31-1 From Elsevier: Buck's 2021 *ICD-10-CM for Hospitals*, St. Louis, 2021, Elsevier.

31-2 From Elsevier: Buck's 2021 *ICD-10-CM for Hospitals*, St. Louis, 2021, Elsevier.

31-3 From Elsevier: Buck's 2021 *ICD-10-CM for Hospitals*, St. Louis, 2021, Elsevier.

Part 6 Final Exam answer sheet Copyright © 2021, Elsevier Inc. All rights reserved.

Appendix A

Resources

The most current coding guidelines and code system updates are posted to the Evolve website at ***http://evolve.elsevier.com/Buck/examreview.***

Once registered for your free Evolve resources (using the access code provided on the inside front cover of this text), go to the ***Course Content*** section to reference the following:

Exam Review

Physician Exam (Format A)
Physician Exam (Format B)
Facility Exam (Format C)

Mobile Quick Quizzes

Parts 1, 4, and 5

Coding Tips and Links

ICD-10-CM Official Guidelines for Coding and Reporting
1995 Guidelines for E/M Services

1997 Documentation Guidelines for Evaluation and Management Services
CPT, ICD-10-CM, ICD-10-PCS, and HCPCS Update Links
Study Tips

Content Updates—Student

Some of the CPT code descriptions for physician services include physician extender services. Physician extenders, such as nurse practitioners, physician assistants, and nurse anesthetists, etc., provide medical services typically performed by a physician. Within this educational material the term "physician" may include "and other qualified health care professionals" depending on the code. Refer to the official CPT® code descriptions and guidelines to determine codes that are appropriate to report services provided by nonphysician practitioners.

Appendix B

Answers

Chapter 1—Integumentary System

Anatomy and Terminology Quiz

1. c
2. d
3. a
4. b
5. d
6. c
7. d
8. b
9. c
10. c

Pathophysiology Quiz

1. c
2. c
3. a
4. d
5. b
6. c
7. d
8. b
9. d
10. a

Chapter 2—Musculoskeletal System

Anatomy and Terminology Quiz

1. b
2. c
3. a
4. c
5. a
6. d
7. b
8. d
9. a
10. c

Pathophysiology Quiz

1. d
2. c
3. b

4. a
5. d
6. d
7. a
8. c
9. b
10. d

Chapter 3—Respiratory System

Anatomy and Terminology Quiz

1. b
2. d
3. c
4. a
5. a
6. c
7. c
8. b
9. d
10. d

Pathophysiology Quiz

1. b
2. a
3. d
4. d
5. d
6. a
7. c
8. b
9. a
10. c

Chapter 4—Cardiovascular System

Anatomy and Terminology Quiz

1. d
2. a
3. c
4. a
5. d
6. b
7. d
8. a
9. d
10. d

Pathophysiology Quiz

1. b
2. c
3. c
4. c
5. d
6. a
7. c
8. c
9. a
10. d

Chapter 5—Female Genital System and Pregnancy

Anatomy and Terminology Quiz

1. d
2. a
3. a
4. b
5. c
6. a
7. b
8. b
9. c
10. d

Pathophysiology Quiz

1. b
2. d
3. a
4. c
5. b
6. a
7. a
8. c
9. b
10. c

Chapter 6—Male Genital System

Anatomy and Terminology Quiz

1. c
2. a
3. d
4. b
5. a
6. a
7. a
8. d
9. d
10. b

Pathophysiology Quiz

1. a
2. b

3. d
4. a
5. c
6. b
7. d
8. b
9. a
10. b

Chapter 7—Urinary System

Anatomy and Terminology Quiz

1. c
2. d
3. a
4. c
5. b
6. d
7. c
8. b
9. d
10. a

Pathophysiology Quiz

1. c
2. d
3. d
4. c
5. b
6. c
7. a or c
8. c
9. b
10. c

Chapter 8—Digestive System

Anatomy and Terminology Quiz

1. b
2. d
3. d
4. b
5. c
6. b
7. a
8. c
9. a
10. b

Pathophysiology Quiz

1. c
2. a
3. d
4. b
5. a
6. c
7. a
8. c

9. a
10. a

Chapter 9—Mediastinum and Diaphragm

Anatomy and Terminology Quiz

1. a
2. b
3. d
4. c
5. c
6. b
7. a
8. b
9. a
10. d

Chapter 10—Hemic and Lymphatic System

Anatomy and Terminology Quiz

1. b
2. d
3. a
4. d
5. c
6. c
7. a
8. d
9. b
10. d

Pathophysiology Quiz

1. c
2. a
3. b
4. d
5. b
6. b
7. a
8. a
9. c
10. b

Chapter 11—Endocrine System

Anatomy and Terminology Quiz

1. c
2. d
3. b
4. a
5. d
6. a
7. d
8. a
9. b
10. d

Pathophysiology Quiz

1. a
2. b
3. c
4. a
5. d
6. b
7. a
8. d
9. a
10. c

Chapter 12—Nervous System

Anatomy and Terminology Quiz

1. b
2. a
3. a
4. b
5. b
6. c
7. a
8. d
9. b
10. a

Pathophysiology Quiz

1. a
2. c
3. b
4. d
5. a
6. b
7. a
8. b
9. b
10. c

Chapter 13—Senses

Anatomy and Terminology Quiz

1. d
2. d
3. a
4. a
5. a
6. b
7. c
8. b
9. d
10. a

Pathophysiology Quiz

1. d
2. b
3. c

4. a
5. b
6. a
7. a
8. a
9. b
10. b

PART 2 QUIZ ANSWERS

Chapter 14—Reimbursement Issues

Reimbursement Quiz

1. b
2. a
3. c
4. b
5. d
6. a
7. a
8. b
9. d
10. b

PART 3 QUIZ ANSWERS

Chapter 15—Facility-based Reimbursement Issues

Reimbursement Quiz

1. b
2. d
3. d
4. b
5. d
6. b
7. a
8. b
9. b
10. b

PART 4 PRACTICE EXERCISE ANSWERS AND RATIONALES

Chapter 17—Evaluation and Management (E/M) Section

Practice Exercise 17.1

Professional Service: 99232 (Evaluation and Management, Hospital)

ICD-10-CM: N17.9 (Failure, renal, acute), **I12.9** (Hypertension, kidney, with stage I through stage IV chronic kidney disease), **N18.9** (Failure, renal, chronic), **E86.9** (Depletion, volume NOS), **I73.9** (Disease, peripheral, vascular [occlusive])

Rationale: The service in this inpatient progress note is reported with 99232 because it describes an expanded problem-focused history and examination. The patient has two stable chronic conditions (hypertension and peripheral vascular disease) and acute-on-chronic renal failure that is improving; therefore, the medical decision making is of moderate complexity.

The patient has acute renal failure (N17.9) and chronic renal failure (N18.9), but according to ICD-10-CM Section I.C.9.a.2 of the *Official Guidelines for Coding and Reporting*, the coder is to assign a code from the I12 category to report hypertensive kidney disease, when a hypertensive patient has a condition that is classifiable to N18. You are to assume a cause-and-effect relationship and classify the chronic renal failure with hypertension as hypertensive renal disease (I12.9 and N18.9). The acute renal failure category N17 is not included in the Guideline to assume a cause-and-effect relationship. The acute renal failure would be reported because when you reference the Excludes note following I12, the coder is directed to assign N17.x for acute renal failure. Note that according to ICD-10-CM, Section I.B.8. of the Guidelines, when there is both an acute and chronic condition present, the acute condition is reported first.

The patient also has volume depletion (E86.9), which is reported because the condition contributes to the patient's renal status. The peripheral vascular disease (I73.9) is reported because it was important enough for the physician to mention it in the impression section of the report.

Practice Exercise 17.2

Professional Service: 99214 (Evaluation and Management, Office and Other Outpatient)

ICD-10-CM: A08.4 (Gastroenteritis, viral NEC)

Rationale: Code 99214 reports an office visit for an established patient. The note is titled as a follow-up clinic visit. The patient is established with this provider. The medical decision making is moderate because there are possibly two new problems—gastroenteritis and possible otitis media. Prescription drugs were given—making this a moderate medical decision making.

The diagnosis is viral gastroenteritis reported with A08.4, and because the otitis media was stated as possible, that diagnosis would not be reported.

Practice Exercise 17.3

Professional Service: 99284 (Evaluation and Management Emergency Department)

ICD-10-CM: R11.2 (Vomiting, with nausea), **E86.0** (Dehydration), **C15.9** (Neoplasm, esophagus, Malignant Primary), **C79.51** (Neoplasm, bones, Malignant Secondary), **C78.89** (Neoplasm, stomach, Malignant Secondary)

Rationale: This was a level 4 emergency department service and included a detailed history, comprehensive examination, and moderate decision making level of complexity.

The first-listed diagnosis is the primary reason the patient presented to the emergency department—vomiting and nausea, reported with R11.2. The dehydration was noted in the assessment and was treated and would be reported with E86.0. The underlying condition that is causing these symptoms is the primary malignant neoplasm of the esophagus and is reported with C15.9. She has severe pain due to the metastases being treated with morphine. Assign the codes for these conditions because they were treated. Metastases included bones (C79.51) and stomach (C78.89).

Practice Exercise 17.4

Professional Service: 99391 (Preventive Medicine, Established Patient)

ICD-10-CM: Z00.129 (Examination, child [over 28 days old])

Rationale: This is a routine checkup for an established infant and is considered preventive medicine. When choosing a code from this category, the age of the infant or child and whether the patient is new or established determines the code choice. Code 99391 is assigned for a newborn until 1 year of age.

The diagnosis is a routine health check reported with Z00.129. Note the slightly different terms to locate the correct code. If the infant were seen for a routine health check with abnormal findings or a specific complaint, then report Z00.121 followed by the appropriate code(s) for the abnormal findings.

Practice Exercise 17.5

Professional Service: 99469 (Critical Care Services, Neonatal, Subsequent)

ICD-10-CM: P07.17 (Low birth weight, 1750-1999 grams), **P07.31** (Preterm infant, newborn, with gestation of, 28-31 weeks), **P22.0** (Hyaline, membrane), **P59.9** (Jaundice, newborn), **Q25.0** (Patent ductus arteriosus or Botallo)

Rationale: When a critically ill newborn 30 days of age or less is either born or brought to the hospital and placed in the Neonatal Critical Care Unit, the initial care day is coded with 99468; each additional day is coded with 99469, as long as the baby is considered critically ill.

The diagnosis is preterm infant with a body weight of 1716 kg. Code P07.17 reports the low birth weight between 1750-1999 grams. The preterm gestation is reported with P07.31. The hyaline membrane is reported P22.0. Referencing hyperbilirubinemia of neonate directs the coder to "see Jaundice, newborn." The report does not state that the jaundice is due to preterm delivery (P59.0); therefore, the jaundice is reported with code P59.9. This patient also has patent ductus arteriosus (Q25.0). There is mention of some type of pulmonary valve disorder which could be associated with Noonan syndrome; however, that has not been verified and we do not know what the pulmonary valve disorder is.

Chapter 18—Anesthesia Section

Practice Exercise 18.1

Professional Service: 00840-QK-P2 (Anesthesia, Abdomen, Intraperitoneal), **99100** (Anesthesia, Special Circumstances, Extreme Age)

Rationale: The surgical procedure is an abdominal procedure in which the anesthesia is reported with 00840. HCPCS modifier -QK indicates the anesthesiologist was medically directing two to four concurrent cases. 99100 is added to indicate age over 70, which is a qualifying circumstance that may impact the anesthesia service. -P2 indicates a patient with a mild systemic disease (hypertension).

Practice Exercise 18.2

Professional Service: 00400-AA-QS-P1 (Anesthesia, Integumentary System, Anterior Trunk)

Rationale: The service is an anesthesia service for a procedure to the breast reported with 00400. -AA indicates that the anesthesiologist personally performed the anesthesia service. -P1 indicates a normal healthy patient. This was a monitored anesthesia case (MAC) as noted by modifier -QS.

Practice Exercise 18.3

Professional Service: 00790-QK-P2 (Anesthesia, Abdomen, Intraperitoneal)

Rationale: The service is an abdominal anesthesia service for a procedure of the upper abdomen, reported with 00790. Modifier -QK is added to indicate the anesthesiologist was supervising more than one procedure at the same time. -P2 indicates a patient with a mild systemic disease.

Practice Exercise 18.4

Professional Service: 00902-AA-P3 (Anesthesia, Anus)

Rationale: The service is anesthesia for a procedure of the anus in which a spinal was administered and reported with 00902. -AA indicates that the anesthesiologist personally performed the anesthesia service.

Practice Exercise 18.5

Professional Service: 00211-AA-P5 (Anesthesia, Brain)

Rationale: The service was anesthesia for an intercranial hematoma reported with 00211. -AA indicates that the anesthesiologist personally performed the anesthesia service. -P5 indicates that the patient is not expected to survive without this procedure.

Chapter 19—CPT/HCPCS Level I Modifiers

Practice Exercise 19.1

Professional Service: 49060-78-52 (Drainage, Abscess, Retroperitoneal), **11005-78-51** (Debridement, Skin, Subcutaneous Tissue, Infected)

ICD-10-CM: T81.41XD (Infection, postoperative wound), **K65.4** (Necrosis, fat, peritoneum), **I96** (Necrosis, skin or subcutaneous tissue), **K63.2** (Fistula, abdominal wall)

Rationale: The primary procedure was drainage of an abdominal abscess reported with 49060. Modifier -78 is added to indicate an unplanned return to the operating room. Modifier -52 (reduced services) is added to indicate that the abdomen was already open and it was packed and left open. This patient had debridement (11005) of an abdominal wound, which was necrotic. Modifier -51 is added to 11005 to indicate multiple procedures were performed. Modifier -78 is also added.

This is a life-threatening condition that required extensive debridement of the skin, fat, and the area behind the abdominal contents. The diagnoses codes are: T81.41XD reports the postoperative wound infection, K65.4 reports fat necrosis of abdominal wall, I96 reports the necrosis of the skin, and K63.2 reports the fistula of the abdominal wall between the abdominal cavity and the retroperitoneal area. The ICD-10-CM complication code (T81.41XD) includes the seventh character of "D," indicating a subsequent encounter.

Practice Exercise 19.2

Professional Service: 11404-58 (Excision, Skin, Lesion, Benign)

ICD-10-CM: D23.61 (Neoplasm, skin, arm, Benign)

Rationale: The procedure was re-excision of a benign lesion that measured 1 cm in diameter; the original procedure had 0.5-cm margins. This left a 2-cm incision that the surgeon now re-excised with a 1-cm margin. The total measurement for the re-excision is 4 cm. Modifier -58 is added to indicate that the patient was returned to the operating room during the postoperative period of the first procedure in part two of a two-part procedure.

The pathology report states fibrosis and granulation tissue, and there was no evidence of the Spitz nevus. In cases such as this, when there is excision of additional skin margins, it is acceptable to report the original diagnosis, which in this case is the Spitz nevus, a benign lesion, and reported with D23.61.

Practice Exercise 19.3

Professional Service: 93306-26 (Echocardiography, Transthoracic)

ICD-10-CM: I07.1 (Insufficiency, tricuspid), **I48.91** (Fibrillation, atrial or auricular [established]), **I51.9** (Dysfunction, ventricular)

Rationale: This patient had an echocardiogram and the key to correctly reporting an echocardiogram is to identify whether it was performed transthoracic or transesophageal, and if it was a complete study or follow-up/limited study. The service in this case was a two-dimensional with M-mode recording complete echo—93306 for the real-time image and documentation. Code 93306 includes spectral and color flow Doppler; therefore, 93320 and 93325 are not reported separately. You would add modifier -26 because you are reporting only the physician portion of the procedure.

The patient has valvular disease, and the report indicates the specific type of valvular disease. In this case, tricuspid insufficiency (I07.1), atrial fibrillation (I48.91), and ventricular dysfunction (I51.9).

Practice Exercise 19.4

Professional Service: 99214-24 (Evaluation and Management, Office and Other Outpatient)

ICD-10-CM: O34.32 (Pregnancy, complicated by, incompetent, cervix), **Z87.51** (History personal [of], obstetric complications, pre-term labor)

Rationale: This is an office visit service in which a decision was made to proceed with surgery. Modifier -57 is not assigned as the global period for 59320 (Cerclage, Cervix, Vaginal) has a 0-day global period. Use modifier -24 to indicate that this service is totally separate from the obstetric global package for a complication of the pregnancy. The medical decision making complexity is of a moderate level, reported with 99214.

The diagnosis is incompetent cervix, which is an abnormal cervix with a tendency to dilate prematurely in one who is pregnant, reported with O34.32. Note that ICD-10-CM includes the trimester, which was determined based on the opening statement that patient is 19 weeks 3 days gestation (second trimester). The history of pre-term labor was a factor in the decision to proceed, code Z87.51 is also reported.

Practice Exercise 19.5

Professional Service: 30520 (Septoplasty), **31267-51-50** (Antrostomy, Sinus, Maxillary), **31288-51-50** (Sphenoidotomy, Excision with Nasal/Sinus Endoscopy), **31255-51-50** (Ethmoidectomy, Endoscopic), **30930-51-50** (Turbinate, Fracture, Therapeutic)

ICD-10-CM: J34.2 (Deviation, septum), **J33.9** (Polyp, nasal), **J33.8** (Polyp, sinus), **J32.4** (Pansinusitis), **J34.3** (Hypertrophy, nasal, turbinate)

Rationale: The services are listed in the Procedures Performed section of the report and are supported within the body of the report as: (1) bilateral endoscopic total ethmoidectomy, 31255-50-51; (2) bilateral endoscopic maxillary antrostomy with removal of polyps from maxillary sinus, 31267-50-51; (3) bilateral endoscopic sphenoidotomy, 31288-50-51; (4) septoplasty, 30520; and (5) bilateral inferior turbinate outfracture, 30930-50-51. Note that all procedures except the primary procedure, septoplasty, have modifier -50 to indicate bilateral procedures and modifier -51 to indicate multiple procedures.

The diagnoses are listed in the Postoperative Diagnosis section of the report as: (1) septal deviation, J34.2; (2) bilateral sinonasal polyposis, J33.9 (nasal) and (3) J33.8 (sinus); (4) pansinusitis, J32.4, (5) bilateral inferior turbinate hypertrophy, J34.3; and nasal obstruction. The nasal obstruction is not reported because it is caused by the septal deviation.

Chapter 20—Surgery Section

Practice Exercise 20.1

Professional Service: 11312 (Lesion, Skin, Shaving)

ICD-10-CM: D23.39 (Neoplasm, skin, cheek, Benign)

Rationale: The procedure is a shave excision of a lesion on the cheek that measures 1.6 cm. When reporting lesion removal, first identify the technique used. Shaving involves transverse incision or horizontal slicing and does not involve a full-thickness (through the dermis) excision. The excision codes involve full-thickness excision and generally require suture closure. Also identify the body area on which the lesion is located, the size of the lesion, and whether the lesion is benign or malignant. Note that in the case of shavings, the nature (benign or malignant) does not influence the selection of the CPT code.

In this case, the lesion shaved was benign, as indicated by the pathology report and reported with D23.39.

Practice Exercise 20.2

Professional Service: 19120-RT (Breast, Excision, Lesion)

ICD-10-CM: C50.011 (Neoplasm, breast, female, nipple, Malignant Primary)

Rationale: This patient presents for excision of a tumor of the right breast (19120-RT). The tumor is submitted for frozen section, which is an analysis performed by the pathologist during the procedure (intraoperatively).

The results of the frozen section were carcinoma of the right breast nipple (C50.011).

Practice Exercise 20.3

Professional Service: 15574-F7 (Pedicle Flap, Formation), **15120-51** (Split, Grafts)

ICD-10-CM: S68.622A (Amputation, traumatic, finger, transphalangeal, partial, middle), **W31.9XXA** (External Cause Index, Contact with, machinery)

Rationale: While working on machinery, this patient amputated the tip of her middle finger. A flap was formed from the ulnar aspect of the hand to place over the defect of the right middle finger (15574-F7). Modifier -F7 indicates the middle finger of the right hand. The split-thickness graft is reported with 15120 with modifier -51.

The diagnosis is traumatic amputation of the finger reported with S68.622A. Note that the ICD-10-CM code descriptions specify a traumatic, partial (tip) amputation of each specific finger of the right and left hand. The external cause code W31.9xxA is reported to indicate the injury was sustained while working on machinery. The seventh character "A" indicates the initial encounter for the injury.

Practice Exercise 20.4

Professional Service: 12002-F7 (Closure)

ICD-10-CM: S61.212A (Laceration, finger[s], middle, right), **W45.8XXA** (External Cause Index, Contact [accidental] with, arrow, not thrown, projected or falling)

Rationale: The patient presents with multiple lacerations of the finger that total 6 cm for which simple repair is performed (12002). Modifier -F7 is added to indicate the middle right finger.

Code S61.212A reports a laceration of the right finger. S61.212A reports the specific finger and laterality (side) and includes the seventh character of "A," to indicate the initial

encounter. An external cause code (W45.8XXA) is reported to indicate how the finger was injured (due to arrow).

Practice Exercise 20.5

Professional Service: 11005-58 (Debridement, Skin, Subcutaneous Tissue, Infected)

ICD-10-CM: K65.4 (Necrosis, fat, abdominal wall), **I96** (Necrosis, skin or subcutaneous tissue NEC), **T81.83XD** (Fistula, postoperative, persistent)

Rationale: The patient returns to the operating room for additional debridement of the abdominal wound (11005). Modifier -58 indicates returning to the operating room for a related procedure by the same physician during the postoperative period.

The diagnoses are necrosis of the abdominal wall fat (K65.4), necrosis of the skin/subcutaneous tissue (I96), and postoperative fistula (T81.83XD). The complication code (T81.83XD) includes the seventh character of "D," indicating a subsequent encounter.

Practice Exercise 20.6

Professional Service: 20610-LT (Injection, Joint)

ICD-10-CM: M75.52 (Bursitis, shoulder)

Rationale: This is an injection into the shoulder without guidance, which is considered a major joint. The main code 20600 states arthrocentesis, aspiration, and/or injection small joint. This was an injection, so the area is correct, but the small joints are listed in parentheses after 20600 as fingers and toes. The indented codes that follow 20600 indicate shoulder, as included in 20610.

In the ICD-10-CM Index, under bursitis, subacromial instructs the coder to *see* bursitis, shoulder. There is no specific reporting for the different structures within the shoulder. Report code M75.52, which is bursitis of the left shoulder.

Practice Exercise 20.7

Professional Service: 29898-RT (Arthroscopy, Surgical, Ankle)

ICD-10-CM: M19.071 (Osteoarthritis, ankle), **M25.771** (Osteophyte, ankle), **M79.9** (Disorder, soft tissue, ankle)

Rationale: The service is an arthroplasty of the right ankle by means of a scope, not an open surgical procedure as would be reported with 27700-27703. The arthroscopic procedures are located in the Endoscopy/Arthroscopy category of codes (29800-29999). When locating the service in the index of the CPT, the main term *Arthroplasty* directs the coder to the incisional procedures. The main term *Arthroscopy* directs the coder to the correct surgical and diagnostic arthroscopic procedure codes. Codes 29894-29898 are the correct range, and the code to report the services in this case is 29898, with modifier -RT to indicate right.

The first diagnosis in the Postoperative Diagnoses section of the report is osteoarthritic change of the ankle. ICD-10-CM code M19.071 includes the sixth character "1," indicating right side.

The second postoperative diagnosis is osteophytic spurring. In ICD-10-CM reference in the Index, Osteophyte, ankle M25.77-. The sixth character "1" indicates the right side.

The third postoperative diagnosis is impinging soft tissue, but when referencing the Index of the ICD-10-CM, the only entry under impingement is of the soft tissue between the teeth. With no more specific entry, the coder would reference a general term, such as "Disorder, soft tissue." In ICD-10-CM, referencing "Disorder, soft tissue, ankle" leads to code M79.9.

Practice Exercise 20.8

Professional Service: 25210-LT (Carpal Bone, Excision), **25310-51-LT** (Tendon, Transfer, Wrist)

ICD-10-CM: M18.12 (Osteoarthritis, primary, hand joint, first carpometacarpal joint)

Rationale: This is an arthroplasty of the patient's carpometacarpal joint. The trapezium, one of the carpal bones, was removed in pieces (25210). The flexor carpi radialis (FCR) tendon was transferred to the site and threaded through bone. This was harvested through two incisions at the distal wrist and in the forearm. The report states that the underlying FCR tendon was preserved and later it was cut at the floor of the thumb and transferred through the hole at the base of the first metatarsal and pinned to the second metatarsal (25310). The report is difficult to read because it appears that the "harvested" FCR is removed; however, it is just separated and the proximal end was left intact. Code 25447 involves the insertion of a prosthesis; therefore, it is not correct. Modifier -LT is appended to both procedures to indicate the procedure was performed on the left wrist. Modifier -51 indicates 25210 is a second procedure during the same session.

The patient has degenerative arthritis. For ICD-10-CM the coder is directed to "*see osteoarthritis.*" Code M18.12 reports localized osteoarthritis, as indicated by the reporting of the specific joint, carpometacarpal (hand).

Practice Exercise 20.9

Professional Service: 27355-RT (Excision, Cyst, Femur)

ICD-10-CM: D16.21 (Neoplasm, bone, femur, right side, Benign)

Rationale: This is an excision of a bone tumor of the femur. You would not use code 27328 because this code reports a procedure of the muscle of the thigh, and the tumor in this case was in the bone, reported with 27355, with -RT to indicate the right leg.

The diagnosis is a benign neoplasm (per the pathology report) of the long bone (D16.21). The femur, or thigh bone, is the longest bone in the leg. It would not be correct to report D16.31 because this is for the short bones of the leg, such as the tibia or fibula.

Practice Exercise 20.10

Professional Service: 27327-LT (Excision, Tumor, Knee)

ICD-10-CM: D21.22 (Neoplasm, connective tissue, knee, Benign)

Rationale: This mass is in the subcutaneous tissue of the patient's knee, reported with 27327, with -LT added to indicate left side. You would not use code 27328 because this code is for deeper than subcutaneous.

The pathology report indicated a benign mass of the bursa, and when referencing "Neoplasm" in the Index of the ICD-10-CM, subterm *bursa,* the coder is directed to the subterm *connective tissue.* D21.22 reports a benign tumor of the connective tissue of the knee. The fifth character of "2" designates the left knee.

Practice Exercise 20.11

Professional Service: 36217-RT (Insertion, Catheter, Brachiocephalic Artery), **36216-59-LT** (Insertion, Catheter, Brachiocephalic Artery), **36215-59-LT** (Insertion, Catheter, Brachiocephalic Artery)

ICD-10-CM: I61.1 (Hemorrhage, intracranial [nontraumatic], intracerebral, hemisphere, cortical [superficial])

Rationale: You were given instructions to assign the codes for the catheterizations only. When reporting catheterizations of the carotid and peripheral arteries, carotids in this case, you need to know where the catheter tip is being placed. The arteries are listed by family and by order—the deeper the vessel, the higher the order. In this case, the third-order vessel is reported first (right internal carotid artery), the second-order vessel is reported second (left vertebral artery), and the first-order vessel (left common carotid artery) is reported last. Modifier -59 is added to 36215 and 36216 to indicate the catheterizations are in different families than 36217. Modifiers -RT and -LT indicate right or left vessels.

The procedure is being performed because the patient has an intracranial hemorrhage, reported with I61.1. The temporal lobe is a cerebral lobe which is noted under I61.1 in the ICD-10-CM Tabular; therefore, the reference in the Index is Hemorrhage, intracranial, intracerebral, hemisphere, cortical, I61.1.

Practice Exercise 20.12

Professional Service: 36580 (Vein, Catheterization, Replacement)

ICD-10-CM: Z49.01 (Preparatory care for subsequent treatment NEC, for dialysis), **N18.6** (Disease, renal, end stage [ESRD])

Rationale: The service is a venous catheter replacement by means of a percutaneous approach reported with 36580.

In ICD-10-CM, first locate dependence on dialysis and then reference the notes in the Tabular under Z99.2, Excludes to locate the adjustment code Z49.01. The code description for Z49.01 includes removal or replacement of the dialysis catheter. This is also found in the Index under "Preparatory care for subsequent treatment NEC, for dialysis." The diagnosis is stated as end-stage renal failure and reported with N18.6.

Practice Exercise 20.13

Professional Service: 36558 (Insertion, Catheter, Venous), **77001-26** (Fluoroscopy, Venous Access Device), **99152, 99153** (Sedation, Moderate)

ICD-10-CM: C34.90 (Neoplasm, lung, lobe NEC, Malignant Primary)

Rationale: The service was the placement of a Port-a-Cath, which is a catheter that is inserted into a large central vein, such as the jugular in this case, with a pump attached to the other end of the catheter. The small pump (about the size of three silver dollars stacked) is a port or reservoir implanted under the skin. The pump is used to infuse various substances by means of a reservoir. The substance is infused over time. In this case, the pump is being used for chemotherapy administration, and the insertion is reported with 36558. Codes 36555 and 36556 report temporary pump or port placement, 36557 and 36558 report a port or pump that is level with the skin by placing it under the skin. Codes 36560 and 36561 report ports or pumps that extend outside the skin and are not often used.

The physician fluoroscopic guidance service is reported with 77001. Modifier -26 is added to indicate that only the professional component of the service is being provided. Conscious sedation was provided as indicated in the report and was assigned code 99144 (30 minutes) and 99145 (15 minutes) because the patient was over age 5 and the sedation lasted 45 minutes.

The diagnosis is stated as primary lung cancer, reported with C34.90.

Practice Exercise 20.14

Professional Service: 36217-RT (Catheterization, Thoracic Artery), **36218-RT** (Catheterization, Thoracic Artery), **36215-51-LT** (Catheterization, Thoracic Artery)

ICD-10-CM: I65.23 (Occlusion, artery, carotid)

Rationale: 36200 (Insertion, Catheter, Aorta) is bundled into 36217-RT (Catheterization, Thoracic Artery), which reports the selective catheterization of the RT vertebral artery. 36218-RT (Catheterization, Thoracic Artery) reports the selective catheterization of the right common carotid artery, which is a second order; therefore, the add-on code is assigned for the additional second or third order in the same family.

36215-51-LT (Catheterization, Thoracic Artery) reports the selective catheterization of the left carotid artery. Modifier -51 is placed to indicate an additional procedure.

The Clinical Symptoms section of the report indicates carotid artery stenosis, and the Impression statement in the third item (30-40% diameter narrowing of the carotid bulb on right) and the fourth item (complete occlusion of the left internal carotid artery) support stenosis of the carotid artery, reported with I65.23. Further, ICD-10-CM 5th character of "3" indicates both carotid arteries have stenosis/occlusion.

Practice Exercise 20.15

Professional Service: 36247-RT (Catheterization, Legs), **37211** (Transcatheter Therapy, Infusion), **75710-59-26-RT** (Angiography, Leg Artery)

ICD-10-CM: T82.392A (Complication, extremity artery [bypass] graft, mechanical, obstruction, femoral artery), **I74.3** (Thrombosis, thrombotic, leg, arterial)

Rationale: The service is a selective catheter placement of the arterial system of the second order for a diagnostic right extremity angiogram (36246-RT, 75710-59-26-RT) followed by catheter placement for infusion of tissue plasminogen activator (tPA). The catheters are placed in the common femoral through the Gore-Tex graft (36247) to below the knee. A coaxial system is one in which catheters are placed into the vessel on each side of the clot to release tPA to dissolve/lyse the clot. 36247 replaces 36246 as it is the highest order. The tPA is a thrombolytic drug used for arterial thrombotic occlusion. The infusion (37211) has a radiology component included. Modifier -59 is required on the diagnostic extremity angiogram to indicate that it was completely separate from the thrombolytic procedure. The patient returns in the morning so that the interventional radiologist can determine the extent to which the procedure was successful.

The reason for the service is a complication due to a Gore-Tex graft that is reported with T82.392A. Note that ICD-10-CM code includes seventh character "A" to indicate the first encounter for this condition. The patient has a complete occlusion of the peripheral artery of the lower extremity, reported with I74.3.

Practice Exercise 20.16

Professional Service: 43752 (Placement, Orogastric Tube)
ICD-10-CM: K31.84 (Gastroparesis)

Rationale: The service is placement of an orogastric tube (43752), known as CORFLO placement. The tube is placed to ensure that the patient receives proper nutrition. The KUB (kidneys, ureter, bladder) would be reported separately by the radiologist.

The patient has gastroparesis (K31.84).

Practice Exercise 20.17

Professional Service: 49440 (Gastrostomy Tube, Placement, Percutaneous, Nonendoscopic), **49446-51** (Gastrostomy Tube, Conversion to Gastrojejunostomy Tube), **76942-26** (Ultrasound, Guidance, Needle Biopsy)

ICD-10-CM: E46 (Malnutrition)

Rationale: This patient required placement of a feeding tube for nutritional support. Code 49440 is assigned to report the percutaneous placement of the feeding tube. The notes following 49440 state, "For conversion to a gastrojejunostomy tube at the time of initial gastrostomy tube placement, use 49440 in conjunction with 49446," which is the second procedure. Modifier -51 is appended to the second procedure, 49446-51. Ultrasound guidance 76942-26 was used to locate the edge of the liver to assist with needle placement for the catheter. Modifier -26 is added to indicate that only the professional service was provided. The fluoroscopic guidance is included in codes 49440 and 49446 and is not reported separately.

This procedure was performed because the patient is malnourished, E46.

Practice Exercise 20.18

Professional Service: 49000-78 (Laparotomy, Exploration)

ICD-10-CM: N99.72 (Complication, intraoperative, puncture or laceration [accidental], genitourinary organ or structure, during procedure on other organ)

Rationale: This patient had a laparoscopy the day before this procedure. After discharge, the patient presents to the emergency department with abdominal pain and is taken to the operating room where she was found to have a large amount of urine in her peritoneal cavity. During her previous surgery the urinary bladder had been punctured. Report 49000 for the exploratory laparotomy because this is the portion of the service that Dr. Martinez performed. Add modifier -78 to indicate the return to the operating room for a related procedure during the postoperative period. The cystorrhaphy (51860) was performed by Dr. Smithson, who dictated the note separately for the cystorrhaphy and intestinal adhesiolysis (44005).

The postoperative complication of the puncture of the urinary bladder is reported with N99.72.

Practice Exercise 20.19

Professional Service: 44640-22 (Repair, Intestines, Small, Fistula), **44120-51** (Excision, Intestines, Small)

ICD-10-CM: K63.2 (Fistula, intestine)

Rationale: A fistula is an abnormal communication between two epithelialized surfaces. An intestinal fistula is an abnormal anatomic connection between a part (or multiple parts) of the intestinal lumen and the lumen of another epithelialized structure or the skin. The goal of the procedure was to restore the continuity of the gastrointestinal tract and restore function to the other involved structures. There were multiple intestinal fistulas repaired and reported with 44640. The report stated that the procedure took significantly more time than would typically be required, which directs the assignment of modifier -22, increased procedural service.

The colon is the large intestine and the small bowel is the small intestine. The small intestine was resected and reported with 44120 with modifier -51 to indicate multiple procedures.

The diagnosis is K63.2 (fistula of the intestine).

Practice Exercise 20.20

Professional Service: 43117-62 (Esophagectomy, Partial), **47100** (Biopsy, Liver), **47000-59-53-51** (Biopsy, Liver), **44015** (Jejunostomy, Insertion, Catheter)

ICD-10-CM: K22.711 (Barrett's esophagus, with dysplasia, high grade), **D18.03** (Hemangioma, intra-abdominal)

Rationale: The report states that a wedge biopsy (47100) was performed on a liver mass on the right lobe of the liver. The pathology report was returned with a diagnosis of hemangioma, which is a benign neoplasm.

The report states that if the cancer has not spread to the liver, an esophagogastrectomy using the Ivor-Lewis technique (43117, partial esophagectomy) will be performed. Dr. White is a co-surgeon with Dr. Sanchez because Dr. White performed the mobilization of the stomach and the pyloroplasty for the abdominal portion of the procedure and closed the abdomen. Dr. Sanchez then performed

a thoracotomy for the remainder of the procedure. Co-surgery refers to a single surgical procedure that requires the skill of two surgeons of different specialties to perform parts of the same procedure. It could be that the two surgeons perform different procedures, in which case it is not co-surgery. Co-surgery has been performed if the procedure performed is part of and would be reported using a single surgical code. Each surgeon dictates his part of the procedure and reports 43117-62. Modifier -62 is appended for co-surgeon and each surgeon will be paid 62.5% of the procedure. Dr. White also performed the jejunostomy (44015). Code 44015 is an add-on code when the jejunostomy is performed during another procedure; therefore, modifier -51 is not reported.

Before the open biopsy, the physician attempted to perform a percutaneous biopsy of a lesion on the liver (47000), which was terminated after the start of the procedure because the patient was unable to hold his breath. Since the lesion was very close to the diaphragm, the surgeon elected to discontinue the procedure and take the patient to the operating room. An open wedge biopsy of the liver was performed and is reported with 47100, which is an add-on code when performed with another open procedure. Modifier -59 is required because 47000 is mutually exclusive of 47100. Since 47000 was performed earlier than the abdominal procedure, modifier -59 denotes that the percutaneous biopsy was performed at a different session than 47100. The surgeon elected to terminate the procedure; therefore, modifier -52 (reduced procedure) is also added to 47000-59-52. The liver biopsy was a staged procedure in that a frozen section was performed to rule out metastasis to the liver. The frozen section showed hemangioma. Had the FS showed metastasis, the procedure would have been cancelled.

Code K22.711 is reported for Barrett's syndrome, as is stated in the Postoperative Diagnosis section of the report. Code D18.03 (Hemangioma, intra-abdominal structures) is reported for the liver biopsy because this is indicated in the pathology report. You would not report C15.9 (Malignant neoplasm of the esophagus) because it states possible malignancy and you cannot report possible or rule-out conditions.

Practice Exercise 20.21

Professional Service: 50280-RT (Excision, Cyst, Kidney)

ICD-10-CM: N28.1 (Cyst, kidney [acquired])

Rationale: The procedure was the excision of a cyst on the right kidney, which is reported with 50280. Modifier -RT is added to indicate that the procedure was on the right side.

The diagnosis is stated in the Postoperative Diagnosis section of the report as renal cyst, reported with N28.1.

Practice Exercise 20.22

Professional Service: 50541-RT (Kidney, Cyst, Ablation)

ICD-10-CM: N28.1 (Cyst, kidney [acquired])

Rationale: This service was a laparoscopic cyst removal reported with 50541 with modifier -RT to indicate the right side. The biopsy is included in the ablation code and is not reported separately.

The diagnosis is cyst of the kidney (N28.1) and is confirmed by the pathology report.

Practice Exercise 20.23

Professional Service: 58150 (Hysterectomy, Abdominal, Total)

ICD-10-CM: N92.0 (Menorrhagia [primary]), **D25.9** (Fibroid, uterus)

Rationale: This patient had a total abdominal hysterectomy with bilateral removal of tubes and ovaries. The report indicates this was an open abdominal approach (58150).

Code N92.0 is assigned to report menorrhagia and is listed as the first diagnosis in the Preoperative Diagnoses section of the report. The leiomyomas are listed as the second diagnosis in the Preoperative Diagnoses section and are reported with D25.9. When referencing the Index of the ICD-10-CM under "Fibroid, uterus," the coder is directed to D25.9.

Practice Exercise 20.24

Professional Service: 59515 (Cesarean Delivery, Postpartum Care)

ICD-10-CM: O45.93 (Pregnancy, complicated by, premature separation of placenta, unspecified), **O60.14X0** (Pregnancy, complicated by, preterm labor third trimester, with third trimester preterm delivery), **Z37.0** (Outcome of delivery, single, liveborn)

Rationale: This patient presents for an emergency cesarean section in which the OB surgeon will then follow the patient postpartum (59515).

Code O45.93 reports the premature separation of the placenta for unspecified reasons (i.e., coagulation defect in mother), occurring in the third trimester. The onset of preterm labor complicating pregnancy is reported with O60.14X0. The seventh character "0" denotes single gestation. The outcome of delivery is reported on the mother's record with Z37.0 for single liveborn.

Practice Exercise 20.25

Professional Service: 56630-RT (Vulvectomy, Radical)

ICD-10-CM: D07.1 (Neoplasm, labium, majus, Ca in situ)

Rationale: The vulvectomy, radical/partial is the excision of a portion of the labia, reported with 56630. We are not told the size of the lesion, only that it was located at the 11 o'clock position of the right labia majora and that a 1 cm margin was taken on all sides. Even a 1 cm margin on two sides would lead to an area of 2 cm (based on size of lesion and the narrowest margin × 2). A partial radical vulvectomy involves removal of less than 80% of the vulvar area and a radical procedure involves removal of the skin and deep subcutaneous tissue. The report does indicate that "running locked suture of 2-0 Vicryl was then placed in the deeper tissues." This is correctly coded with 56630. It would not be appropriate to use the excision of malignant lesions

codes (11620-11626) and the intermediate repair codes (12041-12047) because deeper tissue was involved. Modifier -RT indicates the vulvectomy was performed on the right only.

The lesion, which was sent to pathology, was returned with a diagnosis of Neoplasia III, which is carcinoma in situ of the labia majora, reported with D07.1.

The ICD-10-CM Neoplasm Table for "Neoplasm, labia [skin], majora, Ca in situ" indicates D07.0. When you reference the Tabular, you will see Carcinoma in situ of endometrium. The correct code is D07.1 (Carcinoma in situ of vulva). The Tabular lists severe dysplasia of vulva, which is noted in the Postoperative Diagnosis of the report.

Practice Exercise 20.26

Professional Service: 61313-RT (Craniotomy, Surgery)

ICD-10-CM: I61.1 (Hemorrhage, intracranial [nontraumatic], intracerebral, hemisphere, cortical [superficial])

Rationale: This patient had a craniotomy for evacuation of an intracerebral hematoma (supratentorial), 61313. Modifier -RT indicates the surgery was performed on the right temporal lobe. If this procedure was infratentorial, it would be much more extensive, and the physician service would be reported with infratentorial codes.

The diagnosis is stated as a nontraumatic intracerebral hematoma of the right temporal lobe, reported with I61.1. In the ICD-10-CM Index, Hematoma, brain (traumatic), nontraumatic, refers you to "see Hemorrhage, intracranial."

Practice Exercise 20.27

Professional Service: 61154-RT (Burr Hole, Skull, Drainage, Hematoma)

ICD-10-CM: I62.01 (Hemorrhage, intracranial [nontraumatic], subdural [nontraumatic], acute)

Rationale: This patient had a nontraumatic subdural hematoma drained through burr holes, which were drilled into the frontal and posterior parietal areas of the right cranium (61154). Code 61154 represents evacuation and/or drainage of either a subdural (under the dura) or extradural (on top of the dura) hematoma. This was a unilateral procedure, so the modifier -RT is appended to indicate the right side.

The diagnosis is stated as a nontraumatic subacute subdural hematoma, reported with I60.9.

Practice Exercise 20.28

Professional Service: 64721-LT (Carpal Tunnel Syndrome, Decompression)

ICD-10-CM: G56.02 (Syndrome, carpal tunnel)

Rationale: Carpal tunnel release is performed on this patient (64721), in which the physician decompresses the median nerve by freeing the nerve inside the carpal tunnel of the wrist. Modifier -LT indicates the procedure was performed on the left wrist.

The diagnosis is stated as carpal tunnel syndrome, reported with G56.02. Note the fifth character "2" indicates the left side.

Practice Exercise 20.29

Professional Service: 63709-78 (Repair, Spinal Cord, Cerebrospinal Fluid Leak)

    ICD-10-CM: G97.82 (Pseudomeningocele, postprocedural [spinal])

    Rationale: A pseudomeningocele is an abnormal collection of cerebrospinal fluid (CSF) without a membrane (dura) surrounding it. A leak in the dura causes the CSF to build in the extradural space or the tissues. This leak was a complication of a previous procedure. The previous incision was reopened. Repair of pseudomeningocele is performed on this patient for whom the physician repairs an opening in the dura with a fat graft which was taken from the same area; therefore, it is included in the procedure. After the repair the surgeon noticed another leak, and he performed a partial hemilaminectomy of L5 on the left and closed the leak. A hemilaminectomy involves removing lamina and part of the spinal process (63709). Code 63709 describes this procedure as it states repair of pseudomeningocele, with laminectomy. Had the surgeon stopped after the repair of the first leak, you would have reported 63707 for a repair of a pseudomeningocele without laminectomy. Modifier -78 indicates that the patient has returned to the operating room for a related procedure during the postoperative period.

    The diagnosis is postprocedural spinal pseudomeningocele (G97.82).

Practice Exercise 20.30

Professional Service: 63047 (Laminectomy, with Facetectomy), **63048 x 2** (Laminectomy, with Facetectomy)

    ICD-10-CM: M48.061 (Stenosis, spinal, lumbar region), **M43.16** (Spondylolisthesis, lumbar region)

    Rationale: This patient had a bilateral laminectomy with foraminotomy for spinal stenosis that was indicated on an MRI. The first segment is reported with 63047; each additional segment is reported with 63048 (this code is submitted times the number of segments involved, in this case, two). The additional segments are L4 and L5. Modifier -50 is not reported because the description in the CPT for these codes states unilateral or bilateral. Code 63048 is an add-on code; therefore, modifier -51 is not required.

    The diagnosis is stated as spinal stenosis, reported with M48.061, and grade 1 spondylolisthesis of L4-5 level, reported with M43.16.

Chapter 21—Radiology Section

Practice Exercise 21.1

Professional Service: 70450-26 (CT Scan, without Contrast, Head)

    ICD-10-CM: R41.82 (Alteration [of], Altered, mental status)

    Rationale: This is stated as a noncontrast CT scan of the head (70450). Modifier -26 is appended to indicate the physician portion only.

    Code R41.82 indicates an altered mental status.

Practice Exercise 21.2

Professional Service: 76705-26 (Ultrasound, Abdomen)

    ICD-10-CM: E80.6 (Disorder, bilirubin excretion)

    Rationale: This is an ultrasound of the gallbladder, which is an organ located in the right upper abdomen. The physician states that it is a limited ultrasound. Code 76705 specifies that this code is for a single organ ultrasound. You would not use code 76700 because this code describes a complete ultrasound.

    The indication for the ultrasound was elevation of the patient's bilirubin (E80.6).

Practice Exercise 21.3

Professional Service: 78452-26 (Stress Tests, Myocardial Perfusion Imaging)

    ICD-10-CM: R07.9 (Pain, chest), **I25.10** (Disease, heart, ischemic, atherosclerotic), **Z95.2** (Status, organ replacement, by artificial or mechanical device or prosthesis of, heart, valve)

    Rationale: This report is the professional radiologic component of a Cardiolite stress test reported by the radiologist. Modifier -26 would be added to the codes indicating the radiologist's portion of the procedure. Code 78452 reports the SPECT imaging portion of the stress test with multiple studies. Although the stress study and at rest study were performed on separate days, 78452 is reported only once. Note that the code range 78451-78454 contains imaging codes that require careful reading to ensure the correct code has been assigned.

    The reason for the encounter was chest pain (R07.9). The report indicates that the patient has arteriosclerotic coronary artery disease (I25.10) and that he has had an aortic and mitral valve replacement (Z95.2). These diagnoses are reported as they may be related to the cause of the chest pain.

Practice Exercise 21.4

Professional Service: 76506-26 (Echoencephalography, Intracranial)

    ICD-10-CM: P07.17 (Low birthweight, 1750-1999 grams), **P07.30** (Preterm, newborn, infant)

    Rationale: The service was an ultrasound of the head (76506) to examine the brain. The radiology technologist performs the ultrasound to detect intracranial abnormalities, determine ventricular size, and define cerebral contents. The examination (76506) includes all the various imaging methods performed, such as B-scan, A-scan, and real-time. Modifier -26 indicates the professional component.

    The diagnosis is preterm newborn with body weight between 1750 and 1999 grams (P07.17). Patient indicated to be preterm; however, gestational weeks not specified, code P07.30 is correctly reported.

Practice Exercise 21.5

Professional Service: 74455-26 (Urethrocystography)

    ICD-10-CM: Q62.0 (Hydronephrosis, congenital)

Rationale: Voiding cystourethrogram (74455) is a radiologic examination of the urethra and bladder to evaluate the voiding function. Modifier -26 indicates the professional component.

The clinical symptoms and diagnosis for this examination indicate congenital hydronephrosis (Q62.0).

Chapter 22—Pathology and Laboratory Section

Practice Exercise 22.1

Professional Service: 88304 (Pathology, Surgical, Gross and Micro Exam, Level III)

ICD-10-CM: M51.26 (Displacement, intervertebral disc, lumbar region)

Rationale: Intervertebral disc is listed in the 88304 code description. This includes any intervertebral disc, whether lumbar, thoracic, sacral, or cervical. When reporting this code for payment of service, a word of caution is that 88304 does not mean level 4 pathology; it means level 3 pathology. There is no CPT code 88303. The pathologic findings are fragments of fibrocartilage, consistent with herniated disc L3-4.

When referencing the Index in the ICD-10-CM under the term "Hernia disc," the coder is directed to "*see Displacement intervertebral disc.*" Reference "Displacement" in the Index with the subterm "*intervertebral disc, lumbar*" directs the coder to M51.26.

Practice Exercise 22.2

Professional Service: 88307 (Pathology, Surgical, Gross and Micro Exam, Level V)

ICD-10-CM: N80.0 (Adenomyosis), **N83.01** (Cyst, follicular [ovarian]), **D25.1** (Leiomyoma, uterus, intramural), **N87.9** (Dysplasia, cervix)

Rationale: The specimen taken in this case was the uterus, fallopian tubes, and ovaries. Code 88305 would initially seem to be the right code because it reports the uterus, fallopian tubes, and ovaries, which is the case here. However, under uterus in the description for 88305, it states "for prolapse," which was not stated in this case. Code 88307 states uterus, with or without tubes and ovaries, other than neoplastic/prolapse, which is correct.

This patient had a total hysterectomy due to menorrhagia. The pathology report indicates more definitive diagnoses of adenomyosis (N80.0) and follicular cyst (N83.01), so the menorrhagia would not be reported. Dysplasia of the cervix is reported with N87.9. The proliferating endometrium is included in N80.0 and not reported separately. Also reported are multiple intramural leiomyomata (D25.1).

Practice Exercise 22.3

Professional Service: 88307 (Pathology, Surgical, Gross and Micro Exam, Level V)

ICD-10-CM: O41.143 (Placentitis)

Rationale: This is a pathologic examination of a third-trimester placenta. The description for 88307 states "placenta, third trimester." Third trimester is the last 3 months of a woman's pregnancy. This woman is 31 weeks pregnant. You would not report 88305 because the code description states "placenta, other than third trimester." There was one specimen, as the umbilical cord is attached to the placenta. There is only one report describing the placenta and the umbilical cord; therefore, only one unit is reported for 88307.

The diagnosis is mild early placentitis reported with ICD-10-CM code O41.1430. The 6th character indicates the third trimester. The seventh character "0" indicates single gestation and multiple gestations where the fetus is unspecified. You would not report code O45.93, which reports placental abruption, because the code description states possible abruption, and in the findings no abruption was seen. Remember, although this is an inpatient, you are reporting the professional services of the physician and you cannot report possible or rule-out diagnoses; only facility coders report possible or rule-out diagnoses.

Practice Exercise 22.4

Professional Service: 88304 (Pathology, Surgical, Gross and Micro Exam, Level III)

ICD-10-CM: M48.02 (Stenosis, spinal, cervical region)

Rationale: Listed under the code description for 88304 is intervertebral disc.

Code M48.02 reports stenosis of the cervical spine.

Practice Exercise 22.5

Professional Service: 88304 (Pathology, Surgical, Gross and Micro Exam, Level III)

ICD-10-CM: I61.9 (Hemorrhage, intracranial, intracerebral [nontraumatic])

Rationale: Listed in the code description for 88304 is hematoma; this is the only code that lists hematoma. Nowhere in the description of the code does it state cerebral hematoma. Even though this hematoma was located in the patient's brain, you would still report 88304 because the specimen was the hematoma, not brain tissue.

In the ICD-10-CM Index, referencing "Hematoma, brain, non-traumatic" indicated I61.9 and also directs the coder to "*see Hemorrhage, brain,*" which in turn lists "*see Hemorrhage, intracranial, intracerebral,*" reported with I61.9. Although intracerebral hemorrhage is not specifically stated, review of ICD-10-CM category I61 reveals terms *intracerebral* and *cerebral* can be used interchangeably.

Chapter 23—Medicine Section

Practice Exercise 23.1

Professional Service: 93458-26 (Catheterization, Cardiac, Left Heart, with Ventriculography)

ICD-10-CM: I25.110 (Arteriosclerosis, coronary [artery], native vessel, with angina pectoris, unstable)

Rationale: This patient is having a left heart catheterization (LHC) and coronary artery angiography. The placement of the catheter into the left side of the heart and the injection of contrast and the selective catheterization of the coronary arteries followed by the injection of contrast is reported with 93458. All components of the cardiac catheterization (placement, injection, imaging) are reported with 93458. Modifier -26 is added to indicate only the physician portion of this procedure is being reported.

ICD-10-CM code I25.110 reports the coronary artery disease and includes the unstable angina in one combination code.

Practice Exercise 23.2

Professional Service: 93971-26-LT (Duplex Scan, Venous Studies, Extremity)

ICD-10-CM: Z01.810 (Examination, pre-procedural, cardiovascular), **I25.811** (Arteriosclerosis, coronary [artery], native coronary artery), **R07.9** (Pain, chest)

Rationale: This patient is in need of a bypass procedure on his heart. Before this can be performed, the lower extremity veins need to be mapped to see whether they can be used as bypass grafts. You would not code 93970 because this is for a complete bilateral study and the service was a unilateral service. It states specifically in the note that only the left side was assessed, so you would use code 93971, which is for just one side. You would then add -26 to indicate that only the professional component was provided and -LT to indicate the left side.

The patient has atherosclerotic heart disease of the native coronary arteries (I25.811) and chest pain (R07.9). Z01.810 (Examination, preoperative, cardiovascular) indicates that this is a preoperative examination to assess the veins in the lower extremities before the patient's bypass procedure.

Practice Exercise 23.3

Professional Service: 93971-26 (Duplex Scan, Venous Studies, Extremity)

ICD-10-CM: M79.606 (Pain, limb, lower), **M79.89** (Swelling, leg)

Rationale: This is an ultrasound on the veins of the leg that is performed as a diagnostic test to rule out deep vein thrombosis. The procedure in this report was performed bilaterally and is reported with 93970; however, the ultrasound was a limited study, so rather than 93970, you would report 93971 because that code description indicates a unilateral or limited study. Modifier -26 is assigned to indicate that only the professional component is being reported.

Outpatient coders do not report rule out diagnoses, rather, you report the presenting symptoms, which in this case are leg pain (M79.606) and leg swelling (M79.89). Note that the ICD-10-CM code for leg pain could be more specific if the portion of the leg, such as thigh or calf, had

been documented. The ICD-10-CM code also could specify the side, left or right. Although bilateral is implied by the study of both legs, bilateral leg pain is not stated in the medical documentation. Studies are often completed on both limbs for comparison purposes.

Practice Exercise 23.4

Professional Service: 93970-26 (Duplex Scan, Venous Studies, Extremity), **76700-26** (Ultrasound, Abdomen)

ICD-10-CM: M79.89 (Swelling, leg), **R06.9** (Abnormal/abnormality/abnormalities, breathing), **R18.8** (Ascites [abdominal])

Rationale: Code 93970 reports the ultrasound of both legs that was performed to diagnose deep vein thrombosis (DVT). Modifier -26 is added to indicate that only the professional component of the service is being reported. An ultrasound of the abdomen was performed (76700) and modifier -26 is added to indicate the professional component of the service. The ultrasound included the liver, spleen, bile ducts, gallbladder, pancreas, kidneys, and abdominal aorta, which is a complete examination reported with 76700.

The diagnosis is M79.89 (swelling of the legs to rule out DVT) and R06.8 (difficulty breathing). The ascites was diagnosed and is reported with R18.8. The ICD-10-CM code for leg pain could be more specific if the portion of the leg, such as thigh or calf, had been documented, as well as the side, left or right; though bilateral is implied, it is not stated. Further, the difficulty breathing is classified as an abnormality of breathing in the Index. When referencing the Index of the ICD-10-CM under the main term "Breathing, labored," the coder is directed to "*see* Hyperventilation." You must then review the codes in the R06 range to determine the most appropriate code.

Practice Exercise 23.5

Professional Service: 90966 (Dialysis, End Stage Renal Disease)

ICD-10-CM: N18.6 (Disease, renal, end stage [ESRD]), **D63.1** (Anemia, in, end stage renal disease)

Rationale: This patient is on home peritoneal dialysis and presents for a monthly checkup. The patient's age is not stated. Usually peritoneal dialysis is performed by the patient at his/her home. The patient is over 20 years of age. The code for the office evaluation is 90966 (Dialysis, End Stage Renal Disease). Although 90945 reports a physician evaluation of a patient one time during dialysis, this would not be the correct code to report because the patient is not receiving dialysis at the time of this visit.

The patient is receiving dialysis for end-stage renal disease N18.6. Code D63.1 is also reported for the anemia in end-stage renal disease because the physician is managing this condition.

Appendix C

Medical Terminology

ablation	removal or destruction by cutting, chemicals, or electrocautery
abortion	termination of pregnancy
absence	without
actinotherapy	treatment of acne using ultraviolet rays
adenoidectomy	removal of adenoids
adipose	fatty
adrenals	glands, located at the top of the kidneys, that produce steroid hormones
albinism	lack of color pigment
allograft	homograft, same species graft
alopecia	condition in which hair falls out
amniocentesis	percutaneous aspiration of amniotic fluid
amniotic sac	sac containing the fetus and amniotic fluid
A-mode	one-dimensional ultrasonic display reflecting the time it takes a sound wave to reach a structure and reflect back; maps the structure's outline
anastomosis	surgical connection of two tubular structures, such as two pieces of the intestine
aneurysm	abnormal dilation of vessels, usually an artery
angina	sudden pain
angiography	radiography of the blood vessels
angioplasty	procedure in a vessel to dilate the vessel opening
anhidrosis	deficiency of sweat
anomaloscope	instrument used to test color vision
anoscopy	procedure that uses a scope to examine the anus
antepartum	before childbirth
anterior (ventral)	in front of
anterior segment	those parts of the eye in the front of and including the lens (cornea, iris, ciliary body, aqueous humor)
anteroposterior	from front to back
antigen	a substance that produces a specific response
aortography	radiographic recording of the aorta
apex cardiography	recording of the movement of the chest wall over the end of the heart
aphakia	absence of the lens of the eye
apicectomy	excision of a portion of the temporal bone
apnea	cessation of breathing
arthrocentesis	injection and/or aspiration of joint
arthrodesis	surgical immobilization of joint
arthrography	radiography of joint
arthroplasty	reshaping or reconstruction of joint
arthroscopy	use of scope to view inside joint
arthrotomy	incision into a joint
articular	pertains to joint
asphyxia	lack of oxygen
aspiration	use of a needle and a syringe to withdraw fluid
assignment	Medicare's payment for the service, which participating physicians agree to accept as payment in full
asthma	shortage of breath caused by contraction of bronchi
astigmatism	condition in which the refractive surfaces of the eye are unequal
atelectasis	incomplete expansion of lung, collapse

atherectomy	removal of plaque by percutaneous method
atrophy	wasting away
audiometry	hearing test
aural atresia	congenital absence of the external auditory canal
auscultation	listening to sounds within the body
autograft	from patient's own body
avulsion	ripping or tearing away of part either surgically or accidentally
axillary nodes	lymph nodes located in the armpit
bacilli	plural of bacillus, a rod-shaped bacterium
barium enema	radiographic contrast medium
beneficiary	person who benefits from health or life insurance
bifocal	two focuses in eyeglasses, one usually for close work and the other for improvement of distance vision
bilaminate skin	skin substitute usually made of silicone-covered nylon mesh
bilateral	occurring on two sides
biliary	refers to gallbladder, bile, or bile duct
bilobectomy	surgical removal of two lobes of a lung
biofeedback	process of giving a person self-information
biometry	application of a statistical measure to a biologic fact
biopsy	removal of a small piece of living tissue for diagnostic purposes
block	frozen piece of a sample
brachytherapy	therapy using radioactive sources that are placed inside the body
bronchiole	smaller division of bronchial tree
bronchography	radiographic recording of the lungs
bronchoplasty	surgical repair of the bronchi
bronchoscopy	inspection of the bronchial tree using a bronchoscope
B-scan	two-dimensional display of tissues and organs
bulbocavernosus	muscle that constricts the vagina in a female and the urethra in a male
bulbourethral	gland with duct leading to the urethra
bundle of His	muscular cardiac fibers that provide the heart rhythm to the ventricles; blockage of this rhythm produces heart block
bundled codes	one code that represents a package of services
bunion	hallux valgus, abnormal increase in size of metatarsal head that results in displacement of the great toe
burr	drill used to create an entry into the cranium
bursa	fluid-filled sac that absorbs friction
bursitis	inflammation of bursa (joint sac)
bypass	to go around
calcaneal	pertaining to the heel bone
calculus	concretion of mineral salts, also called a stone
calycoplasty	surgical reconstruction of a recess of the renal pelvis
calyx	recess of the renal pelvis
cancellous	lattice-type structure, usually of bone
cardiopulmonary	refers to the heart and lungs
cardiopulmonary bypass	blood bypasses the heart through a heart-lung machine
cardioversion	electrical shock to the heart to restore normal rhythm
carotid body	located on each side of the common carotid artery, often a site of tumor
cartilage	connective tissue
cataract	opaque covering on or in the lens
catheter	tube placed into the body to put fluid in or take fluid out
caudal	same as inferior; away from the head, or the lower part of the body
causalgia	burning pain
cauterization	destruction of tissue by the use of cautery
cavernosa	connection between the cavity of the penis and a vein
cavernosography	radiographic recording of a cavity, e.g., the pulmonary cavity or the main part of the penis
cavernosometry	measurement of the pressure in a cavity, e.g., the penis
central nervous system	brain and spinal cord

cervical	pertaining to the neck or to the cervix of the uterus
cervix uteri	rounded, cone-shaped neck of the uterus
cesarean	surgical opening through abdominal wall for delivery
cholangiography	radiographic recording of the bile ducts
cholangiopancreatography	radiographic recording of the biliary system or pancreas
cholecystectomy	surgical removal of the gallbladder
cholecystoenterostomy	creation of a connection between the gallbladder and intestine
cholecystography	radiographic recording of the gallbladder
cholesteatoma	tumor that forms in middle ear
chondral	referring to the cartilage
chordee	condition resulting in the penis being bent downward
chorionic villus sampling	CVS, biopsy of the outermost part of the placenta
circumflex	a coronary artery that circles the heart
Cloquet's node	also called a gland; it is the highest of the deep groin lymph nodes
closed fracture repair	not surgically opened with/without manipulation and with/without traction
closed treatment	fracture site that is not surgically opened and visualized
coccyx	caudal extremity of vertebral column
collagen	protein substance of skin
Colles' fracture	fracture at lower end of radius that displaces the bone posteriorly
colonoscopy	fiberscopic examination of the entire colon that may include part of the terminal ileum
colostomy	artificial opening between the colon and the abdominal wall
component	part
computed axial tomography	CAT or CT, procedure by which selected planes of tissue are pinpointed through computer enhancement, and images may be reconstructed by analysis of variance in absorption of the tissue
conjunctiva	the lining of the eyelids and the covering of anterior sclera
contraction	drawn together
contralateral	opposite side
cordectomy	surgical removal of the vocal cord(s)
cordocentesis	procedure to obtain a fetal blood sample; also called a percutaneous umbilical blood sampling
corneosclera	cornea and sclera of the eye
corpectomy	removal of vertebrae
corpora cavernosa	the two cavities of the penis
corpus uteri	uterus
crackle	abnormal sound when breathing (heard on auscultation)
craniectomy	permanent, partial removal of skull
craniotomy	opening of the skull
cranium	that part of the skeleton that encloses the brain
curettage	scraping of a cavity using a spoon-shaped instrument
curette	spoon-shaped instrument used to scrape a cavity
cutdown	incision into a vessel for placement of a catheter
cyanosis	bluish discoloration
cystocele	herniation of the bladder into the vagina
cystography	radiographic recording of the urinary bladder
cystolithectomy	removal of a calculus (stone) from the urinary bladder
cystolithotomy	cystolithectomy
cystometrogram	CMG, measurement of the pressures and capacity of the urinary bladder
cystoplasty	surgical reconstruction of the bladder
cystorrhaphy	suture of the bladder
cystoscopy	use of a scope to view the bladder
cystostomy	surgical creation of an opening into the bladder
cystotomy	incision into the bladder
cystourethroplasty	surgical reconstruction of the bladder and urethra
cystourethroscopy	use of a scope to view the bladder and urethra
dacryocystography	radiographic recording of the lacrimal sac or tear duct sac
dacryostenosis	narrowing of the lacrimal duct
debridement	cleansing of or removal of dead tissue from a wound

deductible	amount the patient is liable for before the payer begins to pay for covered services
delayed flap	pedicle of skin with blood supply that is separated from origin over time
delivery	childbirth
dermabrasion	planing of the skin by means of sander, brush, or sandpaper
dermatologist	physician who treats conditions of the skin
dermatoplasty	surgical repair of skin
dialysis	filtration of blood
dilation	expansion
discectomy	removal of a vertebral disc
discography	radiographic recording of an intervertebral joint
dislocation	placement in a location other than the original location
distal	farther from the point of attachment or origin
diverticulum	protrusion in the wall of an organ
Doppler	ultrasonic measure of blood movement
dosimetry	scientific calculation of radiation emitted from various radioactive sources
drainage	free flow or withdrawal of fluids from a wound or cavity
duodenography	radiographic recording of the duodenum or first part of the small intestine
dysphagia	difficulty swallowing
dysphonia	speech impairment
dyspnea	shortness of breath, difficult breathing
dysuria	painful urination
echocardiography	radiographic recording of the heart or heart walls or surrounding tissues
echoencephalography	ultrasound of the brain
echography	ultrasound procedure in which sound waves are bounced off an internal organ and the resulting image is recorded
ectopic	pregnancy outside the uterus (i.e., in the fallopian tube)
edema	swelling due to abnormal fluid collection in the tissue spaces
elective surgery	nonemergency procedure
electrocardiogram	ECG, written record of the electrical action of the heart
electrocautery	cauterization by means of heated instrument
electrocochleography	test to measure the eighth cranial nerve (hearing test)
electrode	lead attached to a generator that carries the electrical current from the generator to the atria or ventricles
electroencephalogram	EEG, written record of the electrical action of the brain
electromyogram	EMG, written record of the electrical activity of the skeletal muscles
electronic claim submission	claims prepared and submitted via a computer
electronic signature	identification system of a computer
electro-oculogram	EOG, written record of the electrical activity of the eye
electrophysiology	study of the electrical system of the heart, including the study of arrhythmias
embolectomy	removal of blockage (embolism) from vessel
emphysema	air accumulated in organ or tissue
encephalography	radiographic recording of the subarachnoid space and ventricles of the brain
endarterectomy	incision into an artery to remove the inner lining so as to eliminate disease or blockage
endomyocardial	pertaining to the inner and middle layers of the heart
endopyelotomy	procedure involving the bladder and ureters, including the insertion of a stent into the renal pelvis
endoscopy	inspection of body organs or cavities using a lighted scope that may be inserted through an existing opening or through a small incision
enterolysis	releasing of adhesions of intestine
enucleation	removal of an organ or organs from a body cavity
epicardial	over the heart
epidermolysis	loosening of the epidermis
epidermomycosis	superficial fungal infection
epididymectomy	surgical removal of the epididymis
epididymis	tube located at the top of the testes that stores sperm
epididymography	radiographic recording of the epididymis
epididymovasostomy	creation of a new connection between the vas deferens and epididymis

epiglottidectomy	excision of the covering of the larynx
episclera	connective covering of the sclera
epistaxis	nosebleed
epithelium	surface covering of internal and external organs of the body
erythema	redness of skin
escharotomy	surgical incision into necrotic (dead) tissue
eventration	protrusion of the bowel through an opening in the abdomen
evisceration	pulling the viscera outside of the body through an incision
evocative	tests that are administered to evoke a predetermined response
exenteration	removal of an organ all in one piece
exophthalmos	protrusion of the eyeball
exostosis	bony growth
exstrophy	condition in which an organ is turned inside out
extracorporeal	occurring outside of the body
false aneurysm	sac of clotted blood that has completely destroyed the vessel and is being contained by the tissue that surrounds the vessel
fasciectomy	removal of a band of fibrous tissue
Federal Register	official publication of all "Presidential Documents," "Rules and Regulations," "Proposed Rules," and "Notices"; government-instituted national changes are published in the *Federal Register*
fee schedule	services and payment allowed for each service
femoral	pertaining to the bone from the pelvis to knee
fenestration	creation of a new opening in the inner wall of the middle ear
fissure	cleft or groove
fistula	abnormal opening from one area to another area or to the outside of the body
fluoroscopy	procedure for viewing the interior of the body using x-rays and projecting the image onto a television screen
fracture	break in a bone
free full-thickness graft	graft of epidermis and dermis that is completely removed from donor area
fulguration	use of electrical current to destroy tissue
fundoplasty	repair of the bottom of the bladder
furuncle	nodule in the skin caused by *Staphylococci* entering through hair follicle
ganglion	knot
gastrointestinal	pertaining to the stomach and intestine
gastroplasty	operation on the stomach for repair or reconfiguration
gastrostomy	artificial opening between the stomach and the abdominal wall
gatekeeper	a physician who manages a patient's access to health care
glaucoma	eye diseases that are characterized by an increase of intraocular pressure
globe	eyeball
glottis	true vocal cords
gonioscopy	use of a scope to examine the angles of the eye
Group Practice Model	an organization of physicians who contract with a Health Maintenance Organization to provide services to the enrollees of the HMO
grouper	computer used to input the principal diagnosis and other critical information about a patient and then provide the correct DRG code
Health Maintenance Organization	HMO, a health care delivery system in which an enrollee is assigned a primary care physician who manages all the health care needs of the enrollee
hematoma	mass of blood that forms outside the vessel
hemodialysis	cleansing of the blood outside of the body
hemolysis	breakdown of red blood cells
hemoptysis	bloody sputum
hepatography	radiographic recording of the liver
hernia	organ or tissue protruding through the wall or cavity that usually contains it
histology	study of structure of tissue and cells
homograft	allograft, same species graft
hormone	chemical substance produced by the body's endocrine glands
hydrocele	sac of fluid
hyperopia	farsightedness; eyeball is too short from front to back

hypogastric	lowest middle abdominal area
hyposensitization	decreased sensitivity
hypothermia	low body temperature; sometimes induced during surgical procedures
hypoxemia	low level of oxygen in the blood
hypoxia	low level of oxygen in the tissue
hysterectomy	surgical removal of the uterus
hysterorrhaphy	suturing of the uterus
hysterosalpingography	radiographic recording of the uterine cavity and fallopian tubes
hysteroscopy	visualization of the canal and cavity of the uterus using a scope placed through the vagina
ichthyosis	skin disorder characterized by scaling
ileostomy	artificial opening between the ileum and the abdominal wall
ilium	portion of hip
imbrication	overlapping
immunotherapy	therapy to increase immunity
implantable defibrillator	surgically placed device that directs an electrical shock to the heart to restore rhythm
incarcerated	regarding hernias, a constricted, irreducible hernia that may cause obstruction of an intestine
incise	to cut into
Individual Practice Association	IPA, an organization of physicians who provide services for a set fee; Health Maintenance Organizations often contract with the IPA for services to their enrollees
inferior	away from the head or the lower part of the body; also known as caudalingual
inguinofemoral	referring to the groin and thigh
inofemoral	referring to the groin and thigh
internal/external fixation	application of pins, wires, and/or screws placed externally or internally to immobilize a body part
intracardiac	inside the heart
intramural	within the organ wall
intramuscular	into a muscle
intrauterine	inside the uterus
intravenous	into a vein
intravenous pyelography	IVP, radiographic recording of the urinary system
introitus	opening or entrance to the vagina from the uterus
intubation	insertion of a tube
intussusception	slipping of one part of the intestine into another part
invasive	entering the body, breaking skin
iontophoresis	introduction of ions into the body
ischemia	deficient blood supply due to obstruction of the circulatory system
island pedicle flap	contains a single artery and vein that remain attached to origin temporarily or permanently
isthmus	connection of two regions or structures
isthmus, thyroid	tissue connection between right and left thyroid lobes
isthmusectomy	surgical removal of the isthmus
jaundice	a condition in which excessive bilirubin causes the skin and whites of the eyes to appear yellowish
jejunostomy	artificial opening between the jejunum and the abdominal wall
joint	the place at which two bones attach
jugular nodes	lymph nodes located next to the large vein in the neck
keloid	a fibrous growth that forms at the site of a scar
keratomalacia	softening of the cornea associated with a deficiency of vitamin A
keratoplasty	surgical repair of the cornea
ketones	compounds that are carbon-based by-products of fatty acid metabolism; excess ketone bodies in urine may indicate diabetes mellitus
kidney	organs that filter blood and balance the levels of water, salt, and minerals in the blood
kidney stones	formations of minerals and salt that may form in the urine
Kock pouch	surgical creation of a urinary bladder from a segment of the ileum
kyphosis	humpback
labyrinth	inner connecting cavities, such as the internal ear
labyrinthitis	inner ear inflammation
lacrimal	related to tears
lamina	flat plate

laminectomy	surgical excision of the lamina
laparoscopy	exploration of the abdomen and pelvic cavities using a scope placed through a small incision in the abdominal wall
laryngeal web	congenital abnormality of connective tissue between the vocal cords
laryngectomy	surgical removal of the larynx
laryngography	radiographic recording of the larynx
laryngoplasty	surgical repair of the larynx
laryngoscope	fiberoptic scope used to view the inside of the larynx
laryngoscopy	direct visualization and examination of the interior of larynx with a laryngoscope
laryngotomy	incision into the larynx
lateral	away from the midline of the body (to the side)
lavage	washing out
leukoderma	depigmentation of skin
leukoplakia	white patch on mucous membrane
ligament	fibrous band of tissue that connects cartilage or bone
ligation	binding or tying off, as in constricting the blood flow of a vessel or binding fallopian tubes for sterilization
lipocyte	fat cell
lipoma	fatty tumor
lithotomy	incision into an organ or a duct for the purpose of removing a stone
lithotripsy	crushing of a stone by sound waves or force
lobectomy	surgical excision of lobe of the lung
lordosis	anterior curve of spine
lumbodynia	pain in the lumbar area
lunate	one of the wrist (carpal) bones
lymph node	station along the lymphatic system
lymphadenectomy	excision of a lymph node or nodes
lymphadenitis	inflammation of a lymph node
lymphangiography	radiographic recording of the lymphatic vessels and nodes
lymphangiotomy	incision into a lymphatic vessel
lysis	releasing
magnetic resonance imaging	MRI, procedure that uses nonionizing radiation to view the body in a cross-sectional view
Major Diagnostic Categories	MDC, the division of all principal diagnoses into 25 mutually exclusive principal diagnosis areas within the DRG system
mammography	radiographic recording of the breasts
Managed Care Organization	MCO, a group that is responsible for the health care services offered to an enrolled group of persons
manipulation	movement by hand
manipulation or reduction	alignment of a fracture or joint dislocation to its normal position
mastoidectomy	removal of the mastoid bone
Maximum Actual Allowable Charge	MAAC, limitation on the total amount that can be charged by physicians who are not participants in Medicare
meatotomy	surgical enlargement of the opening of the urinary meatus
medial	toward the midline of the body
Medical Volume Performance Standards	MVPS, government's estimate of how much growth is appropriate for nationwide physician expenditures paid by the Part B Medicare program
Medicare Economic Index	MEI, government mandated index that ties increases in the Medicare prevailing charges to economic indicators
Medicare Fee Schedule	MFS, schedule that listed the allowable charges for Medicare services; was replaced by the Medicare reasonable charge payment system
Medicare Risk HMO	a Medicare-funded alternative to the standard Medicare supplemental coverage
melanin	dark pigment of skin
melanoma	tumor of epidermis, malignant and black in color
Ménière's disease	condition that causes dizziness, ringing in the ears, and deafness
M-mode	one-dimensional display of movement of structures
modality	treatment method

Mohs surgery or Mohs micrographic surgery	removal of skin cancer in layers by a surgeon who also acts as pathologist during surgery
monofocal	eyeglasses with one vision correction
multipara	more than one pregnancy
muscle	organ of contraction for movement
muscle flap	transfer of muscle from origin to recipient site
myasthenia gravis	syndrome characterized by muscle weakness
myelography	radiographic recording of the subarachnoid space of the spine
myopia	nearsightedness; eyeball too long from front to back
myringotomy	incision into tympanic membrane
nasal button	synthetic circular disk used to cover a hole in the nasal septum
nasopharyngoscopy	use of a scope to visualize the nose and pharynx
National Provider Identifier	NPI, a 10-digit number assigned to a physician by Medicare
nephrectomy, paraperitoneal	kidney transplant
nephrocutaneous fistula	a channel from the kidney to the skin
nephrolithotomy	removal of a kidney stone through an incision made into the kidney
nephrorrhaphy	suturing of the kidney
nephrostolithotomy	creation of an artificial channel to the kidney
nephrostolithotomy, percutaneous	procedure to establish an artificial channel between the skin and the kidney
nephrostomy	creation of a channel into the renal pelvis of the kidney
nephrostomy, percutaneous	creation of a channel from the skin to the renal pelvis
nephrotomy	incision into the kidney
neurovascular flap	contains artery, vein, and nerve
noninvasive	not entering the body, not breaking skin
nuclear cardiology	diagnostic specialty that uses radiologic procedures to aid in diagnosis of cardiologic conditions
nystagmus	rapid involuntary eye movements
ocular adnexa	orbit, extraocular muscles, and eyelid
olecranon	elbow bone
Omnibus Budget Reconciliation Act of 1989	OBRA, act that established new rules for Medicare reimbursement
oophorectomy	surgical removal of the ovary(ies)
opacification	area that has become opaque (milky)
open fracture repair	surgical opening (incision) over or remote opening as access to a fracture site
open treatment	fracture site that is surgically opened and visualized
ophthalmodynamometry	test of the blood pressure of the eye
ophthalmology	body of knowledge regarding the eyes
ophthalmoscopy	examination of the interior of the eye by means of a scope, also known as fundoscopy
optokinetic	movement of the eyes to objects moving in the visual field
orchiectomy	castration; removal of the testes
orchiopexy	surgical procedure to release undescended testes and fixate them within the scrotum
order	shows subordination of one thing to another; family or class
orthopnea	difficulty in breathing, needing to be in erect position to breathe
orthoptic	corrective; in the correct place
osteoarthritis	degenerative condition of articular cartilage
osteoclast	absorbs or removes bone
osteotomy	cutting into bone
otitis media	noninfectious inflammation of the middle ear; serous otitis media produces liquid drainage (not purulent) and suppurative otitis media produces purulent (pus) matter
otoscope	instrument used to examine the internal and external ear
oviduct	fallopian tube
papilledema	swelling of the optic disc (papilla)
paraesophageal hiatal hernia	hernia that is near the esophagus
parathyroid	produces a hormone to mobilize calcium from the bones to the blood

paronychia	infection around nail
Part A	Medicare's Hospital Insurance; covers hospital/facility care
Part B	Medicare's Supplemental Medical Insurance; covers physician services and durable medical equipment that are not paid for under Part A
participating provider program	Medicare providers who have agreed in advance to accept assignment on all Medicare claims, now termed Quality Improvement Organizations (QIO)
patella	knee cap
pedicle	growth attached with a stem
Peer Review Organizations	PROs, groups established to review hospital admission and care
pelviolithotomy	pyeloplasty
penoscrotal	referring to the penis and scrotum
percussion	tapping with sharp blows as a diagnostic technique
percutaneous	through the skin
percutaneous fracture repair	repair of a fracture by means of pins and wires inserted through the fracture site
percutaneous skeletal fixation	considered neither open nor closed; the fracture is not visualized, but fixation is placed across the fracture site under x-ray imaging
pericardiocentesis	procedure in which a surgeon withdraws fluid from the pericardial space by means of a needle inserted percutaneously
pericardium	membranous sac enclosing heart and ends of great vessels
perineum	area between the vulva and anus; also known as the pelvic floor
peripheral nerves	12 pairs of cranial nerves, 31 pairs of spinal nerves, and autonomic nervous system; connects peripheral receptors to the brain and spinal cord
peritoneal	within the lining of the abdominal cavity
peritoneoscopy	visualization of the abdominal cavity using one scope placed through a small incision in the abdominal wall and another scope placed in the vagina
pharyngolaryngectomy	surgical removal of the pharynx and larynx
phlebotomy	cutting into a vein
phonocardiogram	recording of heart sounds
photochemotherapy	treatment by means of drugs that react to ultraviolet radiation or sunlight
physics	scientific study of energy
pilosebaceous	pertains to hair follicles and sebaceous glands
placenta	a structure that connects the fetus and mother during pregnancy
plethysmography	determining the changes in volume of an organ part or body
pleura	covers the lungs and lines the thoracic cavity
pleurectomy	surgical excision of the pleura
pleuritis	inflammation of the pleura
pneumonocentesis	surgical puncturing of a lung to withdraw fluid
pneumonolysis	surgical separation of the lung from the chest wall to allow the lung to collapse
pneumonostomy	surgical procedure in which the chest cavity is exposed and the lung is incised
pneumonotomy	incision of the lung
pneumoplethysmography	determining the changes in the volume of the lung
posterior (dorsal)	in back of
posterior segment	those parts of the eye behind the lens
posteroanterior	from back to front
postpartum	after childbirth
Preferred Provider Organization	PPO, a group of providers who form a network and who have agreed to provide services to enrollees at a discounted rate
priapism	painful condition in which the penis is constantly erect
primary care physician	PCP, physician who oversees a patient's care within a managed care organization
primary diagnosis	chief complaint of a patient in outpatient setting
primipara	first pregnancy
prior approval	also known as a prior authorization, the payer's approval of care
proctosigmoidoscopy	fiberscopic examination of the sigmoid colon and rectum
Professional Standards Review Organization	PSRO, voluntary physicians' organization designed to monitor the necessity of hospital admissions, treatment costs, and medical records of hospitals
prognosis	probable outcome of an illness

prostatotomy	incision into the prostate
Provider Identification Number	PIN, assigned to physicians by payers for use in claims submission
pyelography	radiographic recording of the kidneys, renal pelvis, ureters, and bladder
qualitative	measuring the presence or absence of
Quality Improvement Organizations	QIO, consists of a national network of 53 entities that work with consumers, physicians, hospitals, and caregivers to refine care delivery systems
quantitative	measuring the presence or absence of and the amount of
rad	radiation-absorbed dose, the energy deposited in patient's tissues
radiation oncology	branch of medicine concerned with the application of radiation to a tumor site for treatment (destruction) of cancerous tumors
radiograph	film on which an image is produced through exposure to x-radiation
radiologist	physician who specializes in the use of radioactive materials in the diagnosis and treatment of disease and illness
radiology	branch of medicine concerned with the use of radioactive substances for diagnosis and therapy
rales	coarse sounds on inspiration, also known as crackles (heard on auscultation)
real time	two-dimensional display of both the structures and the motion of tissues and organs, with the length of time also recorded as part of the study
reduction	replacement to normal position
Relative Value Unit	RVU, unit value that has been assigned for each service
Resource-Based Relative Value Scale	RBRVS, scale designed to decrease Medicare expenditures, redistribute physician payment, and ensure quality health care at reasonable rates
resource intensity	refers to the relative volume and type of diagnostic, therapeutic, and bed services used in the management of a particular illness
retrograde	moving backward or against the usual direction of flow
rhinoplasty	surgical repair of nose
rhinorrhea	nasal mucous discharge
salpingectomy	surgical removal of the uterine tube
salpingostomy	creation of a fistula into the uterine tube
scan	mapping of emissions of radioactive substances after they have been introduced into the body; the density can determine normal or abnormal conditions
sclera	outer covering of the eye
scoliosis	lateral curve of the spine
sebaceous gland	secretes sebum
seborrhea	excess sebum secretion
sebum	oily substance
section	slice of a frozen block
segmentectomy	surgical removal of a portion of a lung
septoplasty	surgical repair of the nasal septum
serum	blood from which the fibrinogen has been removed
severity of illness	refers to the levels of loss of function and mortality that may be experienced by patients with a particular disease
shunt	an artificial passage
sialography	radiographic recording of the salivary duct and branches
sialolithotomy	surgical removal of a stone of the salivary gland or duct
sinography	radiographic recording of the sinus or sinus tract
sinusotomy	surgical incision into a sinus
skeletal traction	application of pressure to the bone by means of pins and/or wires inserted into the bone
skin traction	application of pressure to the bone by means of tape applied to the skin
skull	entire skeletal framework of the head
somatic nerve	sensory or motor nerve
specimen	sample of tissue or fluid
spirometry	measurement of breathing capacity
splenectomy	excision of the spleen
splenography	radiographic recording of the spleen
splenoportography	radiographic procedure to allow visualization of the splenic and portal veins of the spleen
split-thickness graft	all epidermis and some of dermis

spondylitis	inflammation of vertebrae
Staff Model	a Health Maintenance Organization that directly employs the physicians who provide services to enrollees
steatoma	fat mass in sebaceous gland
stem cell	immature blood cell
stereotaxis	method of identifying a specific area or point in the brain
strabismus	extraocular muscle deviation resulting in unequal visual axes
stratified	layered
stratum (strata)	layer
subcutaneous	tissue below the dermis, primarily fat cells that insulate the body
subluxation	partial dislocation
subungual	beneath the nail
superior	toward the head or the upper part of the body; also known as cephalic
supination	supine position
supine	lying on the back
Swan-Ganz catheter	a catheter that measures pressure in the heart
sympathetic nerve	part of the peripheral nervous system that controls automatic body function and nerves activated under stress
symphysis	natural junction
synchondrosis	union between two bones (connected by cartilage)
tachypnea	quick, shallow breathing
tarsorrhaphy	suturing together of the eyelids
Tax Equity and Fiscal Responsibility Act	TEFRA, act that contains language to reward cost-conscious health care providers
tendon	attaches a muscle to a bone
tenodesis	suturing of a tendon to a bone
tenorrhaphy	suture repair of tendon
thermogram	written record of temperature variation
third-party payer	insurance company or entity that is liable for another's health care services
thoracentesis	surgical puncture of the thoracic cavity, usually using a needle, to remove fluids
thoracic duct	collection and distribution point for lymph, and the largest lymph vessel located in the chest
thoracoplasty	surgical procedure that removes rib(s) and thereby allows the collapse of a lung
thoracoscopy	use of a lighted endoscope to view the pleural spaces and thoracic cavity or to perform surgical procedures
thoracostomy	incision into the chest wall and insertion of a chest tube
thoracotomy	surgical incision into the chest wall
thromboendarterectomy	procedure to remove plaque or clot formations from a vessel by percutaneous method
thymectomy	surgical removal of the thymus
thymus	gland that produces hormones important to the immune response
thyroglossal duct	connection between the thyroid and the tongue
thyroid	part of the endocrine system that produces hormones that regulate metabolism
thyroidectomy	surgical removal of the thyroid
tinnitus	ringing in the ears
titer	measure of a laboratory analysis
tocolysis	repression of uterine contractions
tomography	procedure that allows viewing of a single plane of the body by blurring out all but that particular level
tonography	recording of changes in intraocular pressure in response to sustained pressure on the eyeball
tonometry	measurement of pressure or tension
total pneumonectomy	surgical removal of an entire lung
tracheostomy	creation of an opening into trachea
tracheotomy	incision into trachea
traction	application of pressure to maintain normal alignment
transcutaneous	entering by way of the skin
transesophageal echocardiogram	TEE, echocardiogram performed by placing a probe down the esophagus and sending out sound waves to obtain images of the heart and its movement
transmastoid	creates an opening in the mastoid for drainage antrostomy

transplantation	grafting of tissue from one source to another
transseptal	through the septum
transtracheal	across the trachea
transureteroureterostomy	surgical connection of one ureter to the other ureter
transurethral resection of prostate	TURP, procedure performed through the urethra by means of a cystoscopy to remove part or all of the prostate
transvenous	through a vein
transvesical ureterolithotomy	removal of a ureter stone (calculus) through the bladder
trephination	surgical removal of a disc of bone
trocar needle	needle with a tube on the end; used to puncture and withdraw fluid from a cavity
tubercle	lesion caused by infection of tuberculosis
tumescence	state of being swollen
tunica vaginalis	covering of the testes
tympanolysis	freeing of adhesions of the tympanic membrane
tympanometry	test of the inner ear using air pressure
tympanostomy	insertion of ventilation tube into tympanum
ultrasound	technique using sound waves to determine the density of the outline of tissue
unbundling	reporting with multiple codes that can be reported with one code
unilateral	occurring on one side
uptake	absorption of a radioactive substance by body tissues; recorded for diagnostic purposes in conditions such as thyroid disease
ureterectomy	surgical removal of a ureter, either totally or partially
ureterocolon	pertaining to the ureter and colon
ureterocutaneous fistula	channel from the ureter to exterior skin
ureteroenterostomy	creation of a connection between the intestine and the ureter
ureterolithotomy	removal of a stone from the ureter
ureterolysis	freeing of adhesions of the ureter
ureteroneocystostomy	surgical connection of the ureter to a new site on the bladder
ureteropyelography	ureter and bladder radiography
ureterotomy	incision into the ureter
urethrocystography	radiography of the bladder and urethra
urethromeatoplasty	surgical repair of the urethra and meatus
urethropexy	fixation of the urethra by means of surgery
urethroplasty	surgical repair of the urethra
urethrorrhaphy	suturing of the urethra
urethroscopy	use of a scope to view the urethra
urography	same as pyelography; radiographic recording of the kidneys, renal pelvis, ureters, and bladder
uveal	vascular tissue of the choroid, ciliary body, and iris
varices	varicose veins
varicocele	swelling of a scrotal vein
vas deferens	tube that carries sperm from the epididymis to the urethra
vasectomy	removal of segment of vas deferens
vasogram	recording of the flow in the vas deferens
vasotomy	incision in the vas deferens
vasorrhaphy	suturing of the vas deferens
vasovasostomy	reversal of a vasectomy
vectorcardiogram	VCG, continuous recording of electrical direction and magnitude of the heart
venography	radiographic recording of the veins and tributaries
vertebrectomy	removal of vertebra
vertigo	dizziness
vesicostomy	surgical creation of a connection of the viscera of the bladder to the skin
vesicovaginal fistula	creation of a tube between the vagina and the bladder
vesiculectomy	excision of the seminal vesicle
vesiculography	radiographic recording of the seminal vesicles
vesiculotomy	incision into the seminal vesicle
viscera	an organ in one of the large cavities of the body

volvulus	twisted section of the intestine
vomer	flat bones of the nasal septum
xanthoma	tumor composed of cells containing lipid material, yellow in color
xenograft	different species graft
xeroderma	dry, discolored, scaly skin
xeroradiography	photoelectric process of radiographs

Appendix D

Combining Forms

abdomin/o	abdomen	celi/o	abdomen
acetabul/o	hip socket	cephal/o	head
acr/o	height/extremities	cerebell/o	cerebellum
aden/o	in relationship to a gland	cerebr/o	cerebrum
adenoid/o	adenoids	cervic/o	neck/cervix
adip/o	fat	chol/e	gall/bile
adren/o, adrenal/o	adrenal gland	cholangio/o	bile duct
albin/o	white	cholecyst/o	gallbladder
albumin/o	albumin	choledoch/o	common bile duct
alveol/o	alveolus	cholester/o	cholesterol
ambly/o	dim	chondr/o	cartilage
amni/o	amnion	chori/o	chorion
an/o	anus	clavic/o, clavicul/o	clavicle (collar bone)
andr/o	male	col/o	colon
andren/o	adrenal gland	colp/o	vagina
andrenal/o	adrenal gland	coni/o	dust
angi/o	vessel	conjunctiv/o	conjunctiva
ankyl/o	bent, fused	cor/o, core/o	pupil
aort/o	aorta	corne/o	cornea
aponeur/o	tendon type	coron/o	heart
appendic/o	appendix	cortic/o	cortex
aque/o	water	cost/o	rib
arche/o	first	crani/o	cranium (skull)
arter/o, arteri/o	artery	crin/o	secrete
arthr/o	joint	crypt/o	hidden
atel/o	incomplete	culd/o	cul-de-sac
ather/o	plaque	cutane/o	skin
atri/o	atrium	cyan/o	blue
audi/o	hearing	cycl/o	ciliary body
aut/o	self	cyst/o	bladder
axill/o	armpit	dacry/o	tear
azot/o	urea	dacryocyst/o	pertaining to the lacrimal sac
balan/o	glans penis	dent/i	tooth
bi/o	life	derm/o, dermat/o	skin
bil/i	bile	diaphragmat/o	diaphragm
bilirubin/o	bile pigment	dips/o	thirst
blephar/o	eyelid	disc/o	intervertebral disc
brachi/o	arm	diverticul/o	diverticulum
bronch/o	bronchus	duoden/o	duodenum
bronchi/o	bronchus	dur/o	dura mater
bronchiol/o	bronchiole	encephal/o	brain
burs/o	fluid-filled sac in a joint	enter/o	small intestine
calc/o, calc/i	calcium	eosin/o	rosy
cardi/o	heart	epididym/o	epididymis
carp/o	carpals (wrist bones)	epiglott/o	epiglottis
cauter/o	burn	episi/o	vulva
cec/o	cecum	erythr/o, erythem/o	red

esophag/o	esophagus	mamm/o	breast
essi/o, esthesi/o	sensation	mandibul/o	mandible (lower jawbone)
estr/o	female	mast/o	breast
femor/o	thighbone	maxill/o	maxilla (upper jawbone)
fet/o	fetus	meat/o	meatus
fibul/o	fibula	melan/o	black
galact/o	milk	men/o	menstruation, month
gangli/o	ganglion	mening/o, meningi/o	meninges
ganglion/o	ganglion	menisc/o, menisci/o	meniscus
gastr/o	stomach	ment/o	mind
gingiv/o	gum	metacarp/o	metacarpals (hand)
glomerul/o	glomerulus	metatars/o	metatarsals (foot)
gloss/o	tongue	metr/o	uterus, measure
gluc/o	sugar	metr/i	uterus
glyc/o	sugar	mon/o	one
glycos/o	sugar	muc/o	mucus
gonad/o	ovaries and testes	my/o, muscul/o	muscle
gyn/o	female	myc/o	fungus
gynec/o	female	myel/o	bone marrow, spinal cord
hepat/o	liver	myring/o	ear drum
herni/o	hernia	myx/o	mucus
heter/o	different	nas/o	nose
hidr/o	sweat	nat/a, nat/i	birth
home/o	same	natr/o	sodium
hormon/o	hormone	necr/o	death
humer/o	humerus (upper arm bone)	nephr/o	kidney
hydr/o	water	neur/o	nerve
hymen/o	hymen	noct/i	night
hyster/o	uterus	ocul/o	eye
ichthy/o	dry/scaly	olecran/o	olecranon (elbow)
ile/o	ileus	olig/o	scant, few
ili/o	ilium (upper pelvic bone)	onych/o	nail
immun/o	immune	oo/o	egg
inguin/o	groin	oophor/o	ovary
ir/o	iris	ophthalm/o	eye
irid/o	iris	opt/o	eye, vision
ischi/o	ischium (posterior pelvic bone)	optic/o	eye
jaund/o	yellow	or/o	mouth
jejun/o	jejunum	orch/i, orch/o, orchi/o, orchid/o	testicle
kal/i	potassium		
kerat/o	hard, cornea	orth/o	straight
kinesi/o	movement	oste/o	bone
kyph/o	hump	ot/o	ear
lacrim/o	tear	ov/o	egg
lact/o	milk	ovari/o	ovary
lamin/o	lamina	ovul/o	ovulation
lapar/o	abdomen	ox/i, ox/o	oxygen
laryng/o	larynx	oxy/o	oxygen
lingu/o	tongue	pachy/o	thick
lip/o	fat	palat/o	palate
lith/o	stone	palpebr/o	eyelid
lob/o	lobe	pancreat/o	pancreas
lord/o	curve	papill/o	optic nerve
lumb/o	lower back	patell/o	patella (kneecap)
lute/o	yellow	pelv/i	pelvis (hip)
lymph/o	lymph	pericardi/o	pericardium
lymphaden/o	lymph gland	perine/o	perineum

peritone/o	peritoneum	sperm/o, spermat/o	sperm
petr/o	stone	sphygm/o	pulse
phac/o	eye lens	spir/o	breath
phak/o	eye lens	splen/o	spleen
phalang/o	phalanges (finger or toe)	spondyl/o	vertebra
pharyng/o	pharynx	staped/o	middle ear, stapes
phas/o	speech	staphyl/o	clusters
phleb/o	vein	steat/o	fat
phren/o	mind, diaphragm	ster/o, stere/o	solid, having three dimensions
phys/o	growing	stern/o	sternum (breast bone)
pil/o	hair	steth/o	chest
pituitar/o	pituitary gland	stomat/o	mouth
pleur/o	pleura	strept/o	twisted chain
pneumat/o	lung/air	synovi/o	synovial joint membrane
pneumon/o	lung/air	tars/o	tarsal (ankle)
poli/o	gray matter	ten/o	tendon
polyp/o	polyp	tend/o, tendin/o	tendon (connective tissue)
pont/o	pons	test/o	testicle
proct/o	rectum	thorac/o	thorax
prostat/o	prostate gland	thromb/o	clot
psych/o	mind	thym/o	thymus gland
pub/o	pubis	thyr/o, thyroid/o	thyroid gland
pulmon/o	lung	tibi/o	shin bone
pupill/o	pupil	toc/o	childbirth
py/o	pus	tonsill/o	tonsil
pyel/o	renal pelvis	top/o	place
pylor/o	pylorus	tox/o, toxic/o	poison
quadr/i	four	trache/o	trachea
rachi/o	spine	trich/o	hair
radi/o	radius (lower arm)	tympan/o	eardrum
radic/o, radicul/o	nerve root	uln/o	ulna (lower arm bone)
rect/o	rectum	ungu/o	nail
ren/o	kidney	ur/o	urine
retin/o	retina	ureter/o	ureter
rhin/o	nose	urethr/o	urethra
rhiz/o	nerve root	urin/o	urine
rhytid/o	wrinkle	uter/o	uterus
rube/o	red	uve/o	uvea
sacr/o	sacrum	uvul/o	uvula
salping/o	uterine tube, fallopian tube	vagin/o	vagina
scapul/o	scapula (shoulder)	valv/o, valvul/o	valve
scler/o	sclera	vas/o, vascul/o	vessel
scoli/o	bent	ven/o	vein
seb/o	sebum/oil	ventricul/o	ventricle
semin/i	semen	vertebr/o	vertebra
sept/o	septum	vesic/o	bladder
sial/o	saliva	vesicul/o	seminal vesicles
sigmoid/o	sigmoid colon	vitre/o	glass/glassy
sinus/o	sinus	vulv/o	vulva
somat/o	body	xanth/o	yellow
son/o	sound	xer/o	dry

Appendix E

Prefixes

a-	not	neo-	new
an-	not	nulli-, nulti-	none
ante-	before	oxy-	sharp, oxygen
audi-	hearing	pan-	all
bi-	two	para-	beside
brady-	slow	per-	through
de-	lack of	peri-	surrounding
dys-	difficult, painful	poly-	many
ecto-	outside	post-	after
endo-	in	primi-	first
epi-	on/upon	pseudo-	false
eso-	inward	quadri-	four
eu-	good/normal	retro-	behind
exo-	outward	sub-	under
extra-	outside	supra-	above
hemi-	half	sym-	together
hyper-	excess, over	syn-	together
hypo-	under	tachy-	fast
in-	into	tetra-	four
inter-	between	tri-	three
intra-	within	tropin-	act upon
meta-	change, after	uni-	one
multi-	many		

Appendix F

Suffixes

-agon	assemble
-algesia	pain sensation
-algia	pain
-ar	pertaining to
-arche	beginning
-ary	pertaining to
-asthenia	weakness
-blast	embryonic
-capnia	carbon dioxide
-cele	hernia
-centesis	puncture to remove (drain)
-chezia	defecation
-clast, -clasia, -clasis	break
-coccus	spherical bacterium
-cyesis	pregnancy
-desis	fusion
-dilation	widening, expanding
-drome	run
-dynia	pain
-eal	pertaining to
-ectasis	stretching
-ectomy	removal
-edema	swelling
-emia	blood
-esthesis	feeling
-gram	record
-graph	recording instrument
-graphy	recording process
-gravida	pregnancy
-ia	condition
-iatrist	physician specialist
-iatry	medical treatment
-ical	pertaining to
-ictal	pertaining to
-in	a substance
-ine	a substance
-itis	inflammation
-listhesis	slipping
-lithiasis	condition of stones
-lysis	separation
-malacia	softening
-megaly	enlargement
-meta	change
-meter	measurement; instrument that measures
-metry	measurement of
-oid	resembling
-oma	tumor
-omia	smell
-one	hormone
-opia	vision
-opsy	view of
-orrhexis	rupture
-osis	condition
-oxia	oxygen
-para	woman who has given birth
-paresis	incomplete paralysis
-parous	to bear
-penia	deficient
-pexy	fixation
-phagia	eating
-phonia	sound
-phylaxis	protection
-physis	to grow
-plasty	repair
-plegia	paralysis
-pnea	breathing
-poiesis	production
-poly	many
-porosis	passage
-retro	behind
-rrhagia	bursting of blood
-rrhaphy	suture
-rrhea	discharge
-schisis	split
-sclerosis	hardening
-scopy	to examine
-spasm	contraction of muscle
-steat/o	fat
-stenosis	blockage, narrowing
-stomy	opening
-thorax	chest
-tocia	labor
-tom/o	to cut
-tome	an instrument that cuts
-tomy	cutting, incision
-tripsy	crush
-tropia	to turn
-tropin	act upon
-uria	urine
-version	turning

Appendix G

Abbreviations

ABG	arterial blood gas
ABN	Advanced Beneficiary Notice; used by CMS to notify beneficiary of payment of provider services
ACL	anterior cruciate ligament
AD	right ear
AFB	acid-fast bacillus
AFI	amniotic fluid index
AGA	appropriate for gestational age
AGCUS	atypical glandular cells of undetermined significance
AKA	above-knee amputation
ANS	autonomic nervous system
APCs	Ambulatory Payment Classifications, patient classification that provides a payment system for outpatients
ARDS	adult respiratory distress syndrome
ARF	acute renal failure
ARM	artificial rupture of membrane
AS	left ear
ASCUS	atypical squamous cells of undetermined significance
ASCVD	arteriosclerotic cardiovascular disease
ASD	atrial septal defect
ASHD	arteriosclerotic heart disease
AU	both ears
AV	atrioventricular
BCC	benign cellular changes
BiPAP	bi-level positive airway pressure
BKA	below-knee amputation
BP	blood pressure
BPD	biparietal diameter
BPH	benign prostatic hypertrophy
BPP	biophysical profile
BUN	blood urea nitrogen
BV	bacterial vaginosis
bx	biopsy
C1-C7	cervical vertebrae
ca	cancer
CABG	coronary artery bypass graft
CBC	complete blood (cell) count
CF	conversion factor, national dollar amount that is applied to all services paid on the Medicare Fee Schedule basis
CHF	congestive heart failure
CHL	crown-to-heel length
CK	creatine kinase
CMS	Centers for Medicare and Medicaid Services, formerly HCFA, Health Care Financing Administration
CNM	certified nurse midwife
CNS	central nervous system
COB	coordination of benefits, management of payment between two or more third-party payers for a service
COPD	chronic obstructive pulmonary disease
CPAP	continuous positive airway pressure
CPD	cephalopelvic disproportion
CPK	creatine phosphokinase
CPP	chronic pelvic pain
CSF	cerebrospinal fluid
CTS	carpal tunnel syndrome
CVA	cerebrovascular accident, stroke
CVI	cerebrovascular insufficiency
D&C	dilation and curettage
D&E	dilation and evacuation
derm	dermatology
DHHS	Department of Health and Human Services
DLCO	diffuse capacity of lungs for carbon monoxide
DRGs	Diagnosis Related Groups, disease classification system that relates the types of inpatients a hospital treats (case mix) to the costs incurred by the hospital
DSE	dobutamine stress echocardiography
DUB	dysfunctional uterine bleeding
ECC	endocervical curettage
EDC	estimated date of confinement
EDD	estimated date of delivery
EDI	electronic data interchange, exchange of data between multiple computer terminals
EEG	electroencephalogram
EFM	electronic fetal monitoring
EFW	estimated fetal weight
EGA	estimated gestational age
EGD	esophagogastroduodenoscopy
EGJ	esophagogastric junction
EMC	endometrial curettage
EOB	explanation of benefits, remittance advice

EPO	Exclusive Provider Organization, similar to a Health Maintenance Organization except that the providers of the services are not prepaid but rather are paid on a fee-for-service basis
EPSDT	Early and Periodic Screening, Diagnosis, and Treatment
ERCP	endoscopic retrograde cholangiopancreatography
ERT	estrogen replacement therapy
ESRD	end-stage renal disease
FAS	fetal alcohol syndrome
FEF	forced expiratory flow
FEV_1	forced expiratory volume in 1 second
FEV_1:FVC	maximum amount of forced expiratory volume in 1 second
FHR	fetal heart rate
FI	fiscal intermediary, financial agent acting on behalf of a third-party payer
FRC	functional residual capacity
FSH	follicle-stimulating hormone
FVC	forced vital capacity
fx	fracture
GERD	gastroesophageal reflux disease
GI	gastrointestinal
H or E	hemorrhage or exudate
HCFA	Health Care Financing Administration, now known as Centers for Medicare and Medicaid Services (CMS)
HCVD	hypertensive cardiovascular disease
HD	hemodialysis
HDL	high-density lipoprotein
HEA	hemorrhage, exudate, aneurysm
HHN	handheld nebulizer
HJR	hepatojugular reflux
H&P	history and physical (examination)
HPV	human papillomavirus
HSG	hysterosalpingogram
HSV	herpes simplex virus
I&D	incision and drainage
IO	intraocular
IOL	intraocular lens
IPAP	inspiratory positive airway pressure
IRDS	infant respiratory distress syndrome
IVF	in vitro fertilization
IVP	intravenous pyelogram
JBP	jugular blood pressure
KUB	kidneys, ureter, bladder
L1-L5	lumbar vertebrae
LBBB	left bundle branch block
LEEP	loop electrosurgical excision procedure
LGA	large for gestational age
LLQ	left lower quadrant
LP	lumbar puncture
LUQ	left upper quadrant
LVH	left ventricular hypertrophy
MAT	multifocal atrial tachycardia

MDI	metered dose inhaler
MI	myocardial infarction
MRI	magnetic resonance imaging
MSLT	multiple sleep latency testing
MVV	maximum voluntary ventilation
NCPAP	nasal continuous positive airway pressure
NSR	normal sinus rhythm
OA	osteoarthritis
OD	right eye
OS	left eye
OU	each eye
PAC	premature atrial contraction
PAT	paroxysmal atrial tachycardia
PAWP	pulmonary artery wedge pressure
PCWP	pulmonary capillary wedge pressure
PEAP	positive end-airway pressure
PEEP	positive end-expiratory pressure
PEG	percutaneous endoscopic gastrostomy
PERL	pupils equal and reactive to light
PERRL	pupils equal, round, and reactive to light
PERRLA	pupils equal, round, and reactive to light and accommodation
PFT	pulmonary function test
pH	symbol for acid/base level
PICC	peripherally inserted central catheter
PID	pelvic inflammatory disease
PND	paroxysmal nocturnal dyspnea
PNS	peripheral nervous system
PROM	premature rupture of membranes
PSA	prostate-specific antigen
PST, PSVT	paroxysmal supraventricular tachycardia
PT	prothrombin time
PTCA	percutaneous transluminal coronary angioplasty
PTT	partial thromboplastin time
PVC	premature ventricular contraction
RA	remittance advice, explanation of services
RA	rheumatoid arthritis
RBBB	right bundle branch block
RDS	respiratory distress syndrome
REM	rapid eye movement
RLQ	right lower quadrant
RSR	regular sinus rhythm
RUQ	right upper quadrant
RV	respiratory volume
RVG	*Relative Value Guide*
RVH	right ventricular hypertrophy
RVS	relative value studies, list of procedures with unit values assigned to each
RV:TLC	ratio of respiratory volume to total lung capacity
SHG	sonohysterogram
sp gr	specific gravity
SROM	spontaneous rupture of membranes
subcu, subq, SC, SQ	subcutaneous
SUI	stress urinary incontinence

SVT	supraventricular tachycardia	UA	urinalysis
T1-T12	thoracic vertebrae	UCR	usual, customary, and reasonable—third-party payers' assessment of the reimbursement for health care services: usual, that which would ordinarily be charged for the service; customary, the cost of that service in that locale; and reasonable, as assessed by the payer
TAH	total abdominal hysterectomy		
TEE	transesophageal echocardiography		
TENS	transcutaneous electrical nerve stimulation		
TIA	transient ischemic attack		
TLC	total lung capacity		
TLV	total lung volume		
TM	tympanic membrane	UPJ	ureteropelvic junction
TMJ	temporomandibular joint	URI	upper respiratory infection
TPA	tissue plasminogen activator	UTI	urinary tract infection
TSH	thyroid-stimulating hormone	V/Q	ventilation/perfusion scan
TST	treadmill stress test	VBAC	vaginal birth after cesarean
TURBT	transurethral resection of bladder tumor	WBC	white blood (cell) count
TURP	transurethral resection of prostate		

Appendix H

Further Text Resources

Anatomy and Physiology

Book Title	Author	Imprint	Copyright Date	ISBN-13
Medical Terminology & Anatomy for Coding, 3rd Edition	Shiland	Mosby	2018	978-0-323-42795-1
The Anatomy and Physiology Learning System, 4th Edition	Applegate	Saunders	2011	978-1-4377-0393-1
Gray's Anatomy for Students, 3rd Edition	Drake, Vogl, Mitchell	Churchill Livingstone	2014	978-0-702-05131-9
Anthony's Textbook of Anatomy and Physiology, 20th Edition	Thibodeau, Patton	Mosby	2012	978-0-323-09600-3

Coding

Book Title	Imprint	Copyright Date	ISBN-13
Buck's Step-by-Step Medical Coding, 2021 Edition	Elsevier	2021	978-0-323-70926-2
Buck's 2021 ICD-10-CM for Hospitals	Elsevier	2021	978-0-323-76282-3
Buck's 2021 ICD-10-CM for Physicians	Elsevier	2021	978-0-323-76280-9
Buck's 2021 ICD-10-PCS	Elsevier	2021	978-0-323-76281-6
Buck's 2021 HCPCS Level II	Elsevier	2021	978-0-323-76279-3
Buck's The Next Step: Advanced Medical Coding and Auditing, 2021/2022 Edition	Elsevier	2021	978-0-323-76277-9
Buck's Simulated Medical Coding Internship, 2021/2022 Edition	Elsevier	2021	978-0-323-79254-7
Practice Management with Auditing for Coders Powered by SimChart® for the Medical Office	Elsevier	2016	978-0-323-43011-1
ICD-10-CM/PCS Coding: Theory and Practice, 2021/2022 Edition	Elsevier	2021	978-0-323-76414-8

Pathophysiology

Book Title	Author	Imprint	Copyright Date	ISBN-13
Pathology for the Health Professions, 5th Edition	Damjanov	Saunders	2017	978-0-323-35721-0
Essentials of Human Diseases and Conditions, 6th Edition	Frazier, Drzymkowski	Saunders	2016	978-0-323-22836-7
Gould's Pathophysiology for the Health Professions, 5th Edition	VanMeter, Hubert	Saunders	2015	978-1-4557-5411-3
Introduction to Human Anatomy and Physiology, 4th Edition	Solomon	Saunders	2016	978-0-323-23925-7
The Human Body in Health and Illness, 5th Edition	Herlihy	Saunders	2014	978-1-4557-7234-6
The Human Body in Health and Disease, 7th Edition	Thibodeau, Patton	Mosby	2017	978-0-323-40211-8

Medical Terminology

Book Title	Author	Imprint	Copyright Date	ISBN-13
The Language of Medicine, 11th Edition	Chabner	Saunders	2017	978-0-323-37081-3
Mastering Healthcare Terminology, 5th Edition	Shiland	Mosby	2016	978-0-323-29858-2
Jablonski's Dictionary of Medical Acronyms & Abbreviations, 6th Edition	Jablonski	Saunders	2008	978-1-4160-5899-1
Exploring Medical Language, 10th Edition	LaFleur Brooks, LaFleur Brooks	Mosby	2018	978-0-323-39645-5
Building a Medical Vocabulary: With Spanish Translations, 9th Edition	Leonard	Saunders	2015	978-1-4557-7268-1
Quick & Easy Medical Terminology, 7th Edition	Leonard	Saunders	2014	978-1-4557-4070-3
Mosby's Dictionary of Medicine, Nursing & Health Professions, 10th Edition		Mosby	2017	978-0-323-22205-1
Dorland's Illustrated Medical Dictionary, 32nd Edition		Saunders	2011	978-1-4160-6257-8

Computers & Electronic Health Record

Book Title	Author	Imprint	Copyright Date	ISBN-13
SimChart® for the Medical Office		Elsevier	2014	978-0-323-24195-3
SimChart® for the Medical Office: Learning the Medical Office Workflow, 2017 Edition		Elsevier	2017	978-0-323-49792-3
The Electronic Health Record for the Physician's Office with SimChart® for the Medical Office, 2nd Edition	Pepper		2017	978-0-323-51146-9
Computerized Medical Office Procedures: A Worktext, 4th Edition	Larsen	Saunders	2014	978-1-4557-2620-2

Medical Transcription

Book Title	Author	Imprint	Copyright Date	ISBN-13
Medical Transcription Guide: Do's and Don'ts, 3rd Edition	Diehl	Saunders	2005	978-0-7216-0684-2
Medical Transcription: Techniques and Procedures, 7th Edition	Diehl	Saunders	2012	978-1-4377-0439-6

Professionalism

Book Title	Author	Imprint	Copyright Date	ISBN-13
Job Readiness for Health Professionals: Soft Skills Strategies for Success, 2nd Edition		Elsevier	2016	978-0-323-43026-5
Health Careers Today, 6th Edition	Gerdin	Mosby	2016	978-0-323-28050-1
Career Development for Health Professionals: Success in School and on the Job, 4th Edition	Haroun	Saunders	2016	978-0-323-31126-7

Basic Math

Book Title	Author	Imprint	Copyright Date	ISBN-13
Saunders Math Skills for Health Professionals, 2nd Edition	Hickey	Saunders	2016	978-0-323-32248-5

Medical Billing/Insurance

Book Title	Author	Imprint	Copyright Date	ISBN-13
Health Insurance Today: A Practical Approach, 5th Edition	Beik	Saunders	2015	978-0-323-18817-3
Insurance Handbook for the Medical Office, 14th Edition	Fordney	Saunders	2017	978-0-323-31625-5

Law and Ethics

Book Title	Author	Imprint	Copyright Date	ISBN-13
Legal and Ethical Issues for Health Professions, 3rd Edition		Elsevier	2015	978-1-4557-3366-8

Appendix I

Pharmacology Review

Generic Name	Registered Brand or Trade Name	Therapeutic Use/Medication Action
ANTI-ATTENTION DEFICIT HYPERACTIVITY DISORDER		
atomoxetine	Strattera	Attention Deficit Hyperactivity Disorder (ADHD) therapy
AMNESIC		
diazepam	Valium	amnesic, antianxiety, anticonvulsant, antipain, anti-tremor agent, sedative-hypnotic, skeletal muscle relaxant adjunct
lorazepam	Ativan	amnesic, antianxiety, anticonvulsant, antiemetic, antipanic, anti-tremor, sedative-hypnotic, skeletal muscle relaxant
ANALGESIC		
acetaminophen-codeine	Phenaphen with Codeine	analgesic
acetaminophen-codeine	Tylenol with Codeine	analgesic
celecoxib	Celebrex	analgesic, antirheumatic NSAID
fentanyl	Duragesic	analgesic
fentanyl	Actiq	analgesic, anesthetic adjunct
fentanyl	Sublimaze	analgesic, anesthetic adjunct
hydrocodone	Hycodan	analgesic
hydrocodone-acetaminophen	Lortab	analgesic
hydrocodone-acetaminophen	Vicodin	analgesic
ibuprofen	Advil	analgesic
ibuprofen	Motrin	analgesic
naproxen	Aleve	analgesic, nonsteroid anti-inflammatory, antidysmenorreal, antigout, antipyretic, antirheumatic, vascular headache prophylactic and suppressant
naproxen	Naprosyn	analgesic, nonsteroid anti-inflammatory, antidysmenorreal, antigout, antipyretic, antirheumatic, vascular headache prophylactic and suppressant
oxycodone	OxyContin	analgesic
oxycodone-acetaminophen	Endocet	analgesic
oxycodone-acetaminophen	Percocet	analgesic
oxycodone-acetaminophen	Tylox	analgesic
propoxyphene-acetaminophen	Darvocet-N 100	analgesic
tramadol	Ultram	analgesic
tramadol-acetaminophen	Ultracet	analgesic
ANTI HIV AIDS		
efavirenz	Sustiva	anti HIV AIDS
emtricitabine	Emtriva	anti HIV AIDS
tenofovir	Viread	anti HIV AIDS

Generic Name	Registered Brand or Trade Name	Therapeutic Use/Medication Action
ANTI-IMPOTENCE		
sildenafil	Viagra	impotence, anti-erectile dysfunction
ANTI-PARKINSONISM		
cabergoline	Dostinex	anti-parkinsonism, anti-migraine headache
ANTIPROSTATIC HYPERTROPHY		
finasteride	Propecia	benign prostatic hyperplasia therapy, hair growth stimulant
finasteride	Proscar	benign prostatic hyperplasia therapy, hair growth stimulant
tamsulosin HCL	Flomax	benign prostatic hyperplasia therapy
ANTIACNE		
ethinyl estradiol-norethindrone	Estrostep Fe	antiacne, antiendometriotic, systemic contraceptive, estrogen-progestin, gonadotropin inhibitor
ethinyl estradiol-norethindrone	Femhrt	antiacne, antiendometriotic, systemic contraceptive, estrogen-progestin, gonadotropin inhibitor
ethinyl estradiol-norethindrone	Loestrin Fe	antiacne, antiendometriotic, systemic contraceptive, estrogen-progestin, gonadotropin inhibitor
ethinyl estradiol-norethindrone	Ovcon	antiacne, antiendometriotic, systemic contraceptive, estrogen-progestin, gonadotropin inhibitor
ethinyl estrodiol-norgestinmate	Ortho Tri-Cyclen	antiacne, antiendometriotic, systemic contraceptive, estrogen-progestin, gonadotropin inhibitor
ANTIADRENERGIC		
metoprolol	Lopressor	antiadrenergic, antianginal, antianxiety, antiarrhythmic, antihypertensive, anti-tremor, hypertrophic cardiomyopathy, MI therapy
metoprolol succinate	Toprol XL	antiadrenergic, antianginal, antianxiety, antiarrhythmic, antihypertensive, anti-tremor, hypertrophic cardiomyopathy, MI therapy
propranolol	Inderal	antiadrenergic, antianginal, antianxiety, antiarrhythmic, antihypertensive, anti-tremor, hypertrophic cardiomyopathy, MI prophylactic, MI therapy, neuroleptic-induced akathisia therapy
timolol	Blocadren	antiadrenergic, antianginal, antianxiety, antiarrhythmic, systemic antiglaucoma, antihypertensive, anti-tremor, hypertrophic cardiomyopathy, MI prophylactic
ANTIANGINAL		
diltiazem	Cardizem	antianginal, antiarrhythmic, antihypertensive
diltiazem	Dilacor	antianginal, antiarrhythmic, antihypertensive
felodipine	Plendil	antianginal, antihypertensive
isosorbide mononitrate	Imdur	antianginal
isosorbide mononitrate	Ismo	antianginal
nifedipine	Procardia	antianginal, antihypertensive
nitroglycerin	Minitran	antianginal, congestive heart failure (CHF), vasodilator
nitroglycerin	Nitrolingual	antianginal, CHS, vasodilator
nitroglycerin	Nitrostat	antianginal, CHS, vasodilator
verapamil	Isoptin	antianginal, antiarrhythmic, antihypertensive, hypertrophic cardiomyopathy therapy vascular headache prophylactic
verapamil	Verelan	antianginal, antiarrhythmic, antihypertensive, hypertrophic cardiomyopathy therapy vascular headache prophylactic
verapamil	Calan	antianginal, antiarrhythmic, antihypertensive, hypertrophic cardiomyopathy therapy, vascular headache prophylactic
verapamil	Covera HS	antianginal, antiarrhythmic, antihypertensive, hypertrophic cardiomyopathy therapy, vascular headache prophylactic

Generic Name	Registered Brand or Trade Name	Therapeutic Use/Medication Action
ANTIANXIETY		
alprazolam	Xanax	antianxiety
buspirone	BuSpar	antianxiety
escitalopram oxalate	Lexapro	antianxiety, antidepressant
paroxetine HCL	Paxil	antianxiety, antidepressant, antiobsessional, antipanic, posttraumatic stress disorder, social anxiety disorder agent
sertraline	Zoloft	antianxiety, antidepressant, antiobsessional, antipanic, posttraumatic stress disorder, premenstrual dysphoric disorder therapy
ANTIARRHYTHMIC		
digoxin	Digitek	antiarrhythmic, cardiotonic
digoxin	Lanoxicaps	antiarrhythmic, cardiotonic
digoxin	Lanoxin	antiarrhythmic, cardiotonic
phenytoin	Dilantin	antiarrhythmic, anticonvulsant, trigeminal neuralgic antineuralgic, skeletal muscle relaxant
ANTIASTHMATIC		
budesonide	Pulmicort	antiasthmatic
fluticasone-salmeterol	Advair Diskus	antiasthmatic, inhalation anti-inflammatory, bronchodilator
ipratropium bromide	Atrovent	antiasthmatic bronchodilator
lipatropium-albuterol	Combivent	antiasthmatic bronchodilator
montelukast sodium	Singular	antiasthmatic, leukotriene receptor antagonist
salmeterol maleate	Serevent	antiasthmatic
zafirlukast	Accolate	antiasthmatic
ANTIBACTERIAL		
amoxicillin	Trimax	systemic antibacterial
amoxicillin-clavulanate	Augmentin	systemic antibacterial
azithromycin	Zithromax	systemic antibacterial
cefadroxil	Duricef	systemic antibacterial
cefdinir	Omnicef	systemic antibacterial
cefluroximine axetil	Ceflin	systemic antibacterial
cefprozil	Cefzil	systemic antibacterial
cephalexin	Keflex	systemic antibacterial
ciprofloxacin	Ciloxan	ophthalmic antibacterial
ciprofloxacin	Cipro	systemic antibacterial
clarithromycin	Biaxin	systemic antibacterial, antimycobacterial
clindamycin	Cleocin	systemic antibacterial
doxycycline	Vibramycin	systemic antibacterial, antiprotozoal
levofloxacin	Levaquin	systemic antibacterial
metronidazole	Flagyl	systemic antibacterial
minocycline	Minocin	systemic antibacterial
moxifloxacin	Avelox	systemic antibacterial
moxifloxacin	Vigamox	ophthalmic antibacterial
mupirocin	Bactroban	topical antibacterial
nitrofurantoin	Macrodantin	systemic antibacterial
nitrofurantoin monohydrate	Macrobid	systemic antibacterial
ofloxacin	Floxin	systemic antibacterial

Generic Name	Registered Brand or Trade Name	Therapeutic Use/Medication Action
penicillin V	Veetids	systemic antibacterial
sulfamethoxazole-trimethoprim	Bactrim	systemic antibacterial, antiprotozoal
sulfamethoxazole-trimethoprim	Cotrim	systemic antibacterial, antiprotozoal
sulfamethoxazole-trimethoprim	Septra DS	systemic antibacterial, antiprotozoal
trimethoprim	Bactrim	systemic antibacterial

ANTICOAGULANT

dipyridamole/ASA	Aggrenox	anticoagulant
warfarin	Coumadin	anticoagulant

ANTICONVULSANT

clonazepam	Klonopin	anticonvulsant
divalproex sodium	Depakote	anticonvulsant, antimanic, migraine headache prophylactic
gabapentin	Neurontin	anticonvulsant, antineuralgic
lamotrigine	Lamictal	anticonvulsant
levetiracetam	Keppra	anticonvulsant
oxcarbazepine	Trileptal	anticonvulsant
tiagabine	Gabitril	anticonvulsant
topiramate	Topamax	anticonvulsant, antimigraine headache
zonisamide	Zonegran	anticonvulsant

ANTIDEMENTIA

donepezil	Aricept	antidementia
galantamine HBr	Reminyl	antidementia-mild/moderate Alzheimer's
rivastigmine tartrate	Exelon	antidementia of Parkinson's

ANTIDEPRESSANT

amitriptyline	Elavil	antidepressant
bupropion	Zyban	antidepressant, smoking cessation
bupropion HCL	Wellbutrin	antidepressant, smoking cessation
citalopram hydrobromide	Celexa	antidepressant
doxepin	Sinequan	antidepressant
fluoxetine	Prozac	antidepressant, antiobsessional agent
fluoxetine	Sarafem	antidepressant, antiobsessional, antibulimic agent
mirtazapine	Remeron	antidepressant
trazodone	Desyrel	antidepressant, antineuralgic
venlafaxine HCL	Effexor	antidepressant, antianxiety agent

ANTIDIABETIC

doxazosin mesylate	Diabinese	antidiabetic
glimepiride	Amaryl	antidiabetic
glipizide	Glucotrol	antidiabetic
glyburide	DiaBeta	antidiabetic
glyburide	Glynase	antidiabetic
glyburide	Micronase	antidiabetic
glyburide-metformin	Glucovance	antidiabetic
insulin	Nolog	antidiabetic
insulin	Novolin	antidiabetic
insulin glargine	Lantus	antidiabetic

Generic Name	Registered Brand or Trade Name	Therapeutic Use/Medication Action
insulin lispro	Humalog	antidiabetic
metformin HCL	Glucophage	antihyperglycemic
miglitol	Glyset	antidiabetic
NPH isophane insulin	Humulin N	antidiabetic
NPH regular insulin	Humulin 70/30	antidiabetic
pioglitazone	Actos	antidiabetic
repaglinide	Prandin	antidiabetic
rosiglitazone	Avandia	antidiabetic

ANTIEMETIC

meclizine	Antivert	antiemetic, antivertigo
promethazine	Phenergan	antiemetic, antihistaminic, H1 receptor, antivertigo, sedative-hypnotic

ANTIENDOMETRIOTIC

ethinyl estradiol-desogestrel	Cyclessa	antiendometriotic, systemic contraceptive, gonadotropin inhibitor
ethinyl estradiol-desogestrel	Desogen	antiendometriotic, systemic contraceptive, gonadotropin inhibitor
ethinyl estradiol-desogestrel	Kariva	antiendometriotic, systemic contraceptive, gonadotropin inhibitor
ethinyl estradiol-desogestrel	Mircette	antiendometriotic, systemic contraceptive, gonadotropin inhibitor
ethinyl estradiol-desogestrel	Ortho-Cept	antiendometriotic, systemic contraceptive, gonadotropin inhibitor
ethinyl estradiol-levonorgestrel	Levlen	antiendometriotic, systemic postcoital contraceptive, systemic contraceptive, estrogen progestin, gonadotropin inhibitor
ethinyl estradiol-levonorgestrel	Nordette	antiendometriotic, systemic postcoital contraceptive, systemic contraceptive, estrogen-progestin, gonadotropin inhibitor
ethinyl estradiol-levonorgestrel	Seasonale	antiendometriotic, systemic postcoital contraceptive, systemic contraceptive, estrogen-progestin, gonadotropin inhibitor
ethinyl estradiol-levonorgestrel	Tri-Levlen	antiendometriotic, systemic postcoital contraceptive, systemic contraceptive, estrogen-progestin, gonadotropin inhibitor
ethinyl estradiol-levonorgestrel	Triphasil	antiendometriotic, systemic postcoital contraceptive, systemic contraceptive, estrogen-progestin, gonadotropin inhibitor
ethinyl estradiol-levonorgestrel	Trivora-28	antiendometriotic, systemic postcoital contraceptive, systemic contraceptive, estrogen-progestin, gonadotropin inhibitor
ethinyl estradiol-norgestrel	Lo/Ovral	antiendometriotic, systemic postcoital contraceptive, systemic contraceptive, estrogen-progestin, gonadotropin inhibitor
ethinyl estradiol-norgestrel	Low-Ogestrel	antiendometriotic, systemic postcoital contraceptive, systemic contraceptive, estrogen-progestin, gonadotropin inhibitor
ethinyl estradiol-norgestrel	Ovral	antiendometriotic, systemic postcoital contraceptive, systemic contraceptive, estrogen-progestin, gonadotropin inhibitor

ANTIFUNGAL

clotrimazole	Mycelex Cream	antifungal
clotrimazole-betamethasone	Lotrisone	antifungal, corticosteroid
econazole	Sporanox	antifungal
econazole	Spectazole Cream	antifungal
fluconazole	Diflucan	systemic antifungal
griseofulvin	Grifulvin	antifungal
itraconazole	Sporanox	antifungal
ketoconazole	Nizoral	antifungal
miconazole	Monistat Derm	cream antifungal
terbinafine	Lamisil	antifungal
terconazole	Terazol	vaginal antifungal cream, suppositories

Generic Name	Registered Brand or Trade Name	Therapeutic Use/Medication Action
ANTIGLAUCOMA		
bimatoprost	Lumigan Ophthalmic	antiglaucoma solution
brimonidine	Alphagan P	antiglaucoma solution
dorzolamide/timolol maleate	Cosopt	decreases ocular hypertension
latanoprost	Xalatan	antiglaucoma
latanoprost	Xalatan Ophthalmic	antiglaucoma, ocular antihypertensive
timolol	Timoptic	ophthalmic antiglaucoma
ANTIGOUT		
allopurinol	Zyloprim	antigout agent
ANTIHISTAMINE		
cetirizine	Zyrtec	antihistamine, H1 receptor
cetirizine-pseudoephedrine	Zyrtec-D	antihistamine, H1 receptor-decongestant
desloratadine	Clarinex	antihistamine, H1 receptor
fexofenadine	Allegra	antihistamine, H1 receptor
fexofenadine-pseudoephedrine	Allegra D	antihistamine, H1 receptor-decongestant
hydrocodone-chlorpheniramine	Tussionex	antihistamine, H1 receptor antitussive
hydroxyzine	Vistaril	antihistamine
loratadine	Claritin	antihistamine
olopatadine	Patanol	ophthalmic antihistamine, H1 receptor, mask cell stabilizer, antiallergic
promethazine-codeine	Prometh with Codeine	antihistamine, H1 receptor-antitussive
ANTIHYPERCALCEMIC		
furosemide	Lasix	antihypercalcemic, antihypertensive, renal disease diagnostic aid, diuretic
ANTIHYPERLIPIDEMIC		
atorvastatin	Lipitor	antilipidemic, statin
colesevelam	WelChol	antihyperlipidemic
ezetimibe	Zetia	antihyperlipidemic
fenofibrate	TriCor	antihyperlipidemic
fluvastatin sodium	Lescol	antihyperlipidemic
gemfibrozil	Lopid	antihyperlipidemic
lovastatin	Mevacor	antihyperlipidemic
pravastatin sodium	Pravachol	antihyperlipidemic, HMG-CoA reductase inhibitor
simvastatin	Zocor	antihyperlipidemic, HMG-CoA reductase inhibitor
ANTIHYPERTENSIVE		
amlodipine/atorvastatin	Caduet	antihypertensive, calcium channel blocker
amlodipine-benazepril HCL	Lotrel	antihypertensive, calcium channel blocker
amlodipine-besylate	Norvasc	antihypertensive, calcium channel blocker
atenolol	Tenormin	antihypertensive
benazepril	Lotensin	antihypertensive, ACE inhibitor
bepridil	Vascor	antihypertensive, calcium channel blocker
candesartan	Atacand	antihypertensive
captopril	Capoten	antihypertensive, ACE inhibitor
carvedilol	Coreg	antihypertensive
clonidine	Duraclon	antihypertensive

Generic Name	Registered Brand or Trade Name	Therapeutic Use/Medication Action
clonidine HCL	Catapres	antihypertensive
doxazosin	Cardura	antihypertensive, alpha blocker
enalapril	Vasotec	antihypertensive, vasodilator, ACE inhibitor
fosinopril sodium	Monopril	antihypertensive, vasodilator, ACE inhibitor
hydrochlorothiazide	Esidrix	antihypertensive, diuretic, antiurolithic
irbesartan	Avapro	antihypertensive
irbesartan-hydrochlorothiazide	Avalide	antihypertensive
lisinopril	Prinivil	antihypertensive, vasodilator
lisinopril	Zestril	antihypertensive, vasodilator, ACE inhibitor
losartan potassium	Cozaar	antihypertensive, angiotensin II-receptor antagonist
losartan-hydrochlorothiazide	Hyzaar	antihypertensive
perindopril	Coversyl	antihypertensive, vasodilator, ACE inhibitor
prazosin	Minipress	antihypertensive, alpha blocker
prazosin/polythiazide	Minizide	antihypertensive, alpha blocker
quinapril	Accupril	antihypertensive, vasodilator, ACE inhibitor
ramipril	Altace	antihypertensive, vasodilator, ACE inhibitor
spironolactone	Aldactone	antihypertensive, antihypokalemic, hyperaldosteronism diagnostic aid, diuretic, aldosterone antagonist
terazosin	Hytrin	antihypertensive, benign prostatic hyperplasia
trandolapril	Mavik	antihypertensive, vasodilator, ACE inhibitor
travoprost	Travatan	antihypertensive, reducing intraocular pressure
triamterene-hydrochlorothiazide	Dyazide	antihypertensive, antihypokalemia, diuretic
triamterene-hydrochlorothiazide	Maxzide	antihypertensive, antihypokalemia, diuretic
valsartan	Diovan	antihypertensive
valsartan-hydrochlorothiazide	Diovan HCT	antihypertensive
verapamil/trandolapril	Tarka	antihypertensive, calcium channel blocker

ANTIHYPOKALEMIC

potassium chloride	Klor-Con	antihypokalemic, electrolyte replenisher

ANTI-INFLAMMATORY (NONSTEROID)

diclofenac	Arthrotec	anti-inflammatory, analgesic
hydroxychloroquine	Plaquenil	systemic anti-inflammatory
mesalamine	Asacol	anti-inflammatory in colon/rectum
piroxicam	Feldene	anti-inflammatory, analgesic
tolmetin	Tolectin	anti-inflammatory, analgesic
triamcinolone	Azmacort	inhalation anti-inflammatory, antiasthmatic
valdecoxib	Bextra	nonsteroidal anti-inflammatory, antirheumatic, antidysmenorrheal

ANTIMETASTATIC

bicalutamide	Casodex	antimetastatic—used with LHRH-A to treat advanced prostate cancer

ANTIMIGRAINE

eletriptan HBr	Relpax	antimigraine
sumatriptan	Imitrex	antimigraine

Generic Name	Registered Brand or Trade Name	Therapeutic Use/Medication Action
ANTINEOPLASTIC		
conjugated estrogen	Enjuvia	antineoplastic, systemic estrogen, osteoporosis prophylactic, ovarian hormone therapy agent
conjugated estrogen	Premarin	antineoplastic, systemic estrogen, osteoporosis prophylactic, ovarian hormone therapy agent
levothyroxine sodium	Synthroid	antineoplastic, thyroid function diagnostic aid, thyroid hormone
levothyroxine T4	Levothroid	antineoplastic, thyroid function diagnostic aid, thyroid hormone
ANTIPSYCHOTIC		
olanzapine	Zyprexa	antipsychotic
quetiapine	Seroquel	antipsychotic
risperidone	Risperdal	antipsychotic
thiothixene	Navane	antipsychotic
ziprasidone	Geodon	antipsychotic
ANTIRHEUMATIC		
meloxicam	Mobic	antirheumatic (NSAID)
ANTISEIZURE		
ethosuximide	Zarontin	antiseizure
ANTISPASMOTIC		
oxybutynin chloride	Ditropan XL	urinary tract antispasmodic
tolterodine tartrate	Detrol	urinary bladder antispasmodic
ANTITHROMBOTIC		
clopidogrel bisulfate	Plavix	antithrombotic, platelet aggregation inhibitor
ANTIULCER		
esomeprazole magnesium	Nexium	gastric acid pump inhibitor, antiulcer
lansoprazole SR	Prevacid	gastric acid pump inhibitor, antiulcer
misoprostol	Cytotec	gastric acid pump inhibitor, antiulcer
omeprazole SA	Prilosec	gastric acid pump inhibitor, antiulcer
pantoprazole	Protonix	gastric acid pump inhibitor, antiulcer
rabeprazole	AcipHex	gastric acid pump inhibitor, antiulcer
ranitidine	Zantac	histamine H2-receptor antagonist, antiulcer, gastric acid secretion inhibitor
ANTIVIRAL		
acyclovir	Zovirax	systemic antiviral
ribavirin	Rebetol	antiviral
ribavirin	Copegus	antiviral
valacyclovir	Valtrex	systemic antiviral
ANTIWRINKLE (TOPICAL)		
tretinoin	Retin-A	antiwrinkle cream
BRONCHODILATOR		
albuterol	Proventil	bronchodilator
albuterol	Ventolin	bronchodilator
BONE RESORPTION INHIBITOR		
alendronate sodium	Fosamax	bone resorption inhibitor
calcitonin-salmon	Miacalcin	bone resorption inhibitor
raloxifene sodium	Evista	selective estrogen receptor modulator, osteoporosis prophylactic
risedronate sodium	Actonel	bone resorption inhibitor

Generic Name	Registered Brand or Trade Name	Therapeutic Use/Medication Action
CATHARTIC		
polyethylene glycol	MiraLax	hyperosmotic laxative
CENTRAL NERVOUS SYSTEM STIMULANT		
dextroamphetamine-amphetamine	Adderall	CNS stimulant, ADHD therapy
methylphenidate	Concerta	CNS stimulant, ADHD therapy
methylphenidate	Metadate	CNS stimulant, ADHD therapy
methylphenidate	Ritalin	CNS stimulant, ADHD therapy
CONTRACEPTIVE		
ethinyl estradiol-drospirenone	Yasmin	systemic contraceptive
ethinyl estradiol-norelgestromin	Ortho Evra	systemic contraceptive
ENZYME		
pancrelipase	Pancrease	pancreatic enzyme replacement
HEMOPOIETIC		
erythropoietin	Epogen	hematopoietic
erythropoietin	Procrit	hematopoietic
HORMONE		
conjugated estrogen-medroxyprogesterone	Premphase	estrogen-progestin, osteoporosis prophylactic, ovarian hormone therapy
conjugated estrogen-medroxyprogesterone	Prempro	estrogen-progestin, osteoporosis prophylactic, ovarian hormone therapy
estrogen conjugated	Premarin	hormone replacement—estrogen
IMMUNE ENHANCER		
pimecrolimus	Elidel	immunomodulator
NEOPLASTIC		
anastrozole	Arimidex	chemotherapeutic-hormone receptor-positive
SEDATIVE		
temazepam	Restoril	sedative-hypnotic
zolpidem tartrate	Ambien	sedative-hypnotic
SKELETAL MUSCLE RELAXANT		
carisoprodol	Soma	skeletal muscle relaxant
chlorzoxazone	Parafon Forte DSC	skeletal muscle relaxant
cyclobenzaprine	Flexeril	skeletal muscle relaxant
metaxalone	Skelaxin	skeletal muscle relaxant
STEROIDS		
fluticasone	Flonase	steroidal nasal anti-inflammatory, nasal corticosteroid
fluticasone	Flovent	steroidal nasal anti-inflammatory, nasal corticosteroid
methylprednisolone	Medrol	steroidal anti-inflammatory, corticoid, steroid, immunosuppressant
mometasone furoate	Nasonex	nasal steroid anti-inflammatory, nasal corticosteroid
prednisone	Deltasone	systemic steroidal anti-inflammatory, cancer chemotherapy antiemetic, corticosteroid immunosuppressant
tobramycin-dexamethasone	TobraDex	ophthalmic corticosteroid, steroidal anti-inflammatory, antibacterial
triamcinolone	Nasacort AQ	nasal steroid anti-inflammatory, nasal corticosteroid
VITAMIN		
niacin	Niacor	nutritional supplement, vitamin

Index

Page numbers followed by "*f*" indicate figures, "*b*" indicate boxes, and "*t*" indicate tables

A

Abbreviations
   ICD-10-CM, 250
   medical (*See* Medical abbreviations)
Abdominal hysterectomy, 221–222*b*
Abduction, 19
Abductor muscles, 21
Ablation, 30*b*
   skin, subcutaneous, and accessory
      structures, 192
ABN. *See* Advance beneficiary notice (ABN)
Abnormal heart rhythms, 43
Abortion, 49*b*, 55–56, 220
   methods, 56
Abruptio placentae, 54, 55*f*
Abscess
   brain, 110
   perirectal, 179*b*
Absence, 4*b*
Absorption atelectasis, 32
Accessory organs
   digestive system, 74–76
   female genital system, 46, 47*f*
   ICD-10-CM chapter 12, diseases of skin
      and subcutaneous tissue, 259
   male genital system, 58, 58*f*
Accessory sinuses, 27, 202
Accounts receivable (AR), 149
Acetabulum, 15
Achilles tendon, 19*f*, 21
Acne vulgaris, 9, 192
Acromegaly, 100
ACS. *See* Acute coronary syndrome (ACS)
ACTH. *See* Adrenocorticotropic hormone
   (ACTH)
Actinic keratosis, 12
Active immunization, 239
Active wound care management, 243–244
Acute coronary syndrome (ACS), 39*b*
Acute inflammatory polyneuropathy, 108
Acute lymphocytic leukemia (ALL), 93–94
Acute myelogenous leukemia (AML), 93
Acute necrotizing fasciitis, 11
Acute pericarditis, 44
Acute poststreptococcal glomerulonephritis
   (APSGN), 71
Acute pyelonephritis, 70–71, 70*f*
Acute renal failure, 69, 172*b*
Acute respiratory failure, 32
Acute respiratory infection, 258

Addison's disease, 101
Adduction, 19
Adductor magnus, 19*f*
Adductors of thigh, 20*f*
Adenocarcinoma, 53
Adenoidectomy, 30*b*
Adenomyosis, 52
ADH. *See* Antidiuretic hormone (ADH)
Adipose, 4*b*
Adjacent tissue transfer, 191–193, 191*f*
Adrenal cortex, 96
Adrenal medulla, 96, 102
Adrenals, 96, 97*f*, 98*b*
   disorders of, 101–102
Adrenocorticotropic hormone (ACTH), 96
Adult respiratory distress syndrome (ARDS), 32
Advance beneficiary notice (ABN), 128*b*,
   130*f*, 153*b*
Advance care planning, 171
Albinism, 4*b*
Alcoholic liver, 85
ALL. *See* Acute lymphocytic leukemia (ALL)
Allergen immunotherapy, 241–242
Allergic contact dermatitis, 8
Allergy and clinical immunology, medicine
   section, 241–242
Allergy testing, 241
Allografts, 4*b*, 191
Alopecia, 4*b*
Alphabetic index
   ICD-10-CM, 249, 250, 252
   ICD-10-PCS, 267
ALS. *See* Amyotrophic lateral sclerosis (ALS)
Alternative laboratory platform testing
   modifier, 183
Alveolar ducts, 27
Alzheimer's disease, 106
Amblyopia, 118
Ambulatory blood pressure monitoring, 208
Ambulatory patient groups (APGs), 137
Ambulatory payment classifications
   (APCs), 137–138, 138*f*
   ambulatory surgical procedures, 142
   CA modifier, 140
   device-dependent procedures, 141
   discounting, 141
   includes some items/services that
      contribute to cost of the service but
      Medicare does not usually reimburse
      separately, 138

Ambulatory payment classifications
   (APCs) *(Continued)*
   inpatient-only procedures with status
      indicator "C," 141
   observation status, 142
   outlier adjustments, 141
   outpatient code editor (OCE), 142
   Outpatient Prospective Payment System
      (OPPS), 138–142, 139*f*
   pass-through codes, 138, 141*f*
   payment rate and co-insurance, 138, 140*f*
   payment status indicators (SI), 138–142
   structure, 138
   transitional pass-through payments for
      certain devices and items, 140–141
Ambulatory surgical procedures, 142
Amenorrhea, 50–51
AML. *See* Acute myelogenous leukemia
   (AML)
Amnesics, 335–343*t*
Amniocentesis, 49*b*, 219
Amniotic sac, 49*b*
A-mode, 230
Amphiarthrosis, 17
Ampulla of Vater, 76
Amyotrophic lateral sclerosis (ALS), 107
Analgesia, 176
   patient-controlled, 176
Analgesics, 335–343*t*
Anastomosis, 39*b*, 78*b*
Anatomic pathology, pathology and
   laboratory section, 236
Anatomy and terminology
   cardiovascular system, 35–38, 40
   digestive system, 74–76, 78–79
   endocrine system, 96–99
   female genital system, 46–47, 47*f*, 50
   further text resources, 332
   hemic and lymphatic system, 89, 91–92
   integumentary system, 2–5
   male genital system, 58, 58*f*, 60
   mediastinum and diaphragm, 87, 87*f*
   musculoskeletal system, 14–21, 23
   nervous system, 103–104, 106
   respiratory system, 27, 31
   senses, 114–115, 118
   urinary system, 66, 69
Ancillary service, 128*b*, 153*b*
Androgen hypersecretion, 102
And/with, ICD-10-CM, 250

Anemia, 92–93
  aplastic, 92
  hemolytic, 92
  ICD-10-CM chapter 2, neoplasms, 256
  iron deficiency, 92
  pernicious, 92
  sickle cell, 92–93
Anesthesia
  introduction/injection of, 224
  by surgeon modifier, 181
  unusual, 180
Anesthesia section, 176–179
  analgesia, 176
  anesthesia formula, 176–177
  anesthesiologist, 176
  B is for base units, 176
  breast biopsy, 178*b*
  Certified Registered Nurse Anesthetist
      (CRNA), 176
  conversion factors, 177
  incision and drainage of perirectal
      abscess, 179*b*
  intracerebral hematoma, 179*b*
  methods of anesthesia, 176
  M is for modifying unit, 176
  moderate (conscious) sedation, 176
  modifiers, 177
  for multiple surgical procedures, 177
  patient-controlled analgesia (PCA), 176
  perforated appendicitis, 177–178*b*
  physical status modifiers, P1-P6,
      176–177
  qualifying circumstances codes, 177
  takedown colostomy and
      cholecystectomy, 178*b*
  T is for time, 176
  uses of, 176
Anesthesiologist, 176
Aneurysm, 39*b*, 42, 110, 205
Angina, 39*b*
Angiography, 39*b*, 209–210*b*, 212*b*, 229
Angioma, 112
Angioplasty, 39*b*, 205
Anhidrosis, 4*b*
Ankylosing spondylitis, 25
Answers, quiz, 297–300
Antepartum, 49*b*
Antepartum care, 219
Anterior pituitary, 96
  disorders of, 99–100
Anterior segment, 117*b*
Antiacne medications, 335–343*t*
Antiadrenergic medications, 335–343*t*
Antianginal medications, 335–343*t*
Antianxiety medications, 335–343*t*
Antiarrhythmic medications, 335–343*t*
Antiasthmatic medications, 335–343*t*
Anti-attention deficit hyperactivity disorder
      medications, 335–343*t*
Antibacterial medications, 335–343*t*
Anticoagulant medications, 335–343*t*
Antidementia medications, 335–343*t*

Antidepressant medications, 335–343*t*
Antidiabetic medications, 335–343*t*
Antidiuretic hormone (ADH), 96
Antiemetic medications, 335–343*t*
Antiendometriotic medications, 335–343*t*
Antifungal medications, 335–343*t*
Antiglaucoma medications, 335–343*t*
Antigout medications, 335–343*t*
Antihistamine medications, 335–343*t*
Anti HIV AIDS medications, 335–343*t*
Antihypercalcemic medications, 335–343*t*
Antihyperlipidemic medications, 335–343*t*
Antihypertensive medications, 335–343*t*
Antihypokalemic medications, 335–343*t*
Anti-impotence medications, 335–343*t*
Anti-inflammatory medications, 335–343*t*
Antimetastatic medications, 335–343*t*
Antimigraine medications, 335–343*t*
Antineoplastic medications, 335–343*t*
Anti-Parkinsonism medications, 335–343*t*
Antiprostatic hypertrophy medications,
      335–343*t*
Antipsychotic medications, 335–343*t*
Antirheumatic medications, 335–343*t*
Antiseizure medications, 335–343*t*
Antispasmotic medications, 335–343*t*
Antithrombotic medications, 335–343*t*
Antiulcer medications, 335–343*t*
Antiviral medications, 335–343*t*
Antiwrinkle medications, 335–343*t*
Anus, 46, 58, 58*f*, 74
Aorta, 36
Aortic regurgitation (AR), 44
Aortic valve, 36
  stenosis of, 44
Aortogram, 211*b*
APCs. *See* Ambulatory payment
      classifications (APCs)
Apex, tongue, 75*f*
APGs. *See* Ambulatory patient groups (APGs)
Apicectomy, 117*b*
Aplastic anemia, 92
Apnea, 30*b*, 32
Aponeurosis of biceps, 20*f*
Appendices, CPT, 160
Appendicitis, 82
  perforated, 177–178*b*
Appendicular skeleton, 15–16
APSGN. *See* Acute poststreptococcal
      glomerulonephritis (APSGN)
Arachnoid, 104, 112
Arms
  bones of, 16
  muscles of, 20
Arterial grafting for coronary artery bypass,
      204
Arterial mechanical thrombectomy, 206
Arteries, 35, 36*f*
  cardiovascular in surgery section,
      204–206, 205*f*
  heart, 37*f*
Arthritis, 25

Arthrocentesis, 22*b*, 196
Arthrodesis, 22*b*, 197
Arthrography, 22*b*
Arthroplasty, 22*b*, 198–199*b*
  fascial sling, 199*b*
Arthroscopy, 22*b*, 198
Arthrotomy, 22*b*
Articular, 22*b*
Articulations, 17
Ascending colon, 76*f*
Asphyxia, 30*b*
Aspiration, 22*b*, 32
Assignment, 128*b*, 153*b*
Assistant surgeon modifier, 182
Assistant surgeon (when qualified resident
      surgeon not available) modifier, 182
Asthma, 30*b*
Astigmatism, 117*b*, 118
Astrocytes, 103
Astrocytoma, 112
Atelectasis, 30*b*, 32
Atherectomy, 39*b*
Atherosclerosis, 41, 109
Atopic dermatitis, 7–8
Atrial fibrillation, 43
Atrioventricular block, 43
Atrioventricular node, 36
Atrophy, 6, 6*f*, 22*b*
Attending physician, 128*b*, 153*b*, 168
Auditory system subsection, 225
Aural atresia, 117*b*
Auricle, 16*f*
Auscultation, 30*b*, 39*b*
Autogenous grafts, 197
Autograft, 4*b*
Autonomic nervous system (ANS), 103,
      104
  nervous system subsection, 224
Avulsion, 4*b*
Axial skeleton, 14–15
Axillary nodes, 90*f*, 91*b*
Axon, 103, 103*f*

B
Bacilli, 30*b*
Bacterial infections
  active immunizations against, 239
  cystitis, 70
  female genital system, 51–52
  skin, 10–11
Balanitis, 62
Barr procedure, 195–196
Bartholin's gland, 46
Basal cell carcinoma, 12
Basic math, further text resources on, 333
Basophilia, 93
Basophils, 35
B cells, 93, 95
Behavioral disorders, ICD-10-CM chapter
      5, mental, behavioral, and
      neurodevelopmental disorders, 257

Beneficiary, 128b, 153b
Beneficiary and Family Centered Care (BFCC), 125
Benign prostatic hyperplasia (BPH), 63
Benign tumors
    female genital system, 52
    skin, 12
        subcutaneous, and accessory structures, 189–190
BFCC. See Beneficiary and Family Centered Care (BFCC)
Biceps brachii, 20, 20f
Biceps femoris, 19f, 21
Bicuspid valve, 36
Bilateral procedure modifier, 181
Bile, 74–76
Biliary, 78b
Bilobectomy, 30b, 202
Biofeedback, 240
Biopsy, 4b
    bone and muscle, 196
    breast, 178b
    male genital system subsection, 216
    skin, subcutaneous, and accessory structures, 189, 193
Birthday rule, 128b, 153b
Birthing room attendance and resuscitation services, 170
B is for base units (anesthesia), 176
Blepharitis, 117b
Blepharoplasty, 191
Blepharotomy, 224
Blood
    composition, 35
    dialysis, 240–241
    function is to maintain a constant environment, 35
    ICD-10-CM chapter 3, diseases of the blood and blood-forming organs and certain disorders involving the immune mechanism, 256
    types, 35
    See also Vessels
Body of sternum, 17f
Bone/joint studies subsection, 230
Bone marrow, 209
Bone resorption inhibitors, 335–343t
Bones
    appendicular skeleton, 15–16
    arm, 16
    classification of, 14
    cranial, 14–15
    disorders of, 24
    ear, 15, 16f
    face, 15
    flat, 14
    hyoid, 15
    ICD-10-CM chapter 13, diseases of musculoskeletal system and connective tissue, 259
    irregular, 14

Bones (Continued)
    joints, 17
    leg, 15–16
    long, 14
    middle ear, 15
    sesamoid, 14
    short, 14
    shoulder, girdle, pelvic girdle, and extremities, pelvis, 15
    skull, 14, 15f, 16f
    spine, 15, 17f
    structure, 14–17, 14f
    thorax, 15, 17f
    tumors of, 25–26, 200b
Bony wall, ear, 16f
Brachialis, 20
Brachioradialis, 20
Brachytherapy, 231
    intracoronary, 207
Bradycardia, 43
Brain
    abscess of, 110
    congenital neurologic disorders, 108, 109f
    functions of, 103
    hemispheres, 104
    hypothalamus, 97
    lobes, 104
    mental disorders, 108
    nervous system subsection, 223–224
    parts of, 103–104, 104f
    traumatic brain injury (TBI), 111
    tumors, 111–112
    vascular disorders, 109–110
Brainstem, 103, 104f
Breast, 46, 47f
    biopsy of, 178b
    cancer of, 53
    procedures, 192–193
    wide excision, 193–194b
Breast mammography subsection, 230
Breech presentation, 56f
Bribery, 127, 151
Broad ligament, 47f
Bronchi, 202
Bronchial thermoplasty, 202
Bronchiectasis, 32
Bronchioles, 27, 28f, 30b
Bronchiolitis, 32
Bronchitis, chronic, 33
Bronchodilators, 335–343t
Bronchoplasty, 30b
Brow presentation of fetus, 56f
B-scan, 230
Buccinator, 19
Buerger's disease, 42
Bulbocavernosus, 68b
Bulbourethral, 58, 58f, 68b
Bulla, 5, 6f
Bundle of His, 36, 39b
Bunion, 22b
Burkitt's lymphoma, 94

Burns
    ICD-10-CM chapter 20, external causes of morbidity, 263
    local treatment, 191–192
    Lund-Browder Classification Method, 192, 192f
Burr, 105b
Burr holes, parietal, 225–226b
Bursa, 17, 200b
Bursitis, 22b, 25
Bypass, 39b

C
CABG. See Coronary artery bypass graft (CABG)
CAD. See Coronary artery disease (CAD)
Calcaneus, 16
Calculus, 68b, 72
Calycoplasty, 68b
Calyx, 68b
Cancer
    bladder, 72
    brain and spinal cord, 111–112
    breast, 53
    cervix, 53
    colorectal, 83–84
    esophagus, 80
    fallopian tubes, 54
    gastric, 81
    liver, 84
    mouth, 79
    ovary, 53–54
    pancreas, 86
    penis, 63
    prostate, 63, 64, 64f
    radiation oncology subsection, 230–231
    scrotum, 61
    testes, 61
    uterus, 53
    vagina, 54
    vulva, 54
    See also Neoplasms; Tumors
Candidiasis, 12, 51, 79
Canker sore, 79
Capillaries, 35
Cardiac catheterization, 189, 207, 244–245b
Cardiac/heart muscle, 18
Cardiac valves, 204
Cardiography, 207
Cardiology coding terminology, 203
Cardiomyopathies, 44
Cardiovascular in medicine section, 206–208, 241
    cardiac catheterization, 189
    cardiography, 207
    cardiovascular monitoring services, 207
    echocardiography, 207
    EP system of heart, 208
    implantable, insertable, and wearable cardiac device evaluations, 207

Cardiovascular in medicine section (*Continued*)
  intracardiac electrophysiologic procedures/studies, 208
  intracoronary brachytherapy, 207
  noninvasive physiologic studies and procedures, 208
  other procedures, 208
  peripheral arterial disease (PAD) rehabilitation, 208
  therapeutic services and procedures, 207
Cardiovascular in radiology section, 208, 209–210*b*, 210–211*b*, 212*b*
Cardiovascular in surgery section, 203–206
  angioplasty, 205
  arteries and veins subheading, 204–206, 205*f*
  cardiac valves, 204
  coronary artery bypass graft (CABG), 204
  electrophysiologic operative procedures, 204
  embolectomy and thrombectomy, 205
  endovascular repair of abdominal aortic aneurysm, 205
  endovascular repair of iliac aneurysm, 205
  endovascular revascularization, 206
  extracorporeal life support services, 204
  extracorporeal membrane oxygenation, 204
  heart/pericardium, 203–204
  noncoronary bypass grafts, 205
  pacemaker or implantable defibrillator, 203–204
  repair arteriovenous fistula, 205
  subcutaneous cardiac rhythm monitor, 204
  transcatheter procedures, 206
  vascular families like a tree, 205
  vascular injection procedures, 205–206
  venous reconstruction, 205
Cardiovascular monitoring services, 207
Cardiovascular system, 35–45
  anatomy and terminology, 35–38, 40
  blood, 35
  cardiomyopathies, 44
  combining forms, 38*b*
  congenital heart defects, 44
  heart, 35–36
  heart disorders, 43
  heart wall disorders, 44
  medical abbreviations, 39*b*
  medical terms, 39*b*
  pathophysiology, 41–44, 41*f*
  prefixes, 38*b*
  quiz, 40, 45
  suffixes, 38*b*
  valvular heart disease, 43–44
  vascular disorders, 41–43, 41*f*
  vessels, 35, 36*f*, 37*f*
Cardiovascular system subsection, 203
  cardiology coding terminology, 203

Cardiopulmonary, 39*b*
Cardiopulmonary bypass, 39*b*
Care, types of, 168
Care management services, 171
Care plan oversight services, 169–170
Carotid body, 223
Carpals, 16, 18*f*
Carpal tunnel syndrome, 22*b*, 226*b*
Case management services, 169
Casts and strapping, 198
CAT. *See* Computed axial tomography (CAT or CT)
Cataract, 117*b*, 119–120, 120*f*, 224
Category II codes-supplemental tracking codes, CPT, 159
Category III codes-new technology, CPT, 160
Cathartic medications, 335–343*t*
Catheter, 30*b*, 210–211*b*
Cauda equina, 104*f*
Causalgia, 4*b*
Cauterization, 30*b*
Cavernosa, 59*b*
Cavernosography, 59*b*
Cavernosometry, 59*b*
CC. *See* Chief complaint (CC); Complications or comorbidities (CC)
Cecum, 74, 76*f*
Celiac disease, 81
Cell body, 103, 103*f*
Cells, nervous system, 103, 103*f*
Cellulitis, 10
Centers for Medicare and Medicaid Services (CMS), 123, 130*f*, 137
  Table of Risk, 164, 165*f*
Central nervous system (CNS), 103–104, 105*b*
  assessments/tests, medicine section, 242
  disorders of, 109–112
  divisions of, 103–104
  stimulants, 335–343*t*
  vascular disorder, 109–110
Central venous access (CVA) procedures, 206
Cerebellum, 103, 104*f*
Cerebral hematoma, 111, 179*b*, 238*b*
Cerebrospinal fluid (CSF), 104, 224
Cerebrovascular accident (CVA), 109–110
Cerebrum, 103, 104*f*
Certified Registered Nurse Anesthetist (CRNA), 128*b*, 153*b*, 176
Cervical cerclage preoperative examination, 186*b*
Cervical dilator, 219
Cervical spinal stenosis, 238*b*
Cervical vertebrae, 15, 17*f*, 18*f*, 104
Cervix, 46, 47*f*, 218
  cancer of, 53
Cesarean, 49*b*
Cesarean section, 222*b*
CF. *See* Contributory factors (CF)
Chalazion, 117*b*

Chambers, heart, 35
Charge description master, 150–151, 150*f*, 153*b*
Chemical peel, 191
Chemistry, pathology and laboratory section, 235
Chemotherapy, medicine section, 243
CHF. *See* Congestive heart failure (CHF)
Chief complaint (CC), 162
Childbirth
  cesarean delivery, 49*b*, 222*b*
  delivery/birthing room attendance and resuscitation services, 170
  ICD-10-CM chapter 15, pregnancy, childbirth, and the puerperium, 261
  vaginal delivery, 55
  See also Delivery
Chiropractic services, 244
Chlamydia, 51–52
Cholangiography, 78*b*
Cholangitis, 85
Cholecystectomy, 78*b*, 178*b*
Cholecystitis, 85
Cholecystoenterostomy, 78*b*
Cholelithiasis, 85, 85*f*
Cholesteatoma, 117*b*
Chondral, 22*b*
Chondroblastoma, 26
Chondrosarcoma, 26
Chordee, 59*b*
Chorea, 107
Chorionic villus sampling, 49*b*
Choroid, 114
Chromosomal abnormalities, ICD-10-CM chapter 17, congenital malformations, deformations, and chromosomal abnormalities, 262
Chronic bronchitis, 33
Chronic care management services, 171
Chronic glaucoma, 120
Chronic kidney disease, ICD-10-CM chapter 9, diseases of circulatory system, 258
Chronic lymphocytic leukemia (CLL), 94
Chronic myelogenous leukemia (CML), 94
Chronic obstructive pulmonary disease (COPD), 33
Chronic pyelonephritis, 71
Chronic renal failure, 69–70, 172*b*
Cicatrix, 7
Circulatory system, ICD-10-CM chapter 9, diseases of, 257–258
Circumduction, 19
Circumflex, 39*b*
Cirrhosis, 85
Cistema chyli, 90*f*
Clavicle, 16, 17*f*, 18*f*
"Clean claim," 128*b*
Cleft lip and palate, 79, 79*f*
Clinical brachytherapy, 231
Clitoris, 46

CLL. *See* Chronic lymphocytic leukemia (CLL)
Cloquet's nodes, 91*b*
Closed fracture repair, 22*b*, 196
Closed fractures, 23
Closed treatment, 22*b*
Closure. *See* Repair (closure)
CML. *See* Chronic myelogenous leukemia (CML)
CMS. *See* Centers for Medicare and Medicaid Services (CMS)
CMS-1500, 157, 158*f*, 183*f*
    ICD-10-CM on, 249, 249*f*
    Medicare, 124, 124*f*
CNS. *See* Central nervous system (CNS)
Coarctation of aorta (CoA), 44
Coccygeal vertebrae, 104
Coccyx, 15, 17*f*
Cochlea, 16*f*
Code, if applicable, any causal condition first, ICD-10-CM, 250
Coding
    E/M, 161, 167
    further text resources, 332
    HCPCS, 247
    introduction to CPT, 157
    outpatient, 265–266
    radiology component, 228
Coding tips and links resources, 296
Co-insurance, APC, 138, 140*f*, 153*b*
Coinsurance compliance plan, 128*b*
Cold sores, 11, 79
Collagen, 4*b*
Colles' fracture, 22*b*
Colon, digestive system, 74, 76*f*
Colon, ICD-10-CM, 250
Colonoscopy, 78*b*, 212
Colorectal cancer, 83–84
Colostomy, 78*b*
    takedown, 178*b*
Combined arterial-venous grafting, 204
Combining forms, 324–326
    cardiovascular system, 38*b*
    digestive system, 77*b*
    endocrine system, 97*b*
    female genital system, 48*b*
    hemic and lymphatic system, 89*b*
    integumentary system, 3*b*
    male genital system, 59*b*
    musculoskeletal system, 21*b*
    nervous system, 104*b*
    respiratory system, 28*b*
    senses, 116*b*
    urinary system, 67*b*
Complete fractures, 23
Complex chronic care management services, 171
Complex wound repair, 190
Compliance plan, 153*b*
Complications or comorbidities (CC), 143–144, 147
Comprehensive examination, 164, 164*f*

Comprehensive history, 163
Computed axial tomography (CAT or CT), 228, 229
    cranial, 232*b*
Computers and electronic health record, further text resources on, 333
Concurrent care, 128*b*, 153*b*
Conduction system of heart, 36, 38*f*
    irregularities of, 43
Conductive hearing loss, 120–121
Condyle, 17
Condyloid process, 15*f*
Congenital cataract, 119
Congenital disorders
    cleft lip and cleft palate, 79, 79*f*
    heart, 44
    ICD-10-CM chapter 17, congenital malformations, deformations, and chromosomal abnormalities, 262
    neurologic, 108, 109*f*
    urinary system, 72–73
Congenital heart defects, 44
Congenital neurologic disorders, 108
Congestive heart failure (CHF), 43
Conization, 218
Conjunctiva, 114, 117*b*
Conjunctivitis, 119
Connective tissue, ICD-10-CM chapter 13, diseases of musculoskeletal system and, 259
Conn's syndrome, 101–102
Constrictive pericarditis, 44
Consultant physician, 168
Consultations, pathology and laboratory section, 235
Consultation services, 168
Contact dermatitis
    allergic, 8
    irritant, 8
Content updates, 296
Contraceptives, 335–343*t*
Contralateral, 98*b*
Contrast material, radiology, 208, 228
Contributory factors (CF), 162, 166
Controlled hypertension, 258
Contusion, brain, 111
Conversion factors (anesthesia), 177
Coordination of benefits, 128*b*, 153*b*
Coordination of care, 166
Co-payment, 128*b*, 153*b*
Cordectomy, 30*b*
Cordocentesis, 49*b*
Cornea, 114
Coronal suture, 15*f*
Coronary artery bypass graft (CABG), 204
Coronary artery disease (CAD), 41
Coronoid process, 15*f*
Corpora cavernosa, 59*b*
Cor pulmonale, 33
Corpus uteri, 218
Correct coding initiative, 153*b*
Corrosions, 263

Corrugator supercilii, 19
Costal cartilage, 17*f*
Costochondral joint, 17*f*
Cough, 32
Counseling, 166
    risk factor reduction and behavior change intervention, 170
CPT, 157
    appendices of, 160
    category II codes-supplemental tracking codes, 159
    category III codes-new technology, 160
    CMS-1500 health insurance claim form and, 157, 158*f*
    codes, 157
    format, 157–159
    incorrect coding, 157
    index, 160
    introduction to medical coding, 157
    modifiers add information, 159
    one of two levels of codes, 157
    outpatient physician (non-hospital) services, 157
    sections, 159
    semicolon, 159
    symbols, 157
    two types of code descriptions, 159
    types of codes, 157
    unlisted services, 159
CPT/HCPCS level I modifiers, 180–187
    alternative laboratory platform testing, 183
    anesthesia by surgeon, 181
    assistant surgeon, 182
    assistant surgeon (when qualified resident surgeon not available), 182
    bilateral procedure, 181
    cervical cerclage preoperative examination, 186*b*
    decision for surgery, 181
    discontinued procedure, 181
    distinct procedural service, 181–182
    echocardiogram, 185*b*
    ethmoidectomy, sphenoidotomy, and septoplasty, 186–187*b*
    habilitative services, 183
    increased procedural service, 180
    mandated service, 180
    massive debridement, 184*b*
    minimum assistant surgeon, 182
    modifier functions, 180
    multiple modifiers, 183
    multiple procedure-three types, 181
    nevus excision, 185*b*
    postoperative management only, 181
    preoperative management only, 181
    preventive services, 180–181
    procedure performed on infants less than 4 kg modifier, 182
    professional component, 180
    reduced services, 181
    reference (outside) laboratory, 182

CPT/HCPCS level I modifiers *(Continued)*
  rehabilitative services, 183
  repeat clinical diagnostic laboratory test, 183
  repeat procedure/service by another physician or other qualified health care professional, 182
  repeat procedure/service by same physician or other qualified health care professional, 182
  significant, separately identifiable E/M service, by same physician or other qualified health care professional on the same day of the procedure or other service, 180
  staged/related procedure or service by same physician or other qualified health care professional during postoperative period, 181
  surgical care only, 181
  surgical team, 182
  synchronous telemedicine services, 183
  two surgeons, 182
  unplanned return to operating/procedure room by the same physician or other qualified health care professional following initial procedure for a related procedure during postoperative period, 182
  unrelated E/M services by same physician or other qualified health care professional during a postoperative period, 180
  unrelated procedure or service by same physician or other qualified health care professional during postoperative period, 182
  unusual anesthesia, 180
Crackle, 30*b*
Cranial bones, 14–15
Cranial computed tomography, 232*b*
Cranial muscles, 20*f*
Cranial nerves, 104
  tumor, 112
  VIII, 16*f*
Craniectomy, 105*b*, 223
Craniotomy, 105*b*, 223
Cranium, 103–104, 105*b*
Creatinine clearance, 69–70
Cretinism, 100–101
Critical care services, 169
CRNA. *See* Certified Registered Nurse Anesthetist (CRNA)
Crohn's disease, 82
Cross references, ICD-10-CM alphabetic index, 250
Croup, 30*b*
Crust, 5, 6*f*
Cryptorchidism, 60
CSF. *See* Cerebrospinal fluid (CSF)
CT. *See* Computed axial tomography (CAT or CT)

Curettage, 49*b*
Cushing syndrome, 101
Custodial care services, 169
Cutdown, 39*b*
CVA. *See* Cerebrovascular accident (CVA)
Cystic duct, 74–76
Cystitis
  bacterial, 70
  non-bacterial, 70
Cystocele, 49*b*
Cystolithectomy, 68*b*
Cystometrogram, 68*b*
Cystoplasty, 68*b*
Cystorrhaphy, 68*b*
Cystoscopy, 68*b*
Cystostomy, 68*b*
Cystotomy, 68*b*, 214*b*
Cystourethrogram, neonatal, 233*b*
Cystourethroplasty, 68*b*
Cystourethroscopy, 68*b*
Cysts, pilonidal, 190
Cytogenetic studies, pathology and laboratory section, 236
Cytopathology, pathology and laboratory section, 236

D

Dacryocystitis, 117*b*
Dacryostenosis, 117*b*
Data quality, 150–151, 150*f*
Data reviewed, 164
Debridement, 4*b*
  ICD-10-CM chapter 20, external causes of morbidity, 263
  massive, 184*b*
  skin, subcutaneous, and accessory structures, 189, 195*b*
Decision for surgery modifier, 181
Decubitus ulcers, 7, 7*f*, 191
Deductible, 128*b*, 153*b*
Deep inguinal nodes, 90*f*
Deformations, ICD-10-CM chapter 17, congenital malformations, deformations, and chromosomal abnormalities, 262
Dehydration, ICD-10-CM chapter 4, endocrine, nutritional, and metabolic diseases, 257
Delayed flap, 4*b*
Delivery, 49*b*
  cesarean, 49*b*, 222*b*
  E/M codes, 170
  global package and, 219
  twins, 220
  vaginal, 55
  See also Childbirth
Deltoideus, 19*f*, 20*f*
Deltoids, 20
Dementias, 106–108
Dendrites, 103, 103*f*
Denial, 128*b*, 153*b*

Department of Health and Human Services (DHHS), 123, 125, 135
Depression, 108
Dermabrasion, 4*b*, 191
Dermatitis
  allergic contact, 8
  atopic, 7–8
  diaper, 10
  irritant, 7
  irritant contact, 8
  seborrheic, 8
Dermatologic procedures, special, 243
Dermatologist, 4*b*
Dermatoplasty, 4*b*
Dermis, 2, 2*f*
Descending colon, 76*f*
Destruction
  lungs and pleura, 203
  nose, 201
  skin, subcutaneous, and accessory structures, 192
  vulva, perineum, and introitus, 217
Detached retina, 119
Detailed examination, 164, 164*f*
Detailed history, 163
Device-dependent procedures, 141
Diabetes insipidus, 100
Diabetes mellitus, 99–102, 99*f*
  gestational, 99
  ICD-10-CM chapter 4, endocrine, nutritional, and metabolic diseases, 256–257
  insulin-dependent, 99
  non-insulin-dependent, 99, 99*f*
Diagnosis and services, ICD-10-CM, 254
Diagnosis-related groups, 153*b*
Diagnostic radiology subsection, 229
Diagnostic ultrasound subsection, 230
Dialysis, 240–241
  catheter replacement, 210*b*
  renal dialysis progress note, 246*b*
Diaper dermatitis, 10
Diaphragm, 20, 28*f*, 76*f*, 87–88, 87*f*, 209
  lymphatic system and, 90*f*
Diaphragmatic hernia, 80
Diarrhea, 172*b*
Diarthrosis, 17
Diastole, 38
Diencephalon, 103
Digestive system, 74–86, 76*f*
  accessory organs, 74–76
  anatomy and terminology, 74–76, 78–79
  combining forms, 77*b*
  esophageal disorders, 79–80
  esophagus, 28*f*, 74
  gallbladder disorders, 85
  ICD-10-CM chapter 11, diseases of digestive system, 259
  intestinal disorders, 81–84
  large intestine, 74
  liver disorders, 84–85
  medical abbreviations, 77*b*

Digestive system (Continued)
    medical terms, 78b
    mouth, 74, 75f, 115
    oral cavity disorders, 79
    pancreas disorders, 85–86
    pathophysiology, 79–86
    peritoneum, 76
    pharynx or throat, 27, 74
    quiz, 78–79, 86
    salivary glands, 74, 76f
    small intestine, 74
    stomach, 74
    stomach and duodenum disorders, 80–81
    suffixes, 77b
    teeth, 74
Digestive system subsection, 212–213
    cystotomy, 214b
    endoscopy, 212
    gastrojejunostomy placement, 213b
    hemorrhoidectomy and fistulectomy,
        212–213
    hernia codes, 213
    laparoscopy and endoscopy, 212
    orogastric tube placement, 213b
    pyloroplasty, 215b
    small-bowel anastomosis, 214–215b
Dilated cardiomyopathy, 44
Dilation, 49b, 68b
Dilation and curettage (D&C), 56, 220
Diphtheria, 239–240
Diplopia, 118
Discectomy, 105b
Discharge, 168, 169
Discontinued procedure modifier, 181
Discounting, 141
Dislocation, 22b, 24, 196
Distinct procedural service modifier,
    181–182
Diverticulitis, 83
Diverticulosis, 83
Diverticulum, 78b
DME. See Durable medical equipment
    (DME)
Documentation, 128b, 153b
Domiciliary, rest home
    or custodial care services, 169
    or home care plan oversight services, 169
Dorsal surface, tongue, 75f
Drainage, 30b
    See also Incision and drainage
Drug assay, pathology and laboratory
    section, 234
Drugs and chemicals, ICD-10-CM table of,
    251–252, 251f
DUB. See Dysfunctional uterine bleeding
    (DUB)
Duodenum, 74, 76f
    disorders of, 82
Durable medical equipment (DME), 128b,
    154b
Dura mater, 104
Dwarfism, 99, 100f

Dysfunctional uterine bleeding (DUB), 51
Dysmenorrhea, 50, 51
Dysphagia, 78b
Dysphoria, 30b
Dyspnea, 30b
Dysuria, 68b

E
Ear
    auditory system subsection, 225
    external, 16f, 114
    hearing, three divisions of, 114–115
    hearing loss, 120–121
    ICD-10-CM chapter 8, diseases of ear
        and mastoid process, 257
    infections of, 120
    inner, 16f, 115
    middle, 15, 16f, 114–115
    otitis externa, 120
    otorhinolaryngologic services, medicine
        section, 241
Echocardiogram, 185b
Echocardiography, 207
Eclampsia, 54
Ectopic, 49b
Ectopic pregnancy, 55, 56f
Ectropion, 117b
EDD. See Estimated date of delivery
    (EDD)
Edema, 39b
EDI. See Electronic data interchange (EDI)
EIN. See Employer identification number
    (EIN)
Ejaculatory duct, 58, 58f
Electrocautery, 4b
Electrode, 39b
Electroencephalography, 105b
Electronic analysis, 208
Electronic data interchange (EDI), 128b,
    154b
Electrophysiologic operative procedures,
    204
Electrophysiology, 39b, 203
E/M. See Evaluation and management
    (E/M) section
Embolectomy, 39b, 205
Embolism, 42
Emergency department services, 168–169
Emphysema, 30b, 33
Employer identification number (EIN),
    128b, 154b
Empyema, 33
Encephalitis, 110
Encounter form superbill, 128b, 154b
Endarterectomy, 39b
Endocardium, 35
Endocrine glands, 96–97, 97f
Endocrine system, 96–102
    anatomy and terminology, 96–99
    combining forms, 97b
    diabetes mellitus, 99–102, 99f, 256–257

Endocrine system (Continued)
    endocrine glands, 96–97, 97f
    ICD-10-CM chapter 4, endocrine,
        nutritional, and metabolic diseases,
        256–257
    medical terms, 98b
    parathyroid disorders, 101
    pathophysiology, 99–102, 99f
    pituitary disorders, 99–100, 100f
    prefixes, 98b
    quiz, 98–99, 102
    suffixes, 98b
    thyroid disorders, 100–101, 100f
Endocrine system subsection, 223
    thyroid gland, excision category, 223
Endometrial cancer, 53
Endometriosis, 51
Endometrium, 46, 47f
    repair phase, 46
Endopyelotomy, 68b
Endoscopy, 22b, 198, 212
    larynx, 202
    nose, 201
    trachea and bronchi, 202
    vagina, 218
    vulva, perineum, and introitus, 217
Endotracheal anesthesia, 176
Endovascular repair
    of abdominal aortic aneurysm, 205
    of descending thoracic aorta, 204
    of iliac aneurysm, 205
Endovascular revascularization, 206
End stage renal disease physician services,
    240–241
Enterolysis, 78b
Entropion, 117b
Enucleation, 117b
Enzymes, 335–343t
EOB. See Explanation of benefits (EOB)
Eosinophilia, 93
Eosinophils, 35
Ependymal cells, 103
Ependymoma, 112
Epicardial, 39b
Epicardium, 35
Epidermis, 2, 2f
Epidermolysis, 4b
Epidermomycosis, 4b
Epididymectomy, 59b
Epididymis, 58, 58f, 59b
    disorders of, 60–62
Epididymitis, 60
Epididymovasostomy, 59b
Epidural anesthesia, 176
Epiglottidectomy, 30b
Epiglottis, 28f, 74, 75f, 76f
Epilepsies, 110–111
Episclera, 117b
Episiotomies, 220
Epispadias, 62
Epistaxis, 30b
Epithelial tumors, 54

Epithelium, 4b
Eponyms, ICD-10-CM alphabetic index, 250
Epstein-Barr virus, 93
Erosion, 6, 6f
Erysipelas, 10–11
Erythema, 4b
Erythrocytes, 35
Escharotomy, 4b
Esophagitis, 80
Esophagogastroduodenoscopy, 212
Esophagogastroscopy, 212
Esophagoscopy, 212
Esophagus, 28f, 74, 76f
    cancer of, 80
    disorders of, 79–80
    esophagitis, 80
    gastroesophageal reflux disease (GERD), 80
    hernias, 80, 80f
    scleroderma, 79–80
Established patient, 161, 167
Estimated date of delivery (EDD), 47
Estrogen hypersecretion, 102
Ethics, ICD-10-CM, 249
Ethmoid bone, 15, 15f, 16f
Ethmoidectomy, 186–187b
Etiology and manifestation of disease,
    ICD-10-CM alphabetic index, 250
Eustachian tube, 16f, 225
Evacuation abortion, 56
Evaluation and management (E/M) section,
    161–175
    advance care planning, 171
    care management services, 171
    care plan oversight services, 169–170
    case management services, 169
    chief complaint (CC), 162
    clinic visit, diarrhea, 172b
    consultation services, 168
    contributory factors (CF), 162, 166
    counseling risk factor reduction and
        behavior change intervention, 170
    critical care services, 169
    domiciliary, rest home
        or custodial care services, 169
        or home care plan oversight services, 169
    emergency department services, 168–169
    E/M levels divided based on, 161–162
    final status of patient, 168
    four elements of history, 162
    four examination levels, 164, 164f
    four history levels, 163, 163f
    four levels of medical decision making
        (MDM) complexity, 166, 166f
    history of present illness (HPI), 162
    home services, 169
    hospital inpatient services, 168
    hospital observation status, 167–168
    inpatient neonatal intensive care services
        and neonatal critical care services,
        170–171
    integral factors when selecting E/M
        codes, 161

Evaluation and management (E/M) section
    (Continued)
    key components (KC), 161, 162
    levels of 992022-99215 based only on, 161
    levels of E/M service based on, 161
    levels of presenting problem, 167
    medical decision making (MDM)
        complexity, 164
    newborn care, 170
    NICU progress note, ventilator assist, 175b
    non-face-to-face services, 170
    nursing facility services, 169
    other E/M services, 171
    past, family, and/or social history
        (PFSH), 162–163
    patient status, 161
    physician and patient dialogue, 162–171
    place of service, 161
    preventive medicine services, 170
    progress note, acute and chronic renal
        failure, 172b
    prolonged services, 169
    psychiatric collaborative care
        management services, 171
    review of systems (ROS), 162
    selection of level of E/M services,
        167–171
    special E/M services, 170
    time, 167
    transitional care management services, 171
    type of service, 161
    use of E/M code, 167
    vomiting, 173b
    well-child check, 174b
Eventration, 78b
Eversion, 19
Evisceration, 78b
Evocative/suppression testing, pathology
    and laboratory section, 235
Examination levels, four, 164, 164f
Examinations
    facility-based, 293–294
    final, 272, 274
    format A, 274
    physician-based, 271–291
    pre- and post-, 271–272
Exam review, 296
Excessive skin excision, 191
Excision
    bone and muscle biopsies, 196
    bone tumor, 200b
    breast wide, 193–194b
    cervix uteri, 218
    cheek lesion, 193b
    corpus uteri, 218
    excessive skin, 191
    labial, 223b
    larynx, 202
    lungs and pleura, 202
    mass, bursa, 200b
    maternity care and delivery subsection, 219
    nevus, 185b

Excision (Continued)
    nose, 201
    penis, 217
    renal tumor, 220–221b
    skin, subcutaneous, and accessory
        structures, 189
    spur, 198–199b
    thyroid, 223
    trachea and bronchi, 202
    vulva, perineum, and introitus, 217
Excisional biopsy, 193
Excludes, ICD-10-CM, 250
Exenteration, 117b
Exophthalmos, 117b
Exostosis, 117b
Expanded problem-focused examination,
    164, 164f
Expanded problem-focused history, 163
Expiration, 27
Explanation of benefits (EOB), 128b, 154b
Exstrophy, 78b
Extension, 19
Extensor digitorum longus, 20f, 21
Extensor hallucis longus tendon, 20f
Extensors, wrist and finger, 19f, 20f
External acoustic meatus, 15f
External ear, 16f, 114
External fixation, 22b, 196–197
External intercostals, 20
External obliques, 20
External occipital protuberance, 15f
Extracorporeal, 68b
Extracorporeal life support services, 204
Extracorporeal membrane oxygenation, 204
Extracranial nerves, 224
Eye
    cataract, 117b, 119–120, 224
    detached retina, 119
    eye and ocular adnexa subsection, 224
    glaucoma, 120
    ICD-10-CM chapter 7, diseases of eye
        and adnexa, 257
    infections, 119
    layers of, 114, 115f
    macular degeneration, 119
    ophthalmology, medicine section, 241
    visual disturbances, 118–119
Eye and ocular adnexa subsection
    cataracts, 224
    eyelids, 224
Eyelids, 224

F
Face
    bones of, 15
    muscles of, 19, 20f
Face presentation of fetus, 56f
Facility-based examinations, 293–294
    final examination, 294
    pre-examination and post-examination,
        293–294

Facility-based reimbursement, 133–155
    abbreviations, 152*b*
    ambulatory payment classifications
        (APCs), 137–138
    data quality, 150–151, 150*f*
    facility responsibility, 133
    Federal Register, 136–137, 136*f*
    hospital-acquired conditions (HAC),
        149–150
    managed health care, 152
    Medicare, 133–137
    Medicare Severity Diagnosis-Related
        Groups (MS-DRGs), 142–147
    National Correct Coding Initiative
        (NCCI), 137
    population change=reimbursement
        change, 133
    post acute transfer, 147
    Present On Admission indicator (POA),
        148–149
    Prospective Payment Systems (PPS), 137
    quiz, 152
    revenue codes, 150
    terminology, 153–154*b*
Facility indicators, pathology and laboratory
    section, 234
Fallopian tubes, 46, 47*f*, 218
    cancer of, 54
False aneurysm, 39*b*
False or pseudoaneurysm, 42
False ribs, 15
Family history, 162
Fascial sling arthroplasty, 199*b*
Fasciectomy, 22*b*
Fasciocutaneous flaps, 191
Federal Register, 125, 126*f*, 136–137, 136*f*
Fee schedule, 128*b*, 154*b*
Female genital system, 46–57
    accessory organs, 46, 47*f*
    anatomy and terminology, 46–47, 47*f*, 50
    benign lesions, 52
    combining forms, 48*b*
    infection, inflammation, and sexually
        transmitted diseases, 51–52
    malignant lesions, 53–54
    medical abbreviations, 49*b*
    medical terms, 49*b*
    menstrual and hormonal disorders, 50–51
    menstruation, 46–47
    pathophysiology, 50–56
    prefixes, 48*b*
    quiz, 50, 57
    suffixes, 48*b*
    See also Pregnancy
Female genital system subsection, 217–218
    cervix uteri, 218
    corpus uteri, 218
    ovary, 218
    oviduct/ovary, 218
    vagina, 217–218
    in vitro fertilization, 218
    vulva, perineum, and introitus, 217

Femoral hernia, 213
Femur, 15–16, 18*f*
Fenestration, 117*b*
Fetal invasive services, 219
Fibrillation, 43
Fibroids, uterine, 52
Fibula, 15–16, 18*f*
Filiform papillae, 75*f*
Fimbriae, 47*f*
Final examination, 272, 274
Final status of patient, 168
Fissure, 4*b*, 6, 6*f*, 22*b*
Fistula, 39*b*
Fistulectomy, 212–213
Flaps, 191–193, 194*b*
Flat bones, 14
Flexion, 19
Flexor retinaculum, 20*f*
Flexors, wrist and finger, 20*f*
Floating ribs, 15
Floor of mouth, 74
Fluids, eye, 114
Flutter, 43
Focal seizures, 110–111
Follicle-stimulating hormone (FSH), 96
Folliculitis, 10
Follow-up days (FUD), 128*b*, 154*b*
Foramen cecum, 75*f*
Foraminotomy, 227*b*
Forceps, 220
Foreign body removal, respiratory system
    subsection, 201
Foreskin, 58*f*
Format
    CPT, 157–159
    HCPCS, 247
    ICD-10-CM, 249–250
Fractures, 22*b*, 23–24
    classification of, 23–24
    ICD-10-CM chapter 20, external causes
        of morbidity, 263
    treatment, 22*b*, 196
Fraud and abuse, Medicare, 127, 151
Free full-thickness graft, 4*b*
Frontal bone, 14–15, 15*f*, 16*f*
Frontal lobe, 104
FSH. *See* Follicle-stimulating hormone (FSH)
FUD. *See* Follow-up days (FUD)
Fulguration, 78*b*
Full-thickness grafts, 191
Fundoplasty, 68*b*
Fundus
    stomach, 74
    uterus, 46, 47*f*
Fungal infections, 11–12
Fungiform papillae, 75*f*
Furuncles, 4*b*, 10

G

Gallbladder, 74–76, 76*f*
    disorders of, 85

Gallbladder ultrasound, 232*b*
Gallstones, 85, 85*f*
Ganglion, 22*b*
Gastric cancer, 81
Gastritis, 80–81
Gastrocnemius, 19*f*, 20*f*, 21
Gastrocnemius tendon, 19*f*
Gastroenterology, 241
Gastroesophageal reflux disease (GERD),
    80
Gastrointestinal, 78*b*
Gastrojejunostomy placement, 213*b*
Gastroplasty, 78*b*
Gastrostomy, 78*b*
General anesthesia, 176
Generalized seizures, 111
Genetic counseling, medicine section, 242
Genital herpes, 52
Genital warts, 52
Genitourinary system, ICD-10-CM chapter
    14, diseases of, 259–260
Geometric Mean Length of Stay (GMLOS),
    147
GERD. *See* Gastroesophageal reflux disease
    (GERD)
Germ cell tumors, 112
Gestation, 47, 219
Gestational diabetes mellitus, 99
GH. *See* Growth hormone (GH)
Gigantism, 99, 100*f*
Glabella, 15*f*, 16*f*
Gland(s)
    adrenal, 96, 97*f*, 101–102
    endocrine, 96–97, 97*f*
    parathyroid, 91*b*, 96, 97*f*, 101
    pineal, 97, 97*f*
    pituitary, 96, 97*f*, 99–100, 100*f*
    prostate, 58, 58*f*, 63–64
    salivary, 74, 76*f*
    sebaceous, 3
    sudoriferous, 3
    thymus, 96–97, 97*f*
    thyroid, 96, 97*f*, 100–101, 100*f*
Glaucoma, 117*b*, 120
Glia, 103
Glioblastoma, 111
Gliomas, 111–112
Global package and delivery, 219
Glomerular disorders, 71
Glomerulonephritis, 71
Glottis, 30*b*
Gluteus maximus, 19*f*, 20
Gluteus medius, 20
Gluteus minimus, 20
Goiter, 100–101, 100*f*
Gonadal stromal tumors, 54
Gonorrhea, 52
Gout, 25
    ICD-10-CM chapter 4, endocrine,
        nutritional, and metabolic
        diseases, 257
GPN. *See* Group provider number (GPN)

Gracilis, 19*f*, 21
Grafts
  musculoskeletal system subsection, 197
  noncoronary bypass, 205
  skin, 191–193, 191*f*
Granulocytosis, 93
Graves' disease, 100
Group provider number (GPN), 128*b*, 154*b*
Growth hormone (GH), 96
Guidance for vascular access, 206
Guillain-Barré syndrome, 108
Gums, 75*f*
Gustatory sense, 115

H

Habilitative services modifier, 183
HAC. *See* Hospital-acquired conditions (HAC)
Hamstring muscles, 21
Hard palate, 28*f*, 75*f*
Hashimoto's thyroiditis, 101
Haustra, 76*f*
HAV. *See* Hepatitis A (HAV)
HBV. *See* Hepatitis B (HBV)
HCG. *See* Human chorionic gonadotropin (HCG)
HCPCS coding, 157, 247
  format, 247
  level II modifiers, 159
  national level II index, 247
  one of two levels of codes, 157, 247
  table of drugs, 247
  temporary codes, 247
HCPCS level II modifiers, 183–184
  examples, 183
  for selective identification of subsets of distinct procedural services, 183–184
HCV. *See* Hepatitis C (HCV)
HDV. *See* Hepatitis D (HDV)
Head
  muscles of, 19–20
  trauma to, 111
  ultrasound of, 233*b*
Health behavior assessment and intervention, 242
Health Insurance Portability and Accountability Act of 1996 (HIPAA), 123, 125, 133
Health maintenance organization (HMO), 127, 128*b*, 152
Health status, ICD-10-CM chapter 21, factors influencing health status and contact with health services, 263–264
Hearing, 114–115
  loss of, 120–121
Heart, 35–36, 37*f*
  cardiac muscle, 18
  chamber walls, 35
  conduction system, 36, 38*f*
  disorders of, 43
  four chambers, 35

Heart *(Continued)*
  heart wall disorders, 44
  major blood vessels, 36
  pericardium, 36
  septa, 35–36
  valves, 36
  vascular disorders of, 41–43, 41*f*
Heartbeat, 38
Heart block, 43
Heart disease
  ICD-10-CM chapter 9, diseases of circulatory system, 257
  valvular, 43–44
Heart disorders, 43
  abnormal heart rhythms, 43
  congenital, 44
  congestive heart failure (CHF), 43
  heart wall disorders, 44
  infective endocarditis, 43
  pericarditis, 43
  rheumatic fever/rheumatic heart disease, 43
  valvular heart disease, 43–44
Heart/pericardium, cardiovascular in surgery section, 203–204
Heart wall disorders, 44
Heat cataract, 119
Helicobacter pylori, 81
Hemangioblastoma, 112
Hematology and coagulation, pathology and laboratory section, 235
Hematoma, 4*b*, 39*b*
  anesthesia for intracerebral, 179*b*
  cerebral, 111, 238*b*
  intracerebral, 225*b*
Hematopoietic organ, 89
Hematopoietic progenitor cell (HPC), 209
Hemic and lymphatic system, 89–95, 90*f*
  anatomy and terminology, 89, 91–92
  anemia, 92–93
  basophilia, 93
  chronic lymphocytic leukemia (CLL), 94
  combining forms, 89*b*
  eosinophilia, 93
  granulocytosis, 93
  hematopoietic organ, 89
  infectious mononucleosis, 93
  leukemia, 93–94
  leukocytopenia, 93
  leukocytosis, 93
  lymph, 89
  lymphadenopathy, 94
  lymph organs, 89
  lymph vessels, 89
  malignant lymphoma, 94
  medical terms, 91*b*
  monocytosis, 93
  myeloma, 95
  pathophysiology, 92–95
  prefixes, 89*b*
  quiz, 91–92, 95
  suffixes, 91*b*

Hemic and lymphatic system subsection, 208–209
  divisions, 208
  general, 209
  lymph nodes and lymphatic channels subheading, 209
  spleen subheading, 208
Hemispheres, brain, 104
Hemodialysis service, 240
Hemolysis, 39*b*
Hemolytic anemia, 92
Hemopoietic medications, 335–343*t*
Hemoptysis, 30*b*, 32
Hemorrhage, nasal, 201
Hemorrhoidectomy, 212–213
Hepatic duct, 74–76
Hepatitis, viral, 84–85
Hepatitis A (HAV), 84
Hepatitis B (HBV), 84
Hepatitis C (HCV), 84
Hepatitis D (HDV), 84
Hepatitis E (HEV), 84
Hepatitis G, 84
Hernia, 213
  hiatal, 78*b*, 80, 80*f*
Herpes simplex
  canker sore, 79
  cold sores, 11, 79
Herpes simplex 2, 52
Herpes zoster, 11
HEV. *See* Hepatitis E (HEV)
HHPPS. *See* Home Health Prospective Payment System (HHPPS)
Hiatal hernia, 78*b*, 80
High-complexity MDM, 166
High-severity presenting problem, 167
History, four elements of, 162
History levels, four, 163, 163*f*
History of present illness (HPI), 162
HMO. *See* Health maintenance organization (HMO)
Hodgkin disease, 94
Home care plan oversight services, 169
Home Health Prospective Payment System (HHPPS), 149
Home services, 169
Homograft, 4*b*
Hordeolum, 117*b*, 119
Hormone(s), 98*b*, 335–343*t*
  androgen, 102
  estrogen, 102
  female genital system disorders of, 50–51
  human chorionic gonadotropin (HCG), 47
  ovaries and, 46
  parathyroid, 101
  pituitary gland, 96
Hospital-acquired conditions (HAC), 149–150
Hospital discharge services, 168
Hospital inpatient services, 168
Hospital observation status, 167–168

Hospital outpatient, 154b

Hospital payment monitoring system (HPMS), 154b

HPC. See Hematopoietic progenitor cell (HPC)

HPI. See History of present illness (HPI)

HPMS. See Hospital payment monitoring system (HPMS)

HTN. See Hypertension (HTN)

Human chorionic gonadotropin (HCG), 47, 97

Human immunodeficiency syndrome (HIV)
ICD-10-CM chapter 1, certain infectious and parasitic diseases, 255
Kaposi's sarcoma and, 13

Humerus, 16, 18f

Huntington's disease, 107

Hydatidiform mole, 55

Hydration, therapeutic, prophylactic, diagnostic injections and infusions, and chemotherapy and other highly complex drug or highly complex biologic agent administration, medicine section, 242–243

Hydrocele, 61, 61f, 68b

Hydrocephalus, 108

Hydromyelia, 109f

Hydronephrosis, 72

Hymen, 46

Hyoid bone, 15

Hypercapnia, 32

Hyperaldosteronism, 101–102

Hyperbilirubinemia, 84

Hypercortisolism, 101

Hyperextension, 19

Hyperopia, 117b, 118

Hyperparathyroidism, 101

Hyperpituitarism, 99, 100

Hypertension (HTN), 41, 41f
controlled, 258
ICD-10-CM chapter 9, diseases of circulatory system, 257, 258
pulmonary, 258
secondary, 258
transient, 258
uncontrolled, 258

Hypertensive cerebrovascular disease for secondary pulmonary hypertension, 258

Hypertensive chronic kidney disease, 257–258

Hypertensive crisis, 258

Hypertensive heart and chronic kidney disease, 258

Hypertensive retinopathy, 258

Hyperthermia, 231

Hyperthyroidism, 100

Hypertrophic cardiomyopathy, 44

Hypertrophy of right ventricle, 44

Hyperventilation, 32

Hypodermis, 2, 2f

Hypomenorrhea, 51

Hypoparathyroidism, 101

Hypopituitarism, 99

Hypospadias, 62

Hypotension, 41–42

Hypothalamus, 97, 103, 104f

Hypothyroidism, 100–101

Hypoventilation, 32

Hypoxemia, 32, 39b

Hypoxia, 32, 39b

Hysterectomy, 49b, 221–222b

Hysterorrhaphy, 49b

Hysteroscopy, 49b, 218

I

IBD. See Inflammatory bowel disease (IBD)

ICD-10-CM
abbreviations, 250
alphabetic index, 249, 250
and/with, 250
chapter 1, certain infectious and parasitic diseases, 255
chapter 2, neoplasms, 256
chapter 3, diseases of the blood and blood-forming organs and certain disorders involving the immune mechanism, 256
chapter 4, endocrine, nutritional, and metabolic diseases, 256–257
chapter 5, mental, behavioral, and neurodevelopmental disorders, 257
chapter 6, diseases of nervous system, 257
chapter 7, diseases of eye and adnexa, 257
chapter 8, diseases of ear and mastoid process, 257
chapter 9, diseases of circulatory system, 257–258
chapter 10, diseases of respiratory system, 258
chapter 11, diseases of digestive system, 259
chapter 12, diseases of skin and subcutaneous tissue, 259
chapter 13, diseases of musculoskeletal system and connective tissue, 259
chapter 14, diseases of genitourinary system, 259–260
chapter 15, pregnancy, childbirth, and the puerperium, 261
chapter 16, certain conditions originating in the perinatal period, 261–262
chapter 17, congenital malformations, deformations, and chromosomal abnormalities, 262
chapter 18, symptoms, signs, and abnormal clinical and laboratory findings, not elsewhere classified, 262

ICD-10-CM (Continued)
chapter 19, injury, poisoning, and certain other consequences of external causes, 262
chapter 20, external causes of morbidity, 262–263
chapter 21, factors influencing health status and contact with health services, 263–264
on CMS-1500, 249, 249f
code, if applicable, any causal condition first, 250
colon, 250
diagnosis and services, 254
diagnosis codes, 157
ethics, 249
format, 249–250
general guidelines, 253
includes, excludes, use additional code, 250
introduction to, 249
italicized type, 250
late effects (sequela), 254
OGCR Section IV, diagnostic coding and reporting guidelines for outpatient services, 265–266
overview of, 249–252
parentheses, 250
placeholder, 249
punctuation, 250
7th character, 249
steps to diagnosis coding, 253–254
table of drugs and chemicals, 251–252, 251f
table of neoplasms, 251, 251f
tabular list, 249, 252
using, 249, 253–254

ICD-10-PCS, 267–269
alphabetic index, 267
bundling, 268
guidelines, 267–268
index, 267
table of contents, 267
tabular list, 267, 268f, 269f

Ichthyosis, 4b

Idiopathic polyneuritis, 108

IHD. See Ischemic heart disease (IHD)

Ileostomy, 78b

Ileum, 74, 76f
Meckel's diverticulum, 82

Iliac nodes, 90f

Iliopsoas, 21

Iliotibial tract, 19f

Ilium, 15, 18f

Imbrication, 78b

Immune enhancers, 335–343t

Immune globulins, 239

Immune system, ICD-10-CM chapter 3, diseases of the blood and blood-forming organs and certain disorders involving the immune mechanism, 256

Immunizations, 239
  active, 239
  administration of, 239
  passive, 239
  See also Vaccines
Immunology, pathology and laboratory
    section, 235
Impetigo, 10
Implantable, insertable, and wearable
    cardiac device evaluations, 207
Implantable defibrillator, 39*b*, 203–204
Improper union, 24
Incarcerated, 78*b*
Incise, 4*b*
Incisional biopsy, 193
Incision and drainage
  lungs and pleura, 202
  nose, 201
  skin, subcutaneous, and accessory
      structures, 189
  trachea and bronchi, 202
  vulva, perineum, and introitus, 217
Includes, ICD-10-CM, 250
Incomplete abortion, 56, 220
Incomplete fractures, 23
Increased procedural service modifier, 180
Incus, 15, 16*f*
Index
  CPT, 160
  ICD-10-CM, 250
  ICD-10-PCS, 267
Induced abortion, 220
Infections
  appendicitis, 82, 177–178*b*
  bone, 24
  ear, 120
  encephalitis, 110
  eye, 119
  female genital system, 51–52
  helicobacter pylori, 81
  hepatitis, 84–85
  ICD-10-CM chapter 1, certain infectious
      and parasitic diseases, 255
  ICD-10-CM chapter 10, diseases of
      respiratory system, 258
  ICD-10-CM chapter 20, external causes
      of morbidity, 263
  infectious arthropathies, 259
  infectious mononucleosis, 93
  mouth, 79
  Reye's syndrome associated with, 110
  skin, 10–12
  upper respiratory, 33
  urinary tract, 70–71
Infectious arthritis, 25
Infective endocarditis, 43
Inferior concha, 16*f*
Inferior vena cava, 36
Inflammatory bowel disease (IBD), 82
Inflammatory disorders
  appendicitis, 82, 177–178*b*
  diverticulitis, 83

Inflammatory disorders *(Continued)*
  esophagitis, 80
  female genital system, 51–52
  gallbladder, 85
  gastritis, 80–81
  infective endocarditis, 43
  inflammatory bowel disease (IBD), 82
  integumentary system, 7–10
  pancreatitis, 85–86
  pericarditis, 43
  peritonitis, 82
  thrombophlebitis, 42
  ulcerative colitis, 83, 83*f*
Influenza vaccine, 240
Infraorbital foramen, 16*f*
Infraspinatus, 19*f*
Infundibulum, 47*f*
Infusion, 242–243
Ingestion challenge testing, 241
Inguinal hernia, 213
Inguinofemoral, 91*b*
Initial and continuing intensive care
    services, 170–171
Initial hospital care, 168
Initial nursing facility assessment, 169
Initial observation care, 168
Injection
  anesthetic agent, 224
  hydration, therapeutic, prophylactic,
      diagnostic injections and infusions,
      and chemotherapy and other highly
      complex drug or highly complex
      biologic agent administration,
      242–243
  intra-amniotic, 56, 220
  steroid, 198*b*
  vascular injection procedures, 205–206
Injuries
  burn, 191–192, 263
  cerebral hematoma, 111, 179*b*, 238*b*
  ICD-10-CM chapter 7, diseases of eye
      and adnexa, 257
  ICD-10-CM chapter 19, injury,
      poisoning, and certain other
      consequences of external causes, 262
  musculoskeletal system, 23–24
  spinal cord, 111
Inner ear, 16*f*, 115
Inpatient, 154*b*, 167–168
  ICD-10-PCS, reporting inpatient
      procedures, 267–269
  noncovered hospital expenses, 135
Inpatient neonatal and pediatric critical
    care, 170
Inpatient neonatal intensive care services
    and neonatal critical care services,
    170–171
Inpatient-only procedures with status
    indicator "C," 141
Inpatient Psychiatric Facility (IPF), 150
Inpatient Rehabilitation Facility (IRF), 150
Insertion, venous access, 206

Inspiration, 27
Insula lobe, 104
Insulin, 76
Insulin-dependent diabetes mellitus, 99
Insurance, further text resources on, 334
Integumentary system, 2–13
  anatomy and terminology, 2–3
  combining forms, 3*b*
  epidermis and dermis, 2
  glands, 3
  inflammatory disorders, 7–10
  layers, 2, 2*f*
  lesions and other abnormalities, 5–7, 6*f*
  medical abbreviations, 3*b*
  medical terms, 4*b*
  nails, 2–3
  pathophysiology, 5–13
  prefixes, 3*b*
  quiz, 4–5, 13
  skin infections, 10–12
  skin tumors, 12–13
  special dermatologic procedures,
      medicine section, 243
  suffixes, 3*b*
Integumentary system subsection, 189–193
  adjacent tissue transfer, flaps, and grafts,
      191–193, 191*f*
  excision, cheek lesion, 193*b*
  introduction, 190
  minimal debridement, 195*b*
  nails, 190
  pilonidal cyst, 190
  right breast wide excision, 193–194*b*
  skin, subcutaneous, and accessory
      structures, 189–190
  thenar flap coverage, 194*b*
Intercostals, 20
Intercostal space, 17*f*
Intermediate wound repair, 190
Internal fixation, 22*b*
Internal intercostals, 20
Internal jugular and subclavian trunks, 90*f*
Internal obliques, 20
Intersex surgery subsection, 217
Interventional radiologist, 228–229
Intestines
  disorders of, 81–84
  large, 74, 83–84
  small, 74, 81–83
Intra-amniotic injections, 56, 220
Intracardiac, 39*b*
Intracardiac electrophysiologic procedures/
    studies, 208
Intracerebral hematoma, 225*b*
Intracoronary brachytherapy, 207
Intramural, 30*b*
Intramural destruction, 201
Intravenous hydration, 242–243
Introduction and removal
  anesthetic agent, 224
  bone and muscle, 196–197
  central venous access device, 206

Introduction and removal (Continued)
  cervical dilator, 219
  corpus uteri, 218
  kidney, 216
  larynx, 202
  lens, 224
  lesion injections, 190
  lungs and pleura, 202, 203
  nose, 201
  penis, 217
  skin, subcutaneous, and accessory
    structures, 189
  trachea and bronchi, 202
  vagina, 217–218
Introitus, 49b, 217
Intubation, 30b
Intussusception, 78b
Invalid claim, 128b, 154b
Invasive, 39b
Inversion, 19
In vitro fertilization, 218
IPF. See Inpatient Psychiatric Facility (IPF)
IRF. See Inpatient Rehabilitation Facility
  (IRF)
Iron deficiency anemia, 92
Irregular bones, 14
Irreversible ischemia, 41
Irritant contact dermatitis, 8
Irritant dermatitis, 7
Ischemia, 41
Ischemic heart disease (IHD), 41
Ischium, 15, 18f
Island pedicle flap, 4b
Islets of Langerhans, 76
Isthmus, 98b
  thyroid, 98b
Isthmusectomy, 98b
Italicized type, ICD-10-CM, 250
Itching, 10

J

Jaundice, 84
Jejunostomy, 78b
Jejunum, 74, 76f
Joints
  bones of, 17
  disorders of, 25
  ICD-10-CM chapter 13, diseases of
    musculoskeletal system and
    connective tissue, 259
Jugular nodes, 91b

K

Kaposi's sarcoma, 12–13
KC. See Key components (KC)
Keloids, 7
Keratitis, 119
Keratoacanthoma, 12
Keratomalacia, 117b
Keratoplasty, 117b

Keratoses, 12
Key components (KC), 161, 162
Kickbacks, 127, 151
Kidneys, 66, 67f, 221b
  introduction, 216
  tumor excision, 220–221b
Kidney stones, 72
Kock pouch, 68b
Kyphosis, 22b

L

Labial excision, 223b
Labia majora, 46
Labia minora, 46
Laboratory testing, human
    immunodeficiency virus, 255
Labyrinth, 117b
Labyrinthitis, 117b
Lacrimal, 117b
Lacrimal bone, 15, 15f, 16f
Lambda, 15f
Lambdoid suture, 15f
Lamina, 22b
Laminectomy, 105b
  with foraminotomy, 227b
Landry's ascending paralysis, 108
Laparoscopy, 78b, 212, 218
Large intestine, 74
  disorders of, 83–84
Laryngeal web, 30b
Laryngectomy, 30b
Laryngopharynx, 28f
Laryngoplasty, 30b
Laryngoscope, 30b
Laryngoscopy, 30b
Laryngotomy, 30b, 202
Larynx, 27, 28f
Last menstrual period (LMP), 47
Late effects, ICD-10-CM, 254
Lateral malleolus, 16
Latissimus dorsi, 19f, 20
Lavage, 30b
Law and ethics, further text resources on,
    334
Layers, skin, 2, 2f
LCDs. See Local coverage determinations
    (LCDs)
Left colonic flexure, 76f
Legs
  bones of, 15–16
  muscles of, 20–21
  ultrasound of, 246b
Leiomyomas, 52
Lens, 114
  removal and replacement, 224
Lesions, 5–7, 6f
  calculating size of, 190f
  female genital system benign, 52
  female genital system malignant, 53–54
  injections, 190

Lesions (Continued)
  shaving of, 189
  skin, subcutaneous, and accessory
    structures removal, 193
Leukemia, 93–94
Leukocytes, 35
Leukocytopenia, 93
Leukocytosis, 93
Leukoderma, 4b
Leukoplakia, 4b
Level II HCPCS modifiers, 159
LH. See Luteinizing hormone (LH)
Lichen planus, 9
Ligaments, 18, 22b
  disorders of, 25
  sprains and strains, 24
Ligation, 49b
Linea alba, 20f
Lingual follicles, 75f
Lingual frenulum, 75f
Lingual tonsil, 75f
Lipocyte, 4b
Lipoma, 4b
Lips, 75f
Lithotomy, 78b
Lithotripsy, 78b
Liver, 74–76, 76f
  cancer of, 84
  cirrhosis, 85
  disorders of, 84–85
  jaundice, 84
LMP. See Last menstrual period (LMP)
Lobectomy, 30b, 98b, 202, 223
Lobes, brain, 104
Local anesthesia, 176
Local coverage determinations (LCDs), 124
Localized myocardial ischemia, 41
Long bones, 14–17, 14f
Longissimus capitis, 20
Lordosis, 22b, 24
Lou Gehrig's disease, 107
Low-complexity MDM, 166
Lower extremities. See Legs
Lower respiratory infection (LRI), 33
Lower respiratory tract (LRT), 27, 28f
Low-severity presenting problem, 167
Lumbar disc herniation, 237b
Lumbar vertebrae, 15, 17f, 18f, 104
Lumbodynia, 22b
Lund-Browder Classification Method, 192,
    192f
Lungs, 27, 28f, 202–203
Luteinizing hormone (LH), 96
Lymph, 89
Lymphadenectomy, 91b, 209
Lymphadenitis, 91b, 94
Lymphadenopathy, 94
Lymphangiography, 91b
Lymphangiotomy, 91b
Lymphangitis, 91b, 94
Lymph nodes, 90f, 91b
Lymphocytes, 35

Lymphoma, malignant, 94
Lymph organs, 89
Lymph vessels, 89
Lysis, 22*b*

M

MAC. *See* Monitored anesthesia care (MAC)
Macular degeneration, 119
Macule, 5, 6*f*
Magnetic resonance imaging (MRI), 228, 229
Major complications for comorbidities (MCC), 143–144, 147
Major Diagnostic Categories (MDCs), 142, 143*f*, 144*f*
    pre-, 144–146, 145*f*, 146*f*, 147*f*, 148*f*
    surgical classes in, 143
Malabsorption conditions, 81–82
Male genital system, 58–65
    accessory organs, 58, 58*f*
    anatomy and terminology, 58, 58*f*, 60
    androgen hypersecretion, 102
    combining forms, 59*b*
    disorders of, 60–64
    essential organs, 58
    medical abbreviations, 59*b*
    medical terms, 59*b*
    pathophysiology, 60–65
    quiz, 60, 64–65
    suffixes, 59*b*
    testes, 97, 97*f*
Male genital system subsection, 216–217
    biopsy codes, 216
    penis, 217
Malignant lymphoma, 94
Malignant melanoma, 12
Malignant tumors, skin, 12–13
    subcutaneous, and accessory structures, 189–190
Malleus, 15, 16*f*
Managed care organizations, 127, 152
Managed health care, 127, 152
Management options, 164
Mandated service modifier, 180
Mandible, 15, 15*f*, 16*f*, 18*f*
Manipulation, 22*b*, 196
    vagina, 218
Manubrium of sternum, 17*f*
Marsupialization, 217
Mass, excision of, 200*b*, 221*b*
Masseter, 20
Mastication, 19
Mastoidectomy, 117*b*
Mastoid process, 15*f*
    ICD-10-CM chapter 8, diseases of ear and mastoid process, 257
Maternity care and delivery subsection, 218–220
    abortion services, 220
    antepartum and fetal invasive services, 219
    delivery of twins, 220

Maternity care and delivery subsection (*Continued*)
    episiotomies and use of forceps, 220
    excision, 219
    gestation, 219
    global package and delivery, 219
    physician provides only portion of global routine care, delivery, 220
    postpartum care, 219
    repair, 219
    routine global obstetric care, 219
Math, further text resources on, 333
Maxilla, 15, 15*f*, 16*f*, 18*f*
MCC. *See* Major complications for comorbidities (MCC)
MDCs. *See* Major Diagnostic Categories (MDCs)
Meatotomy, 59*b*
Mechanoreceptors, 115
Meckel's diverticulum, 82
Medial malleolus, 16
Median glossoepiglottic fold, 75*f*
Median sulcus, 75*f*
Mediastinum, 87–88, 87*f*
Mediastinum and diaphragm subsection, 209
Medical abbreviations, 329–331*t*
    cardiovascular system, 39*b*
    digestive system, 77*b*
    female genital system, 49*b*
    integumentary system, 3*b*
    male genital system, 59*b*
    musculoskeletal system, 22*b*
    nervous system, 105*b*
    reimbursement, 152*b*
    respiratory system, 29*b*
    senses, 116*b*
    urinary system, 67*b*
Medical billing/insurance, further text resources on, 334
Medical decision making (MDM)
    complexity, 164
    four levels, 166, 166*f*
Medical genetics, medicine section, 242
Medical necessity and frequency limitations, Medicare, 124
Medical record, 128*b*, 154*b*
Medical team conferences, 169
Medical terms, 311–323*t*
    cardiovascular system, 39*b*
    digestive system, 78*b*
    endocrine system, 98*b*
    female genital system, 49*b*
    further text resources, 333
    hemic and lymphatic system, 91*b*
    integumentary system, 4*b*
    male genital system, 59*b*
    musculoskeletal system, 22*b*
    nervous system, 105*b*
    reimbursement, 128*b*
    respiratory system, 30*b*
    senses, 117*b*
    urinary system, 68*b*

Medical transcription, further text resources on, 333
Medicare, 123–125, 133–137
    basic structure, 123, 133–135
    beneficiary pays, 124
    coverage, 124
    electronic transactions, 125
    Federal Register and, 125, 126*f*, 136–137, 136*f*
    fraud and abuse, 127, 151
    funding, 124, 135
    getting bigger all the time, 133
    hospital-acquired conditions (HAC), 149–150
    Medicare pays, 124
    Medicare Severity Diagnosis-Related Groups (MS-DRGs), 142–147
    National Correct Coding Initiative (NCCI), 125, 137
    National Fee Schedule (NFS), 126
    National Provider Identification (NPI), 124
    Office of the Inspector General (OIG) and, 127, 151–152
    officiating office, 123, 135
    Part A: Hospital and Institutional Care Coverage, 123, 133–135
    Part A: Hospital Inpatient, 124–125
    Part B: Supplemental—nonhospital, 123, 125, 135
    Part C: Medicare Advantage Organizations (MAO) plans, 123, 135
    Part D: Prescription Drug Plan (PDP), 123, 135
    participating providers, 124, 124*f*
    post acute transfer, 147
    Present On Admission indicator (POA), 148–149
    Prospective Payment Systems (PPS), 137
    Quality Improvement Organizations (QIO) and, 125
    Relative Value Units (RVUs), 126–127
    Resource-Based Relative Value Scale (RBRVS) and, 125–127
    those covered by, 123, 133
    unbundling, 125, 137
Medicare Administrative Contractors, 154*b*
Medicare Severity Diagnosis-Related Groups (MS-DRGs), 142–147, 154*b*
    classification, 144–146
    further defined by a particular set of patient attributes defined in the Uniform Hospital Discharge Data Set (UHDDS), 142–143, 144*f*
    MCC and CC, 143–144, 147
    post acute transfer, 147
    Pre-Major Diagnostic Categories (Pre-MDCs), 144–146, 145*f*, 146*f*, 147*f*, 148*f*
    reimbursement monitoring, 149
    selection if no surgical procedure is performed is based on, 146–147

Medicare Severity Diagnosis-Related Groups (MS-DRGs) (Continued)
structure of, 142–143, 143f
surgical classes in each MDC defined in a hierarchical order, 143
system based on, 142
system of classifying patients into groups by related diagnoses, 142
Medicine section, 239–246
allergy and clinical immunology, 241–242
biofeedback, 240
cardiac catheterization, 244–245b
cardiovascular in medicine section, 241
chemotherapy and other highly complex drug or highly complex biologic agent administration, 243
dialysis, 240–241
education and training for patient self-management, 244
extremities ultrasound, 246b
gastroenterology, 241
health behavior assessment and intervention, 242
hydration, therapeutic, prophylactic, diagnostic injections and infusions, and chemotherapy and other highly complex drug or highly complex biologic agent administration, 242–243
immune globulins, 239
immunization administration, 239
immunizations, 239
medical genetics and genetic counseling, 242
moderate (conscious) sedation, 244
neurology and neuromuscular procedures, 242
non-face-to-face nonphysician services, 244
noninvasive vascular diagnostic studies, 241
ophthalmology, 241
osteopathic and chiropractic services, 244
photodynamic therapy, 243
physical medicine and rehabilitation, 243–244
psychiatry, 240
pulmonary, 241
renal dialysis progress note, 246b
saphenous vein mapping, 245b
special dermatologic procedures, 243
special ophthalmologic services, 241
special otorhinolaryngologic services, 241
special services, procedures, and reports, 244
vaccines, toxoids, 239–240
venous ultrasound, 245b
Medulla oblongata, 103, 104, 104f
Medulloblastoma, 112
Melanin, 4b
Melanocyte-stimulating hormone (MSH), 96

Melanoma, 4b
malignant, 12
Ménière's disease, 117b, 121
Meninges, 104, 104f, 108
nervous system subsection, 223–224
Meningioma, 112
Meningocele, 108, 109f
Menometrorrhagia, 51
Menorrhagia, 51, 237b
Menorrhea, 51
Menstruation, 46–47
disorders of, 50–51
proliferation phase, 46
secretory phase, 46
Mental disorders, 108
depression, 108
ICD-10-CM chapter 5, mental, behavioral, and neurodevelopmental disorders, 257
schizophrenia, 108
Mental foramen, 16f
Mental protuberance, 15f
Merkel cell carcinoma, 13
Metabolic diseases, ICD-10-CM chapter 4, endocrine, nutritional, and metabolic diseases, 256–257
Metacarpals, 16, 18f
Metatarsals, 16, 18f
Metrorrhagia, 51
MG. See Myasthenia gravis (MG)
MI. See Myocardial infarction (MI)
Microbiology, pathology and laboratory section, 235
Microglia, 103
Midbrain, 103
Middle concha, 16f
Middle ear, 114–115
bones of, 15, 16f
Minimal presenting problem, 167
Minimum assistant surgeon modifier, 182
M is for modifying unit (anesthesia), 176
Missed abortion, 56, 220
Mitochondrion, 103f
Mitral regurgitation (MR), 44
Mitral valve stenosis, 44
M-mode, 230
Mobile quick quizzes, 296
Moderate-complexity MDM, 166
Moderate (conscious) sedation, 176, 244
Moderate-severity presenting problem, 167
Modifiers
anesthesia, 177
CA, 140
CPT, 159
CPT/HCPCS level I, 180–187
HCPCS level II, 183–184
Mohs surgery/Mohs micrographic surgery, 4b, 192
Molecular pathology, pathology and laboratory section, 235
Moles, 12
Monitored anesthesia care (MAC), 176

Monocytes, 35
Monocytosis, 93
Morbidity, ICD-10-CM chapter 20, external causes of morbidity, 262–263
Motor neuron disease (MND), 107
Mouth, 74, 75f, 76f
cancer of, 79
cleft lip and palate, 79, 79f
disorders of, 79
infections, 79
sense of taste, 115
ulceration, 79
MRI. See Magnetic resonance imaging (MRI)
MS. See Multiple sclerosis (MS)
MS-DRGs. See Medicare Severity Diagnosis-Related Groups (MS-DRGs)
MSH. See Melanocyte-stimulating hormone (MSH)
Multianalyte assays with algorithmic analyses, pathology and laboratory section, 235
Multipara, 49b
Multiple modifiers, 183
Multiple myeloma, 26, 95
Multiple procedure-three types modifier, 181
Multiple sclerosis (MS), 107
Muscle flap, 4b, 191
Muscle(s), 19f
action of, 18–21
arm, 20
cardiac/heart, 18
disorders of, 25
functions of, 17
leg, 20–21
movement of, 19
names of, 19–21, 19f, 20f
respiratory, 20
smooth/visceral, 18
tendons and ligaments, 18
terms of movement, 19
tissue types, 17–18
trunk, 20
tumors of, 26
Muscular dystrophy, 25
Musculoskeletal system, 14–26
anatomy and terminology, 14–21
appendicular skeleton, 15–16
arm bones, 16
bone disorders, 24
bone tumors, 25–26
classification of bones, 14
combining forms, 21b
cranial bones, 14–15
face bones, 15
hyoid bone, 15
ICD-10-CM chapter 13, diseases of musculoskeletal system and connective tissue, 259
injuries, 23–24
joint bones, 17

Musculoskeletal system (*Continued*)
  joint disorders, 25
  leg bones, 15–16
  medical abbreviations, 22*b*
  medical terms, 22*b*
  middle ear bones, 15
  muscle functions, 17
  muscle tissue types, 17–18
  muscular system, 17, 19*f*, 20*f*
  pathophysiology, 23–26
  prefixes, 21*b*
  quiz, 23, 26
  shoulder, girdle, pelvic girdle, and
      extremities, pelvis, 15
  skeletal system, 14, 18*f*
  skull, 14, 15*f*, 16*f*
  spine, 15, 17*f*
  structure, 14–17, 14*f*
  suffixes, 22*b*
  tendon, muscle, and ligament
      disorders, 25
  thorax, 15, 17*f*
Musculoskeletal system subsection,
    195–198
  arthrodesis, 197
  arthroplasty and spur excision, 198–199*b*
  casts and strapping, 198
  endoscopy/arthroscopy, 198
  excision of mass, bursa, 200*b*
  fascial sling arthroplasty, 199*b*
  fracture treatment, 196
  grafts, 197
  other procedures, 197
  replantation, 197
  soft tissue tumors, 197
  spine and spinal instrumentation,
      197–198, 198*f*
  steroid injection, 198*b*
  subheading "general," 196
  subsequent subheadings, 197–198
  wound exploration, 196
Myasthenia gravis (MG), 107
Mycoses, 11–12
Myelin sheath, 103
Myelocystocele, 109*f*
Myeloma, 26, 95
Myelomeningocele, 108, 109*f*
Myocardial infarction (MI), 41
Myocardium, 35
Myocutaneous flaps, 191
Myometrium, 46, 47*f*
Myopia, 117*b*, 118
Myringotomy, 117*b*, 225
Myxedema, 101

N

Nails, 2–3, 190
Narrow-angle glaucoma, 120
Nasal bone, 15, 15*f*, 16*f*
Nasal button, 30*b*
Nasal conchae, 15, 16*f*, 27, 28*f*

Nasal hemorrhage, 201
Nasal spine, 15*f*
Nasion, 15*f*
Nasopharynx, 28*f*
National Correct Coding Initiative (NCCI),
    125, 137, 154*b*
National Fee Schedule (NFS), 126
National Level II Index, HCPCS, 247
National Provider Identification (NPI), 124,
    128*b*, 154*b*
Nature of presenting problem, 166
NCCI. *See* National Correct Coding
    Initiative (NCCI)
Neck, muscles of, 19–20
Neonatal cystourethrogram, 233*b*
Neoplasms
  ICD-10-CM chapter 2, neoplasms, 256
  ICD-10-CM table of, 251, 251*f*
  See also Cancer; Tumors
Neoplastic medications, 335–343*t*
Nephrocutaneous fistula, 68*b*
Nephrolithiasis, 72
Nephrolithotomy, 68*b*
Nephrorrhaphy, 68
Nephrosclerosis, 72
Nephrostomy, 68*b*
Nephrotic syndrome, 71
Nerves
  cranial and spinal, 104
  ICD-10-CM chapter 20, external causes
      of morbidity, 263
  optic, 114
Nervous system, 103
  anatomy and terminology, 103–104, 106
  autonomic, 103, 104
  cells, 103, 103*f*
  central nervous system (CNS) disorders,
      109–112
  combining forms, 104*b*
  congenital neurologic disorders, 108
  dementias, 106–108
  divisions of central nervous system,
      103–104
  ICD-10-CM chapter 6, diseases of
      nervous system, (257 *See also*
      Central nervous system (CNS))
  medical abbreviations, 105*b*
  medical terms, 105*b*
  mental disorders, 108
  pathophysiology, 106–113
  peripheral, 103–104
  prefixes, 105*b*
  quiz, 106, 112–113
  suffixes, 105*b*
Nervous system subsection, 223–224
  extracranial nerves, peripheral nerves, and
      autonomic nervous system, 224
  skull, meninges, and brain, 223–224
  spine and spinal cord, 224
Neurodevelopmental disorders, ICD-10-CM
    chapter 5, mental, behavioral, and
    neurodevelopmental disorders, 257

Neurology and neuromuscular procedures,
    medicine section, 242
Neurons, 103
Neurovascular flap, 4*b*
Neutron beam treatment delivery, 231
Neutrophils, 35
Nevi, 12
  excision, 185*b*
Newborn care, 170
New patient, E/M codes, 161, 167
NFS. *See* National Fee Schedule (NFS)
NICU progress note, ventilator assist, 175*b*
Nociceptors, 115
Nodule, 5, 6*f*
Noncoronary bypass grafts, 205
Noncovered services, 128*b*, 154*b*
Non-face-to-face nonphysician services, 244
Non-face-to-face services, 170
Non-Hodgkin lymphoma, 94
Non-insulin-dependent diabetes
    mellitus, 99
Noninvasive, 39*b*
Noninvasive physiologic studies and
    procedures, 208
Noninvasive vascular diagnostic studies, 241
Nonobstetric curettage, 219
Nonsegmental spinal instrumentation, 197
Nonviral hepatitis, 85
Nose, 27, 28*f*
  respiratory system subsection, 201
  sense of smell, 115
Notes, ICD-10-CM alphabetic index, 250
Nuclear cardiology, 39*b*, 203
Nuclear medicine subsection, 231
Nucleus, cell, 103*f*
Nursing facility discharge services, 169
Nursing facility services, 169
Nutrition, ICD-10-CM chapter 4,
    endocrine, nutritional, and metabolic
    diseases, 256–257
Nutritional degenerative disease, 106
Nystagmus, 118–119

O

Obliquus externus, 19*f*, 20, 20*f*
OBRA. *See* Omnibus Budget Reconciliation
    Act of 1986 (OBRA)
Observation status, 142
Obstruction
  intestinal, 82–83
  urinary tract, 71–72
Occipital bone, 14–15, 15*f*
Occipital lobe, 104
Occipitofrontalis, 19
OCE. *See* Outpatient code editor (OCE)
Ocular adnexa, 115*f*, 117*b*
  eye and ocular adnexa subsection, 224
  ICD-10-CM chapter 7, diseases of eye
      and adnexa, 257
Office of the Inspector General (OIG), 127,
    151–152

OGCR Section IV, diagnostic coding and reporting guidelines for outpatient services, 265–266
OIG. *See* Office of the Inspector General (OIG)
Olecranon, 16
Olfactory sense receptors, 115
Oligodendrocytes, 103
Oligodendrocytoma, 112
Oligomenorrhea, 51
Omnibus Budget Reconciliation Act of 1986 (OBRA), 137
Oophorectomy, 49*b*
Open fracture repair, 22*b*, 196
Open fractures, 23
Operating microscope subsection, 225
Ophthalmology, 241
Ophthalmoscopy, 117*b*
OPPS. *See* Outpatient Prospective Payment System (OPPS)
Optic foramen, 16*f*
Optic nerve, 114
Oral cavity. *See* Mouth
Orbicularis oculi, 19
Orbicularis oris, 19
Orchiectomy, 59*b*
Orchiopexy, 59*b*
Orchitis, 60
Order, 39*b*
Organ or disease-oriented panels, pathology and laboratory section, 234
Orofacial cleft, 79, 79*f*
Orogastric tube placement, 213*b*
Oropharynx, 28*f*
Orthopnea, 30*b*, 32
Orthostatic hypotension, 41–42
Osteitis deformans, 24
Osteoarthritis, 22*b*, 25
Osteoclast, 22*b*
Osteoma, 26
Osteomalacia, 24
Osteomyelitis, 24
Osteopathic services, 244
Osteoporosis, 24
Osteosarcoma, 26
Osteotomy, 22*b*
OT. *See* Oxytocin (OT)
Otitis externa, 120
Otitis media, 117*b*
Otorhinolaryngologic services, 241
Otoscope, 117*b*
Ototoxic hearing loss, 121
Outlier adjustment, 141
Outpatient
    E/M codes, 161
    hospital, 154*b*
Outpatient code editor (OCE), 142
Outpatient coding, 265–266
Outpatient Prospective Payment System (OPPS), 138–142, 139*f*
Ovaries, 46, 47*f*, 97, 97*f*, 218
    cancer of, 53–54

Ovaries *(Continued)*
    endocrine system subsection, 223
    uterus, bilateral tubes, and ovaries, pathology and laboratory section, 237*b*
Overriding aorta, 44
Oviducts. *See* Fallopian tubes
Ovulation, 46
Oxytocin (OT), 96

P
Pacemaker, 203–204
PAD. *See* Peripheral arterial disease (PAD)
Paget's disease, 24
Pain
    analgesia for, 176
    appendicitis, 82
    gallstones, 85, 85*f*
    ICD-10-CM chapter 6, diseases of nervous system, 257
Palate, 15, 28*f*
Palatine tonsil, 75*f*
Palatoglossal arch, 75*f*
Palatopharyngeal arch, 75*f*
Pancreas, 76, 76*f*, 96, 97*f*
    cancer of, 86
    disorders of, 85–86
    endocrine system subsection, 223
Pancreatic cancer, 86
Pancreatic cells, 76
Pancreatitis, 85–86
Papanicolaou (Pap) smear, 53
Papilledema, 117*b*
Papule, 5, 6*f*
Papulosquamous disorders, 8
Paraesophageal hernia, 78*b*, 80, 80*f*
Paranasal sinuses, 27
Paraphimosis, 62
Parasitic diseases, ICD-10-CM chapter 1, certain infectious and, 255
Parasympathetic system, 104
Parathyroid, 91*b*, 96, 97*f*
    disorders of, 101
Parietal burr holes, 225–226*b*
Parentheses, ICD-10-CM, 250
Parietal bone, 14–15, 15*f*, 16*f*
Parietal lobe, 104
Parietal pericardium, 36
Paring or cutting, skin, subcutaneous, and accessory structures, 189
Parkinson's disease, 107
Parotid gland, 74, 76*f*
Partial seizures, 110–111
Passive immunization, 239
Pass-through codes, 138, 141*f*
Past, family, and/or social history (PFSH), 162–163
Patella, 15–16, 18*f*, 20*f*
Patellar tendon, 20*f*
Patent ductus arteriosus (PDA), 44
Pathology and laboratory section, 234–238
    anatomic pathology, 236

Pathology and laboratory section *(Continued)*
    cerebral hematoma, 238*b*
    cervical disc, 238*b*
    chemistry, 235
    consultation levels, 235
    consultations, 235
    cytogenetic studies, 236
    cytopathology, 236
    drug assay, 234
    evocative/suppression testing, 235
    facility indicators, 234
    hematology and coagulation, 235
    immunology, 235
    L3-4 disc, 237*b*
    microbiology, 235
    molecular pathology, 235
    more consultation codes, 235
    multianalyte assays with algorithmic analyses, 235
    organ or disease-oriented panels, 234
    pathology and laboratory, 234
    pathology/laboratory caution, 234
    placenta, 237–238*b*
    rules of panels, 234
    surgical pathology, 236
    therapeutic drug assays, 234–235
    tissue typing, 235
    transfusion medicine, 235
    urinalysis, 235
    uterus, bilateral tubes, and ovaries, 237*b*
Pathology/laboratory caution, pathology and laboratory section, 234
Pathophysiology
    cardiovascular system, 41–44, 41*f*
    digestive system, 79–86
    endocrine system, 99–102, 99*f*
    female genital system, 50–56
    further text resources, 332
    hemic and lymphatic system, 92–95
    integumentary system, 5–13
    male genital system, 60–65
    musculoskeletal system, 23–26
    nervous system, 106–113
    respiratory system, 32–33
    senses, 118–121
    urinary system, 69–73
Patient-controlled analgesia (PCA), 176
Patient status, E/M codes, 161, 167–168
Patient training, 243, 244
Payment rate, APC, 138, 140*f*
Payment status indicators (SI), 138–142
PCA. *See* Patient-controlled analgesia (PCA)
PDA. *See* Patent ductus arteriosus (PDA)
Pectoralis major, 20, 20*f*
Pediatric critical care patient transport, 170
Pedicle, 4*b*
Pelvic girdle, 15
Pelvic inflammatory disease (PID), 51
Pelvis, 15

Penis, 58, 58f
  cancer of, 63
  destruction, 217
  disorders of, 62–63
  excision, 217
  introduction, 217
  repair, 217
Penoscrotal, 59b
Peptic ulcers, 81
Percussion, 30b
Percutaneous, 22b
Percutaneous fracture repair, 22b, 196
Percutaneous skeletal fixation, 22b
Perforated appendicitis, 177–178b
Pericardial cavity, 36
Pericardial effusion, 44
Pericardiocentesis, 39b
Pericarditis, 43
  acute, 44
  constrictive, 44
Pericardium, 36, 39b
  cardiovascular in surgery section,
    203–204
Perimetrium, 46, 47f
Perinatal period, ICD-10-CM chapter 16,
    certain conditions originating in the,
    261–262
Perineum, 46, 49b, 217
Peripheral arterial disease (PAD), 42
  rehabilitation, 208
Peripheral nerves, 105b, 224
Peripheral nervous system (PNS),
    103–104
Perirectal abscess, 179b
Peritoneum, 76
  peritonitis, 82
Peritonitis, 82
Pernicious anemia, 92
Peroneus brevis, 19f, 20f, 21
Peroneus longus, 19f, 20f, 21
Peroneus tertius, 21
Perpendicular plate of ethmoid, 16f
Pertussis, 30b
Peyronie's disease, 62
PFSH. See Past, family, and/or social history
    (PFSH)
Phalanges, 16, 18f
Pharmacology review, 335–343t
Pharyngolaryngectomy, 30b
Pharynx, 27, 74, 76f
Phimosis, 62
Phlebitis, 42
Photodynamic therapy, 243
Physical medicine and rehabilitation,
    medicine section, 243–244
Physical status modifiers, P1-P6
    (anesthesia), 176–177
Physician and patient dialogue, 162–171
Physician-based examinations, 271–291
  final, 272
  pre-examination and post-examination,
    271–272

Physician-based reimbursement, 123–131,
    128b
  Medicare, 123–125
  physician responsibility, 123
  population changing=reimbursement
    change, 123
  quiz, 130–131
  terminology, 128b
Physician provides only portion of global
    routine care, delivery, 220
Physician status, 168
Pia mater, 104
PID. See Pelvic inflammatory disease (PID)
Pilonidal cyst, 190
Pilosebaceous, 4b
PIN. See Provider identification number (PIN)
Pineal gland, 97, 97f
  endocrine system subsection, 223
Pineal region tumors, 112
Pink eye, 119
Pinna, 16f
Pituitary gland, 96, 97f
  disorders of, 99–100, 100f
  endocrine system subsection, 223
  tumor, 112
Pityriasis rosea, 9
PKD. See Polycystic kidney disease (PKD)
Placeholder, ICD-10-CM, 249
Placenta, 49b, 97, 237–238b
  formation, 47
Placenta previa, 54, 55f
Place of service, E/M codes, 161
Planes of body, 228, 229f
Plantaris, 19f
Plaque, 5, 6f
Plasma, 35
Plethysmography, 59b, 208
Pleura, 30b, 202–203
Pleuracentesis, 30b
Pleural effusion, 33
Pleurectomy, 30b
Pleurisy, 33
Pleuritis, 30b
Pleurocentesis, 30b
PMS. See Premenstrual syndrome (PMS)
Pneumocentesis, 30b
Pneumococcal vaccine, 240
Pneumoconiosis, 33
Pneumolysis, 30b
Pneumonia, 30b, 33
Pneumonocentesis, 30b
Pneumonolysis, 30b
Pneumonotomy, 30b
Pneumothorax, 32–33
Pneumotomy, 30b
PNS. See Peripheral nervous system (PNS)
POA. See Present On Admission indicator
    (POA)
Point of service (POS), 127, 128b, 152
Poisoning, ICD-10-CM chapter 19, injury,
    poisoning, and certain other
    consequences of external causes, 262

Poliomyelitis, 108
Poliovirus vaccine, 239–240
Polycystic kidney disease (PKD), 72–73
Polymenorrhea, 51
Polymyositis, 25
Polyps, nasal, 201
Pons, 103, 104f
Population changing, 123, 133
Portion of rhomboideus, 19f
POS. See Point of service (POS)
Post acute transfer, 147
Posterior pituitary, 96, 100
Posterior segment, 117b
Post-examination, 271–272
Postoperative management only
    modifier, 181
Postpartum, 49b
Postpartum care, 219
Postpartum curettage, 219
Postpolio syndrome (PPS), 108
PPO. See Preferred provider organization
    (PPO)
PPS. See Postpolio syndrome (PPS);
    Prospective Payment Systems (PPS)
Pre-examination, 271–272
Preferred provider organization (PPO), 127,
    128b, 152
Prefixes, 327t
  cardiovascular system, 38b
  endocrine system, 98b
  female genital system, 48b
  hemic and lymphatic system, 89b
  integumentary system, 3b
  musculoskeletal system, 21b
  nervous system, 105b
  respiratory system, 29b
  senses, 116b
  urinary system, 67b
Pregnancy, 46–57
  abortion of, 55–56
  abruptio placentae in, 54, 55f
  eclampsia in, 54
  ectopic, 55, 56f
  gestation, approximately 266 days, 47
  gestational diabetes mellitus in, 99
  human immunodeficiency virus and, 255
  hydatidiform mole in, 55
  ICD-10-CM chapter 15, pregnancy,
    childbirth, and the puerperium, 261
  ICD-10-CM chapter 16, certain
    conditions originating in the
    perinatal period, 261–262
  malpositions and malpresentations in, 55,
    56f
  menstruation and, 46–47
  placenta formation in, 47
  placenta previa in, 54, 55f
  repair during, 219
  See also Childbirth; Female genital system
Pre-Major Diagnostic Categories (Pre-MDCs),
    144–146, 145f, 146f, 147f, 148f
Premenstrual syndrome (PMS), 51

Premenstruation, 46
Preoperative management only modifier, 181
Presbyopia, 118
Prescription Drug, Improvement, and Modernization Act of 2003, 123, 135
Presenting problem, levels of, 167
Present On Admission indicator (POA), 148–149
Pressure ulcers, 7, 7f, 191
Preventive medicine services, 170
Preventive services modifier, 180–181
Priapism, 59b
Primary adrenal insufficiency, 101
Primary bronchus, 28f
Primary fibromyalgia syndrome, 25
Primigravida, 49b
Primipara, 49b
Prior authorization, 128b, 154b
PRL. See Prolactin (PRL)
Problem-focused examination, 164, 164f
Problem-focused history, 163
Procedure performed on infants less than 4 kg modifier, 182
Proctosigmoidoscopy, 78b, 212
Professional component modifier, 180
Professionalism, further text resources on, 333
Progressive systemic sclerosis, 79–80
Prolactin (PRL), 96
Proliferation phase, 46
Prolonged services, 169
Pronation, 19
Proprioceptors, 115
Prospective Payment Systems (PPS), 137, 149
Prostate gland, 58, 58f, 216
    cancer of, 63, 64, 64f
    disorders of, 63–64
Prostatitis, 63
Prostatomy, 59b
Provider identification number (PIN), 128b, 154b
Pruritus, 10
Pseudomeningocele, 226–227b
Psoriasis, 8–9
Psychiatric collaborative care management services, 171
Psychiatric diagnostic evaluation, 240
Psychiatry, 240
Psychotherapy, 240
Pterion, 15f
Pterygoids, 20
Ptosis, 117b
Pubis, 15, 18f
Pubis symphysis, 15
Puerperium, ICD-10-CM chapter 15, pregnancy, childbirth, and the, 261
Pulmonary artery, 36
    stenosis of, 44
Pulmonary edema, 30b, 32
Pulmonary embolism, 30b, 33

Pulmonary hypertension, 258
Pulmonary services, medicine section, 241
Pulmonary valve, 36
Pulmonary veins, 36
Pulmonic regurgitation (PR), 44
Punctuation, ICD-10-CM, 250
Purkinje fibers, 36
Pustule, 5, 6f
Pyelonephritis
    acute, 70–71, 70f
    chronic, 71
Pyloric sphincter, 74
Pyloric stenosis, 81
Pyloroplasty, 215b

Q
QIN. See Quality Innovation Network (QIN)
Quadratus lumborum, 20
Quadriceps muscles, 21
Qualifying circumstances codes, 177
Quality Improvement Organizations (QIO), 125
Quality Innovation Network (QIN), 125

R
Radiation oncology subsection, 230–231
    clinical brachytherapy, 231
    clinical treatment planning-professional component, 230
    hyperthermia, 231
    medical radiation, physics, dosimetry, treatment devices, and special services, 231
    radiation and neutron beam treatment delivery, 231
    reporting radiation treatment management, 231
    stereotactic radiation treatment delivery, 231
Radiologic guidance subsection, 230
Radiology section, 188–227
    bone/joint studies subsection, 230
    breast mammography subsection, 230
    component coding, 228
    contrast material, 228
    cranial CT, 232b
    diagnostic radiology subsection, 229
    diagnostic ultrasound subsection, 230
    gallbladder ultrasound, 232b
    head ultrasound, 233b
    interventional radiologist, 228–229
    neonatal cystourethrogram, 233b
    nuclear medicine subsection, 231
    planes of body, 228, 229f
    procedures, 228
    radiation oncology subsection, 230–231
    radiologic guidance subsection, 230
    stress test, 232–233b
    subsections, 228

Radius, 16, 18f
Rales, 30b
Ramus, 15f
Raynaud's disease, 42
RBRVS. See Resource-Based Relative Value Scale (RBRVS)
Real-time scan, 230
Rectum, 74, 76f
    ulcerative colitis, 83, 83f
Rectus abdominis, 20, 20f
Rectus femoris, 20f, 21
Reduced services modifier, 181
Reduction, 22b
Reference (outside) laboratory modifier, 182
Referring physician, 168
Regional anesthesia, 176
Rehabilitative services modifier, 183
Reimbursement, 123–131, 128b, 154b
    abbreviations, 152b
    ambulatory payment classifications (APCs), 137–138
    data quality, 150–151, 150f
    facility responsibility, 133
    hospital-acquired conditions (HAC), 149–150
    managed health care, 127, 152
    Medicare, 123–125, 133–137
    National Correct Coding Initiative (NCCI), 125, 137
    physician responsibility, 123
    population changing=reimbursement change, 123, 133
    post acute transfer, 147
    Present On Admission indicator (POA), 148–149
    Prospective Payment Systems (PPS), 137
    quiz, 130–131, 152
    revenue codes, 150
    terminology, 128b, 153–154b
Rejection/denial, 128b, 153b
Relative Value Units (RVUs), 126–127
Remittance advice, 149
Removal. See Introduction and removal
Renal calculi, 72
Renal dialysis progress notes, 246b
Renal failure, 69–70, 172b
Renal mass, 221b
Renal tumor excision, 220–221b
Repair (closure)
    arteriovenous fistula, 205
    central venous access device, 206
    laceration, 194–195b
    larynx, 202
    nose, 201
    penis, 217
    during pregnancy, 219
    skin, subcutaneous, and accessory structures, 190, 194–195b
    trachea and bronchi, 202
    vagina, 218
    venous reconstruction, 205
    vulva, perineum, and introitus, 217

Repeat clinical diagnostic laboratory test modifier, 183

Repeat procedure/service by another physician or other qualified health care professional modifier, 182

Repeat procedure/service by same physician or other qualified health care professional modifier, 182

Replacement
central venous access device, 206
dialysis catheter, 210*b*
lens, 224

Replantation, 197

Resource-Based Relative Value Scale (RBRVS), 125–127, 128*b*

Resource utilization groups (RUGs), 149

Respiration, 27

Respiratory acidosis, 32

Respiratory muscles, 20

Respiratory system, 27–34
anatomy and terminology, 27
combining forms, 28*b*
ICD-10-CM chapter 10, diseases of respiratory system, 258
lower respiratory infection (LRI), 33
lower respiratory tract (LRT), 27, 28*f*
medical abbreviations, 29*b*
medical terms, 30*b*
pathophysiology, 32–33
prefixes, 29*b*
pulmonary diseases and disorders, 32–33
pulmonary disorders signs and symptoms, 32
quiz, 31, 34
suffixes, 29*b*
upper respiratory tract (URT), 27, 28*f*

Respiratory system subsection, 201–203
accessory sinuses, 202
endoscopy, 201
larynx, 202
lungs and pleura, 202–203
multiple procedures, 201
nose, 201
removal of foreign body, 201
repair, 201
trachea and bronchi, 202

Rest home services, 169

Restrictive cardiomyopathy, 44

Restrictive pericarditis, 44

Retina, 114
detached, 119

Revenue codes, 150

Review of systems (ROS), 162

Reye's syndrome, 110

Rheumatic fever, 43

Rheumatic heart disease, 43

Rheumatoid arthritis, 25

Rhinoplasty, 30*b*

Rhinorrhea, 30*b*

Rhomboideus, 19*f*

Rhytidectomy, 191

Ribs, 15, 18*f*

Rickets, 24

Right colonic flexure, 76*f*

Risks, 164, 165*f*

Roof of mouth, 74

Root, tongue, 75*f*

ROS. *See* Review of systems (ROS)

Rotation, 19

Routine global obstetric care, 219

Rugae
stomach, 74
uterus, 47*f*

RUGs. *See* Resource utilization groups (RUGs)

RVUs. *See* Relative Value Units (RVUs)

S

Sacrum, 15, 17*f*, 18*f*, 104

Salivary glands, 74, 76*f*

Salpingectomy, 49*b*

Salpingostomy, 49*b*

Saphenous vein mapping, 245*b*

Sarcoidosis, 30*b*

Sartorius, 20*f*, 21

Scales, 5, 6*f*

Scapula, 16, 18*f*

Scar, 6, 6*f*

Schizophrenia, 108

Schwann cell, 103*f*

Sclera, 114, 117*b*

Scleroderma, 79–80

Scoliosis, 22*b*

Scrotum, 58, 58*f*
cancer of, 61
disorders of, 60–62

Sebaceous glands, 3, 4*b*

Seborrhea, 4*b*

Seborrheic dermatitis, 8

Seborrheic keratosis, 12

Sebum, 4*b*

Secondary bronchi, 28*f*

Secondary hypertension, 258

Secretory phase, 46

Sedatives, 335–343*t*

Segmental bronchi, 27

Segmental spinal instrumentation, 197

Segmentectomy, 30*b*, 202

Seizures, 110–111

Self-limiting or minor presenting problem, 167

Semicircular canals, 16*f*

Semicolon, CPT, 159

Semimembranosus, 19*f*, 21

Seminal vesicle, 58, 58*f*

Semispinalis capitis, 20

Semitendinosus, 19*f*, 21

Senses, 114–121
anatomy and terminology, 114–115, 118
combining forms, 116*b*
ear disorders, 120–121
hearing, three divisions of ear, 114–115
medical abbreviations, 116*b*
medical terms, 117*b*
pathophysiology, 118–121
prefixes, 116*b*

Senses *(Continued)*
quiz, 118, 121
sight: three layers of eye, 114, 115*f*
smell, 115
suffixes, 116*b*
taste, 115
touch, 115
visual disturbances, 118–119

Sensorineural hearing loss, 120–121

Sepsis, 255

Septa, heart, 35–36

Septic abortion, 56, 220

Septic arthritis, 25

Septic shock, 255

Septoplasty, 30*b*, 186–187*b*

Serratus anterior, 20*f*

Sesamoid bones, 14

7*th* character, ICD-10-CM, 249

Seventh cervical vertebra, 19*f*

72-hour rule, 149

Severe sepsis, 255

Sexually transmitted disorders, 51–52

Shaving of lesions, 189

Shingles, 11

Short bones, 14

Shoulder bone, 15

Shoulder presentation of fetus, 56*f*

Shunt, 105*b*

Sialolithotomy, 78*b*

Sickle cell anemia, 92–93

Sight, 114, 115*f*

Sigmoid colon, 74, 76*f*
ulcerative colitis, 83, 83*f*

Sigmoidoscopy, 212

Significant, separately identifiable E/M service, by same physician or other qualified health care professional on the same day of the procedure or other service modifier, 180

Simple wound repair, 190

Simulation, 230

Sinoatrial node, 36

Sinuses, 27, 202

Sinusotomy, 30*b*

Skeletal muscles, 17
relaxants, 335–343*t*

Skeletal system. *See* Musculoskeletal system

Skeletal traction, 22*b*, 24*f*

Skene's gland, 217

Skin
adjacent tissue transfer, flaps, and grafts, 191–193, 191*f*
ICD-10-CM chapter 12, diseases of skin and subcutaneous tissue, 259
infections of, 10–12
inflammatory disorders of, 7–10
integumentary system subsection, 189–190
itching of, 10
sense of touch, 115
tumors of, 12–13
See also Integumentary system

Skin tag removal, 189
Skin traction, 22b, 24f
Skull, 14, 15f, 16f, 18f, 105b
    nervous system subsection, 223–224
    surgery, 224
Small-bowel anastomosis, 214–215b
Small intestine, 74
    disorders of, 81–83
Smell, 115
Smooth/visceral muscle, 18
Social history, 162–163
Soft palate, 75f
Soft tissue tumors, 197
Soleus, 19f, 20f, 21
Somatic nerve, 105b
Somatic nervous system, 103
Special E/M services, 170
Special services, procedures, and reports,
        medicine section, 244
Sphenoid bone, 15, 15f, 16f
Sphenoidotomy, 186–187b
Sphenosquamous suture, 15f
Sphincter, 74
Spina bifida, 24, 108, 109f
Spinal anesthesia, 176
Spinal cord, 104f
    congenital neurologic disorders, 108
    housed within vertebrae from medulla
            oblongata to second lumbar, 104
    injury to, 111
    instrumentation, 197–198, 198f
    nervous system subsection, 224
    tumors, 111–112
    See also Vertebrae
Spinal curvatures, 24
Spinal nerves, 104
Spine
    bones of, 15, 17f
    nervous system subsection, 224
    spinal instrumentation, 197–198, 198f
Spirometry, 30b
Spleen, 208
Splenectomy, 91b, 208
Splenius capitis, 19f, 20
Splenography, 91b
Splenoportography, 91b
Split-thickness graft, 4b, 191
Spondylitis, 22b
Spontaneous abortion, 55, 220
Sprains, 24
Spur excision, 198–199b
Squama of temporal bone, 15f
Squamous cell carcinoma, 12
Squamous part, 15f
Squamous suture, 15f
Staged/related procedure or service by same
        physician or other qualified health care
        professional during postoperative
        period modifier, 181
Stand-alone CPT codes, 159
Standby services, 169
Stapes, 15, 16f

State license number, 128b, 154b
Steatoma, 4b
Stem cell, 91b
Stenosis, 44
    pyloric, 81
Stereotactic radiation treatment delivery,
        231
Stereotaxis, 105b
Sternal angle, 17f
Sternochondral joint, 17f
Sternoclavicular joint, 17f
Sternocleidomastoideus, 19f, 20, 20f
Sternum, 15, 17f, 18f
Steroids, 335–343t
    injection, 198b
Stomach, 74, 76f
    cancer of, 81
    disorders of, 80–81
    gastritis, 80–81
    peptic ulcers, 81
    pyloric stenosis, 81
Strabismus, 117b, 119
Straightforward MDM, 166
Strains, 24
Strapping, 198
Stratified, 4b
Stratum, 4b
Stress test, 232–233b
Striated muscle, 17
Stroke, 109–110
Stye. See Hordeolum
Styloid process, 15, 15f
Subarachnoid space, 104
Subcutaneous cardiac rhythm monitor, 204
Subcutaneous tissue, 2, 2f
    ICD-10-CM chapter 12, diseases of skin
            and subcutaneous tissue, 259
    integumentary system subsection,
            189–190
Sublingual gland, 74, 76f
Subluxation, 22b
Submandibular gland, 74, 76f
Subsequent hospital care, 168
Subsequent nursing facility care codes, 169
Subungual, 4b
Sudoriferous glands, 3
Suffixes, 328t
    cardiovascular system, 38b
    digestive system, 77b
    endocrine system, 98b
    female genital system, 48b
    hemic and lymphatic system, 91b
    integumentary system, 3b
    male genital system, 59b
    musculoskeletal system, 22b
    nervous system, 105b
    respiratory system, 29b
    senses, 116b
    urinary system, 67b
Summary of stay, 168
Superficial destruction, 201
Superficial inguinal nodes, 90f

Superior extensor retinaculum, 20f
Superior peroneal retinaculum, 19f
Superior vena cava, 36
Supination, 19, 22b
Supraorbital foramen, 16f
Surgeon, assistant, 182
Surgery
    anesthesia for multiple procedures, 177
    Mohs micrographic, 4b, 192
    skin replacement, 191
    skull base, 224
Surgery section, 188–227
    abdominal hysterectomy, 221–222b
    angiogram, 209–210b
    aortogram, 211b
    arthroplasty and spur excision, 198–199b
    auditory system subsection, 225
    cardiovascular in medicine section,
            206–208, 241
    cardiovascular in radiology section, 208
    cardiovascular in surgery section,
            203–206
    cardiovascular system subsection, 203
    carpal tunnel, 226b
    catheter placement, 210–211b
    cesarean section, 222b
    cystotomy, 214b
    dialysis catheter replacement, 210b
    digestive system subsection, 212–213
    endocrine system subsection, 223
    excision
        bone tumor, 200b
        cheek lesion, 193b
        labial, 223b
        mass, bursa, 200b
    extremity angiogram, 212b
    eye and ocular adnexa subsection, 224
    fascial sling arthroplasty, 199b
    female genital system subsection,
            217–218
    gastrojejunostomy placement, 213b
    general subsection, 188–189
    hemic and lymphatic system subsection,
            208–209
    integumentary system subsection,
            189–193
    intersex surgery subsection, 217
    intracerebral hematoma, 225b
    laceration repair, 194–195b
    laminectomy with foraminotomy, 227b
    as largest CPT section, 188
    major guideline of surgical packages, 188
    male genital system subsection, 216–217
    maternity care and delivery subsection,
            218–220
    mediastinum and diaphragm subsection,
            209
    minimal debridement, 195b
    musculoskeletal system subsection,
            195–198
    nervous system subsection, 223–224
    notes and guidelines, 188, 189f

Surgery section (Continued)
  operating microscope subsection, 225
  parietal burr holes, 225–226b
  pyloroplasty, 215b
  renal mass, 221b
  renal tumor excision, 220–221b
  repair of pseudomeningocele, 226–227b
  reproductive system procedures, 217
  respiratory system subsection, 201–203
  right breast wide excision, 193–194b
  section format, 188
  separate procedures, 188
  small-bowel anastomosis, 214–215b
  special report, 188
  steroid injection, 198b
  supplies, 188
  thenar flap coverage, 194b
  unlisted procedure codes, 188
  urinary system subsection, 216
Surgical care only modifier, 181
Surgical pathology, pathology and
    laboratory section, 236
Surgical team modifier, 182
Swan-Ganz catheter, 39b
Sweat glands, 3
Symbols, CPT, 157
Sympathetic nerve, 105b
Sympathetic system, 104
Synarthrosis, 17
Synchondrosis, 22b
Synchronous telemedicine services
    modifier, 183
Syphilis, 52
Systole, 38

T
Table headings, ICD-10-CM, 252
Table of drugs, HCPCS, 247
Table of drugs and chemicals, ICD-10-CM,
    251–252, 251f
Table of neoplasms, ICD-10-CM, 251,
    251f
Tabular list
  ICD-10-CM, 249, 252
  ICD-10-PCS, 267, 268f
Tachypnea, 30b, 32
Taenia coli, 76f
Tailbone, 104
Takedown colostomy and cholecystectomy,
    178b
Talus, 16, 18f
Tarsorrhaphy, 117b
Taste, 115
Tax Equity and Fiscal Responsibility Act
    (TEFRA) of 1982, 137
Teeth, 74, 75f
Temporal bone, 14–15
Temporalis, 20
Temporal lines, 15f
Temporal lobe, 104
Temporary codes, HCPCS, 247

Tendons, 18, 22b
  disorders of, 25
  sprains and strains, 24
Tenodesis, 22b
Tenorrhaphy, 22b
Tensor fasciae latae, 20f, 21
Teres major, 19f
Teres minor, 19f
Terminal sulcus, 75f
Terms, ICD-10-CM alphabetic index, 250
Testes, 58, 58f, 97, 97f
  cancer of, 61
  endocrine system subsection, 223
  torsion of, 61, 61f
Tetanus, 239–240
Tetralogy of Fallot, 44
Thalamus, 103, 104f
Thenar flap coverage, 194b
Therapeutic drug assays, pathology and
    laboratory section, 234–235
Thermograms, 208
Thermoreceptors, 115
Thighbone, 15–16
Thigh muscles, 20
Third-party-payer consultations, 168
Thoracentesis, 30b, 202
Thoracic duct, 90f, 91b
Thoracic vertebrae, 15, 17f, 104
Thoracocentesis, 30b
Thoracoplasty, 30b
Thoracoscopy, 30b
Thoracostomy, 30b, 39b
Thoracotomy, 30b, 202
Thorax, 15
Throat, 27, 74
Thrombectomy, 205
  arterial mechanical, 206
  venous mechanical, 206
Thromboangiitis obliterans, 42
Thrombocytes, 35
Thromboendarterectomy, 39b
Thrombophlebitis caused by
    inflammation, 42
Thrombus, 42
Thymectomy, 98b
Thymus, 96–97, 97f, 98b
Thyroglossal duct, 98b
Thyroid, 96, 97f, 98b
  disorders of, 100–101, 100f
  excision, 223
Thyroidectomy, 98b, 223
Thyroid-stimulating hormone (TSH), 96
Thyrotoxicosis, 100
TIA. See Transient ischemic attack (TIA)
Tibia, 15–16, 18f
Tibialis anterior, 20f, 21
Time, 167
Tinea capitis, 12
Tinea corporis, 12
Tinea pedis, 12
Tinea unguium, 12
Tinnitus, 117b

T is for time (anesthesia), 176
Tissue typing, pathology and laboratory
    section, 235
Tocolysis, 49b
Tomography, 228
Tongue, 15, 75f, 76f
Tonsil, 75f
Torsion of testes, 61, 61f
Total pneumonectomy, 30b, 202
Touch, sense of, 115
Tourette syndrome, 107–108
Trachea, 27, 28f, 202
Tracheostomy, 30b
Tracheotomy, 30b
Traction, 22b, 24f, 196
Transcatheter procedures, 206
Transfusion medicine, pathology and
    laboratory section, 235
Transient hypertension, 258
Transient ischemia, 41
Transient ischemic attack (TIA), 109
Transitional care management services, 171
Transitional or vermilion surfaces, mouth, 75f
Transluminal angioplasty, 205
Transmastoid, 117b
Transplantation, 91b
Transtracheal, 30b
Transureteroureterostomy, 68b
Transurethral resection, 59b
Transurethral resection of the prostate
    (TURP), 216
Transvenous, 39b
Transverse colon, 76f
Transversus abdominis, 20
Transvesical ureterolithotomy, 68b
Trapezius, 19f, 20, 20f
Trauma
  head, 111
  wound exploration, 196
Traumatic brain injury (TBI), 111
Traumatic cataract, 120, 120f
Trephination, 105b
Triceps, 19f, 20
Trichomoniasis, 52
Tricuspid regurgitation (TR), 44
Tricuspid valve, 36
Trimesters, 219, 261
Trocar needle, 22b
Trochanter, 15–16
True aneurysm, 42
True ribs, 15
Trunk muscles, 20
TSH. See Thyroid-stimulating hormone (TSH)
Tuberculosis, 30b, 33
Tumescence, 59b
Tumor-node-metastasis (TNM) stages, 64, 64f
Tumors, 5, 6f
  blood vessel, 112
  bone, 25–26, 200b
  brain and spinal cord, 111–112
  cranial nerve, 112
  female genital system, 54

Tumors (Continued)
  medulloblastoma, 112
  meningioma, 112
  muscle, 26
  pineal region, 112
  pituitary, 112
  renal, 220–221b
  skin, 12–13
    subcutaneous, and accessory structures,
      189–190
  soft tissue, 197
  spinal cord, 111–112
  urinary bladder, 72
  Wilms', 73
  See also Cancer; Neoplasms
Tunica vaginalis, 59b
Turbinates, 27, 28f
  excision and resection, 201
TURP. See Transurethral resection of the
      prostate (TURP)
Twins, delivery of, 220
Two surgeons modifier, 182
Tympanic membrane, 16f
Tympanolysis, 117b
Tympanometry, 117b
Tympanostomy, 117b, 225
Type of service, E/M codes, 161

U

UCR. See Usual, customary, and reasonable
      (UCR)
UHDDS. See Uniform Hospital Discharge
      Data Set (UHDDS)
Ulcerative colitis, 83, 83f
Ulcers, 6f, 7
  duodenal, 82
  mouth, 79
  peptic, 81
  pressure, 7, 7f, 191
Ulna, 16, 18f
Ultrasound
  diagnostic ultrasound subsection, 230
  extent of study, 230
  extremities, 246b
  gallbladder, 232b
  head, 233b
  three locations for, 230
  venous, 245b
Unbundling, 125, 137
Uncontrolled hypertension, 258
Uniform Hospital Discharge Data Set
      (UHDDS), 142–143
Unique provider identification number
      (UPIN), 128b
Unlisted services, CPT, 159
Unplanned return to operating/procedure
      room by the same physician or other
      qualified health care professional
      following initial procedure for a related
      procedure during postoperative period
      modifier, 182

Unrelated E/M services by same physician
      or other qualified health care
      professional during a postoperative
      period modifier, 180
Unrelated procedure or service by same
      physician or other qualified health care
      professional during postoperative
      period modifier, 182
Unusual anesthesia modifier, 180
UPIN. See Unique provider identification
      number (UPIN)
Upper extremities. See Arms
Upper respiratory tract (URT), 27, 28f
Ureterectomy, 68b
Ureterocutaneous fistula, 68b
Ureteroenterostomy, 68b
Ureterolithotomy, 68b
Ureterolysis, 68b
Ureteroneocystostomy, 68b
Ureteropyelography, 68b
Ureterotomy, 68b
Ureters, 66
Ureter subheading, 216
Urethra, 58f, 66
  disorders of, 62
Urethritis, 62
Urethrocystography, 68b
Urethromeatoplasty, 68b
Urethropexy, 68b
Urethroplasty, 68b
Urethrorrhaphy, 68b
Urethroscopy, 68b
Urinalysis, pathology and laboratory
      section, 235
Urinary bladder, 58f, 66
  cancer of, 72
  urinary system subsection, 216
Urinary meatus, 46
Urinary system, 66–73
  anatomy and terminology, 66, 69
  combining forms, 67b
  congenital disorders, 72–73
  glomerular disorders, 71
  kidneys, 66, 67f
  medical abbreviations, 67b
  medical terms, 68b
  organs, 66, 66f
  pathophysiology, 69–73
  prefixes, 67b
  quiz, 69, 73
  renal failure, 69–70
  suffixes, 67b
  urinary tract obstructions, 71–72
  vascular disorders, 72
Urinary system subsection, 216
  bladder subheading, 216
  kidney subheading, 216
  ureter subheading, 216
Urinary tract infections (UTI), 70–71
Urodynamics, 216
Use additional code, ICD-10-CM,
      250

Usual, customary, and reasonable (UCR),
      128b, 154b
Uterine fibroids, 52
Uterine tubes. See Fallopian tubes
Uterus, 46, 47f, 218
  bilateral tubes, and ovaries, pathology
      and laboratory section, 237b
  cancer of, 53
UTI. See Urinary tract infections (UTI)
Uveal, 117b
Uvula, 75f

V

V, W, X, Y codes, ICD-10-CM, 252
Vaccines
  influenza, 240
  pneumococcal, 240
  toxoids, 239–240
  See also Immunizations
Vagina, 46, 47f, 217–218
  cancer of, 54
Vaginal delivery, 55
Vaginal suppositories, 56, 220
Vallate papillae, 75f
Valves, heart, 36
Valvular heart disease, 43–44
  stenosis, 44
Valvular regurgitation, 44
Varices, 78b
Varicocele, 59b, 61
Varicose veins, 43, 78b
Vascular dementia, 106
Vascular disorders
  aneurysm, 42, 110
  brain abscess, 110
  cardiovascular system, 41–43, 41f
  central nervous system, 109–110
  cerebrovascular accident (CVA),
      109–110
  coronary artery disease (CAD)/ischemic
      heart disease (IHD), 41
  embolism, 42
  encephalitis, 110
  epilepsies, 110–111
  hypertension, 41, 41f
  hypotension, 41–42
  ischemia, 41
  peripheral arterial disease, 42
  Reye's syndrome, 110
  thrombophlebitis caused by
      inflammation, 42
  thrombus, 42
  transient ischemic attack (TIA), 109
  urinary system, 72
  varicose veins, 43
Vascular families like a tree, 205
Vascular injection procedures, 205–206
Vas deferens, 58, 58f, 59b
Vasectomy, 59b
Vasogram, 59b
Vasorrhaphy, 59b

Vasotomy, 59b
Vasovasostomy, 59b
Vastus intermedius, 21
Vastus lateralis, 20f, 21
Vastus medialis, 20f, 21
Veins, 35, 37f
   cardiovascular in surgery section,
      204–206, 205f
   varicose, 43, 78b
Venous grafting only for coronary artery
      bypass, 204
Venous mechanical thrombectomy, 206
Venous reconstruction, 205
Venous ultrasound, 245b
Ventral surface, tongue, 75f
Ventricle, brain, 104, 104f
Ventricular fibrillation, 43
Ventricular septal defect, 44
Vermiform appendix, 76f, 82, 177–178b
Verrucae, 11
Vertebrae, 15, 17f, 18f, 104
   injury to, 111
   spinal cord housed within, 104
   See also Spinal cord
Vertebrectomy, 105b
Vertex presentation, 56f
Vertigo, 117b
Vesical neck, 216
Vesicle, 5, 6f
Vesicostomy, 68b
Vesicovaginal fistula, 49b
Vesiculectomy, 59b
Vesiculotomy, 59b
Vessels
   atherosclerosis of, 41
   circulatory system, 35, 36f, 37f
   heart, 36

Vessels (Continued)
   ICD-10-CM chapter 20, external causes
      of morbidity, 263
   lymph, 89
   tumors of, 112
   See also Blood
Vestibule
   mouth, 75f
   nasal, 28f
Viral hepatitis, 84–85
Viral infections
   active immunizations against, 239
   Epstein-Barr, 93
   female genital system, 52
   hepatitis, 84–85
   Reye's syndrome and, 110
   skin, 11–12
Visceral pericardium, 36
Vision, 114, 115f
   disturbances of, 118–119
Vitamins, 335–343t
   nutritional degenerative disease, 106
Voice box, 27
Volvulus, 78b
Vomer, 15, 16f
Vomiting, 173b
Vulva, 46, 217
   cancer of, 54
Vulvectomy, 217

W

Warts, 11
   genital, 52
Well-child check, 174b
Wheal, 5, 6f
Whitmore-Jewett stages, 64, 64f

Wilms' tumor, 73
Windpipe, 27
Womb. See Uterus
Wounds
   active wound care management, medicine
      section, 243–244
   exploration, 196
   grouping of wound repair, 190
   ICD-10-CM chapter 20, external causes
      of morbidity, 263
   repair factors, 190
   types of repair of, 190

X

Xanthelasma, 117b
Xanthoma, 4b
Xenografts, 4b, 191
Xeroderma, 4b
Xiphoid process, 17f

Y

Yeast. See Candidiasis

Z

Z codes
   ICD-10-CM chapter 2, neoplasms, 256
   ICD-10-CM chapter 21, factors
      influencing health status and
      contact with health services,
      263–264
Zygomatic bone, 15, 15f, 16f
Zygomatic process of temporal bone,
   15, 15f
Zygomaticus, 19

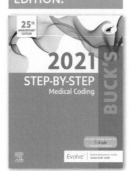

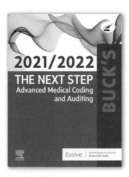
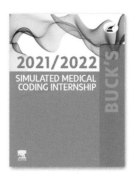
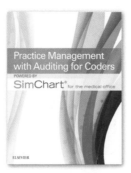
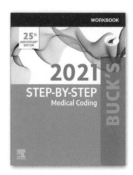